MDMayer MD

W.B. SAUNDERS COMPANY 1985
Philadelphia London Toronto Mexico City
Rio de Janeiro Sydney Tokyo

Surgery of the LARYNX

BYRON J. BAILEY, M.D.
Editor
Wiess Professor and Chairman
Department of Otolaryngology
The University of Texas Medical Branch
Galveston, Texas

HUGH F. BILLER, M.D.
Co-editor
Professor and Chairman
Department of Otolaryngology
Mt. Sinai School of Medicine
New York, New York

W. B. Saunders Company: West Washington Square
Philadelphia, PA 19105

1 St. Anne's Road
Eastbourne, East Sussex BN21 3UN, England

1 Goldthorne Avenue
Toronto, Ontario M8Z 5T9, Canada

Apartado 26370—Cedro 512
Mexico 4, D.F., Mexico

Rua Coronel Cabrita, 8
Sao Cristovao Caixa Postal 21176
Rio de Janeiro, Brazil

9 Waltham Street
Artarmon, N.S.W. 2064, Australia

Ichibancho, Central Bldg., 22-1 Ichibancho
Chiyoda-Ku, Tokyo 102, Japan

Library of Congress Cataloging in Publication Data

Main entry under title:

Surgery of the larynx.

1. Larynx—Surgery. I. Bailey, Byron J. II. Biller, Hugh F. [DNLM: 1. Larynx—Surgery. WV 540 S9606]

RF516.S9 1985 617'.533 83–20415

ISBN 0–7216–1472–8

Surgery of the Larynx ISBN 0-7216-1472-8

Last digit is the print number: 9 8 7 6 5 4 3 2 1

CONTRIBUTORS

WILLIAM A. ALONSO, M.D., F.A.C.S.
Clinical Associate Professor of Surgery, Division of Otolaryngology, University of South Florida College of Medicine; Chairman, Department of Otolaryngology and Head and Neck Surgery, St. Joseph's Hospital; Consultant in Head and Neck Surgery, Veterans Administration Hospital and MacDill USAF Regional Hospital, Tampa, Florida.
Management of Acquired Laryngeal Stenosis

BYRON J. BAILEY, M.D.
Wiess Professor and Chairman, Department of Otolaryngology, University of Texas Medical Branch, Galveston, Texas.
Carcinoma in Situ and Microinvasive Carcinoma of the Larynx; Glottic Carcinoma; Glottic Reconstruction; Transglottic Carcinoma and Total Laryngectomy

JOEL MICHAEL BERMAN, M.D.
Clinical Assistant Professor, Department of Otolaryngology, University of Texas Medical Branch, Galveston; Attending, Humana Hospital, Clear Lake, St. John's Hospital, Nassau Bay, Texas.
Surgical Anatomy of the Larynx

HUGH F. BILLER, M.D.
Professor and Chairman, Department of Otolaryngology, Mount Sinai School of Medicine; Chief, Department of Otolaryngology, Mount Sinai Hospital, New York, New York.
Management of Acute Laryngeal Trauma; Congenital Lesions of the Larynx; Supraglottic Cancer

ERIC D. BLOM, Ph.D.
Attending Staff, Methodist Hospital, Indianapolis, Indiana.
Vocal Rehabilitation with Prosthetic Devices

THOMAS C. CALCATERRA, M.D.
Professor, Department of Surgery, University of California at Los Angeles School of Medicine, Los Angeles, California.
Voice Production after Laryngectomy

D. A. CHARLES, M.D.
Assistant Professor, Department of Otolaryngology, University of Toronto; Senior Otolaryngologist, Western Hospital, Toronto, Canada.
Laryngeal Research

WILLIAM D. CLARK, D.D.S., M.D.
Assistant Professor, University of Texas Medical Branch; Active Staff, University of Texas Medical Branch Hospitals; Courtesy Staff, St. Mary's Hospital, Galveston, Texas.
Diagnosis and Staging of Laryngeal Disease

ROGER L. CRUMLEY, M.D.
Clinical Professor, Department of Otolaryngology–Head and Neck Surgery, University of California at San Francisco School of Medicine, San Francisco, California.
Update of Laryngeal Reinnervation

J. M. FREDRICKSON, M.D., M.D.(HON.)
Professor and Chairman, Department of Otolaryngology, Washington University; Chief of Staff, Barnes Hospital and Children's Hospital, St. Louis, Missouri.
Laryngeal Research

RICHARD L. GOODE, M.D.
Professor of Otolaryngology–Head and Neck Surgery, Stanford Medical Center, Stanford; Chief of Otolaryngology, Palo Alto Veterans Administration Medical Center, Palo Alto, California.
Surgery for Aspiration

JOHN K. JONES, M.D., F.R.C.S.(Eng.), F.R.C.S.(C), F.A.C.S.
Clinical Assistant Professor, Baylor College of Medicine; Staff, Texas Children's Hospital, Methodist Hospital, St. Luke's Hospital, Ben Taub Hospital, Houston, Texas.
Pediatric Laryngology

WILLIAM LAWSON, M.D., D.D.S.
Professor of Otolaryngology, Mount Sinai School of Medicine, New York; Chief of Otolaryngology, Bronx Veterans Administration Hospital, Bronx; Attending Otolaryngologist, Mount Sinai Hospital, New York, and Elmhurst General Hospital, Flushing, New York.
Management of Acute Laryngeal Trauma; Congenital Lesions of the Larynx; Supraglottic Cancer

HOWARD L. LEVINE, M.D.
Staff, Department of Otolaryngology and Communicative Disorders, Cleveland Clinic Foundation, Cleveland, Ohio.
Surgical Management of Paralyzed Larynx

PAUL A. LEVINE, M.D.
Assistant Professor of Otolaryngology–Head and Neck Surgery, Stanford Medical Center, Stanford; Assistant Chief of Otolaryngology, Santa Clara Valley Medical Center, San Jose, California.
Surgery for Aspiration

JAMES E. MARKS, M.D.
Professor of Radiology, Mallinckrodt Institute of Radiology, Washington University School of Medicine; Staff, Barnes Hospital and St. Louis Children's Hospital; Consultant, Jewish Hospital and St. Luke's Hospital, St. Louis, Missouri.
Radiation Therapy for Carcinoma of the Larynx

ROGER McNEILL, M.D., F.R.C.S.(C), M.Sc.
Clinical Assistant Professor, University of Texas Medical Branch, Galveston; Private Practice, Cypress-Fairbanks Medical Center, Houston, and Tomball Community Hospital, Tomball, Texas.
Nonsurgical Conditions of the Larynx

HARLAN R. MUNTZ, M.D.
Assistant Professor of Otolaryngology, Washington University School of Medicine; Acting Director, St. Louis Children's Hospital; Otolaryngologist, Barnes Hospital; Associate Otolaryngologist, Hospital of St. Louis; Instructor, St. Louis County Hospital, St. Louis, Missouri.
Surgery of Laryngopharyngeal and Subglottic Carcinoma

ARNOLD M. NOYEK, M.D., F.R.C.S.(C), F.A.C.S.
Professor, Department of Otolaryngology, and Associate Professor, Department of Radiology, University of Toronto; Staff Otolaryngologist, Mount Sinai Hospital and Sunnybrook Medical Centre; Staff Radiologist (Otolaryngology), Mount Sinai Hospital; Consultant, Department of Radiological Sciences, Toronto General Hospital, Toronto, Canada.
Radiologic Evaluation of the Larynx

C. PAINTER, Ph.D.
Professor of Otolaryngology and Director of Speech Science, Department of Otolaryngology, Washington University, St. Louis, Missouri.
Laryngeal Research

FRANK J. PANETTIERE, M.D., F.A.C.P.
Associate Clinical Professor of Medicine and Former Chief of Medical Oncology, University of Arkansas College of Medicine, Little Rock; Consultant in Medical Oncology to the United States Air Force Surgeon General; Attending Staff, St. Mary's–Rogers Memorial Hospital, Rogers; Courtesy and Consultant Staff, Bates Memorial Hospital, Bentonville, and Springdale Memorial Hospital, Springdale, Arkansas.
General Principles of Chemotherapy and Immunotherapy; Chemotherapy and Immunotherapy of Laryngeal Cancer

WILLIAM R. PANJE, M.D.
Professor and Chairman, Department of Otolaryngology–Head and Neck Surgery, University of Chicago Pritzker School of Medicine; Staff, University of Chicago Medical Center, Chicago, Illinois.
The Panje Voice Prosthesis

BRUCE W. PEARSON, M.D., F.R.C.S.(C)
Associate Professor, Mayo Medical School; Staff, St. Mary's Hospital, Rochester, Minnesota.
Near-Total Laryngectomy

CARLOS A. PEREZ, M.D.
Professor of Radiology, Mallinckrodt Institute of Radiology, Washington University School of Medicine; Radiotherapist-in-Chief, Barnes Hospital; Radiotherapist, St. Luke's Hospitals and Missouri Baptist Hospital, St. Louis, Missouri.
Radiation Therapy for Carcinoma of the Larynx

CLARENCE T. SASAKI, M.D.
Professor of Surgery and Chief of Otolaryngology, Yale University School of Medicine; Attending, Yale–New Haven Hospital, New Haven; Consultant, West Haven Veterans Administration Hospital, West Haven; Backus Hospital, Norwich; Wildham Community Hospital, Wildham; St. Mary's Hospital and Waterbury Hospital, Waterbury, Connecticut.
Laryngeal Physiology

DONALD G. SESSIONS, M.D.
Professor of Otolaryngology, Washington University School of Medicine; Assistant Otolaryngologist, Barnes Hospital Group, St. Louis, Missouri.
Surgery of Laryngopharyngeal and Subglottic Carcinoma

HARRY S. SHULMAN, M.D.
Associate Professor, Department of Radiology, University of Toronto; Senior Staff Radiologist, Sunnybrook Medical Centre, Toronto, Ontario.
Radiologic Evaluation of the Larynx

MARK I. SINGER, M.D., F.A.C.S.
Adjunct Associate Professor of Speech Language Pathology, Northwestern University, Evanston, Illinois; Attending Staff, Methodist Hospital of Indiana, Indianapolis, Indiana.
Vocal Rehabilitation with Prosthetic Devices

MARVIN I. STEINHARDT, M.A., M.D., F.R.C.P.(C)
Associate Professor, Department of Radiology, University of Toronto; Staff Radiologist, Department of Radiological Sciences, Mount Sinai Hospital, Toronto, Canada.
Radiologic Evaluation of the Larynx

CHARLES M. STIERNBERG, M.D.
Assistant Professor of Otolaryngology, University of Texas Medical Branch; Staff, University of Texas Medical Branch Hospitals, Galveston, Texas.
Transglottic Carcinoma and Total Laryngectomy

M. STUART STRONG, M.D.
Professor and Chairman, Department of Otolaryngology, Boston University School of Medicine; Chief of Otolaryngology, University Hospital, Boston, Massachusetts.
Endoscopic Surgery of the Larynx

HARVEY M. TUCKER, M.D.
Chairman, Department of Otolaryngology and Communicative Disorders, Cleveland Clinic Foundation, Cleveland, Ohio.
Surgical Management of the Paralyzed Larynx

JOHN A. TUCKER, M.D.
Professor and Chairman, Otorhinolaryngology, and Professor of Anatomy, Hahnemann University; Chief, Section of Pediatric Otolaryngology, St. Christopher's Hospital for Children, Philadelphia, Pennsylvania.
Developmental Anatomy of the Larynx

D. R. VanDEMARK, Ph.D.
Professor, Department of Otolaryngology–Head and Neck Surgery and Speech Pathology–Audiology, University of Iowa; Staff, University of Iowa Hospitals, Iowa City, Iowa.
The Panje Voice Prosthesis

JUDAH ZIZMOR, M.D., F.A.C.R.
Clinical Professor of Radiology, New York University Medical School; Director Emeritus, Department of Radiology, Manhattan Eye, Ear and Throat Hospital New York, New York.
Radiologic Evaluation of the Larynx

PREFACE

"If you wou'd not be forgotten
As soon as you are dead and rotten,
Either write things worth reading,
Or do things worth the writing."

BENJAMIN FRANKLIN (1706–1790)
Poor Richard's Almanack, 1738

Simply put, Hugh Biller and I have tried to generate a book written primarily for and by laryngeal surgeons.

It is our objective to provide the best current views concerning the evaluation and management of laryngeal disorders and neoplasms. We have endeavored to present a broad perspective of the rationale underlying the various forms of therapeutic intervention that are reviewed. Unlike a surgical atlas, this book emphasizes the important, new, scientific information that documents the effectiveness of specific techniques by long-term follow-up of patients.

We have tried to collect between these two covers all that you ever wanted to know about laryngeal surgery, and more.

The Editor and Co-Editor are deeply indebted to a great many individuals who have been patient, tolerant, and hard-working over the past several years. Through their efforts, the vision has now become a reality, and we offer special thanks—

- To our wives, Margi and Dianne, who sustain us;
- To our teachers, Joel J. Pressman, M.D., and Joseph H. Ogura, M.D., who provided the core inspiration;
- To our numerous, treasured professional colleagues who provided the priceless ingredients—the chapters;
- To our medical institutions, the University of Texas Medical Branch at Galveston and the Mount Sinai Medical School, New York City, who were tolerant over the past years of the time and expense invested in preparation of this volume;
- To our illustrator, Tony Pazos, and our manuscript typists, Marilyn Hall, Carol Grunden, and Connie Smith, for working their fingers "to the bone";
- To Lisette Bralow, our Editor at Saunders, for her patience and encouragement;
- And most especially, to Lynn Alperin, our relentless, perfectionistic project foreman and medical editor, without whose dogged persistence there would be no book.

Finally, we wish to acknowledge the generous support that has been provided by the H. C. Wiess family of Houston and the James A. Sartain family of Newton, Texas. Their philanthropy has been invaluable in the achievement of this project.

We hope the information contained in these pages will provide the answers to the questions raised by the disease states we find in our patients. Any value in this regard will be ample reward for the time that all of us have spent.

BYRON J. BAILEY, M.D.

CONTENTS

PART I

INTRODUCTION TO SURGERY OF THE LARYNX

1

Developmental Anatomy of the Larynx

John A. Tucker, M.D.

The first portion of the human respiratory tree to be studied from the viewpoint of development was the larynx. Although Fleischman[1] reported such studies in 1820, the larynx was not described in a closely graded series of specifically staged human embryos until 1972.[2] Common practice has arranged individual human embryos in order of either supposed age or size. Both criteria are unsatisfactory, first, because we cannot determine the precise age of an embryo and, second, because size at any given age varies. Moreover, arrangement by age does not necessarily coincide with morphologic development because some individuals grow more rapidly than others, both prenatally and postnatally. Longer embryos, like taller people, are not necessarily more developed than shorter ones.[3] Also, fixation and shrinkage affect embryonic length.

Embryos are best arranged in *stages,* with these stages designating developmental levels and marking the appearance of specific morphologic features such as eyes and limb buds. Because embryonic length is merely one index of development and does not, in itself, constitute a stage, expressions such as "a 15-mm stage" should be discarded.[3]

THE CARNEGIE SYSTEM

Dr. Franklin P. Mall, first director of the Department of Embryology of the Carnegie Institution of Washington, Washington, DC, originated the practice of staging the human embryo. In 1887, as a medical student at Johns Hopkins University, Dr. Mall acquired the first of what was to become the most important collection of human embryos in the world—the Carnegie Collection. Subsequently, he continued to enlarge his personal collection of human embryos. In 1914, Dr. Mall suggested that the Carnegie Institution of Washington establish the Department of Embryology. The Carnegie Institution did so and named Dr. Mall its first director. Also in that year, Dr. Mall described human embryonic development by stages.

Dr. Geoge L. Streeter, who succeeded Dr. Mall, outlined the present 23-stage Carnegie System in 1942. Realizing that better specimens of the earlier stages would become available as techniques improved, Dr. Streeter concentrated on describing Stages 10 to 23. Since then, Dr. Ronan O'Rahilly has further described Stages 1 to 9 and refined Stages 10 to 23.[4]

The embryonic period proper—the first eight

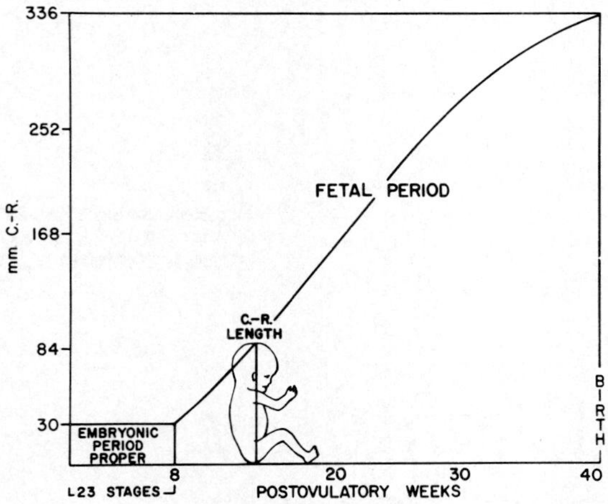

Figure 1–1. The embryonic period proper, the first 8 postovulatory weeks of development, is shown in relation to the fetal period. Fetuses, as well as older embryos, are measured by their crown-rump length, which corresponds to the sitting height postnatally. (From Tucker JA, Tucker GF Jr: Ann Otol Rhinol Laryngol 84:51, 1975.)

postovulatory weeks of development—is contrasted to the fetal period—the last seven months of human development (Fig. 1–1). Fetuses and older embryos are measured by their crown-rump length, which corresponds to the postnatal sitting height.

STAGING OF THE HUMAN EMBRYO
(Table 1–1)

These observations are based on 40 staged and sectioned human embryos in the Carnegie Collection.[3]

Stages 1 to 8—About 19 Days; Length to About 1.4 mm; 0 Pairs of Somites

Staging is based on morphologic appearance of the embryo or its chorion. No sign of the foregut is seen in the early stages, and hence no indication of the respiratory system.

Stage 9—About 20 Days; 1.5 to 2.5 mm; 1 to 3 Pairs of Somites

The first indications of the foregut and of the median pharyngeal groove presaging the respiratory system (including the larynx) are noted at Stage 9 (Fig. 1–2).

Stage 10—About 22 Days; 2 to 3.5 mm; 4 to 12 Pairs of Somites

The neural folds begin to fuse. The respiratory and hepatic primordia appear; the laryngotracheal sulcus is identifiable at the caudal expansion of the median pharyngeal groove (Figs. 1–3 and 1–4).

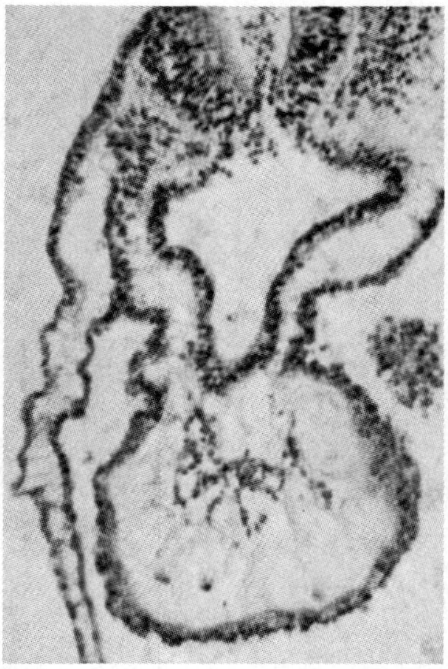

Figure 1–2. Section through the pharynx and heart of a human embryo of Stage 9 (3 weeks), 1.38 mm in length. The median pharyngeal groove can be seen immediately dorsal to the heart. In the heart, the so-called epimyocardial mantle, the cardiac mesenchyme ("jelly"), and the endocardium can be identified. (From O'Rahilly R, Tucker JA: Ann Otol Rhinol Laryngol 82(Suppl 7):14, 1973.)

Stage 11—About 24 Days; 2.4 to 4.5 mm; 13 to 20 Pairs of Somites

The rostral neuropore closes. The respiratory system, including pulmonary primordium, divides into right and left lobes (Fig. 1–5).

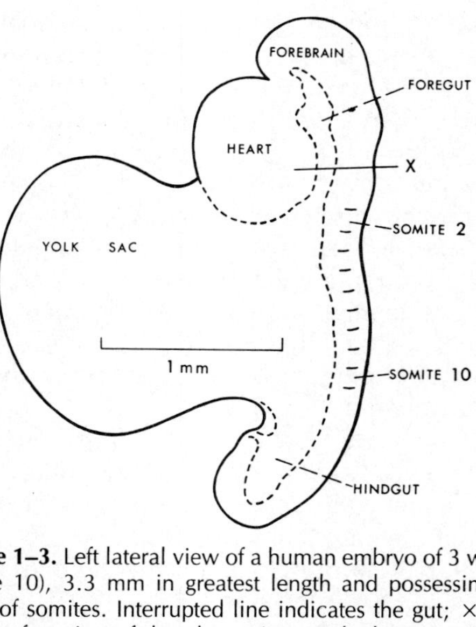

Figure 1–3. Left lateral view of a human embryo of 3 weeks (Stage 10), 3.3 mm in greatest length and possessing 10 pairs of somites. Interrupted line indicates the gut; ×, the plane of section of the photomicrograph shown in Figure 1–4. (From Tucker JA, O'Rahilly R: Ann Otol Rhinol Laryngol 81:521, 1972.)

Table 1–1. DEVELOPMENT OF SOME OF THE MAIN FEATURES OF RESPIRATORY SYSTEM IN RELATION TO STAGING FROM THREE TO SIX POSTOVULATORY WEEKS*

Stage 9	10	11	12	13	14	15	16	17	18
Earliest signs of foregut and median pharyngeal groove	Pharynx								
	Laryngotracheal sulcus				Hypopharyngeal eminence Arytenoid swellings Epithelial lamina	Larynx		Vestibular outgrowth Cricoid condensation	Hyoid chondrification Thyroid condensation Muscular condensation
			Tracheoesophageal septum		Trachea				
	Pulmonary Primordium		Lung bud	R+L Lung buds	R+L Lung buds	Lobar buds		Segmental buds	Some subsegmental buds

*Modified from O'Rahilly R and Boyden EA: Z Anat Entwicklungsgesch 141:237–250, 1973 and from Tucker JA and Tucker GF Jr: Ann Otol Rhinol Laryngol 84:50, 1975.

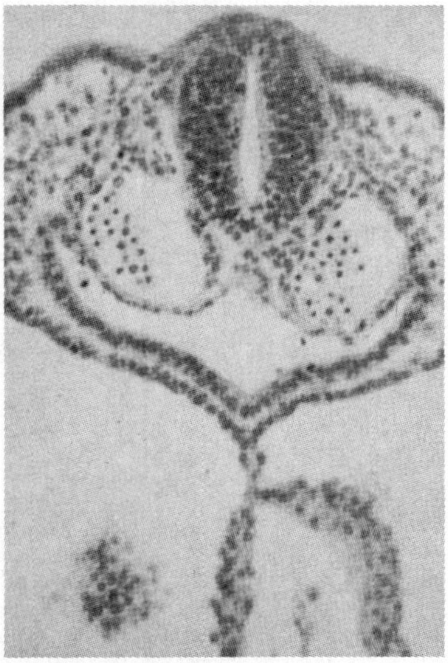

Figure 1–4. Section through the neural tube, dorsal aortae, and pharynx at Stage 10 (3.3 mm). The thick epithelium of the ventral wall of the foregut is noticeable, and the respiratory groove can be seen just dorsal to the dorsal mesocardium and heart. The plane of section is marked × in Figure 1–3. (From O'Rahilly R, Tucker JA: Ann Otol Rhinol Laryngol 82(Suppl 7):14, 1973.)

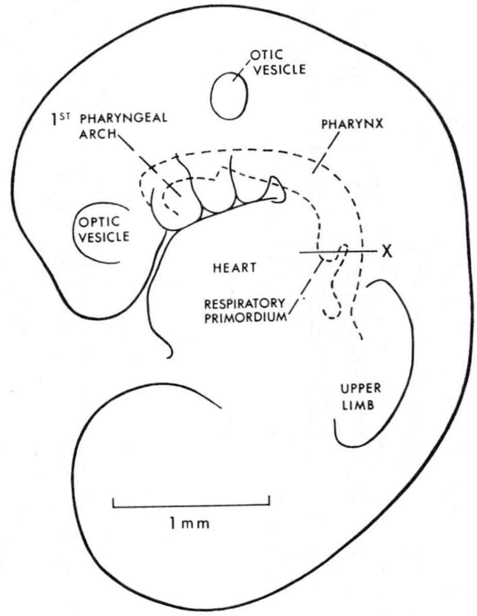

Figure 1–6. Left lateral view of a human embryo of 4 weeks (Stage 13), 4 mm in greatest length and possessing 30 pairs of somites. ×, plane of section of the photomicrograph shown in Figure 1–8. (From Tucker JA, O'Rahilly R: Ann Otol Rhinol Laryngol 81:521, 1972.)

Stage 12—About 26 Days; 3 to 5 mm; 21 to 29 Pairs of Somites

The caudal neuropore closes and the upper limb buds appear. The tracheoesophageal septum first forms from the endodermal proliferation of the lateral walls. Mesoblastic elements of the larynx are massed caudal to the third pharyngeal arch, where the superior laryngeal nerve terminates. A report in 1984 suggests that the trachea and esophagus develop independently rather than by separation of a common lumen into two distinct organs.

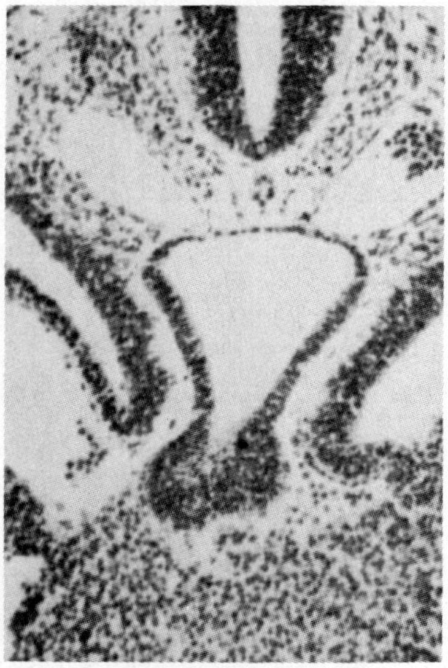

Figure 1–5. Section through the pharynx at Stage 11 (3.1 mm). The apex of the pharyngeal wall (pointing ventrally) shows the division of the respiratory primordium into right and left lobes. The notochord can be seen lying between the pharynx and the neural tube. (From O'Rahilly R, Tucker JA: Ann Otol Rhinol Laryngol 82(Suppl 7):14, 1973.)

Stage 13—About 28 Days; 4 to 6 mm; 30+ Pairs of Somites

Four limb buds are developing. The tracheoesophageal septum is well under way. The endodermal central cells of the tracheoesophageal septum undergo necrosis. Right and left buds of the primary bronchi are distinguishable (Figs. 1–6 to 1–8).

Stage 14—About 32 Days; 5 to 7 mm; 30+ Pairs of Somites

The optic cup forms. The hypopharyngeal eminence, the arytenoid swelling, and the first indication of the aryepiglottic folds appear. The site of the laryngeal inlet is identified. The respiratory groove is transformed into a laryngotracheal conduit as the epithelial lamina of the larynx forms (Fig. 1–9).

Stage 15—About 33 Days; 7 to 9 mm; 30+ Pairs of Somites

Hand plate appears. The hypopharyngeal and vestibulotracheal canals are present. The la-

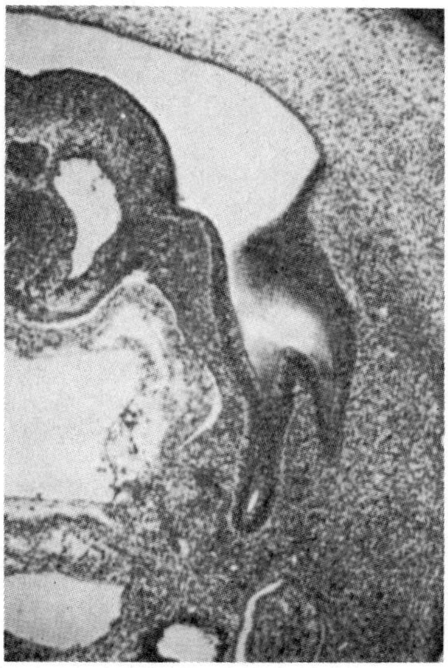

Figure 1–7. Median section through the pharyngeal region at Stage 13 (4.5 mm). The respiratory diverticulum can be seen descending from its origin in the foregut. Its close relationship to the heart is evident. The site of the tracheoesophageal septum is clearly visible. (From O'Rahilly R, Tucker JA: Ann Otol Rhinol Laryngol 82(Suppl 7):15, 1973.)

ryngeal inlet, through active epithelial growth, is Y-shaped. The superior laryngeal nerve has been identified. The lobar bronchial buds are present.

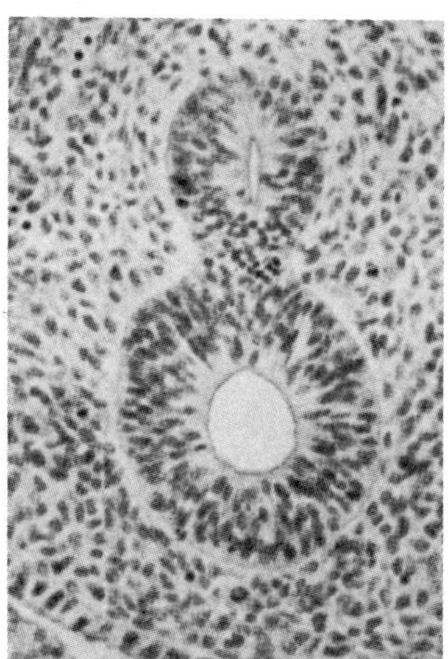

Figure 1–8. The separation of the respiratory canal *(below)* and digestive canal *(above)* at Stage 13 (5.3 mm). In this section at higher magnification, the endodermal cells that divide the originally single foregut tube can be seen. No indication of external pressure is found in this formation of the tracheoesophageal septum. The plane of section is marked × in Figure 1–6. (From O'Rahilly R, Tucker JA: Ann Otol Rhinol Laryngol 82(Suppl 7):15, 1973.)

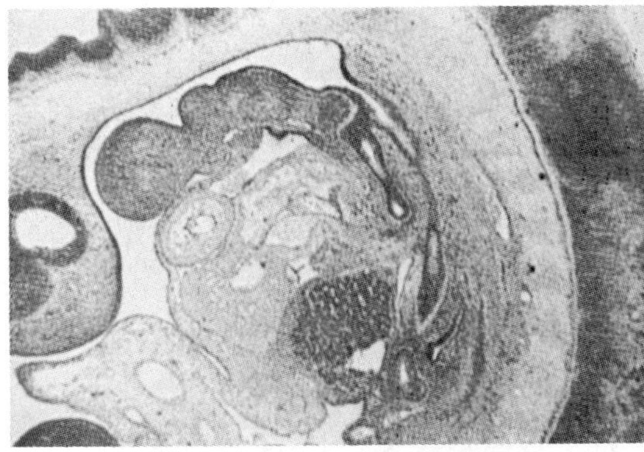

Figure 1–9. Sagittal section near the median plane at Stage 14 (5.85 mm). Portions of the neural tube are visible in the periphery in this low power view, and the heart and liver can be seen near the center. The respiratory tube, now appreciably longer, is evident ventral to the digestive canal and the site of the inlet of the embryonic larynx can be ascertained. (From O'Rahilly R, Tucker JA: Ann Otol Rhinol Laryngol 82(Suppl 7):75, 1973.)

Stage 16—About 37 Days; 8 to 11 mm; 30+ Pairs of Somites

Foot plate appears. Hyoid condensation is beginning. The recurrent laryngeal nerve has been identified. Cases of tracheoesophageal fistula have been recorded (Stages 16 to 19) (Figs. 1–10 and 1–11).

Stage 17—About 41 Days; 11 to 14 mm; 30+ Pairs of Somites

Finger rays appear. A definite larynx is seen. The epiglottis is demarcated from the tongue (Stages 17 to 19). Vestibular outgrowth and cricoid condensation begin.

Stage 18—About 44 Days; 13 to 17 mm; 30+ Pairs of Somites

Toe rays appear on the embryo. The larynx exhibits hyoid chondrification; marked ventral

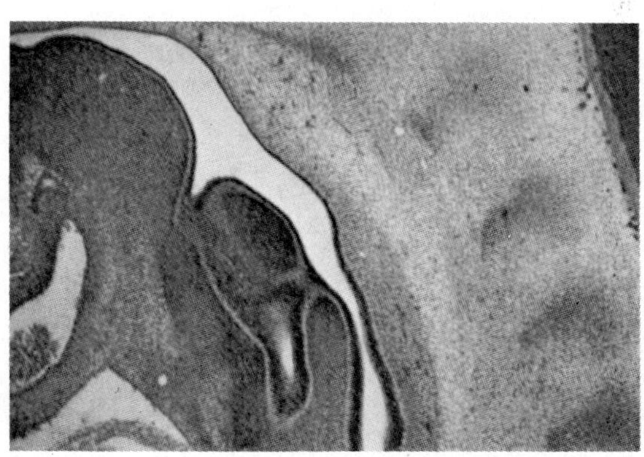

Figure 1–10. Sagittal section at Stage 16 (8.1 mm) shows the epithelial lamina of the larynx. Further details can be seen in Figure 1–11. (From Tucker JA, O'Rahilly R: Ann Otol Rhinol Laryngol 81:520–521, 1972.)

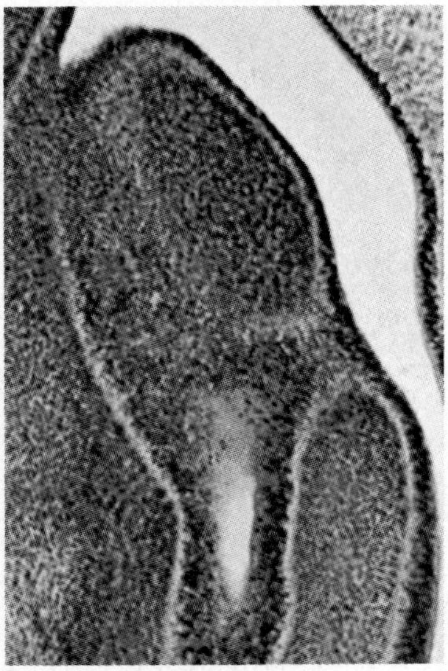

Figure 1–11. High power view of the epithelial lamina of the larynx shown in Figure 1–10. The closed vestibulotracheal canal can be identified on the left-hand side of the lamina and the closed pharyngotracheal canal can be discerned below the lamina on the right-hand side of the photograph. (From Tucker JA, O'Rahilly R: Ann Otol Rhinol Laryngol 81:520–521, 1972.)

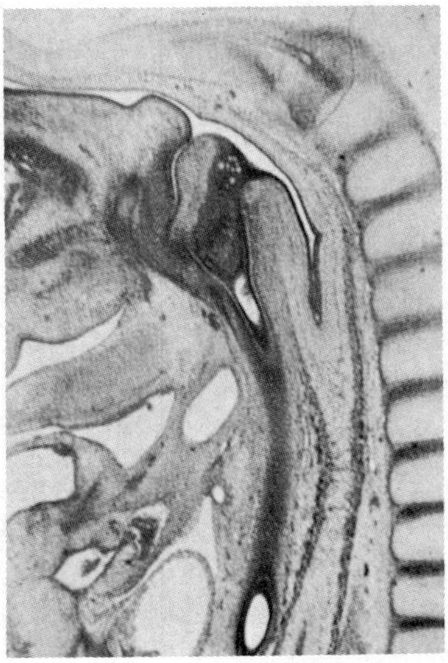

Figure 1–13. Sagittal section, approximately in the median plane, at Stage 19 (18 mm). The vertebral centra can be seen on the right and the base of the skull (containing a part of the notochord) at the top of the photograph. Compare with Figure 1–12. Below the epiglottis, the cartilaginous hyoid condensation is visible. (From Tucker JA, O'Rahilly R: Ann Otol Rhinol Laryngol 81:520–521, 1972.)

cricoid condensations and thyroid lamina condensations appear.[5] Laryngeal musculature condensations are identified (i.e., posterior cricoarytenoid muscle is becoming discrete).

Stage 19—About 48 Days; 16 to 18 mm; 30+ Pairs of Somites

The vallecula is well formed and the epiglottis is clearly demarcated from the base of the tongue. The cartilaginous hyoid condensation is readily identified (Figs. 1–12 and 1–13).

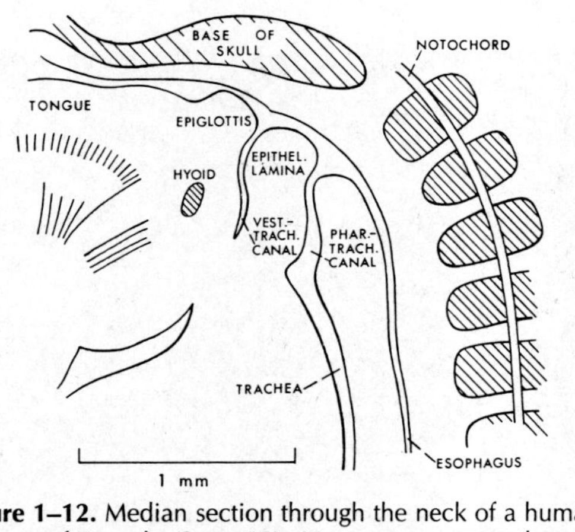

Figure 1–12. Median section through the neck of a human embryo of 7 weeks (Stage 19), 18 mm crown-rump length. Compare with Figure 1–13. (From Tucker JA, O'Rahilly R: Ann Otol Rhinol Laryngol 81:522, 1972.)

Stage 20—About 51 Days; 18 to 22 mm

The base of the skull and the vertebral centra are evident. The remaining stages in the embryonic period are now more subtle (Figs. 1–14 and 1–15).

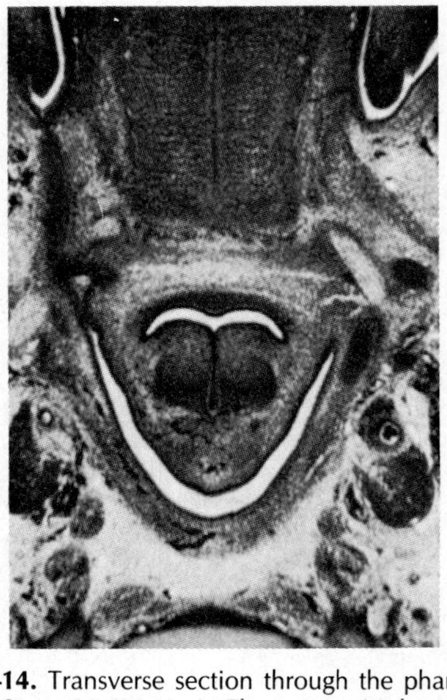

Figure 1–14. Transverse section through the pharynx and larynx at Stage 20 (21 mm). The tongue is shown uppermost. The T-shaped cavity of the larynx is evident and the arytenoid condensations can be determined. The blood vessels have been injected with India ink. (From Tucker JA, O'Rahilly R: Ann Otol Rhinol Laryngol 81:520–521, 1972.)

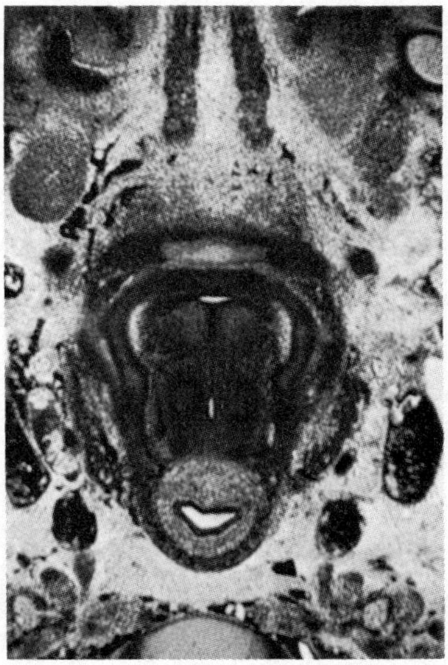

Figure 1–15. Transverse section at Stage 20, taken a little further caudally than that shown in Figure 1–14. The hyoid and thyroid cartilages and the right and left lobes of the thyroid gland can be identified. The blood vessels have been injected with India ink. (From Tucker JA, O'Rahilly R: Ann Otol Rhinol Laryngol 81:520–521, 1972.)

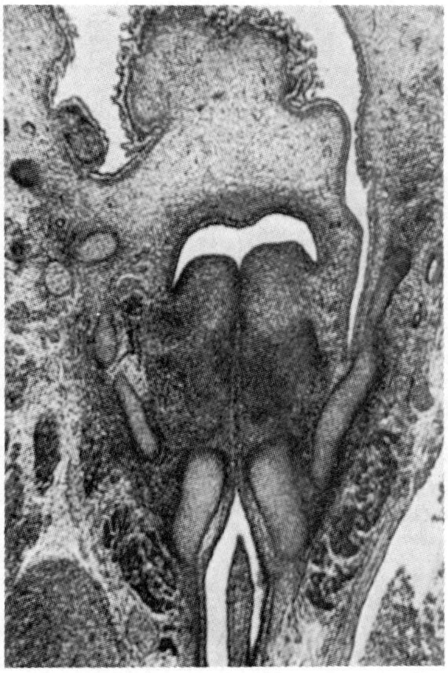

Figure 1–16. Coronal section through the larynx at Stage 21 (22.5 mm). The tongue is shown uppermost. The cartilaginous nodules on the left-hand side are (from above downwards) the hyoid, thyroid (twice), and cricoid. Above the cricoid cartilage bilaterally, muscular condensations (e.g., thyroarytenoid) are present. Lateral to the cricoid cartilage bilaterally, the right and left lobes of the thyroid gland appear as dark areas. Inferolateral to the hyoid cartilage, the hypoglossal nerve is discernible. (From Tucker JA, O'Rahilly R: Ann Otol Rhinol Laryngol 81:520–521, 1972.)

Figure 1–17. Median section through the neck and thorax of a human embryo of 8 weeks (Stage 23), 30 mm crown-rump length, at the end of the embryonic period proper. Compare with Figure 1–18. C, cricoid cartilage; H, hyoid; T, trachea. (From Tucker JA, O'Rahilly R: Ann Otol Rhinol Laryngol 81:522, 1972.)

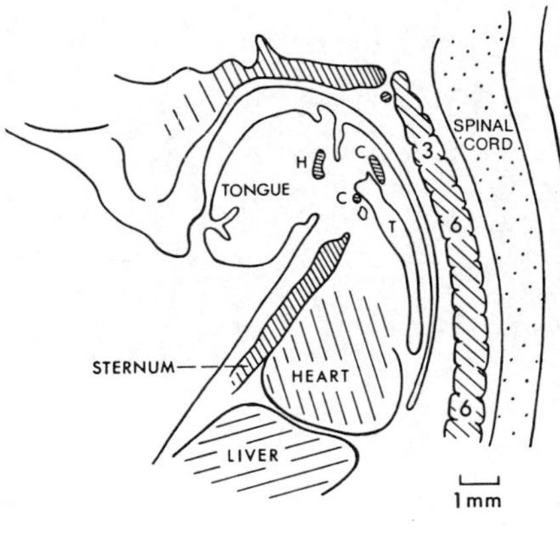

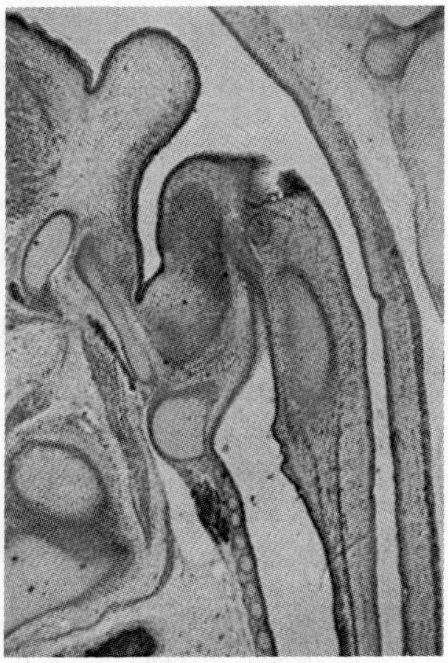

Figure 1–18. Sagittal section through the larynx at Stage 23 (8 weeks), 30 mm. The epiglottis can be seen above. The following cartilaginous elements are visible: hyoid, thyroid lamina, cricoid arch and lamina, and trachea (several rings). In addition, the manubrium sterni and the medial end of a clavicle are evident. The isthmus of the thyroid gland and the thymus appear as dark areas. Compare with Figure 1–17. (From Tucker JA, O'Rahilly R: Ann Otol Rhinol Laryngol 81:520–521, 1972.)

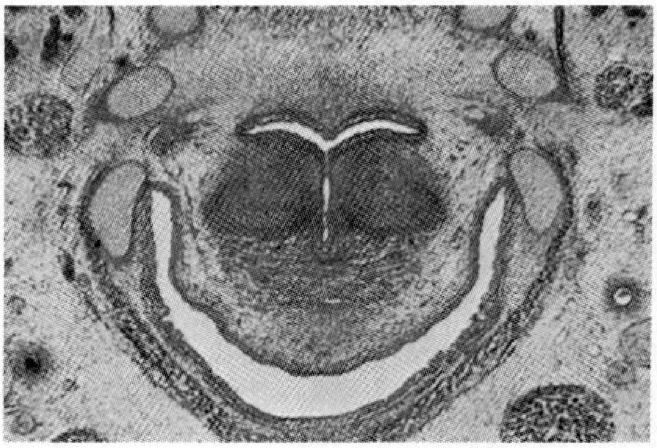

Figure 1–19. Transverse section through the pharynx and larynx of another embryo of Stage 23 (31 mm). The three cartilaginous nodules on each side belong to the styloid, hyoid, and thyroid elements. The vestibule of the larynx, the rostral limit of the arytenoid cartilages, and the transverse arytenoid muscles are clearly shown. (From Tucker JA, O'Rahilly R: Ann Otol Rhinol Laryngol 81:520–521, 1972.)

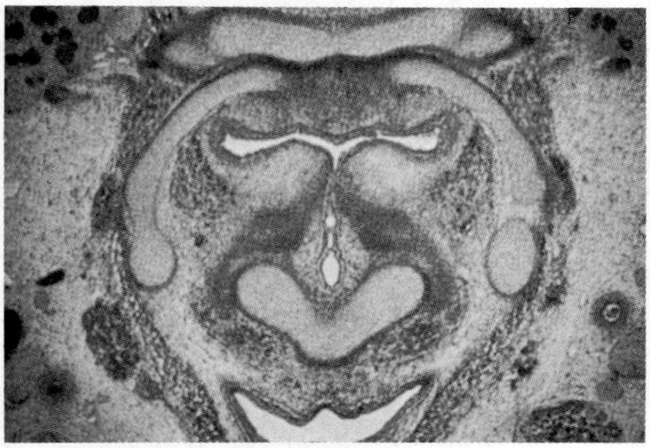

Figure 1–20. Transverse section through the larynx shown in Figure 1–19, taken a little further caudally. The hyoid, thyroid, and cricoid cartilages are evident. The section is just caudal to the arytenoid cartilages and is close to the cricoarytenoid joints. The thyroarytenoid and posterior cricoarytenoid muscles can be detected. (From Tucker JA, O'Rahilly R: Ann Otol Rhinol Laryngol 81:520–521, 1972.)

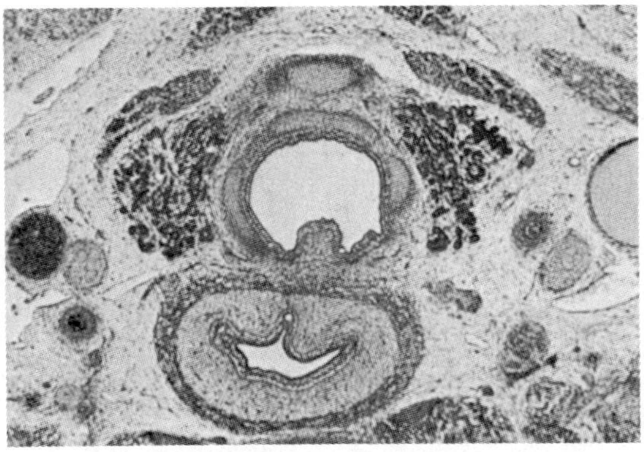

Figure 1–21. Transverse section to demonstrate the rostral limit of the trachea and esophagus at Stage 23. The caudal limit of the arch of the cricoid is shown uppermost and the cartilaginous rings of the trachea are visible. A dorsal folding of the wall of the trachea projects into the lumen. The right and left lobes of the thyroid gland are evident, and several of the nearby muscles can be seen. The mucous, submucous, and muscular coats of the esophagus are readily discernible. (From Tucker JA, O'Rahilly R: Ann Otol Rhinol Laryngol 81:520–521, 1972.)

Stage 21—About 52 Days; 22 to 24 mm
The thyroid gland is identifiable inferolateral to the cricoid cartilage. The cartilaginous nodules are indicated in the hyoid, thyroid, and cricoid section (Fig. 1–16).

Stage 22—About 54 Days; 23 to 28 mm
Arytenoid condensations and the posterior cricoarytenoid muscles are well demonstrated.

Stage 23—About 57 days; 27 to 31 mm
Most features of the adult larynx are recognizable by the end of the embryonic period; however, the epiglottis still contains no sign of cartilage. The vocalis muscle begins to differentiate and is noted for the first time. The histologic degree of development of the intrinsic laryngeal musculature is less advanced than the adjacent musculature in the neck, including the infrahyoid muscle group[6] (Figs. 1–17 to 1–21).

FETAL DEVELOPMENT

Under the Carnegie system of classification, the fetal period begins when bone marrow formation appears in the humerus.

In the third month, the epithelium in the respiratory tract (larynx and trachea) and adjacent portions of the esophagus acquires cilia. The laryngeal ventricle is sharply outlined and the saccule identified. There is a ventral fusion of the thyroid lamina[7] (Figs. 1–22 and 1–23).

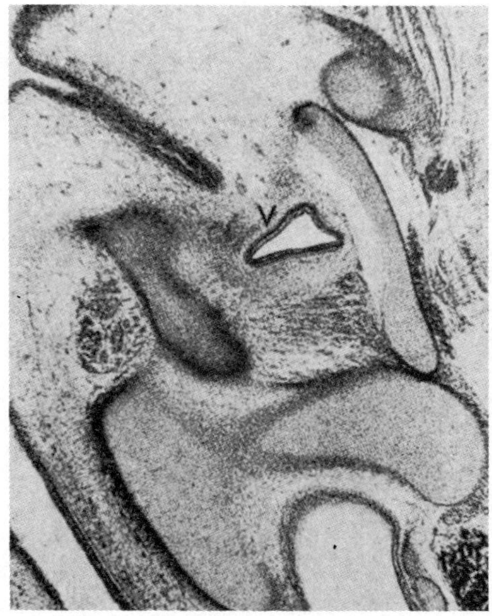

Figure 1–22. Paramedian sagittal section of a third-month (9–12 weeks) fetus, Carnegie Collection Specimen No. 6658, 40 mm in length. The triangular laryngeal ventricle is sharply outlined without glandular development (V). (From Tucker JA, Tucker GF Jr: Ann Otol Rhinol Laryngol 84:52, 1975.)

As for functional development, swallowing is observed at 12 weeks (approximately 75-mm fetal length). Elevation of the tongue and larynx is seen at 13 weeks.

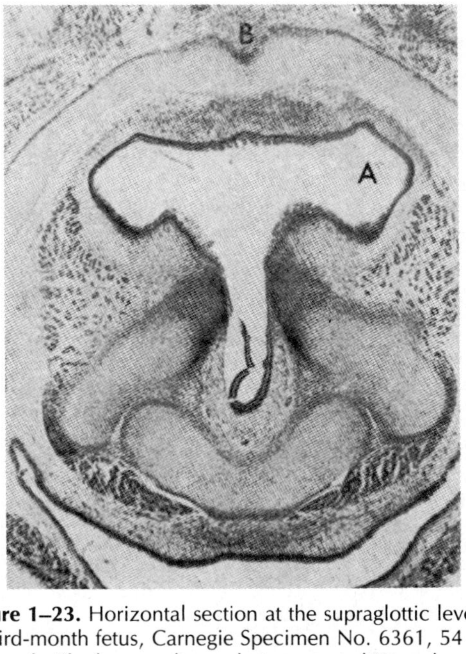

Figure 1–23. Horizontal section at the supraglottic level of a third-month fetus, Carnegie Specimen No. 6361, 54 mm in length. The laryngeal saccule is suggested (A) and ventral fusion of the thyroid laminae is seen (B). (From Tucker JA, Tucker GF Jr: Ann Otol Rhinol Laryngol 84:52, 1975.)

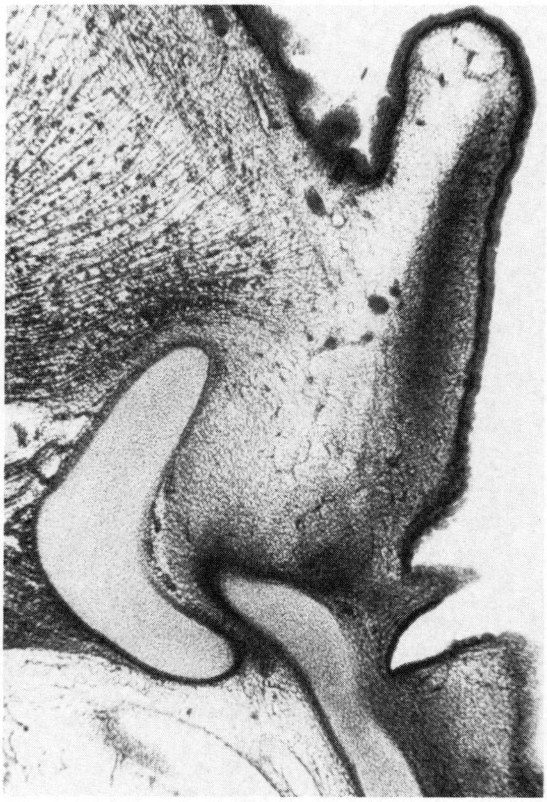

Figure 1–24. Sagittal section of a fourth-month fetus, Carnegie Specimen No. 1455, 78.5 mm in length. No cartilage is as yet demonstrated in the epiglottis. (From Tucker JA, Tucker GF Jr: Ann Otol Rhinol Laryngol 84:52, 1975.)

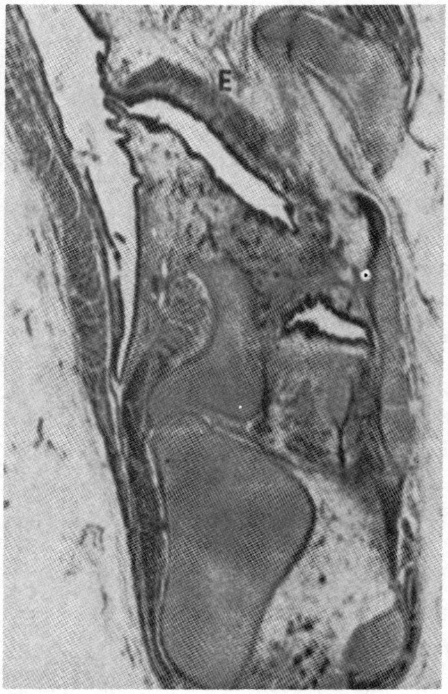

Figure 1–25. Sagittal section of a fifth-month fetus, Laryngeal Institute Specimen No. 411, 140 mm in length. Fibroelastic cartilage is present in the epiglottis (E). (From Tucker JA, Tucker GF Jr: Ann Otol Rhinol Laryngol 84:53, 1975.)

In the fourth month, goblet cells appear. The cilia have now reached the end of the bronchial tree and will reach the terminals of the bronchi at birth. Development of the submucosal glands begins by the fourth month and continues after birth[7] (Fig. 1–24).

In the fifth month, fibroelastic cartilage is present in the epiglottis (Fig. 1–25).

In the sixth month, definitive glandular formation is observed throughout the larynx and the lower respiratory tract (Fig. 1–26).

In the seventh month, elaborate glandular formation is present in the larynx and trachea. Viability, the ability to survive extramaternally, is generally achieved at approximately 24 to 26 postovulatory weeks.[5] Postnatal maturation of the adult trachea includes tracheal enlargement (Fig. 1–27).

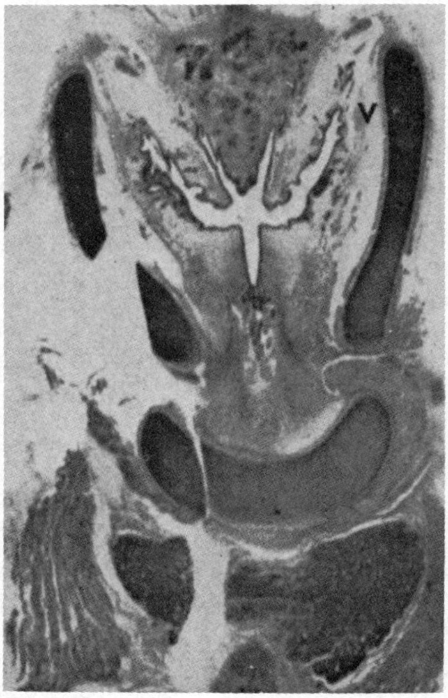

Figure 1–26. Coronal section of a sixth-month fetus, Laryngeal Institute Specimen No. 21, 321 mm in length. Definitive glandular formation in the ventricle and saccule is observed (V). (From Tucker JA, Tucker GF Jr: Ann Otol Rhinol Laryngol 84:53, 1975.)

REFLEX DEVELOPMENT

As noted by Humphrey,[8] mouth opening occurs at 26 mm, swallowing at 75 mm, and

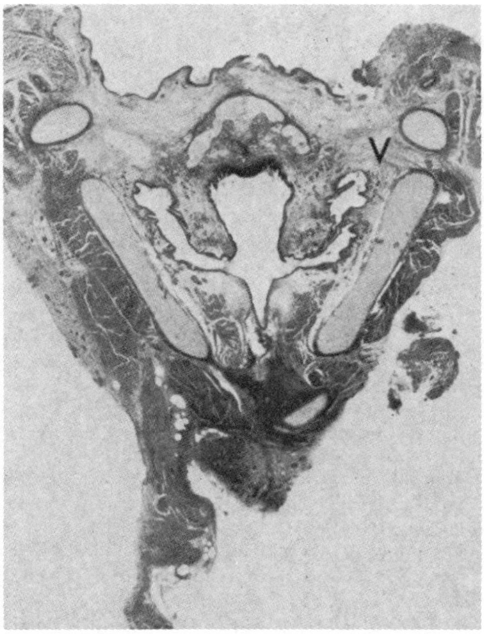

Figure 1–27. Coronal section of a seventh-month fetus, Laryngeal Institute Specimen No. 27, 230.5 mm in length. Elaborate glandular formation is present (V). (From Tucker JA, Tucker GF Jr: Ann Otol Rhinol Laryngol 84:53, 1975.)

elevation of the larynx at approximately 12 weeks. Tongue movements occur at 85.5 mm (approximately 14 weeks of gestation).[8] The combined movements for breathing develop relatively early. At eight weeks, the first reflex elicited from the human fetus appears to be a gasp.[9] Fetal breathing movements occur in utero and are thought to be due to diaphragmatic contraction secondary to phrenic nerve activity. Such movements have been observed as early as 11 weeks[9] and 13 weeks of gestation.[10]

In summary, application of the Carnegie system to the human embryo has provided a detailed, accurate account of the precise sequence of embryologic development. As future fetal staging systems are developed, they should include physiologic milestones of development as well as classic morphologic descriptions.

ANOMALOUS DEVELOPMENT

All true developmental anomalies or teratogenetic effects result from disordered organogenesis. Only by chance does the embryologist have the opportunity to study an abnormally developed embryo. The scientific explanation of anomalies, therefore, becomes a deductive process, correlated to the sequence of normal development.[11]

The most critical period in organogenesis is the stage of the organ primordia. During this time, the greatest potential for differentiation in growth exists. As Smith[12] has noted, the embryo

Table 1–2. ANATOMIC DISTRIBUTION OF CONGENITAL LARYNGEAL ANOMALIES*

Region	Site or Structure	Clinical Name	Associated Problems/Description
Supraglottis		Congenital laryngomalacia	Flaccid larynx Overdeveloped elongated epiglottis with broad base Excessively tubular and short epiglottis Cri du chat syndrome
	Epiglottis	Bifid epiglottis Absence of epiglottis	
	Ventricular band/	Atresia	
	Aryepiglottic fold	"Congenital cyst" Hemangioma	Retention cyst
	Ventricle	Laryngocele	
Glottis	True vocal cords	Webs Atresia	
		Vocal cord sulcus	Absence of arytenoid
Subglottis	Infraglottic and cricoid sites	Stenosis Webs Atresia Cleft Hemangioma	
		Laryngoptosis	Abnormally caudal laryngeal position

*Adapted from Tucker JA et al. Ann Otol Rhinol Laryngol 87:641, 1978.

Table 1–3. CONGENTIAL LARYNGEAL ANOMALIES*

Type of Anomaly	Number of Cases
Laryngomalacia	1,812
Bifid epiglottis	8
Absence of epiglottis	2
Absence of arytenoid	1
Webs	226
Atresia	46
Cysts	62
Laryngocele	8
Subglottic stenosis	348
Clefts	72
Hemangioma	114
Laryngoptosis	9
Total	2,708

*Updated from Tucker JA et al. Ann Otol Rhinol Laryngol 87:638, 1978.

is most sensitive to various noxious agents; indeed, the primordium can be arrested. The degree of embryologic insult is limited to particular organs or organ systems by the specific point of differentiation at the stage when injury occurs. Thus, the organ primordium represents a stage of limited liability, duration, and incidence.[13] The more stages in organogenesis, the greater the chance of anomalous or variant development (e.g., in the case of the supraglottis, normal epiglottic development extends into the fifth fetal month).[6]

Table 1–2 illustrates congenital anomalies by classification into supraglottic, glottic, and subglottic laryngeal locations.[13] Another method of generally classifying laryngeal abnormalities would be to specifically relate the anomaly to the predominant tissue type (i.e., cartilage, muscular, vascular, connective, or epithelial tissues).

A review of 2708 recorded congenital laryngeal anomalies (Table 1–3) illustrates the preponderance of laryngeal abnormality occurring in the supraglottic larynx.[13]

CONCLUSIONS

Our present knowledge of the developmental anatomy of the larynx carries distinct implications for medical practice. The infant larynx has certain fundamental peculiarities of structure that must be considered in examination and treatment.[14]

I would reemphasize, as noted by Holinger et al.,[15] that "an understanding of the embryology of the larynx is necessary for an appreciation of the development of its anomalies."

References

1. Soulie A, Bardier E: Récherchés sur le development du larynx chez l'homme. J Anat Physiol Paris 43:137–240, 1907.
2. Tucker JA, O'Rahilly R: Observations on the embryology of the human larynx. Ann Otol Rhinol Laryngol 81:520–523, 1972.
3. O'Rahilly R, Tucker JA: The early development of the larynx in staged human embryos. Ann Otol Rhinol Laryngol 82(Suppl 7):3–27, 1973.
4. O'Rahilly R: Developmental Stages in Human Embryos, Including a Survey of the Carnegie Collection. Part A: Embryos of the First Three Weeks (Stages 1 to 9). Washington, DC, Carnegie Institution of Washington, 1973.
5. O'Rahilly R, Boyden EA: The timing and sequence of events in the development of the human respiratory system during the embryonic period proper. Z Anat Entwicklungsgesch 141:237–250, 1973.
6. Muller R et al.: The human larynx at the end of the embryonic period proper. Acta Otol 91:323–336, 1981.
7. Tucker JA, Tucker GF Jr: Some aspects of fetal laryngeal development. Ann Otol Rhinol Laryngol 84:49–55, 1975.
8. Humphrey T: The development of mouth opening and related reflex involving the oral area of human fetuses. Alabama J Med Sci 5:126, 1968.
9. Windle WF: Genesis of somatic motor function in mammalian embryos: A synthesizing article. Physiol Zool 17:247, 1944.
10. Dawes GS: Breathing before birth in animals and man. An essay in developmental medicine. New Engl J Med 290:557, 1974.
11. Holinger PH et al.: A correlation of the embryonic development of the trachea and lungs with congenital malformations. Adv Otol Rhinol Laryngol 3:1–40, 1955.
12. Smith EI: The early development of the trachea and esophagus in relation to atresia of the esophagus and tracheoesophageal fistula. Contrib Embryol Carnegie Inst 36:41–57, 1957.
13. Tucker JA et al.: Clinical correlation of anomalies of the supraglottic larynx with staged sequence of normal human laryngeal development. Ann Otol Rhinol Laryngol 87:5, 636–645, 1978.
14. Tucker GF: The infant larynx: Direct laryngoscopic observations. JAMA 99:1899–1902, 1932.
15. Holinger PH et al.: Congenital anomalies of the larynx. Ann Otol Rhinol Laryngol 63:581–606, 1954.

2

Surgical Anatomy of the Larynx

Joel Michael Berman, M.D.

To appreciate the many pathophysiologic processes that may affect the larynx, the otolaryngologist must have a detailed understanding of its rather complex anatomy. The skeleton of the larynx is composed of cartilages, interconnected by ligaments and moved by muscles. It is lined by a mucous membrane continuous with that of the pharynx and the trachea. Until puberty, the larynx of the male differs little in size from that of the female. At puberty, the female larynx increases only slightly, whereas the male larynx undergoes a considerable increase in size of all cartilages with development of the prominent thyroid notch in the midline of the neck. The length of the male rima glottidis is nearly doubled.

The average recorded measurements of the adult larynx are as follows:

	Males	*Females*
Length (in mm)	44	36
Transverse diameter (in mm)	43	41
Anteroposterior diameter (in mm)	36	26

In adult females, the larynx is generally smaller, especially in its length and anteroposterior diameter.

LARYNGEAL SKELETON

Thyroid Cartilage. The thyroid cartilage (Fig. 2–1) is the largest of the laryngeal cartilages. It consists of two flattened quadrilateral alae fused in the midline anteriorly to form an angle of 90 degrees in males and 120 degrees in females. In the male, the fused anterior borders form a projection that can be seen subcutaneously in the front of the neck as the laryngeal eminence or Adam's apple. This eminence is generally absent in females owing to the wider angle subtended by the alae. A small, narrow strip of cartilage, called the intrathyroid cartilage, separates the two alae anteriorly in childhood. The V-shaped thyroid notch is situated just above the laryngeal eminence. The superior and inferior cornua project from the posterior border of each ala. The superior cornu passes upward and backward, ending in a rounded knob to which the lateral thyrohyoid ligament attaches, whereas the shorter inferior cornu articulates on its inner aspect with the cricoid cartilage at the cricothyroid joint.

On the external surface, extending down from the superior thyroid tubercle to the inferior tubercle, is the oblique line to which three muscles (the sternothyroid, the thyrohyoid, and the inferior pharyngeal constrictor) attach. Note

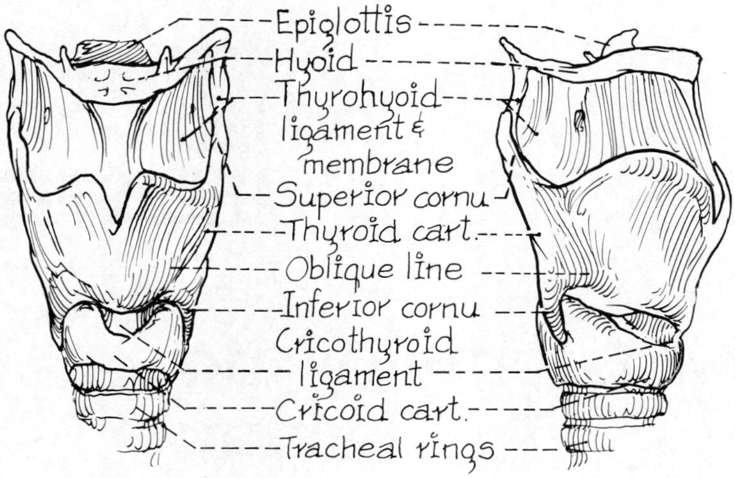

Figure 2–1. Laryngeal skeleton, anterior and lateral projection.

that this line is situated closer to the posterior border of the thyroid cartilage than might be anticipated. The perichondrium covering the external surface of the thyroid laminae adheres firmly to the superior and inferior margins. It blends with the thyrohyoid membrane above but is loosely attached to the smooth outer surface of the cartilage, making preservation of this layer possible during conservation surgical procedures for laryngeal cancer. Internally, the cartilage is lined with mucoperichondrium, except at the anterior commissure where it is deficient. At the anterior junction of the alae and in the angle thus formed, the thyroepiglottic ligament is attached. Below that, on each side, are inserted the vestibular and vocal ligaments that serve as the attachments for the thyroarytenoid, thyroepiglottic, and vocalis muscles.

Morphologically, the thyroid cartilage is composed of hyaline cartilage that ossifies with advancing age. Ossification commences about the 25th year of life and this cartilage may be transformed into bone containing hematopoietic marrow by the seventh decade.

Cricoid Cartilage. Immediately below the thyroid cartilage, and articulating with it, is the cricoid cartilage, which is shaped like a signet ring (Fig. 2–2). It is the only complete cartilaginous ring in the laryngotracheobronchial tree. The cartilage possesses a posterior quadrate lamina and a narrower anterior arch. The lamina measures between 2 cm and 3 cm high with a median vertical ridge on its posterior surface. To the upper part of this ridge are attached two fasciculi of the longitudinal muscle fibers of the esophagus. On each side of

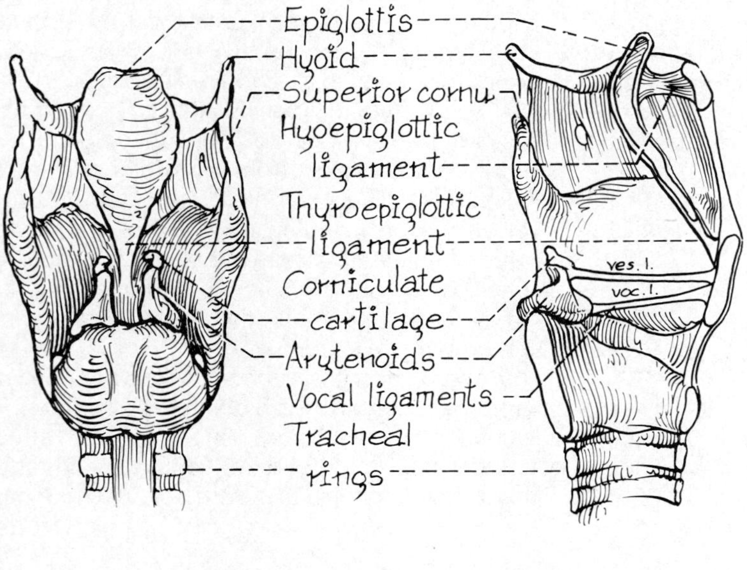

Figure 2–2. Laryngeal skeleton, posterior and sagittal projection.

this ridge, a shallow depression gives rise to the fibers of origin of the posterior cricoarytenoid muscle. A smooth oval convex surface, directed upward and laterally, is present on the superior lateral aspect of the lamina for articulation with the base of the arytenoid cartilage.

The arch of the cricoid narrows anteriorly, measuring between 5 mm and 7 mm, and widens as it approaches the lamina. A prominent articular facet is situated at the junction of the lamina and arch, for articulation with the inferior cornua of the thyroid cartilage.

The upper ring of the trachea is connected to the cricoid by the cricotracheal ligament. The cranial border of the arch gives rise to the cricothyroid ligament in the midline and laterally to the conus elasticus and lateral cricoarytenoid muscles. The internal surface is smooth and is lined with mucous membrane. The cricoid is composed of hyaline cartilage, which undergoes variable ossification with advancing age. This is especially pronounced in the lamina.

Arytenoid Cartilages. The paired arytenoid cartilages (Fig. 2–2) are pyramidal in shape and articulate with the upper and lateral borders of the cricoid lamina. Each has three surfaces, a base, and an apex. The medial surface is smooth and covered by mucous membrane, whereas the posterior surface, also smooth, gives attachment to the transverse arytenoid muscle. The slightly convex and rough anterolateral surface is divided below into two fossae by a crest that runs downward from the apex with a curve to the vocal process. The vestibular ligament attaches to the upper triangular fossa; the vocalis and the lateral cricoarytenoid muscles attach into the lower oblong fossa.

The base is smooth and saddle shaped for articulation with the cricoid lamina. The lateral angle of the base, called the muscular process, projects backward laterally and gives attachment to the posterior cricoarytenoid muscle behind and the lateral cricoarytenoid muscle in front. The anterior angle of the base, called the vocal process, is prolonged forward for attachment of the vocal ligaments. The apex curves backward medially and articulates with, or is sometimes fused with, the corniculate cartilage.

The arytenoid cartilages are composed of hyaline cartilage with a predisposition to ossification in later life.

Corniculate Cartilages. The corniculate cartilages or cartilages of Wrisberg (Fig. 2–2) are composed of fibroelastic cartilage and are conical in shape. They may articulate with or be fused with the medially directed apex of the arytenoid cartilages.

Cuneiform Cartilages. There is one cuneiform cartilage (cartilage of Santorini) in each free margin of the aryepiglottic fold. Club shaped, small, and composed of elastic fibrocartilage, each can be seen in its submucosal situation as a prominence on the aryepiglottic fold just anterior to the corniculate cartilages. A small elastic nodule called the triticeous cartilage is located in each lateral thyrohyoid ligament.

Epiglottic Cartilage. The epiglottis (Fig. 2–2) is a slightly curved, flattened, leaf-shaped sheet of elastic fibrocartilage that never undergoes ossification. The free upper portion is broad and rounded, whereas the attached distal part or stalk, called the petiole, is long and narrow. The petiole is attached by the thyroepiglottic ligament to the inner surface of the thyroid cartilage just below the thyroid notch in the midline. From this attachment, the epiglottis curves upward and backward to overhang the vestibule of the larynx. Mucous membrane extending from the tongue onto the anterior surface of the suprahyoid portion of the epiglottis is raised in the midline to form the median glossoepiglottic fold; lateral reflections of this mucous membrane, passing from the tongue to the lateral pharyngeal wall, form the lateral glossoepiglottic folds. The depression thus formed on each side of the median glossoepiglottic fold is called the vallecula. An elastic ligament, the hyoepiglottic ligament, connects the epiglottis to the hyoid bone in front.

The posterior or laryngeal surface of the epiglottis is smooth and lined by firmly adherent mucous membrane. Numerous mucus-secreting glands lie beneath the mucosa and actually indent the posterior surface of the cartilage. A number of dehiscences are present within the cartilage in which bundles of compound seromucinous glands are situated. These openings provide an important pathway for the spread of supraglottic carcinoma through an intact epiglottis to the preepiglottic space. The tubercle of the epiglottis, a prominence consisting of both cartilage and a condensation of mucous glands, is present on the posterior surface. From each side of the epiglottis, the mucous membrane continues downward toward the arytenoid cartilages, thus forming the aryepiglottic fold.

LARYNGEAL ARTICULATIONS

Cricothyroid Joint. Between the inferior cornu of the thyroid cartilage and the corresponding articulate facet on the cricoid cartilage is a simple synovial joint, reinforced by the anterior, inferior, and prominent posterior cricothyroid ligaments. Rotation of the cricoid cartilage on the thyroid cartilage occurs about an axis passing transversely through the joints.

Cricoarytenoid Joint. Each arytenoid cartilage articulates with the cricoid cartilage by means of a synovial joint that is strengthened by capsular ligaments and by the firm posterior cricoarytenoid ligaments. Two major movements occur concurrently at the cricoarytenoid joint. The first movement occurs through an axis running obliquely through the arytenoid, thereby producing a rotation with either abduction or adduction of the vocal process. The second movement is a complex gliding and tipping motion, either laterally and downward following the slope of the cricoid facet or medially toward the opposite arytenoid cartilage. The cricoarytenoid ligament performs an important function, limiting excessive forward movement of the arytenoid on the cricoid cartilage.

INTRINSIC MUSCLES OF THE LARYNX

All of the intrinsic muscles of the larynx (Fig. 2–3) are paired except for the transverse arytenoid muscle (interarytenoid muscle). They are

1. Muscles that open and close at the glottis: the lateral and posterior cricoarytenoids, and the transverse arytenoid (interarytenoid) muscle.
2. Muscles that control the tension of the vocal ligaments: the thyroarytenoid, the vocalis, and the cricothyroid.
3. Muscles that alter the shape of the inlet of the larynx: the aryepiglottic muscle and thyroepiglottic muscle.

Aryepiglottic Muscle. The free upper edge of the quadrate membrane, the aryepiglottic fold, contains muscle fibers that connect the side of the epiglottis to the muscular process and posterior surface of the opposite arytenoid cartilage. The two muscles thus cross each other like the limbs of the letter X, posterior to the

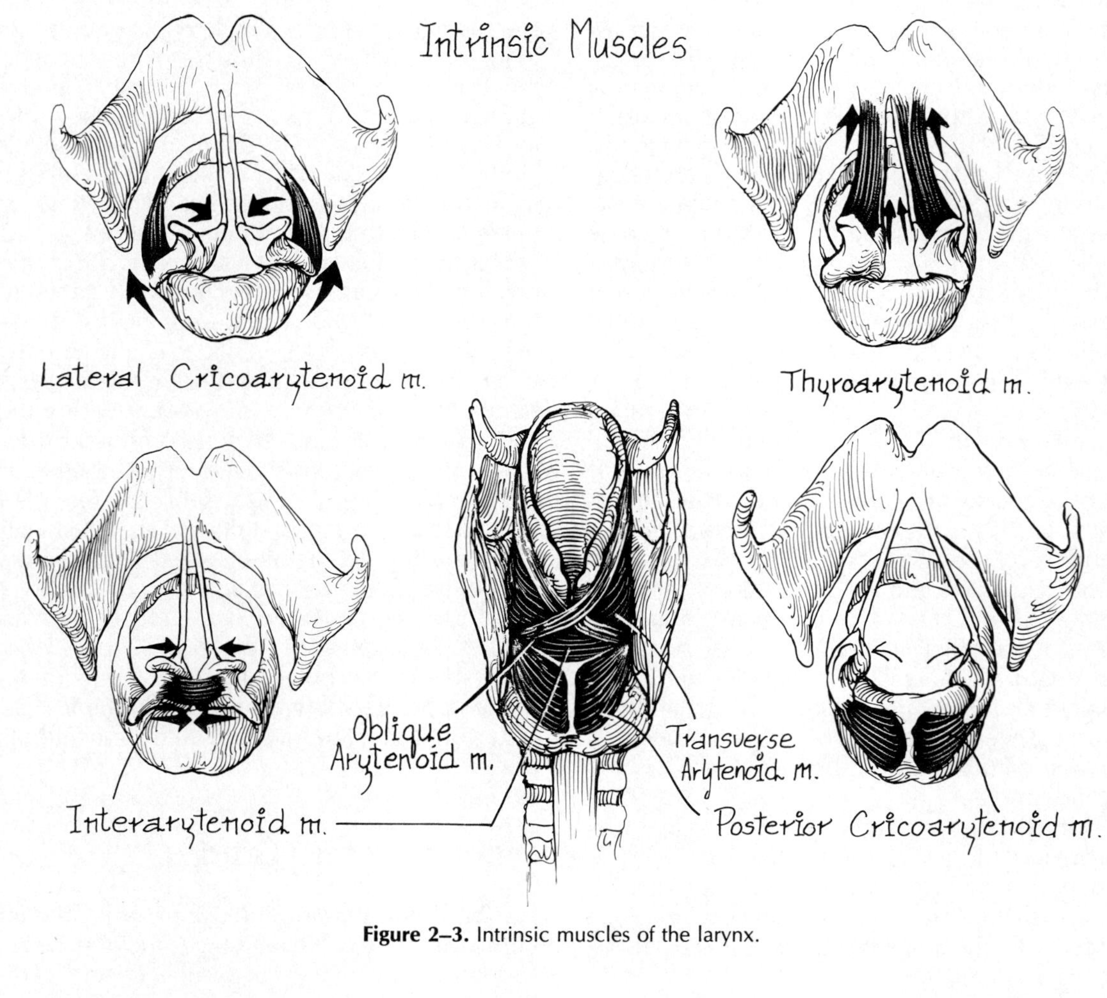

Figure 2–3. Intrinsic muscles of the larynx.

transversely running fibers of the interarytenoid muscle. This portion is sometimes referred to as the oblique arytenoid muscle, but it is more accurate to conceive of this muscle as a single entity that is a complete sphincter of the laryngeal inlet.

Contraction of the oblique arytenoid and interarytenoid muscles apposes the arytenoids to each other and draws down the epiglottis, bringing the tubercle into contact with the arytenoids. Note that the free edge of the aryepiglottic fold in some instances contains no muscle fibers; in these cases, the interarytenoid muscle is well developed.

Posterior Cricoarytenoid Muscle. The posterior cricoarytenoid muscle is the only abductor of the vocal cords and may, therefore, be considered the most important muscle in the larynx. It arises from the lower and medial surface of the back of the cricoid lamina, from which the fibers are directed upward and laterally to be inserted onto the back of the muscular process of the ipsilateral arytenoid. The upper fibers are almost horizontal, the middle fibers are oblique, and the lower fibers are almost vertical. Contraction of the horizontal fibers tends to move the muscular processes toward each other, thereby rotating each arytenoid about its own axis with resulting separation of the vocal processes and the opening of the glottis. The vertical component draws the arytenoids downward on the sloping shoulders of the cricoid lamina, causing separation of the arytenoid without rotation. These movements occur simultaneously, but in man, the lateral gliding displacement constitutes the greater proportion of the total arytenoid movement. The muscle is, therefore, an abductor of the vocal cords. In a secondary action, the muscle braces the arytenoid and prevents the vocal processes from tilting downward.

Lateral Cricoarytenoid Muscle. The lateral cricoarytenoid muscle arises from the upper border of the lateral part of the arch of the cricoid cartilage and is inserted into the anterior surface of the muscular process of the arytenoid cartilage. Traction of the muscle draws the muscular process forward, causing approximation of the vocal processes by rotating the arytenoids. This muscle is, therefore, an adductor of the vocal cords, acting in opposition to the horizontal fibers of the posterior cricoarytenoid muscle.

Interarytenoid Muscle. The interarytenoid muscle is a single muscle that arises from the posterior surface and lateral border of one arytenoid cartilage and is inserted into the corresponding parts of the contralateral arytenoid. It forms a strong mass of transverse fibers, the contraction of which draws the arytenoid cartilages up the sloping shoulders of the cricoid lamina, thereby approximating or adducting the vocal cord without rotation.

Thyroarytenoid Muscle. The thyroarytenoid muscle arises from the back of the inferior part of the angle made by the thyroid alae and from the cricothyroid ligament below this. It forms a broad thin muscle situated lateral to the vocal ligaments and conus elasticus. The muscle fibers pass backward laterally and superiorly to be inserted into the anterolateral surface of the arytenoid cartilage. The lower part of the muscle is thicker and forms a distinct bundle called the vocalis muscle. Fibers of this muscle are inserted into the vocal process of the arytenoid cartilage. The fibers lie parallel to the vocal ligament, to which the muscle adheres. Contraction of the vocalis muscle pulls up portions of the conus elasticus, thereby increasing the vertical depth of the opposing surfaces of the vocal folds.

Numerous fibers of the thyroarytenoid muscles are prolonged into the aryepiglottic fold, which lies outside the quadrate membrane and inserts into the side of the epiglottis. These fibers are sometimes called the thyroepiglottic muscle.

Cricothyroid Muscle. The triangular-shaped cricothyroid muscle arises from the anterior and lateral part of the cricoid arch, from which it fans out in a posterior direction, gaining attachment to the inferior cornua and lower border of the thyroid cartilage. A triangular interval occupied by the conus elasticus separates the medial borders of the paired muscles. Contraction of the muscle rotates the thyroid cartilage about the horizontal axis, which passes through the cricothyroid joints. In this way, the thyroid cartilage is tilted downward toward the relatively fixed cricoid. This increases the distance between the vocal processes and the thyroid cartilage, thus also increasing the tension of the vocal cords. That the cricothyroid has a minor subsidiary action as an adductor of the vocal cords should be appreciated.

Nerve Supply of the Intrinsic Muscles. The recurrent laryngeal nerve supplies all the intrinsic laryngeal muscles except for the cricothyroid muscle, which is supplied by the external branch of the superior laryngeal nerve entering on its lateral surface. Unconfirmed claims suggest that the internal laryngeal nerve may innervate the interarytenoid muscle. That the interarytenoid muscle is the only one with bilateral innervation is also noteworthy. The terminal portion of the recurrent laryngeal nerve passes upward deep to the lower border of the inferior pharyngeal constrictor, immediately behind the cricothyroid joint, and supplies all the other intrinsic muscles. Before entering the larynx, the nerve divides into motor and sensory branches.

LARYNGEAL MEMBRANES

Conus Elasticus. Arising from the cricoid is a fibroelastic membrane (Fig. 2–4) that attaches anteriorly in the midline to the lower border of the thyroid cartilage. This part of the membrane is thick and strong and constitutes the cricothyroid ligament. It is overlapped on each side by the cricothyroid muscle, but it lies in a subcutaneous situation between these muscles at a point where an emergency cricothyrotomy may be performed. Laterally, the conus elasticus is much thinner and extends upward on each side from the upper border of the cricoid cartilage. The conus is attached in front to the inner surface of the thyroid angle and behind to the tip of the vocal process of the arytenoid cartilage. Its free upper border, between these attachments, is slightly thickened and constitutes the vocal ligament. The conus elasticus is lined on its medial surface by mucous membrane of the larynx, whereas the lateral cri-

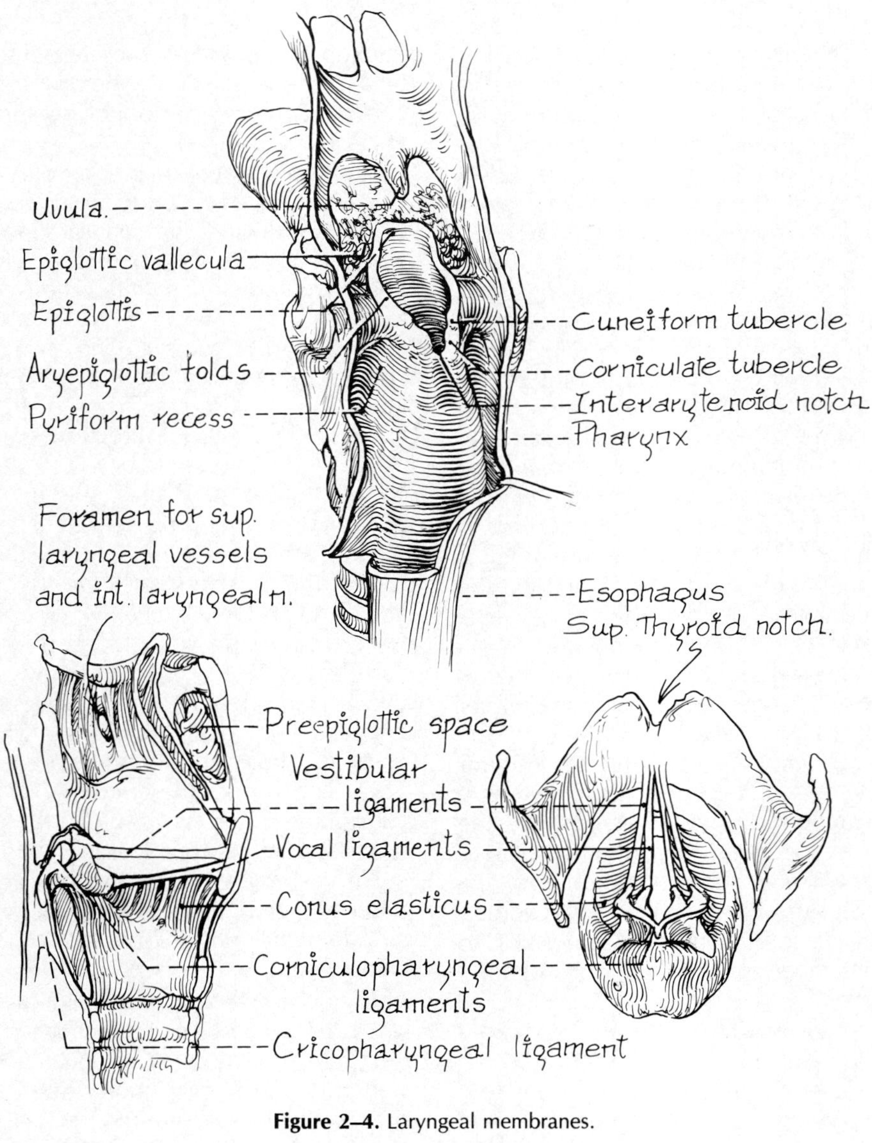

Figure 2–4. Laryngeal membranes.

coarytenoid and thyroarytenoid muscles are intimately related to its lateral surface.

Quadrangular Membrane. The quadrangular membrane is a fibroelastic membrane, less well developed than the conus elasticus, that extends between the arytenoids and epiglottis. Its anterior border is attached to the side of the lower half of the epiglottis, whereas the posterior border is attached to the arytenoid between the vocal process and the corniculate cartilage. Its free lower border, attached anteriorly to the thyroid cartilage, constitutes the vestibular fold (false vocal cord). The upper border, which is longer, forms the aryepiglottic fold containing the tiny cuneiform cartilage.

Thyrohyoid Membrane. The fibroelastic thyrohyoid membrane (Fig. 2–1) is attached below to the superior border of the thyroid cartilage and superior cornua, and above to the upper margin of the posterior surface of the body and greater cornua of the hyoid bone. This membrane is separated from the posterior surface of the body of the hyoid bone by a bursa that facilitates upward movement of the larynx during deglutition. The superior laryngeal vessels and internal laryngeal nerve pierce this membrane. Rounded fibroelastic cords, called the lateral thyrohyoid ligaments, form the posterior borders of the thyrohyoid membrane and connect the tips of the superior cornua with the posterior end of the greater cornua of the hyoid bone. These ligaments sometimes contain small cartilaginous nodules called cartilago triticea.

Mucous Membrane of the Larynx. Lining the interior of the larynx is a mucous membrane. Continuous with the tongue above, the laryngopharynx behind, and the trachea below, this membrane sweeps down from the base of the tongue over the vallecula, where it is loosely attached to the smooth anterior surface of the suprahyoid portion of the epiglottis. Next, the mucosa drapes over the aryepiglottic folds to line the laryngeal vestibule and extends from the free margin of the aryepiglottic folds to the false cords below. The membrane is firmly attached to the posterior surface of the epiglottis and arytenoid cartilages. The laryngeal ventricle, a deep cleft separating the false cords and vocal folds, is prolonged anteriorly to form the laryngeal saccule that lies between the thyroid cartilage and the false cord. The saccule is thought to represent the phylogenetic remnant of the laryngeal air sac of the higher anthropoid apes. Its size varies but normally never extends beyond the upper margin of the thyroid ala. From the ventricle, the mucosa projects over the surface of the vocal ligaments and thyroarytenoid muscle to form the true vocal cord. From this point, the mucosa lines the subglottic portion of the larynx, the upper part being loosely applied to the underlying structures with numerous submucosal glands, whereas the lower portion adheres more firmly to the underlying cricoid cartilage.

Histology. The anterior surface of the suprahyoid epiglottis faces the tongue and is lined by thick stratified squamous epithelium with numerous submucosal glands conforming to the functional need. Over the laryngeal surface of the epiglottis is found low stratified squamous epithelium that adheres firmly to the underlying cartilage. Mucous glands are particularly numerous on the posterior surface of the epiglottis, where they form indentations into the cartilage. Pseudostratified ciliated columnar epithelium covers the inferior portions of the false cords, the ventricles, and the subglottic region. Nonkeratinizing squamous epithelium covers the free margins of the vocal cords. Although the epithelium of the vocal cord closely adheres to the underlying vocal ligament, a potential subepithelial space exists. Called Reinke's space, it runs the length of the vocal cord. This space is limited above and below by the linea arcuata, small indentations in the vocal cord that mark the junction of the squamous and columnar epithelium.

BLOOD SUPPLY OF THE LARYNX

Arteries. The vasculature of the larynx (Fig. 2–5) is divided into superior and inferior segments at the level of the glottis. The superior laryngeal branch of the superior thyroid artery supplies blood to the supraglottic larynx. This artery enters the pyriform fossa with the internal laryngeal nerve by piercing the posteroinferior part of the thyrohyoid membrane.

The lower half of the larynx is supplied by the inferior laryngeal branch of the inferior thyroid artery, which accompanies the recurrent laryngeal nerve beneath the inferior constrictor of the pharynx. Some blood supply to the subglottic region is derived from the cricothyroid branch of the superior thyroid artery and enters through the cricothyroid membrane. Microvascular patterns are rather haphazard but are predominantly circumferential, in contrast to the linear and parallel microvascular arrangement of the vocal cords. In the region of the anterior commissure, a relatively avascular area separates the blood supply of the vocal cords.

Venous Drainage. The superior laryngeal veins (Fig. 2–5) accompany the artery and empty into the superior thyroid vein, which in

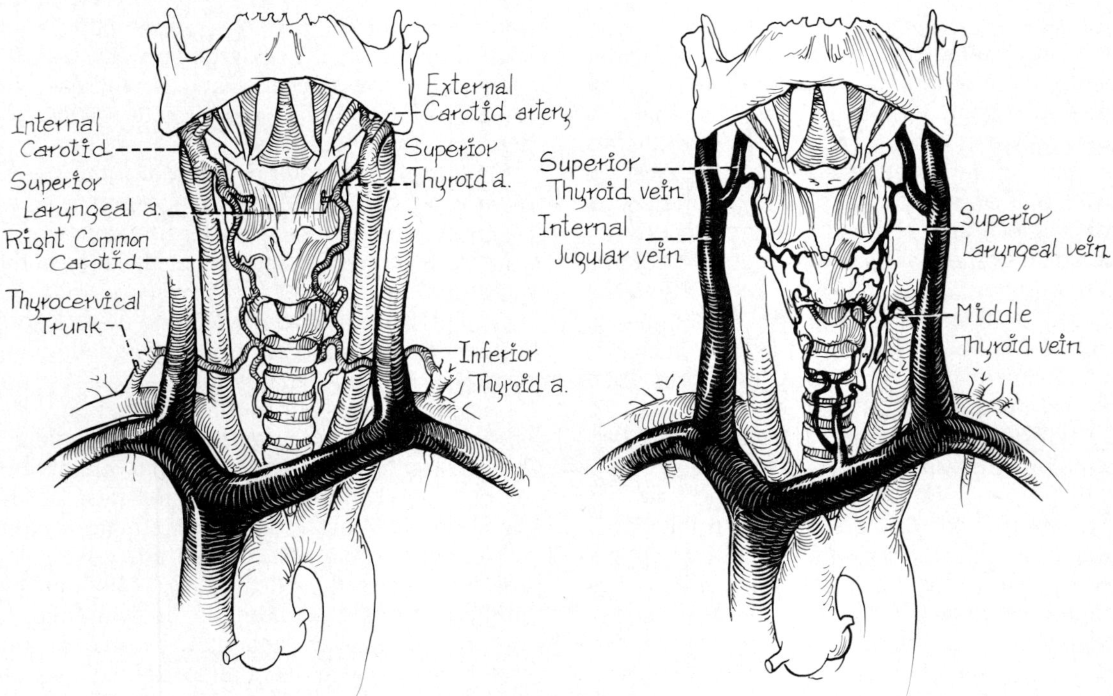

Figure 2–5. Arteries and veins of the larynx.

turn opens into the internal jugular vein. Those veins accompanying the inferior laryngeal artery join the inferior thyroid vein, which opens subsequently into the left brachiocephalic vein.

Lymph Vessels. The lymphatic vessels draining the supraglottic region accompany the superior thyroid artery. These lymphatics drain into the anterosuperior group of deep cervical lymph nodes. This anatomic configuration is important in understanding the feasibility of performing horizontal partial supraglottic laryngectomy.

The subepithelial space of the vocal cords is largely devoid of lymph vessels, accounting for the less frequent occurrence of metastatic nodes in vocal cord carcinoma.

Studies by Welsh et al. and by Pressman et al. revealed that lymphatic drainage of the subglottis is complex. They found that the superficial plexus of lymphatics unites to form three main pedicles, one anterior and two posterolateral. The anterior pedicle pierces the cricothyroid membrane to terminate in the prelaryngeal or Delphian node, which in turn drains through the pretracheal and supraclavicular nodes, following the branches of the inferior thyroid artery. The two posterolateral pedicles pierce the cricotracheal membrane and terminate in the paratracheal nodes, which are continuous with those in the superior mediastinum.

NERVE SUPPLY OF THE LARYNX

The supraglottic larynx is innervated with sensory and secretomotor fibers by the internal laryngeal division of the superior laryngeal branch of the vagus nerve. While the internal branch is probably entirely sensory, some investigators have claimed that motor filaments may innervate the interarytenoid muscle. After perforating the posteroinferior portion of the thyrohyoid membrane above the corresponding artery, this nerve crosses the pyriform fossa and, in this position, may be anesthetized by application of a cocaine or lidocaine (Xylocaine) pledget. The nerve supplies both surfaces of the epiglottis, the aryepiglottic fold, and the vestibule of the larynx to the level of the vocal folds. Motor supply to the cricothyroid muscle is derived from the external division of the superior laryngeal nerve, which enters the muscle on its deep surface.

The recurrent laryngeal nerve supplies both sensory and secretomotor fibers to the lower half of the larynx; this nerve also innervates all the intrinsic muscles of the larynx except for the cricothyroid muscle. The terminal part of the recurrent laryngeal nerve accompanies the laryngeal branch of the inferior thyroid artery and enters the larynx after passing deep to the lower border of the inferior pharyngeal constrictor, immediately behind the cricothyroid joint.

Prior to entering the larynx, the nerve sometimes divides into a motor and sensory branch. This arrangement is of practical importance in extended conservation laryngeal procedures that may accidentally traumatize the nerve. The nerve fibers arise from neurons located in the lower part of the nucleus ambiguus; each neuron supplies approximately 30 muscle fibers.

The sympathetic nerve supply follows the arteries and derives from the superior cervical ganglion for the supraglottic larynx and from the middle cervical ganglion for the sublottis.

LARYNGEAL SPACES

An informed concept of the preepiglottic and paraglottic space is essential to understanding the growth and spread of laryngeal cancer and, thus, to the adequacy of surgical extirpation in conservation procedures for carcinoma of the larynx. These spaces are rarely described in standard anatomic textbooks.

The preepiglottic space, also called the space of Boyer, (Fig. 2–4) is triangular or funnel-shaped on sagittal section. It is bounded by the upper part of the thyroid cartilage and thyrohyoid membrane in front, the hyoepiglottic ligament beneath the floor of the vallecula superiorly, and the epiglottis and quadrangular membrane behind. Lateral extensions of the space merge with the paraglottic space. The preepiglottic space contains adipose and areolar tissue. While lymphatic channels are present, the space is devoid of any lymph nodes. As the anterior boundary of the larynx is considered to be the thyrohyoid membrane, the preepiglottic space should be regarded as being entirely intralaryngeal.

The paraglottic space is bounded by the thyroid cartilage anterolaterally, the conus elasticas inferomedially, and ventricle and quadrangular membrane medially, with the posterior limit being the pyriform fossa mucosa. It contains the vocal muscles (the thyroarytenoid and vocalis) surrounded by the paramycium that separates these muscles from the adipose tissue of the posterior projection of the preepiglottic space. Note that this space is in direct continuity with the paralaryngeal tissues of the neck through the cricothyroid space, presenting an important route for the spread of laryngeal cancer out of the larynx.

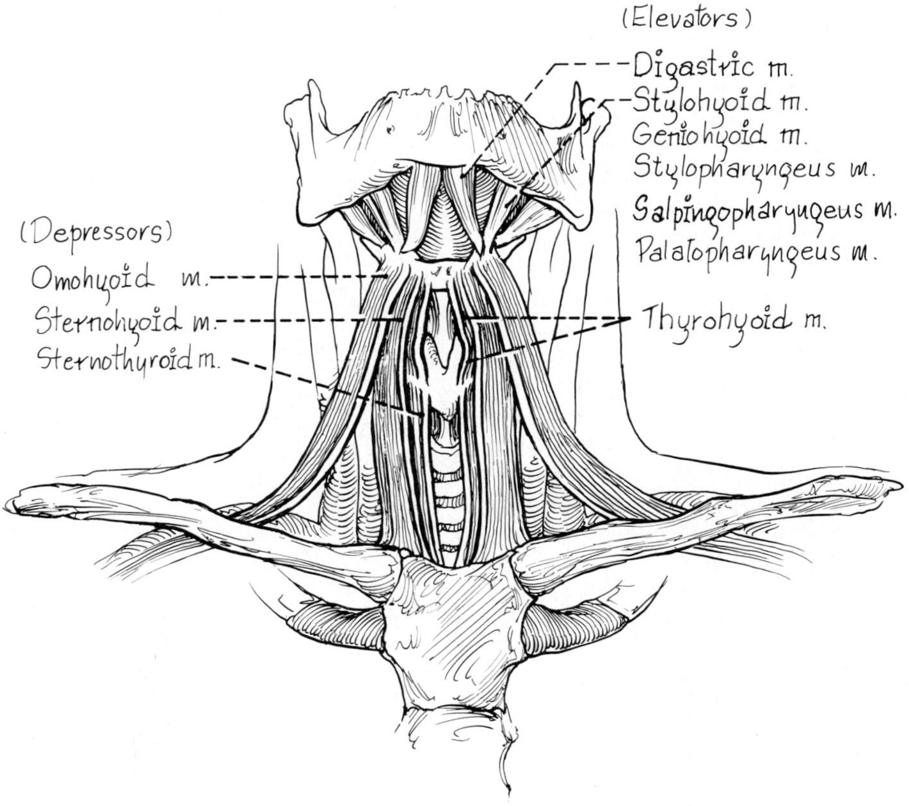

Figure 2–6. Extrinsic muscles of the larynx.

EXTRINSIC MUSCLES OF THE LARYNX

Two groups comprise the extrinsic laryngeal musculature: depressors and elevators (Fig. 2–6). Any muscle that produces elevation of the hyoid bone must elevate the larynx by transmitting its pull to the thyrohyoid membrane. Following elevation of the larynx, return to its position of rest is largely due to elastic recoil of the trachea. The dominant elevator of the hyoid is the mylohyoid; the digastric, stylohyoid, and geniohyoid play secondary roles. Four muscles, the stylopharyngeus, salpingopharyngeus, palatopharyngeus, and thyrohyoid, are the primary elevators of the larynx. Their fibers are inserted chiefly into the posterior border of the laminae and cornua of the thyroid cartilage.

The infrahyoid strap muscles (the sternohyoid, the sternothyroid, and the omohyoid) may be considered laryngeal depressors. For a more detailed and comprehensive description of these muscles, the reader is referred to a standard anatomic textbook (see Suggested Readings).

ANATOMIC REGIONS OF THE LARYNX

Traditionally, and for sound clinical reasons, otolaryngologists have divided the larynx into three anatomic regions: the supraglottis, glottis, and subglottis. According to the 1983 staging manual of the American Joint Committee on Cancer (AJCC), the supraglottis is composed of the epiglottis (both its lingual and laryngeal aspects), aryepiglottic folds, arytenoids, and ventricular bands (false cords). The inferior border of the supraglottis is an arbitrary horizontal plane passing through the apex or lateral angle of the ventricle. The glottis is composed of the true vocal cords, including the anterior and posterior commissures, with the lower boundary taken as a horizontal plane 1 cm below the apex of the ventricle. This point, called the linea arcuata, corresponds roughtly to the insertion of the upper border of the conus elasticus into the free edge of the true vocal cord. The subglottis is the region extending from the lower boundary of the glottis to the lower margin of the cricoid cartilage.

THE INTERIOR OF THE LARYNX

The inlet of the larynx is bounded superiorly by the free edge of the epiglottis and on each side by a fold of mucous membrane, the aryepiglottic fold, extending from the lateral edges of the epiglottis to the arytenoid cartilage. Posteriorly, the inlet is completed by the mucous membrane that passes between the two arytenoid cartilages. In the posterior part of each aryepiglottic fold, the corniculate and cuneiform cartilages form two subtle enlargements.

The vestibule of the larynx lies between the inlet of the larynx and the level of the vestibular fold. Narrowing as it extends downward, it has a longer anterior than posterior wall. The anterior wall consists of the posterior surface of the epiglottis, whereas the posterior wall consists of the mucous membrane covering the anterior surface of the arytenoid cartilages. The lateral wall of this vestibule is formed by the inner aspect of the aryepiglottic fold.

A narrow horizontal slit, called the ventricle (sinus) of the larynx, is located between the ventricular and vocal folds. From the anterior part of the ventricle, a pouch (the saccule of the larynx) extends between the vestibular fold and the inner surface of the thyroid cartilage.

An elongated fissure, known as the rima glottidis, is situated between the vocal cords anteriorly and the vocal processes and base of the arytenoid cartilages posteriorly. About three-fifths of its length is called the intermembraneous part because it lies between the vocal cords; the remainder is termed the intercartilaginous part. The average length of the rima glottidis varies from 23 mm in the male to 16 mm in the female. The true vocal cords are formed by a sharp reflection of the mucous membrane over the vocal ligaments. Because the mucous membrane over the vocal ligaments is closely applied to the ligaments with only a potential subepithelial space, the vocal folds appear as two shiny white cords.

That portion of the larynx extending from the true vocal cord above to a horizontal plane at the level of the lower border of the cricoid cartilage represents the subglottis. It is lined by mucous membrane with numerous submucosal glands.

APPLIED ANATOMY

The anatomic considerations in this chapter pertain to the growth and spread of certain laryngeal carcinomas as well as to the surgical application of conservation laryngectomy procedures.

The conus elasticus, a fibroelastic membrane, acts as a buffer to the inferior spread of glottic tumors; as a result, subglottic extension is a relatively late and serious manifestation of glottic carcinoma.

Because the internal perichondrium is deficient at the anterior commissure, tumors in this region frequently invade deeply into the adjacent thyroid cartilage, possibly accounting for the poor response of these tumors to radiation therapy. Tumors in this region can also extend into the neck through the cricothyroid space. The external perichondrium is much thinner near the midline and becomes thicker laterally.

The paraglottic space of the larynx containing the vocalis muscle is deficient laterally at the cricothyroid space. This becomes an important route for glottic carcinoma spread to the perilaryngeal tissues of the neck. Clinical evaluation of this extension can be difficult, causing some glottic tumors to be understaged. Also, the paraglottic space is in communication with the preepiglottic space and transglottic extension into the supraglottis may occur via this pathway.

Dehiscences in the epiglottic cartilage provide a direct route for spread of epiglottic cancer into the preepiglottic space. During the course of a total or partial horizontal supraglottic laryngectomy, it is important not to violate this space; dissection should be performed in a plane anterior to the thyrohyoid membrane and strap muscles. It is important to avoid resection of a portion of the epiglottis when performing vertical partial laryngectomy because this often results in some degree of aspiration. Tumors confined to the supraglottic region with normal vocal cord mobility can be treated surgically by partial horizontal supraglottic laryngectomy. The reason for this is that lymphatic vessels from this region do not extend to the vocal cords. Furthermore, the nerve supply of the intrinsic muscles enters the larynx from below, so that supraglottic laryngectomy in no way interferes with vocal cord mobility and competence.

Glottic tumors with normal cord mobility and tumors involving the anterior commissure may be treated surgically by various types of vertical hemilaryngectomy and extended frontolateral partial laryngectomy procedures, a family of techniques that remove the paraglottic compartment.

The relationship of important anatomic regions to the topographic anatomy of the cartilaginous portion of the larynx is not constant, but certain approximate anatomic correlations are helpful:

1. The superior margin of the true vocal folds in a male patient is usually immediately inferior to a plane that is located at the midpoint of a line drawn from the most superior extent of the apex of the thyroid notch to the midline of the inferior margin of the thyroid cartilage. This is the usual level of the horizontal cartilage cut made when performing a supraglottic partial laryngectomy. In the female patient, the cartilage cut is made 1 to 2 mm more superiorly.
2. The apex of the pyriform sinus is at the level of a plane that passes horizontally about 1.5 cm superior to the caudal margin of the cricoid cartilage.
3. The vallecula can be entered by a plane of dissection that begins at the superior border of the hyoid bone and angles superiorly at about 30 degrees.
4. The insertion of the vocalis tendons (Broyles' ligament) extends laterally for a distance of approximately 3 mm and can be avoided in vertical partial laryngectomy by a vertical cartilage cut that is 4 to 5 mm from the midline in the case of tumor involving the anterior commissure.

The following approximate dimensions for the average larynx in adult males are based on measurements of fresh total laryngectomy specimens:

1. The total height of the larynx is about 8 cm.
2. The distance from the superior margin of the true vocal fold to the tip of the epiglottis is about 5 cm.
3. The distance from the superior margin of the true vocal fold to the superior margin of the cricoid cartilage is about 2 cm, and the distance to the inferior margin of the cricoid is about 3 cm.
4. The height of the laryngeal ventricle is approximately 1 cm posteriorly and 1.5 cm anteriorly (in the region of the saccule).

These observations concerning topographic anatomy are useful to the surgeon performing conservation surgery or surgery for benign tumors in the larynx.

Suggested Readings

1. American Joint Committee on Cancer: Manual for Staging of Cancer, 2nd ed. Beahrs OH, Myers MH (eds). Philadelphia, JB Lippincott Company, 1983.
2. Anson B (ed): Morris' Human Anatomy, 12th ed. New York, McGraw-Hill Book Company, 1966, pp 1409–1427.
3. Grant JCB: An Atlas of Anatomy, 6th ed. Baltimore, The Williams and Wilkins Company, 1972, plates 621–632.
4. Hollinshead W: Anatomy for Surgeons, 3rd ed. Hagerstown, Md., Harper and Row, 1982.
5. Pernkopf E: Atlas of Topographical and Applied Anat-

omy, Vol. I, Head and Neck, 2nd ed. Baltimore, Urban and Schwarzenberg, 1980, pp 313–339.
6. Pressman JJ et al.: Further studies upon the submucosal compartments and lymphatics of the larynx by the injection of dyes and radioisotopes. Ann Otol Rhinol Laryngol 65:963, 1956.
7. Quiring DP, Warfel JH: The Head, Neck, and Trunk, 2nd ed. Philadelphia, Lea and Febiger, 1960.
8. Romanes GJ (ed): Cunningham's Textbook of Anatomy, 12th ed. Oxford, Oxford University Press, 1981, pp 498–506.
9. Sobotta J, Figge F: Atlas of Human Anatomy, Vol. 2, 9th English ed. New York, Hafner Press, 1974, pp 156–166.
10. Spalteholz W: Hand-Atlas of Human Anatomy. Philadelphia, JB Lippincott Company, 1943.
11. Warwick R, Williams P (eds): Gray's Anatomy, 35th British ed. Philadelphia, WB Saunders Company, 1973, pp 1173–1182.
12. Welsh LW et al.: Analysis of laryngeal compartments. Ann Otol Rhinol Laryngol 71:913, 1962.

3

Laryngeal Physiology

Clarence T. Sasaki, M.D.

The larynx performs three important functions that may be ranked by their importance as (1) protection, (2) respiration, and (3) phonation. A thorough understanding of these priorities appears essential to the management of the myriad diseases besetting this complex organ. This chapter addresses these three functions in terms of phylogeny, structure, and neuromuscular reflex activity as they may apply to surgically induced disturbances of laryngeal function.

PHYLOGENY AND FUNCTION

One may best understand the function of the larynx by an appreciation of its origin, as determined by primitive needs. On the evolutionary time-scale, as animals migrated from an aquatic to a terrestrial existence, major changes to meet the new respiratory requirements obviously became necessary.

According to Negus,[1] these accomplishments appear to be reflected in certain contemporary species of fish that have developed respiratory modifications allowing them to survive on dry land. Notably, the climbing perch *(Anabas scandens)* displays a respiratory diverticulum located above its gills (Fig. 3–1A). In the Indian siluroid fish *(Saccobranchus)*, a long diverticulum leads into an internal air reservoir. Its respiratory structures, however, contain no valves to prevent the entrance of water when an aquatic existence is resumed.

The most primitive larynx has been found in the bichir lungfish *(Polypterus)*, which inhabits the Nile River. Its larynx consists simply of a muscular sphincter to guard against the entrance of water (Fig. 3–1B). The African lungfish *(Protopterus)* possesses, in addition to sphincteric musculature, discrete muscle fibers that act to draw the valvular margins apart, producing active dilatation (Fig. 3–1C). This muscular sphincter, therefore, remains contracted when the fish is waterborne. During periods of drought, the sphincter can be actively opened to allow air to be gulped into the lungs by a swallowing maneuver. This capability obviously provides a tremendous advantage in survival when the supply of water is limited or undependable.

The primitive larynx basically functions as a simple sphincter that protects the lower airway from the intrusion of foreign matter. As respiratory requirements in a terrestrial environment grew, however, the need for adequate ventilation also grew, accompanied by the potential for active dilatation of the primitive sphincter.

To enhance ventilatory flow through the laryngeal aperture, the phylogenetic acquisition of lateral cartilages can be noted in certain amphibians such as the Mexican axolotl *(Amblystoma)*. These lateral cartilages form bars on

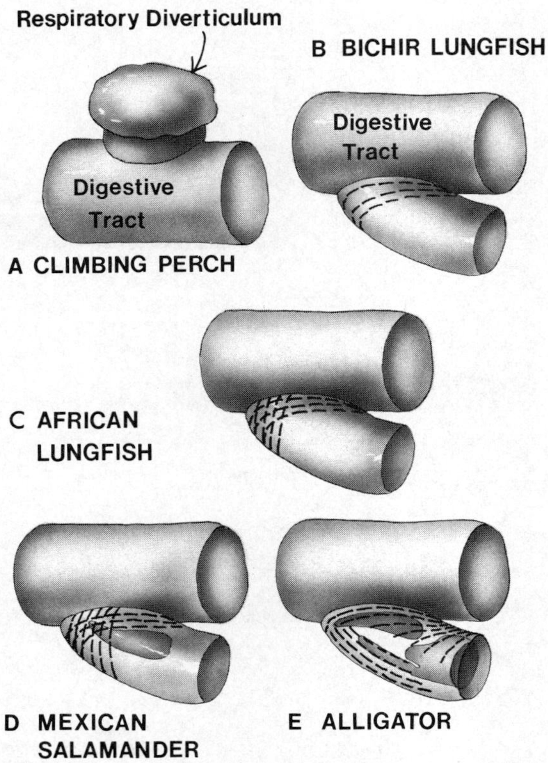

Figure 3–1. Structure and function of the larynx viewed phylogenetically (according to Negus).

either side of the glottis to which the dilator muscles join (Fig. 3–1D). To augment the mechanical advantage of these muscles, a cartilaginous ring (giving origin to the dilator muscles) can be found between the glottis and trachea in other higher vertebrates. Such a configuration is apparent among such reptiles as the alligator (Fig. 3–1E). Therefore, while the lateral cartilages of amphibians share a structural similarity to the arytenoid bodies of humans, the origin of the cartilaginous ring in reptiles can be compared to the acquisition of the cricoid cartilage in other mammals, including man.

Viewed phylogenetically, the primary function of the larynx is, without question, its use as a sphincter that protects the lower airway from the intrusion of liquids and food. Its secondary function, supported by the sequential phylogenetic acquisition of the cricoarytenoid complex, centers about its role in respiration governed by active muscular dilatation of the laryngeal aperture. The third function of the larynx, phonation (best observed in mammals), appears to be a late phylogenetic acquisition and therefore, contrary to prevailing opinion, may be considered of tertiary importance only. According to Negus, phonation is considered the least significant of the three basic functions

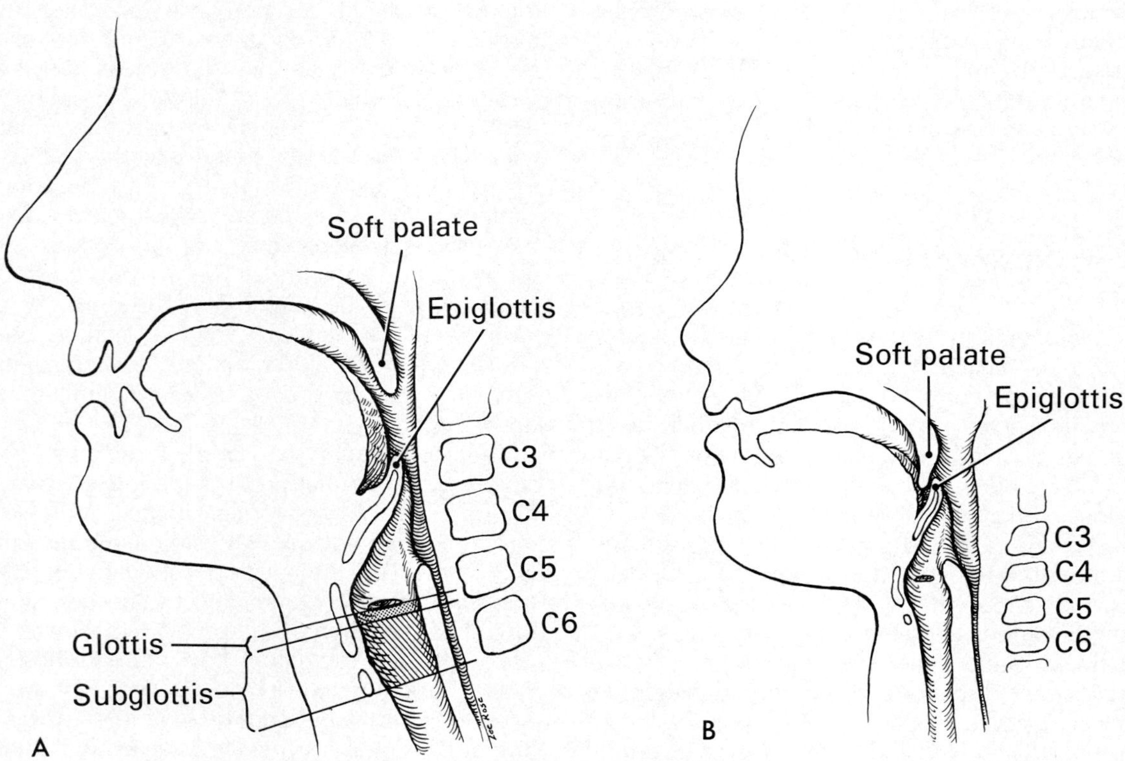

Figure 3–2. Nasolaryngeal relationships. *A,* in the adult. *B,* in the newborn.

ascribed to the larynx, whose primary role remains that of guardian of the lower airway.

STRUCTURE AND FUNCTION

In man, the anatomy of the larynx may be viewed as a functional compromise. The upper airway in adult man traverses the digestive tract in the region of the pharynx. This complicates the sphincteric protection of the lower airway. By sharing a common passageway with the upper digestive system, the larynx is also compromised in its respiratory performance by resultant ventilatory turbulence and, therefore, resistance. Thus, the anatomic configuration in adult man that benefits the phonatory purposes of the larynx simultaneously serves to compromise its sphincteric and respiratory functions. This functional dilemma is successfully resolved at the laryngopharyngeal level by two important organic modifications: (1) structural adaptation and (2) delicate coordination among the three basic laryngeal functions as determined by precisely organized brainstem reflexes.

From a structural point of view, the protective function of the adult human larynx is admittedly precarious by virtue of the low position of the larynx in the neck (Fig. 3–2A). Other mammalian species possess a relatively high-riding larynx, resulting in close approximation to structures of the posterior nasal cavities. The intranarial position of the larynx in such species secures a continuous airway from the nose to the bronchi, thereby decreasing the risk of pulmonary contamination by swallowed matter. This structural modification is exaggerated among certain cetaceans (Fig. 3–3) and herbivores but appears to a lesser degree among carnivores, which use an elongated epiglottis to effect nasolaryngeal connection during deglutition.

The human newborn exhibits similar nasolaryngeal connection by approximation of its epiglottis with the posterior surface of its palate, thus insuring against aspiration by forming a continuous upper and lower airway (Fig. 3–2B). The observation of obligate nasal breathing in the newborn period may be related to this anatomic configuration, which is lost from four to six months postnatally.[2]

In man, the characteristic, flat, shieldlike configuration of the epiglottis serves to direct swallowed food laterally into the pyriform fossae, away from the midline laryngeal aperture (Fig. 3–4). Furthermore, in adult man, elevation of the larynx toward the nasal cavity during the height of deglutition exaggerates this protective function by bringing nose and larynx into an infantile structural relationship for a fraction of a second during the act of swallowing. Implicit in this maneuver is the role of the aryepiglottic folds, which consist of mucous membrane, connective tissue, and muscle extending from the epiglottic framework to the arytenoid bodies posteriorly. These lateral folds act as ramparts of the larynx, causing swallowed matter to pass on either side of the epiglottis along the gutter produced between each fold and the lateral pharyngeal wall. The cartilages of Santorini and Wrisberg, also called the corniculate and cuneiform cartilages, respectively, are contained in the aryepiglottic folds to provide added support and stiffness to these ramparts of the laryngeal aperture. It would appear from a structural perspective alone that the primary role of the supraglottic larynx in adult humans lies in its protection of the lower airway. Surgical removal of part or all of the supraglottic larynx results in compromised protection, even though adequate function may be eventually achieved through reorganization of compensatory neuromuscular reflexes.

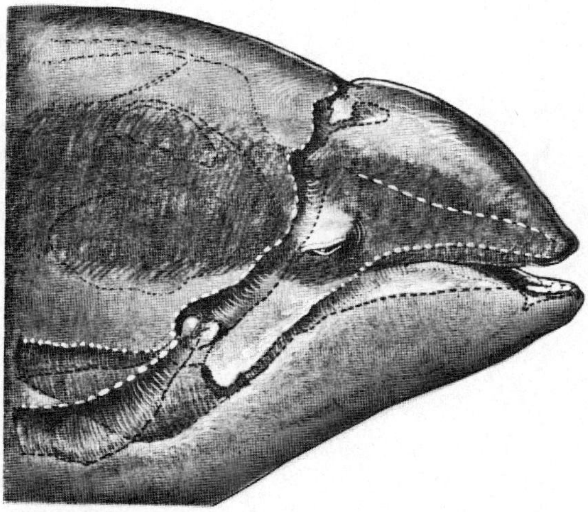

Figure 3–3. Head of a porpoise, showing the intranarial position of its larynx.

In contrast to the role of the supraglottic larynx, the valvular mechanism of the larynx depends on the unique shelflike configuration of its superior and inferior folds (Fig. 3–5). The ventricular folds or false cords, which are located superiorly, act as exit valves preventing the escape of air from the lower respiratory tract. When positioned by muscular contraction, they seal even more tightly as tracheal pressure is increased from below. This feature of adducted false cords occurs independently

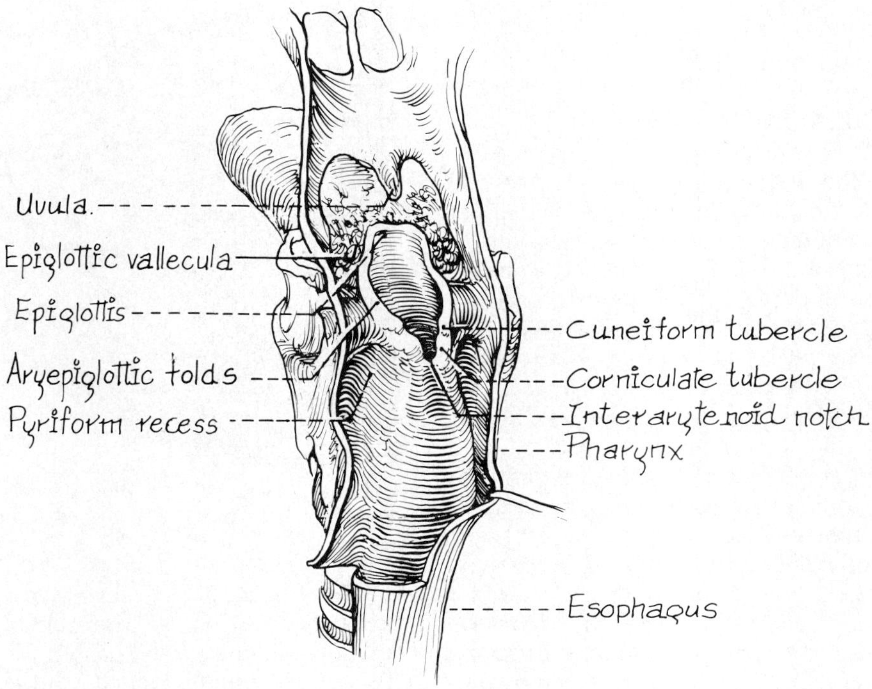

Figure 3–4. Human larynx and pharynx viewed from behind. Note the role of the epiglottis and aryepiglottic folds in directing swallowed matter around the laryngeal inlet into the upper esophaus posteriorly.

of muscle tone, a phenomenon attributable to their unique shape, which is characterized by the downturned direction of their free margins. Such a configuration is made possible by the lateral ventricles and is exaggerated by the superior extension of the laryngeal saccules. Brunton,[3] working with cadaver larynges, demonstrated that closed ventricular bands (closed by valvular action alone without muscular contraction) offered a resistance to a pressure head from below equaling 30 mm Hg. When the pressure head was reversed, however, no resistance was offered by the approximated false cords.

On the other hand, the true cords were shown to behave as a one-way valve in the opposite direction, obstructing the ingress of air and fluids. When passively approximated in the cadaver, the true cords offered little resistance to pressure from below but resisted a pressure head from above exceeding 140 mm Hg. Their ability to resist pressure from above was not influenced by passive closure of the false cords.

The false cords therefore appear to prevent the egress of air from the lungs, and the true cords with their upturned margins are capable of impeding its ingress. These views were confirmed by Lindsay[4] on tomographic analysis of the larynx. It is not surprising, as Chevalier Jackson observed, that expectorative functions of the larynx remain unimpaired in bilateral laryngeal paralysis. In this regard, passive closure of the false cords alone appears essential to effective cough production. Whereas surgical removal of one or both false cords appears to impair effective cough production, expectorative ability may be compensated by the careful reorganization of other conditioned reflexes.

The valvular component of the true cords is implicated in the clinical difficulty experienced in overcoming laryngeal spasm by abrupt pressure peaks of positive pressure ventilation, which only serve to further protectively seal the true cords. When this critical sphincteric characteristic is lost through surgery, it must be structurally reconstructed to reconstitute laryngeal protective function and to prevent aspiration. From a structural perspective, the false cords provide an expectorative function, whereas the true cords assume a protective role in respiration. The loss of either by ablative surgery could result in life-threatening aspiration, a result that may be minimized through structural reconstruction and through the natural compensatory reorganization of neuromuscular reflexes.

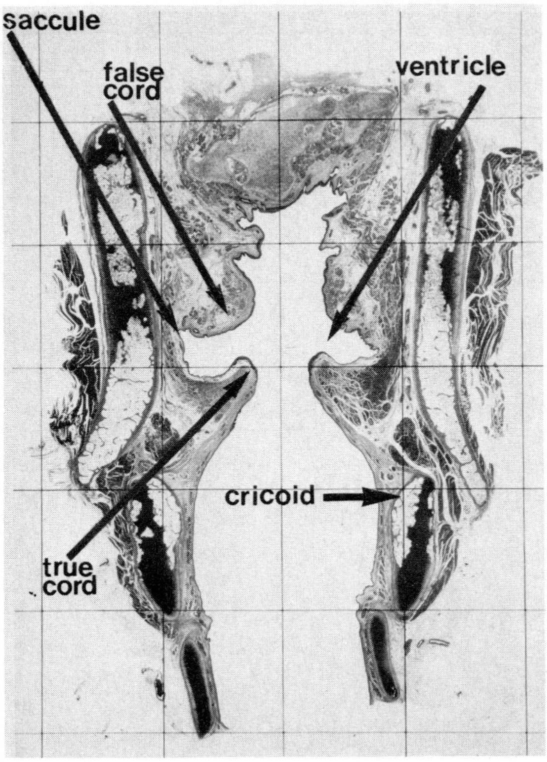

Figure 3–5. Frontal section through the human larynx demonstrating the valvular structure of the false and true cords. (From Kirchner JA, private communication.)

Table 3–1. SENSORY INNERVATION

Nerve	Distribution
Superior laryngeal nerve (internal division)	Supraglottic mucosa Thyroepiglottic joint Cricoarytenoid joint
Superior laryngeal nerve (external division)	Anterior subglottic mucosa Cricothyroid joint
Recurrent laryngeal nerve	Subglottic mucosa Muscle spindles
Nerve of Galen (communicating branch between superior and recurrent nerves)	Aortic arch

NEUROMUSCULAR PHYSIOLOGY

Neuroanatomy

The Afferent System. Sensory nerve fibers to the supraglottic larynx are derived from the internal branch of each superior laryngeal nerve that ipsilaterally innervates the superior mucosal boundary of the larynx to the level of the true vocal cords. Similarly, below the true cords, ipsilateral sensation is mediated by each recurrent laryngeal nerve. Suzuki,[5] however, demonstrated a diamond-shaped area anteriorly in the midline of the subglottic space of the cat that is innervated by both external branches of the superior laryngeal nerve. Afferent impulses from deep muscle receptors and cricothyroid joints also travel cephalad in this external nerve branch. The sensory innervation of the larynx is summarized in Table 3–1.

The density of sensory innervation appears greatest in the laryngeal inlet, an observation consistent with the concept that the aditus serves as a protective zone for the more distal respiratory system. When nerve-staining techniques are used, the laryngeal surface of the epiglottis appears to contain the most compact innervation, while the true cords exhibit lesser degrees of sensory density.[6] Specifically, the posterior half of the true cord is more heavily furnished with touch receptors than its anterior portion. Chemical and thermal receptors appear to be limited to the anterior portions of the supraglottic larynx. In this regard, water chemoreceptors on the epiglottis have been experimentally implicated in the production of prolonged apnea.[7] Furthermore, it has been demonstrated that the respiratory response to water-aerosol inhalation for treatment of croup and other upper airway obstruction may be related to the exquisite sensitivity of these epiglottic mechanoreceptors and chemoreceptors. The effect produced consists of respiratory slowing with associated increase in tidal volume, certainly an effect beneficial to partial upper airway obstruction. This centrally mediated respiratory response appears to be greater early in life than in adulthood.[8]

It is therefore generally agreed that sensory components of the superior laryngeal nerve include representation from (1) mucosal touch receptors, (2) epiglottic chemoreceptors, (3) joint receptors, (4) aortic baroreceptors, and (5) stretch receptors from the intrinsic laryngeal muscles.[9] Afferent impulses are delivered through the ganglion nodosum to the ipsilateral brainstem tractus solitarius. To date, there is no evidence for the crossed projection of laryngeal sensory innervation.

The Efferent System. Motor innervation of the larynx is no less complex (Table 3–2). It is generally agreed that the motor distribution to the intrinsic laryngeal musculature originates in the medullary nucleus ambiguus. Each recurrent laryngeal nerve ipsilaterally innervates all

Table 3–2. MOTOR INNERVATION

Nerve	Distribution	Action
Superior laryngeal nerve	Cricothyroid muscle	Adductor, tensor
Recurrent laryngeal nerve	Thyroarytenoid muscle Lateral cricoarytenoid muscle Interarytenoid muscle Posterior cricoarytenoid muscle	Adductor, isometric tensor Adductor Adductor Abductor
Nerve of Galen (communication branch)	Tracheoesophageal mucosa Tracheal smooth muscle	Autonomic (secretory) Autonomic

muscles except the cricothyroid muscle, which receives its motor impulses from the external division of its ipsilateral superior laryngeal nerve. The interarytenoid muscles, however, receive bilateral motor innervation through both recurrent laryngeal nerves. In man there is no evidence for the crossed projection of laryngeal motor innervation. Nevertheless, there are additional data suggesting that crossed projections may exist between second and third order medullary neurons of the laryngeal reflex arc, although their level of activity appears

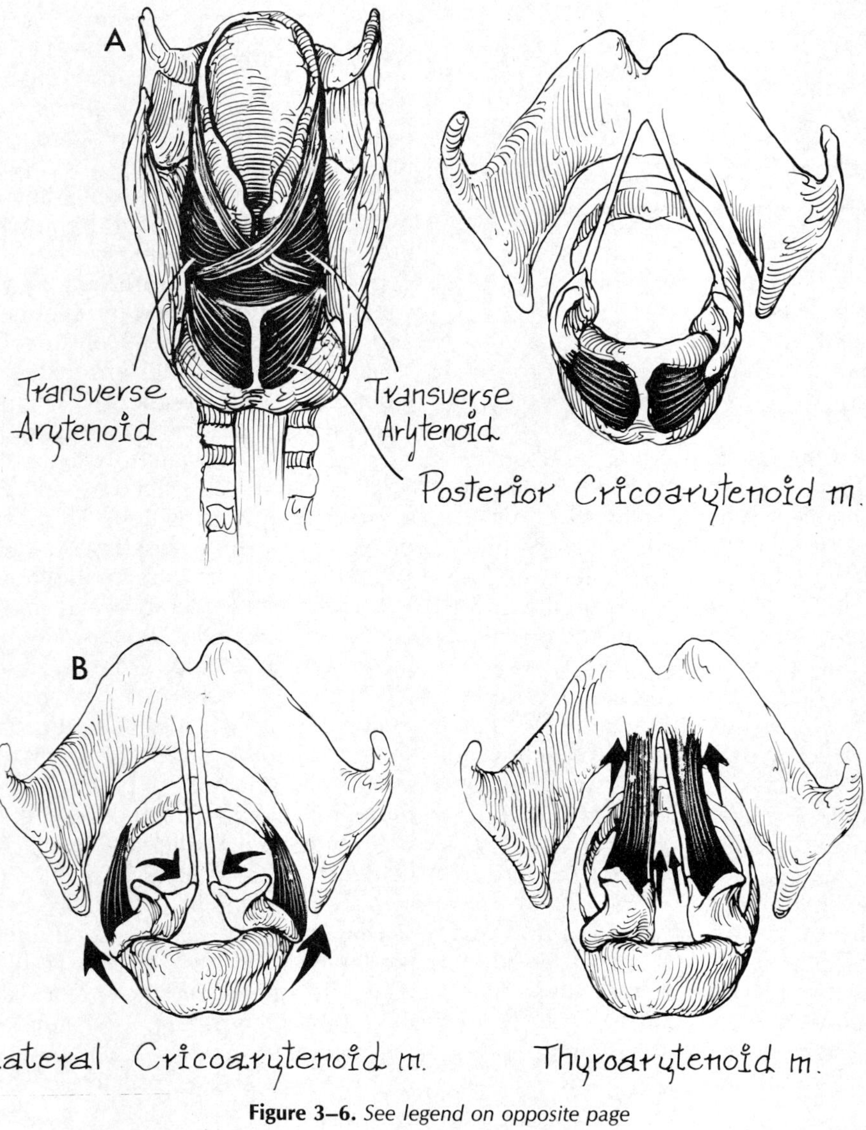

Figure 3–6. *See legend on opposite page*

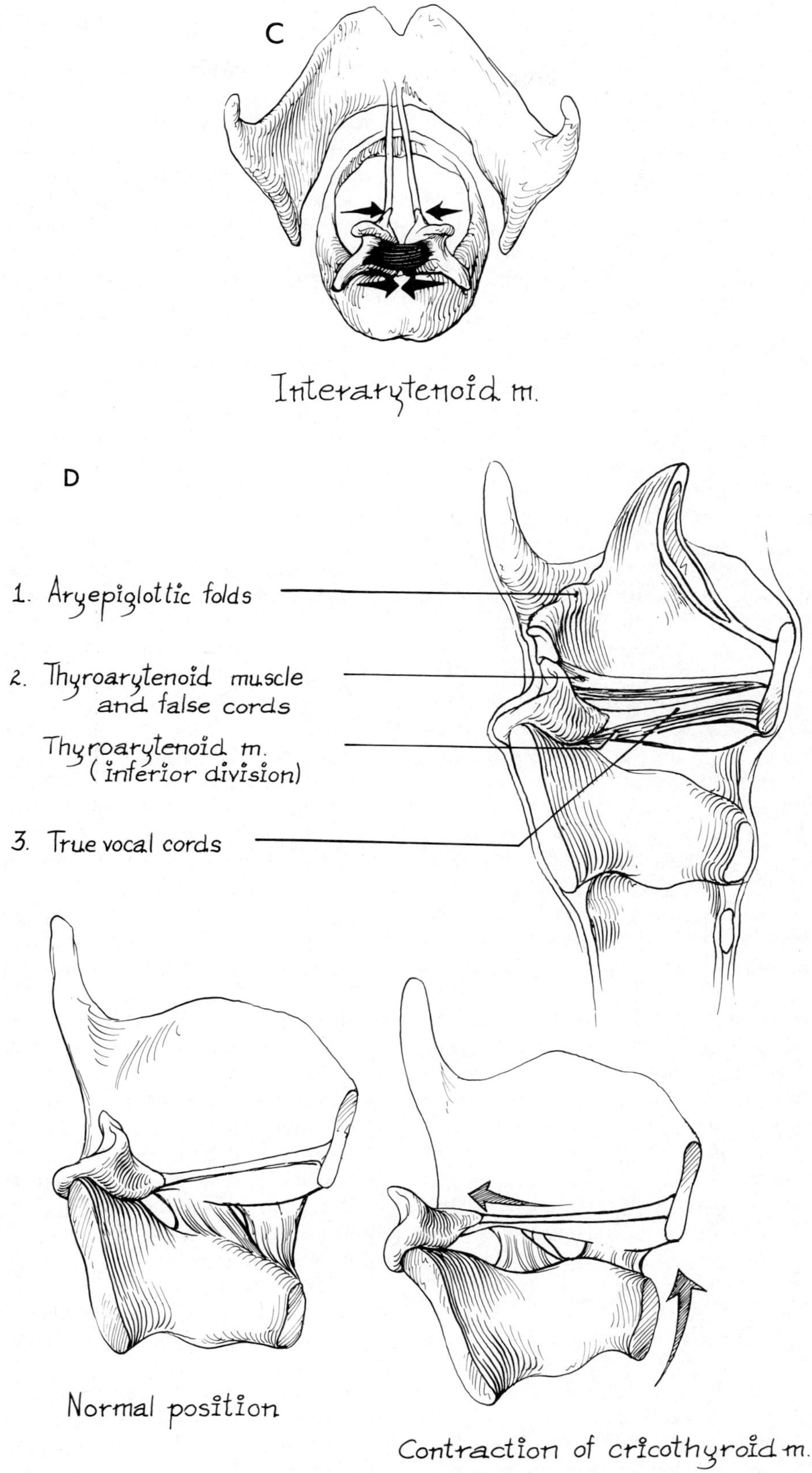

Figure 3–6. Laryngoscopic view of the intrinsic muscles responsible for activating vocal cord position.

species specific—that is, more active in cat than in dog or man.[10]

The intrinsic muscle that widens the glottic chink, as takes place in inspiration, is solely the posterior cricoarytenoid muscle. This muscle extends from the posterior aspect of the cricoid plate to the muscular process of the arytenoid (Fig. 3–6A). By exerting a posterolateral pull on the arytenoid body, it will rotate the vocal fold outward, effecting cord abduction on inspiration. On the other hand, vocal fold adduction results from contraction of all other intrinsic musculature, major contributions arising from the action of thyroarytenoid and lateral cricoarytenoid muscles (Fig. 3–6B). The interarytenoid muscles serve to close the posterior gap in the glottis (Fig. 3–6C), while the cricothyroid muscle adducts and tenses the vocal cord, passively lengthening it by 30 per cent. This is accomplished by shortening the anterior distance between the cricoid and thyroid cartilages, resulting in dorsal and posterior displacement of the posterior cricoid plate. The vocal cord, therefore, undergoes a mechanical stretch displacement resulting in an increase in the anteroposterior diameter of the laryngeal aperture (Fig. 3–6D).

When one cricothyroid muscle is denervated by sectioning the superior laryngeal nerve, the unopposed contraction of the contralateral cricothyroid muscle results in rotation of the posterior commissure toward the inactive side, with foreshortening of the cord on the side of denervation. Unilateral recurrent laryngeal nerve injury results in the paramedian position of that cord because the unopposed action of the ipsilateral cricothyroid muscle, innervated by an intact superior laryngeal nerve, produces cord adduction on the side of recurrent laryngeal nerve injury. This physiologic principle replaces Semon's law, which incorrectly postulates that adductor motor components of the recurrent laryngeal nerve are more resistant to injury than abductor fibers. Knowledge of this mechanism, in terms of unopposed cricothyroid action, represents the basis of superior laryngeal nerve section advocated by Martens[11] in the treatment of bilateral recurrent laryngeal nerve paralysis in man.

Laryngeal Reflexes

Because neurophysiologic study requires the use of invasive techniques, direct human investigation is not generally feasible or therapeutically justifiable. For this reason, with a few exceptions, the bulk of data relating to complex neuromuscular activity of the larynx is necessarily derived from animal experimentation. Despite the obvious limitations of laboratory investigation, several neurophysiologic discoveries stand out as pivotal in our discussion of laryngeal function.

Basic functions of the larynx (protective, respiratory, and phonatory) are derived from a complicated interrelationship of diverse polysynaptic brainstem reflexes. Protective function is entirely reflexive and involuntary. This constitutes one end of a spectrum that is balanced on the other end by respiratory and phonatory performances. These may be initiated voluntarily but regulated involuntarily through an array of feedback reflexes. It is thought that this complex reflex system provides the principal mechanism by which the organism may compensate for structural alterations imposed by disease processes or through necessary ablative surgery.

Neurophysiology of Protective Function. To view the protective function of the larynx neurophysiologically, one needs only to examine the glottic closure reflex. The functional analogue of this simple reflex is to produce protective laryngeal closure during deglutition. In this regard, touch, chemical, and thermal stimulation of the laryngeal aditus is analogous to the electrostimulation of the superior laryngeal nerve, which produces a low threshold evoked action potential in the adductor branches of the recurrent laryngeal nerve. In man, the threshold of the adductor reflex measures 0.5 V and possesses a latency of 25 ms, indicating this to be a polysynaptic brainstem reflex, a view supported by appropriate calculations of central reflex time[10] (Fig. 3–7). Unlike commonly used animal models, man does not possess a crossed adductor reflex. That is, stimulation of one superior laryngeal nerve does not produce simultaneous action potentials in the contralateral adductor musculature. It is therefore possible that unilateral superior laryngeal nerve injury in man may result in failure of ipsilateral cord closure, a condition predisposing to aspiration despite anatomic integrity of both recurrent laryngeal nerves.

Under conditions of health, sphincteric closure of the upper airway produced by bilateral superior laryngeal nerve stimulation results in protective adduction of three muscular tiers within the laryngeal framework. The highest tier occurs at the level of the aryepiglottic folds, which contain the superior-most division of the thyroarytenoid muscle. With reflex contraction

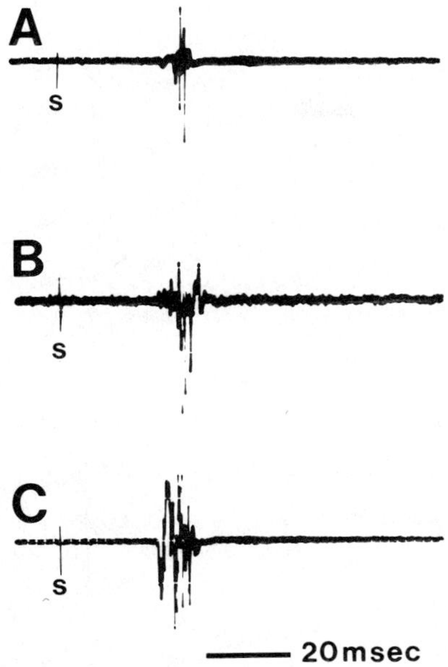

Figure 3–7. Ipsilateral adductor responses evoked by single-shock stimulation of superior laryngeal nerve in three separate patients. *A*, *B*, and *C*; Stimulus, s. In man, no contralateral adductor reflex can be demonstrated.

of these fibers, the aryepiglottic folds approximate to cover the superior inlet of the larynx. At this level, the anterior gap is filled by the epiglottic tubercle and the posterior gap by the arytenoid cartilages, completing the first of three sphincteric tiers of protection.

The second tier of protection occurs at the level of the false cords, consisting of bilateral folds forming the roofs of the laryngeal ventricles. Each fold contains numerous fat cells and mucous glands. Laterally along each fold, however, are fibers of the thyroarytenoid muscle capable of bringing the folds together in reflex response to superior laryngeal nerve stimulation.

The third tier of protection occurs at the level of the true vocal cord, which in man is shelflike with a slightly upturned free border. The inferior division of the thyroarytenoid muscle forms the bulk of this shelf, thus producing the potential for strong reflex protective closure. In conjunction with the passive valvular effect caused by the upturned border of the cord margin, the true vocal cord perhaps represents the most significant of the three barriers to aspiration.

In experiments dealing with direct recurrent laryngeal nerve stimulation, the rapid response of thyroarytenoid contraction appears crucial in effective reflex glottic closure. Hast[12] demonstrates that the thyroarytenoid is one of the fastest of all striated muscles, approaching the medial rectus of the eye in speed of contraction. Thyroarytenoid muscle of the dog contracts in 14 ms, compared with 40 ms for cricothyroid muscle and 44 ms for posterior cricoarytenoid muscle.

Although the glottic closure reflex may be classically elicited by direct superior laryngeal nerve stimulation, other sensory stimuli are also capable of eliciting this vitally basic reflex response. For example, stimulation of all major cranial afferent nerves produces strong laryngeal adductor responses, as will stimulation of other special sensory and spinal somatic sensory nerves. In the cat, reflex action potentials in the adductor branch of the recurrent laryngeal nerve can be elicited by electrostimulation of the optic, acoustic, trigeminal, splanchnic, vagus, radial, and intercostal nerves and the chorda tympani.[13] The susceptibility of this reflex response to such diverse sensory elicitation is unique and emphasizes its primitive role in respiratory protection of the organism from a wide variety of potentially noxious influences.

Physiologic exaggeration of the glottic closure reflex, called laryngospasm, is commonly observed as prolonged glottic closure in response to intense glottic or supraglottic stimulation. In the clinical setting, strong closure is maintained well beyond the cessation of mucosal irritation. This has led some investigators to suggest its similarity to a form of focal seizure initiated by a local sensory aberration or aura. From neurophysiologic analysis, laryngeal spasm consists of prolonged tonic adductor spike activity in the recurrent laryngeal nerve—spike activity bearing no precisely reproducible temporal relationship (latency) to its initiating stimulus[14] (Fig. 3–8). This observation

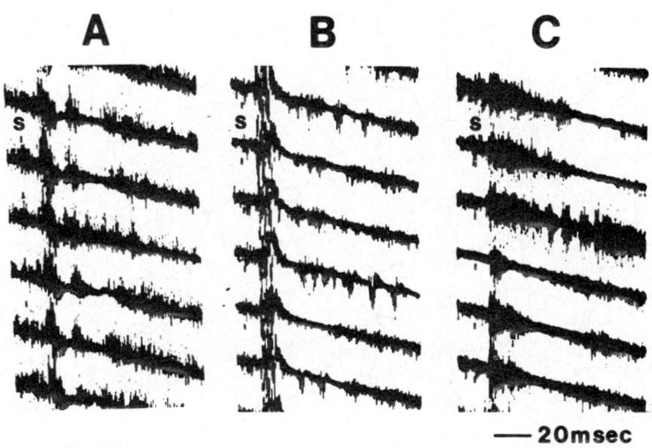

Figure 3–8. Primary evoked responses and random high frequency afterdischarge activity produced by repetitive stimulation of ipsilateral superior laryngeal nerve in dog (0.3 V, 0.1 ms at 8 Hz). Stimulus, s. *A*, Recurrent laryngeal nerve. *B*, Thyroarytenoid muscle. *C*, Lateral cricoarytenoid muscle.

is based on the fact that laryngeal spasm is solely mediated by the superior laryngeal nerve. High-frequency stimulation of other afferent nerves, though capable of eliciting simple glottic closure, produces little of the adductor afterdischarge activity that is characteristic of the exaggerated clinical response called laryngospasm.

In the laboratory production of laryngeal spasm, the output characteristic of the brainstem adductor motoneuron aggregate is strongly modified by the level of barbiturate administration (Fig. 3–9). The deeper the anesthesia, the fewer afterdischarges are elicited by repetitive superior laryngeal nerve electrostimulation. This response is, of course, anticipated since barbiturates not only increase the refractory period of active motoneurons but also impair their synaptic transmission.[15] This explains the marked impairment of motor output function elicited by repetitive superior laryngeal nerve stimulation under heavy barbiturate anesthesia.

Furthermore, the observed adductor motor depression caused by hypoventilation is supported by other experimental data indicating preferential abolition of postsynaptic potentials by hypoxia.[16] This experimental evidence further indicates that in hypoxic states postsynaptic recovery lags behind the presynaptic recovery, producing a net depressive effect on all reflex neural activity. Hypoventilation, therefore, understandably impairs the output capability of the brainstem adductor motor aggregate in response to repetitive superior laryngeal nerve stimulation (Fig. 3–10). Such experimental data seem to support the clinical observation that laryngeal spasm occurs more often in well ventilated rather than cyanotic patients, the spasm often breaking spontaneously as the level of hypoxia increases.

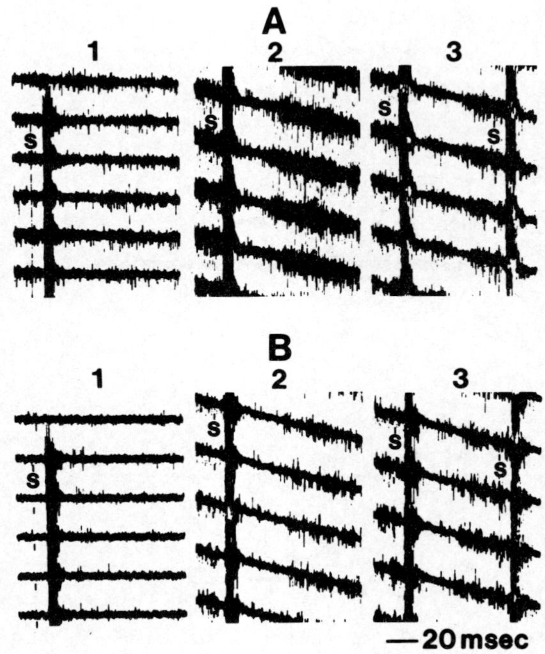

Figure 3–10. Thyroarytenoid responses produced by repetitive superior laryngeal stimulation (0.3 V, 0.1 ms). Stimulus, s. *A,* Hyperventilation. *B,* Hypoventilation. *Column 1,* 1 Hz. *Column 2,* 8 Hz. *Column 3,* 16 Hz. Note reduced afterdischarge activity in the hypoventilated state.

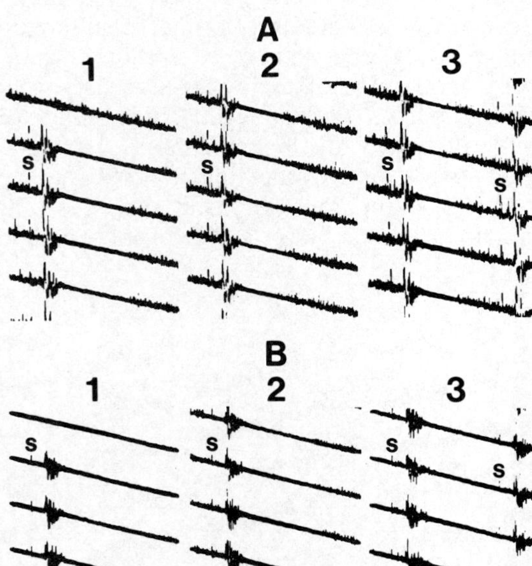

Figure 3–9. Thyroarytenoid responses produced by repetitive superior laryngeal stimulation (0.3 V, 0.1 ms). Stimulus, s. *A,* Light anesthesia with intact corneal reflex. *B,* Deep anesthesia, absent corneal reflex. *Column 1,* 1 Hz. *Column 2,* 8 Hz. *Column 3,* 16 Hz. Note reduced afterdischarge activity in deep anesthesia.

Finally, it should be recognized that superior laryngeal nerve stimulation, aside from the variety of excitatory adductor responses it produces, also exerts an inhibitory effect on the medullary inspiratory motoneurons. Not only does laryngeal abductor activity cease but phrenic activity is also inhibited, resulting in various degrees of reflex apnea.

Neurophysiology of Respiratory Function. Physiologic investigation of laryngeal respiratory function is worthy of brief review. Galen, because of his finding that all respiration ceased after high spinal cord section, is considered the first to demonstrate that the brain controlled breathing. Since then, evidence has shown the medulla to indeed possess an intrinsic respiratory rhythmicity of its own. This is not to say that the medulla alone can initiate and maintain eupneic respiration, for further evidence has indicated that facilitatory and inhibitory impulses from both higher structures and peripheral receptors determine the final level of activity.

The dual importance of central as well as peripheral respiratory control only gradually became apparent, through considerable controversy, during the growth of knowledge of respiratory physiology. The role of the vagus was first appreciated in 1819 when Krimer[17] stimulated this nerve electrically and observed a respiratory effect, thereby establishing the importance of peripheral receptors and pathways in the regulation of breathing. The classic work of Breuer and Hering appeared in 1868.[18, 19] They found that inflation of the lung in expiration stopped breathing and inferred that inflation mechanically stimulated pulmonary nerve endings, resulting in ascending vagal impulses inhibitory to inspiration. The periodic inhibition theory for the origin of normal rhythmic breathing was thus formulated.

Theories governing the chemical control of breathing appeared later, during the mid-19th century, when Kussmaul and Tenner,[20] by occluding the blood vessels to the brain, noted that the "venosity" of the blood produced a stimulus to breathing. Subsequent studies on the chemical control of breathing then centered around its effect on the brainstem and enhanced the apparent importance of central rather than peripheral control of respiration. To Haldane and Priestley,[21] in 1893, must go the credit for the first controlled quantitative studies demonstrating carbon dioxide excess rather than oxygen lack as a sensitive regulator of respiration.

Finally, with the discovery of carotid chemoreceptors, a new outlook on respiratory physiology occurred. Comroe[22] called it "the most important discovery of the last century," for it returned interest to the peripheral receptors and established once and for all the dual importance of central and peripheral control in the maintenance of eupneic respiration.

Admittedly, this rich background in respiratory physiology had been directed at the function of the lower respiratory tract. Studies concerning the respiratory contribution of the larynx did not appear until the mid-20th century. Negus,[1] in 1949, noted that the glottis opened a fraction of a second before air was drawn in by the descent of the diaphragm. In 1969, Suzuki[23] established this activity as a direct effect of the medullary respiratory center,

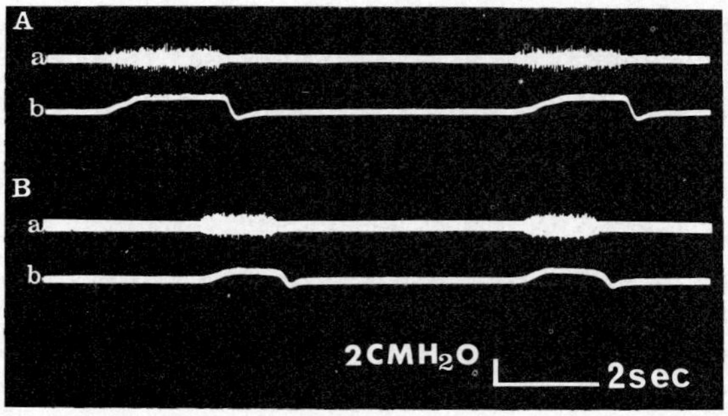

Figure 3–11. Laryngeal abductor activity. *A,* Nose breathing. *B,* Mouth breathing. *Tracing a,* Posterior cricoarytenoid EMG; *tracing b,* intratracheal pressure. Upward deflection represents negative pressure change.

thereby opening the way to further understanding of laryngeal respiratory function in terms of the rich historical background of basic respiratory physiology. Having established that widening of the glottis occurred with rhythmic bursts of activity in the recurrent laryngeal nerve, Suzuki then demonstrated that, like phrenic activity, this rhythmic widening was accentuated by hypercapnia and ventilatory obstruction; it was depressed by hyperventilation and resultant hypocapnia. Just as phrenic activity is modified by ventilatory resistance, it would seem reasonable that glottic widening, influenced by the respiratory center, would be similarly modified.

From a purely structural perspective, because the true vocal cords passively act to obstruct the ingress of air to the lungs, active inspiratory abduction by phasic muscular contraction of the posterior cricoarytenoid appears mandatory to successful ventilation. Using electromyographic techniques on the posterior cricoarytenoid muscle, we can show that phasic inspira-

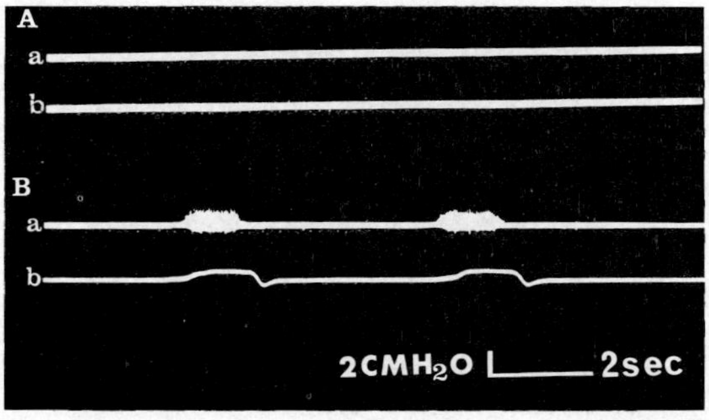

Figure 3–12. Laryngeal abductor activity. *A,* Immediately after tracheostomy. *B,* With tracheostoma partially closed. *Tracing a,* Posterior cricoarytenoid EMG; *tracing b,* intratracheal pressure. Note disappearance of phasic abduction in tracheostomized breathing.

tory abduction is, in fact, synchronous with inspiration[24] (Figs. 3–11 and 3–12). Furthermore, the degree of abductor activity appears to vary directly with ventilatory resistance; it disappears entirely when inspiratory resistance is removed, only to return when resistance to ventilation is reestablished. Because vagotomy abolishes this response, it is felt that the afferent limb for the reflex regulation of phasic inspiratory abduction lies within the ascending vagus nerve.[25] End organ receptors concerned in this reflex presumably lie within the thorax, although their exact nature and location remain unknown.

Pertinent to respiratory laryngeal function is the role of the cricothyroid muscle, known to be a vocal cord adductor and tensor. Neurophysiologic investigation demonstrates that this muscle contracts phasically with inspiration[26] (Fig. 3–13). While its adductor role would appear to be counterproductive to inspiration through narrowing the glottic aperture, its role in lengthening the vocal cord actually enhances the cross-sectional diameter of the glottis by increasing its anteroposterior dimension. Therefore, it would appear that both posterior cricoarytenoid and cricothyroid muscles are driven by the medullary respiratory center, the level of their activity regulated in eupneic breathing by afferent impulses originating in the chest. Posterior cricoarytenoid contraction increases the horizontal diameter of the glottic chink while the anteroposterior diameter is increased by phasic inspiratory contraction of cricothyroid muscle (Fig. 3–14).

The function of the cricothyroid muscle is even more complex than this, for it displays a

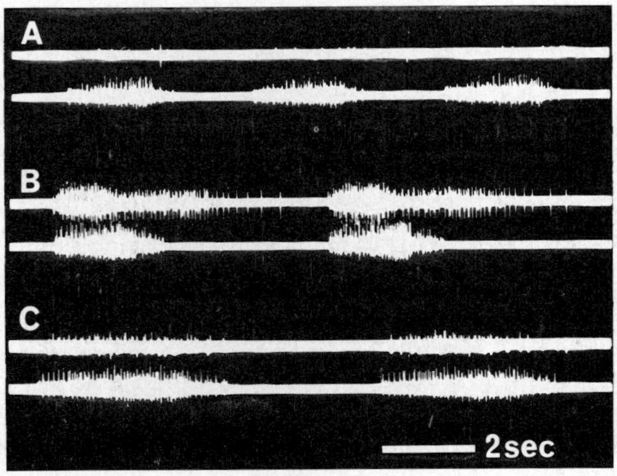

Figure 3–13. Cricothyroid EMG *(upper tracings)* and phrenic EMG *(lower tracings)*. *A*, Quiet breathing. *B*, Expiratory dyspnea. *C*, Inspiratory dyspnea. Cricothyroid, like posterior cricoarytenoid, appears to be an inspiratory muscle.

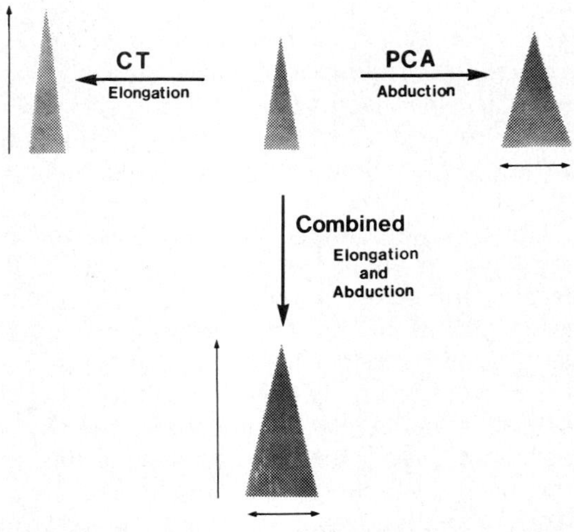

Figure 3–14. Glottic alteration produced by cricothyroid (CT) and posterior cricoarytenoid (PCA) action alone and in combination. Combined muscle action maximizes the cross-sectional area of the laryngeal aperture.

critical role during the expiratory phase of respiration as well. Its expiratory activity, in fact, appears to be its most crucial function in respiration.[27] Its importance is demonstrated by its major role in the overall regulation of breathing resulting from its control of expiratory resistance and flow.

Neurally controlled retardation of expiratory air flow is an essential characteristic of normal breathing. In eupneic states, expiratory flow and duration are principal determinants of respiratory frequency. As others have demonstrated in both animal and human investigations, variations in respiratory rate result primarily from changing the duration of the expiratory phase rather than that of the inspiratory phase of the respiratory cycle. In this regard, cricothyroid contraction in expiration results in vocal elongation, increasing glottic size. Such a mechanical effect reduces airway resistance and shortens expiratory duration. By such a mechanism, the rate of respiration may ultimately be modified using the larynx as the principal effector of this control. In this connection, cricothyroid expiratory activity is a pressure sensitive evoked response influenced by afferent vagal stimuli. Its activity is triggered by the critical threshold of pressure increase with respect to time (Fig. 3–15) and its duration is directly dependent on the duration of positive subglottic pressure. The threshold of cricothyroid activation is reduced in hypercapnia and elevated in hypocapnic states.

Neurophysiology of Phonation. The phonatory function of the larynx is probably the least well understood of its three basic functions.

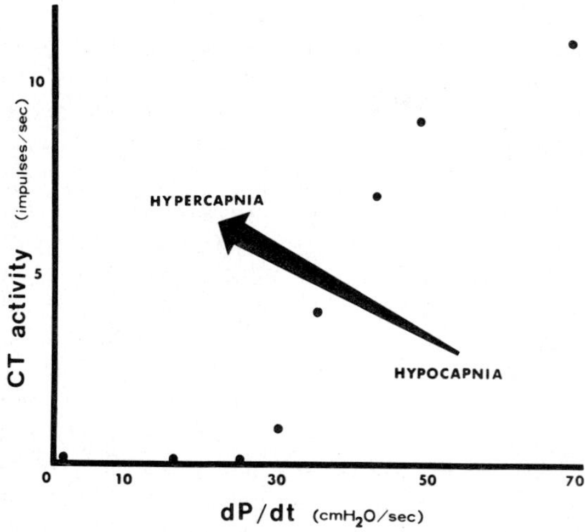

Figure 3–15. The threshold of cricothyroid (CT) elicitation in response to rate of tracheal pressure change measures 30 cm H_2O per s in normocapnia. Hypercapnia reduces cricothyroid threshold whereas hypocapnia raises its threshold.

Because of advances in investigative technique, many established hypotheses based on animal models have been challenged, in large measure because of the advent of more sophisticated technology based on human study. High-speed cinematography, improved endoscopic techniques with use of the laryngeal stroboscope, and direct human electromyographic measurements made possible by hooked wire electrodes are largely responsible for these newer additions.

It is generally agreed that speech results from a fundamental tone produced at the larynx and modified by resonating chambers of the upper aerodigestive tract. Intelligible speech represents the combined effect of the larynx, tongue, palate, and related structures of the oral vestibule. The production of the fundamental tone is accomplished by the vibration of the vocal folds against each other, this vibration being generated by the passage of air between them. That vocal cord vibrations are a passive phenomenon represents the basis of the aerodynamic theory of sound generation. Such a theory finds support in the observation that the completely paralyzed larynx is capable of producing sound, as is the cadaver larynx when subglottic pressure is forcefully increased. Furthermore, phonation ceases when a tracheostomy is performed for diversionary purposes.

The aerodynamic theory of sound production therefore replaces the neurochronaxic theory proposed by Husson,[28] who postulated that the central generation of recurrent laryngeal nerve impulses produced cord vibrations by active contraction of the thyroarytenoid muscles. Each vibration was thought to represent the result of beat-by-beat impulses through the recurrent laryngeal nerve. This theory is no longer accepted.

Although sound production by the larynx may be considered a passive function, the regulation of its acoustic quality is not a passive phenomenon. Rather, vocal cord shaping and positioning are under active neurophysiologic regulation. In this regard, during phonation the vocal folds are positioned near the midline by cord tension provided by the cricothyroid muscles. Additionally, the thyroarytenoid muscle provides finer isometric modification, reflected in final shaping of the vocal folds. When the vocal folds are viewed in the frontal plane during phonation, the effect of shaping may be further appreciated. During the production of high-pitched notes, the folds seen on cross section appear thin, but during low pitches the folds appear to thicken considerably.

The frequency of vibration depends upon (1) the vibratory mass of both cords, (2) their anteroposterior tension, (3) functional damping at high pitches, and (4) subglottic pressure. As pitch increases, the true cords lengthen and tense through the action of the cricothyroid muscles. Although cord lengthening alone might serve to reduce pitch, this effect is offset by cord thinning produced by thyroarytenoid action, which increases the internal tension of the true cord. It must also be recognized that the activity of the extrinsic laryngeal muscles affects pitch by altering the spatial relationship between the cricoid and thyroid cartilages. The sternothyroid muscle is felt to influence pitch in this way.

Only when one considers the wide range of frequency, volume, and esthetic quality observed in the human voice does one recognize the severe limitation of our knowledge regarding phonatory control. The question, "Why is a particular voice esthetically pleasant and another irritating to the ear?" cannot be completely answered by the present state of anatomic and neurophysiologic investigation. Part of the answer lies in the recognition of feedback to the central nervous system, which provides the necessary degree of coordination between the respiratory muscles of the thorax, oropharynx, and larynx. The role of auditory feedback is surely essential in the gross regulation of vocal training. The role of mucosal receptors of the pharynx and larynx is also essential to phonatory regulation, as judged by the impaired vocal qualities of singers whose throats are topically anesthetized. Finally, one needs to recognize other feedback mechanisms arising from within the larynx itself and consisting of (1) mucosal[6] and perichondrial[29] touch receptors, and (2) stretch receptors of the joint capsules.[9] Despite the abundance of experimental data documenting servomechanisms within the larynx, the exact mechanism of their influence on final voice regulation remains unknown. Phonatory control continues to challenge the ingenuity of all laryngologists, whose questions are only beginning to be answered.

NEUROMUSCULAR DYSFUNCTION

Paralysis. Isolated unilateral superior laryngeal nerve injury produces anesthesia of the supraglottic portion of the hemilarynx. Because of associated cricothyroid paralysis, the involved vocal cord appears foreshortened, while the posterior commissure of the larynx rotates toward the side of injury. If it is remembered that the glottic closure reflex produced by stimulation of each superior laryngeal nerve is unilateral adduction, then it becomes obvious that damage to one superior laryngeal nerve abolishes closure activity of its corresponding (ipsilateral) cord, thus resulting in occasional aspiration. Respiratory function, however, is rarely affected by unilateral superior laryngeal nerve injury; phonatory performance is more commonly altered by the loss of cord tension produced by this kind of injury. Bilateral superior laryngeal nerve injury is rare, although a more severe aspiration problem would be expected because of complete supraglottic anesthesia. Compensatory protective mechanisms, under these circumstances, are believed to be provided by the use of the afferent limb of the ninth cranial nerve for protective reconstitution of reflex laryngeal closure.

Isolated recurrent laryngeal nerve injury produces nearly midline positioning of the involved vocal cord because of unopposed action of the ipsilateral cricothyroid muscle. Innervated by an intact superior laryngeal nerve, cricothyroid muscle produces cord adduction on the side of recurrent laryngeal nerve injury. An acute nerve injury may be difficult to diagnose functionally because of the relative absence of symptoms. Aspiration, dyspnea, or dysphonia may go unnoticed because of the relative midline position of the paralyzed cord. As musculature of the denervated vocal cord atrophies, the involved cord may lateralize enough to produce occasional aspiration and hoarseness. On the other hand, bilateral recurrent laryngeal nerve paralysis usually produces airway obstruction because of the unopposed action of both intact cricothyroid muscles. In fact, in the untracheostomized state, severe dyspnea may develop as cricothyroid inspiratory and expiratory activity rises in a crescendo response to ventilatory loading (Fig. 3–16). Note that as ventilatory resistance is removed by tracheostomy, cricothyroid activity on inspiration and expiration may cease to provide intermediate positioning of the paralyzed cords. Attempts to decannulate such a patient, however, will result in resumption of cricothyroid inspiratory and expiratory activity, reproducing bilateral cord adduction and continued dyspnea. Because of the midline position of both cords in this situation, aspiration may be minimal. The absence of hoarseness in bilateral recurrent laryngeal nerve injury should not be misinterpreted as indication of neurologic integrity.

Rare situations involving unilateral superior laryngeal nerve palsy and simultaneous contralateral recurrent laryngeal nerve injury will produce devastating disturbances in laryngeal protective function. Since the glottic closure reflex produced by stimulation of each superior laryngeal nerve elicits an ipsilateral adductor cord reflex, it becomes obvious that neither cord will respond to supraglottic stimulation during the act of deglutition. On the side of superior laryngeal nerve injury, the afferent limb of the reflex is interrupted; on the side of recurrent laryngeal nerve injury, the efferent limb of the reflex has been jeopardized.[30] Rehabilitation of

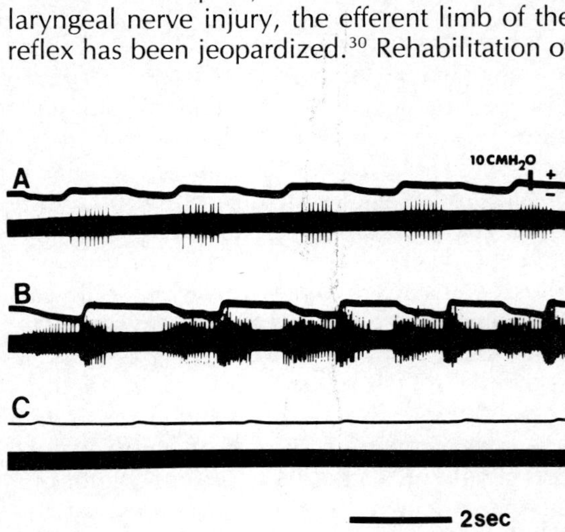

Figure 3–16. Cricothyroid response to ventilatory loading in the spontaneously breathing animal. *Upper tracings,* tracheal pressure; *lower tracings,* cricothyroid EMG. *A,* Untracheostomized, eupneic breathing. *B,* Upper airway obstruction. *C,* Tracheostomized breathing. Note that mild ventilatory loading elicits expiratory activity whereas moderate loading produces inspiratory and expiratory cricothyroid activity.

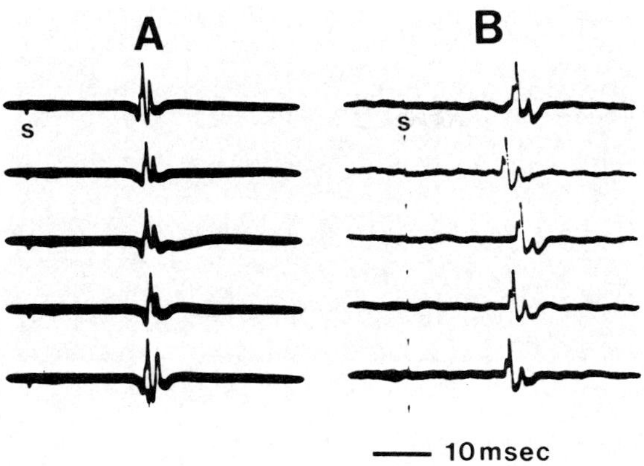

Figure 3–17. Thyroarytenoid action potentials elicited by single-shock stimulus (s) applied to the ipsilateral superior laryngeal nerve. *A*, Control dogs. *B*, Chronically tracheostomized dogs (six to eight months). Note latency shifts in dogs chronically tracheostomized.

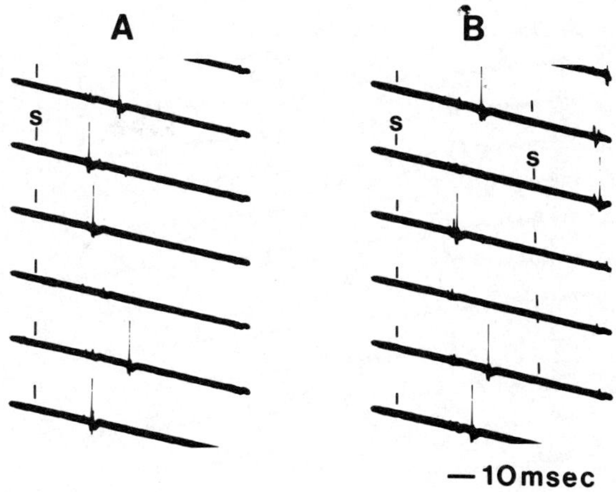

Figure 3–19. Thyroarytenoid action potentials elicited by superior laryngeal stimulation (s) in tracheostomized dogs. *A*, 8 Hz. *B*, 16 Hz. Note latency shifts. No afterdischarge activity is observed.

the swallow mechanism may be especially prolonged as compensatory mechanisms using afferent limbs of the ninth cranial nerve eventually subserve protection of the lower airway.

Tracheostomy. Upper airway obstruction is the most urgent indication for tracheostomy. This lifesaving surgical procedure, however, may be complicated by serious deficiencies in laryngeal function, even when no prior laryngeal pathology exists. Decannulation difficulty because of continued airway obstruction above the tracheostomy may be caused by an array of functional deficiencies produced by the tracheostomy itself, including abductor failure and vocal cord fusion. Chronic aspiration, a defect in protective laryngeal function, may

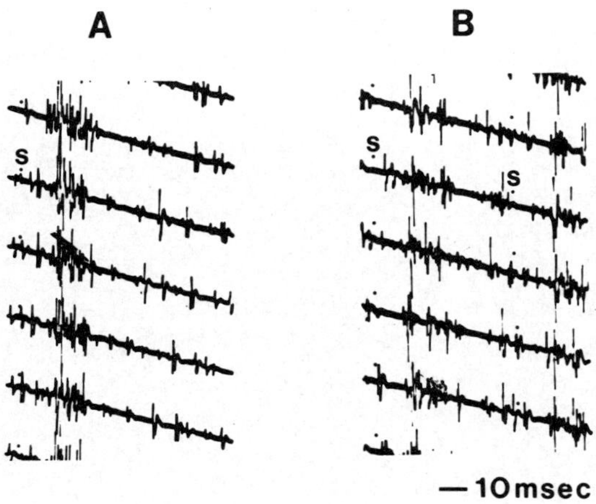

Figure 3–18. Thyroarytenoid action potentials elicited by repetitive stimulation (s) of superior laryngeal nerve in control dogs. *A*, 8 Hz. *B*, 16 Hz. Note numerous afterdischarges following the primary evoked response.

occur in response to tracheostomy well before decannulation is even attempted.

The effect of tracheostomy on an otherwise healthy larynx may be considerably more complex than previously appreciated. The following experimental data provide clues to the mechanism of tracheostomy-related laryngeal dysfunction.

The chronically tracheostomized dog, submitted to neurophysiologic evaluation of protective glottic closure, will develop significant laryngeal incoordination two to eight months after tracheostomy[31] (Fig. 3–17). The threshold of the adductor reflex produced by superior laryngeal nerve electrostimulation nearly doubles after prolonged tracheostomy, while evoked adductor reflexes undergo wide shifts in their latency. These abnormal changes indicate alteration of both central threshold and conduction time. Furthermore, repetitive superior laryngeal nerve stimulation produces marked attenuation of the adductor reflex, reflected in a weakened closure response after long-term tracheostomy (Figs. 3–18 to 3–20). Such changes in the behavior of the medullary adductor motoneurons indicate their susceptibility to surgical modifications in lower respiratory function. These changes may help to explain the onset of aspiration arising from a weakened, ill-coordinated closure response resulting from tracheostomy when no laryngotracheal surgical injury can be found.

Respiratory function of the larynx appears even more susceptible to central alterations when the upper airway is bypassed through tracheostomy. When the electromyographic ac-

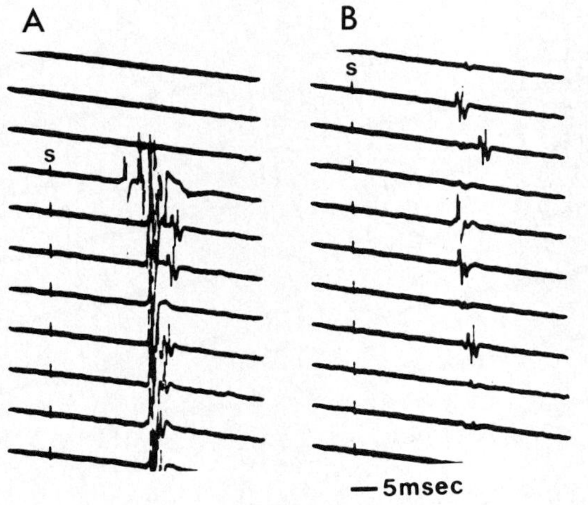

Figure 3–20. Thyroarytenoid action potentials produced by 16 Hz superior laryngeal stimulation (s) in chronically tracheostomized dogs. Primary evoked response attenuates within seconds of stimulus onset. *A,* Onset of stimulus train. *B,* 1 s to 2 s after onset of stimulus train.

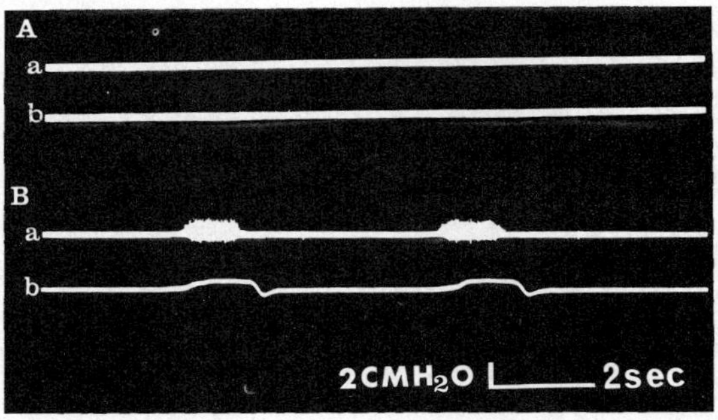

Figure 3–22. Laryngeal abductor activity. *A,* Immediately after tracheostomy. *B,* With tracheostoma partially closed. *Tracing a,* Posterior cricoarytenoid EMG; *tracing b,* intratracheal pressure. Note disappearance of phasic abduction in tracheostomized breathing.

tivity of the posterior cricoarytenoid muscle is measured in the dog before and after tracheostomy, interesting changes in the level of its activity can be observed.[24]

During spontaneous nasal breathing when ventilatory resistance is judged to be maximal (Fig. 3–21A), posterior cricoarytenoid activity also appears to be maximal, corresponding to a negative inspiratory pressure change of 15 mm H_2O. Approximately 3 min after a change to mouth breathing, posterior cricoarytenoid activity decreases, corresponding to a decrease in intratracheal pressure change (Fig. 3–21B). When spontaneous breathing is then shunted through a tracheostomy (Fig. 3–22A), abductor activity not only gradually diminishes but completely disappears. When the tracheostomy is partially occluded and breathing is resumed in part through the upper air passages, posterior cricoarytenoid activity slowly returns (Fig. 3–22B). A week later, although abductor activity is absent with an open tracheostomy, minimal posterior cricoarytenoid activity can be elicited when the tracheostoma is partially occluded (Fig. 3–23).

At four weeks, as expected, no abductor activity can be recorded with an open tracheostomy (Fig. 3–24A). Repeated partial closure of the tracheostoma at this time, however, produces no return in posterior cricoarytenoid activity (Fig. 3–24B). Total stomal closure results in severe laryngeal inspiratory stridor and cyanosis, presumably caused by failure of phasic abductor activity in the posterior cricoarytenoid muscles.

The observations listed below help to explain the difficulty in tracheostomy decannulation when laryngeal abductor activity is temporarily lost. They may also provide insight into the posttracheostomy finding of fused vocal cords when they have been traumatized by previous endotracheal intubation. Such injury may lead

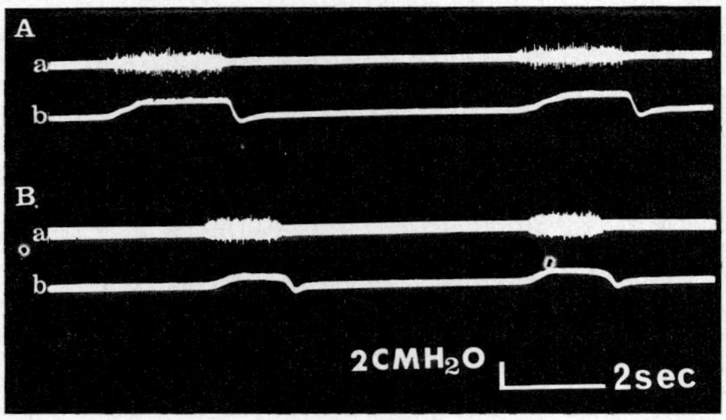

Figure 3–21. Laryngeal abductor activity. *A,* Nose breathing. *B,* Mouth breathing. *Tracing a,* Posterior cricoarytenoid EMG; *tracing b,* intratracheal pressure.

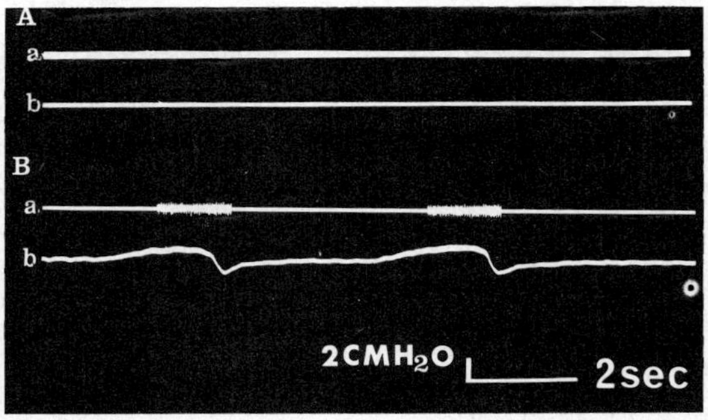

Figure 3–23. Laryngeal abductor activity one week posttracheostomy. *A,* Tracheostoma open. *B,* Tracheostoma partially occluded. *Tracing a,* Posterior cricoarytenoid EMG; *tracing b,* intratracheal pressure.

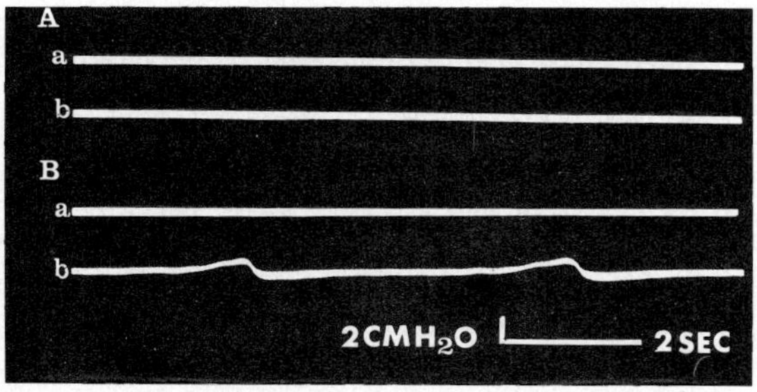

Figure 3–24. Laryngeal abductor activity four weeks post-tracheostomy. *A,* Tracheostoma open. *B,* Tracheostoma partially closed. *Tracing a,* Posterior cricoarytenoid EMG; *tracing b,* intratracheal pressure. No abductor activity could be elicited by increasing ventilatory resistance.

to fusion of the denuded cordal surfaces when they are apposed in the absence of phasic inspiratory abduction.

1. Phasic abductor activity diminishes as ventilatory resistance decreases.
2. The elimination of all measurable ventilatory resistance results in complete cessation of laryngeal abductor activity within 3 to 5 min.
3. The loss of abductor activity persists for as long as airway resistance remains severely reduced.
4. Phasic abductor activity can be reestablished in 3 to 5 min by gradually increasing ventilatory resistance.
5. The longer the duration of reduced resistance, the more difficulty is encountered in reestablishing abductor function once it is lost.

While the effects of tracheostomy on the lower respiratory tract have been studied in great detail, little previous attention has been paid to its influence on the upper respiratory system. It is apparent that tracheostomy bears a greater effect on upper respiratory function than previously appreciated.

RECONSTRUCTIVE SURGERY

The goal of all laryngeal surgery is the complete restoration of function in the following order of importance: (1) protection of the lower airway, (2) respiration, and (3) phonation. Failure to recognize these priorities frequently results in prolonged postoperative recovery, excessive patient expense, and an unnecessary threat to life. Two common surgical procedures will be used to illustrate these reconstructive efforts.

Supraglottic Laryngectomy. When the supraglottic larynx must be surgically resected, the principal dysfunction produced is aspiration. Loss of laryngeal protective function results from the removal of the shieldlike epiglottis and associated aryepiglottic folds, the ramparts of the laryngeal inlet. Even more significant is the interruption of one or both superior laryngeal nerves, producing loss of sensation and abolition of the glottic closure response. The following measures aid in rehabilitating deglutition by preventing aspiration.

1. Laryngeal suspension may be accomplished by preserving the hyoid bone to which the thyroid cartilage may be secured. If the hyoid is resected, the larynx may be suspended from the mandible. This maneuver facilitates deglutition by permitting elevation of the larynx against the tongue base, thus protecting the glottis against intrusion of foreign matter. Excessive and unnecessary resection of the tongue base will jeopardize this compensatory protective measure, while associated injury to the hypoglossal nerve will further adversely affect rehabilitation of the swallow mechanism. In fact, inadvertent hypoglossal injury during supraglottic resection is a serious error in technique and frequently results in total failure of swallow rehabilitation despite an otherwise smooth postoperative course.
2. If the arytenoid cartilage is removed, fixation of the involved vocal cord to the midline cricoid is mandatory for effective reflex glottic closure produced by the pivotal motion of the opposite cord. Attempts to lateralize the involved cord in order to favor respiratory demands will inevitably result in life-threatening aspiration. Midline cord fixation is accomplished principally to reestablish protective function, although this maneuver will rehabilitate phonation as a secondary accomplishment.
3. Cricopharyngeal myotomy will produce a patulous cricopharyngeal sphincter, thus preventing fluids from pooling in the pyriform fossae and spilling into the laryngeal inlet. A posterior midline myotomy will avoid injury to the recurrent laryngeal nerves.
4. Early tracheostomy decannulation may prevent central disorganization of the larynx closure reflex. Subglottic pressure regulation is also reestablished by early decannulation, restoring expectorative laryngeal function in the prevention of aspiration.
5. Weaning from the tracheostomy tube by gradually reducing cannula diameter will assist in the restoration of phasic vocal cord abduction prior to complete decannulation. Tracheostomy decannulation is facilitated in this way by the restoration of the respiratory movements of the cords.

6. Early diet should include semisolid food rather than liquids, which tend to pool in the pyriform fossae and spill into the laryngeal inlet between each attempt at swallowing.

Vertical Hemilaryngectomy. The disabilities produced by resecting one side of the larynx are aspiration, dyspnea, and dysphonia caused by the loss of the false and the true cords. By comparison, aspiration appears to be a less severe problem here than it is after supraglottic resection.

1. In reconstructive efforts to minimize aspiration, replacement of bulk to the aryepiglottic fold reestablishes a barrier to aspiration by restoring stiffness and volume to this laryngeal rampart removed by ablative surgery. Imbedding muscle, cartilage, or bone may effectively reconstruct such a barrier to aspiration.

2. Formation of a pseudocord using perichondrium or strap muscle aids in protective and phonatory function by reestablishing a degree of glottic competence.

3. Early decannulation (a) reestablishes phasic respiratory vocal cord activity, (b) prevents central disorganization of the closure reflex, and (c) reestablishes expectorative function of the larynx.

SUMMARY

Determined by primitive needs, the larynx subserves three basic functions in man: (1) protection of the lower airway, (2) respiratory regulation, and (3) phonation. To a large extent, these functional priorities appear to define the latitudes of surgical prudence.

References

1. Negus VE: The Comparative Anatomy and Physiology of the Larynx. London, Heinemann, 1949.
2. Sasaki CT et al.: Postnatal descent of the epiglottis in man: A preliminary report. Arch Otolaryngol 103:169, 1977.
3. Brunton TL, Cash T: The valvular action of the larynx. J Anat Physiol 17:363, 1883.
4. Lindsay JR: Laryngocele ventricularis. Ann Otol Rhinol Laryngol 49:661, 1940.
5. Suzuki M, Kirchner JA: Afferent nerve fibers in the external branch of the superior laryngeal nerve in the cat. Ann Otol Rhinol Laryngol 77:1059, 1968.
6. Koizumi H: On sensory innervation of larynx in dog. Tohoku J Exp Med 58:199, 1953.
7. Downing SE, Lee JC: Laryngeal chemosensitivity: A possible mechanism for sudden infant death. Pediatrics 55:640, 1975.
8. Sasaki CT, Suzuki M: The respiratory mechanism of aerosol inhalation in treatment of partial airway obstruction. Pediatrics 59:689, 1977.
9. Bowden REM: Innervation of intrinsic laryngeal muscles. *In* Wyke B (ed): Ventilatory and Phonatory Control Systems. London, Oxford University Press, 1974.
10. Sasaki CT, Suzuki M: Laryngeal reflexes in cat, dog, and man. Arch Otolaryngol 102:400, 1976.
11. Martens M: Zur Behandlung von Folgezustanden doppel seitiger Recurrensschadigung. Arch Klin Chir 96:76, 1911.
12. Hast MH: Mechanical properties of the vocal fold muscle. Pract Otorhinolaryngol 29:53, 1967.
13. Suzuki M, Sasaki CT: The effect of various sensory stimuli on reflex laryngeal adduction. Ann Otol Rhinol Laryngol 86:30, 1977.
14. Suzuki M, Sasaki CT: Laryngeal spasm: A neurophysiologic redefinition. Ann Otol Rhinol Laryngol 86:150, 1977.
15. Bishop PO, McLeod JG: Nature of potentials associated with synaptic transmission in lateral geniculate of cat. J Neurophysiol 17:387, 1954.
16. Chang H: Activation of internuncial neurons through collaterals of pyramid fibers at cortical level. J Neurophysiol 18:452, 1955.
17. Krimer, *cited by* Rothschuh KE: Enwichlungsgeschichte Physiologisher Probleme in Tabellenform. Munich, Urban and Schwarzenberg, 1952.
18. Breuer J: Die Selbststeurerung der Atmung durch den Nervus Vagus. Sitzber Akad Wiss Wien 58:909, 1868.
19. Hering E: Die Selbststeurerung der Atmung durch den Nervus Vagus. Sitzber Akad Wiss Wien 57:672, 1868.
20. Kussmaul A, Tenner A: Untersuchungen uber Ursprung und wesen der fallsuchtartigen Zuckungen bei der verblutung sowie der fallsucht uberhaupt. Unters Naturl Mensch Tiere 3:1, 1857.
21. Haldane JS, Priestley JG: Respiration. London, Oxford University Press, 1935.
22. Comroe JH Jr: The hyperpnea of muscular exercise. Physiol Rev 24:319, 1944.
23. Suzuki M, Kirchner JA: The posterior cricoarytenoid as an inspiratory muscle. Ann Otol Rhinol Laryngol 78:849, 1969.
24. Sasaki CT, Fukuda H, Kirchner JA: Laryngeal abductor activity in response to varying ventilatory resistance. Trans Am Acad Ophthalmol Otolaryngol 77:403, 1973.
25. Fukuda H, Sasaki CT, Kirchner JA: Vagal afferent influences on the phasic activity of the posterior cricoarytenoid muscle. Acta Otolaryngol 75:112, 1973.
26. Suzuki M, Kirchner JA, Murakami Y: The cricothyroid as a respiratory muscle. Ann Otol Rhinol Laryngol 79:1, 1970.
27. Horiuchi M, Sasaki CT: Cricothyroid muscle in respiration. Ann Otol Rhinol Laryngol 87:386, 1978.
28. Husson R: Étude des phenomenes physiologiques et acoustiques fondamentaux de la voix chantée. These Fac Sc, Paris, 1950.
29. Gracheva MS: Sensory innervation of locomotor apparatus of the larynx. Fed Proc 22:T 1120, 1963.
30. Suzuki M, Sasaki CT: Initiation of reflex glottic closure. Ann Otol Rhinol Laryngol 85:382, 1976.
31. Sasaki CT, Suzuki M, Horiuchi M, Kirchner JA: The effect of tracheostomy on reflex laryngeal closure. Laryngoscope 87:1428–1433, 1977.

4

Diagnosis and Staging of Laryngeal Disease

William D. Clark, D.D.S., M.D.

The minimum diagnostic evaluation for a laryngeal complaint should include a careful history and complete head and neck examination with special emphasis on use of indirect laryngoscopy, examination of laryngeal function, and palpation of the neck. In the usual case, a reasonable working diagnosis for a laryngeal complaint can be formulated from the history and an office examination. Often, direct laryngoscopy will be required to confirm the diagnosis or effect surgical treatment. Special studies may be useful to confirm a diagnosis and to evaluate the extent or severity of involvement by disease. Thus, they can aid in treatment-planning and offer prognostic information.

HISTORY

The importance of a carefully taken history cannot be overemphasized. The patient should be asked to discuss in detail the presenting complaint. Considerable skill may be required of the laryngologist to guide the patient through an accurate and complete history. Points that should be documented in the history include (1) onset of first related symptom or sign, (2) progression of events leading to the date of the evaluation, and (3) details of prior evaluations or treatments for this complaint.

Once the details of the principal complaints have been obtained, specific inquiry should be made into the numerous signs and symptoms that may be related (Table 4–1). Brewer[1] has listed 33 symptoms and 54 signs that may be early indications of laryngeal disease. Additionally, he has provided the differential diagnosis and suggested the appropriate evaluation for each sign and symptom.

A brief general medical history is in order for all new patient evaluations. The patient should be asked to reveal any chronic uses of drugs, including nonprescription agents. Details of any chronic medical condition should be sought, with specific questioning regarding diabetes mellitus, rheumatoid arthritis, hypertension, pulmonary diseases, heart disease, and tuberculosis. Drug allergies should be documented.

EXAMINATION

A portion of the laryngeal examination should be accomplished during the history-taking by simply listening to the patient talk. Asking the patient to demonstrate a cough and to drink a glass of water will assess the sphincteric function of the larynx. Having the patient breathe rapidly through an open mouth will give clues as to the adequacy of the laryngeal airway.

Table 4–1. AREAS TO QUESTION IN TAKING A LARYNGEAL HISTORY

Past history
- Past laryngeal disorders
- Past laryngeal medical therapy
- Past laryngeal surgical therapy
- Past neck surgery (including thyroid surgery)
- Past neck trauma

Social history
- Use of tobacco products
- Use of alcohol beverages
- Use or abuse of drugs
- Use of voice in vocation
- Use of voice in avocations
- Country of origin
- Travel in foreign countries
- Environmental exposure (dusts, pollutants, infectious diseases, carcinogens)

Review of laryngeal signs and symptoms
- Quality of voice
- Endurance of voice
- Frequency of throat clearing
- Cough precipitated by food or drink
- Ability to produce effective cough
- Adequacy of airway
- Noisy breathing
  - At rest
  - With exertion
- Dyspnea
- Exposure to foreign bodies (or aspiration)

Associated signs and symptoms
- Blood in secretions
- Cough
  - Productive
  - Nonproductive
  - Time of day
  - Hemoptysis
- Throat pain
- Odynophagia
- Ear pain
- Weight loss
- Neck masses
- Fever, chills

A complete head and neck examination is in order for the patient with a laryngeal complaint. The ears should be examined and an estimate of auditory acuity made. The nose should be examined with special interest in signs of allergy, chronic infection, and nasal obstruction.

The oral cavity and oropharynx should be inspected. Signs of mucous membrane dryness or inflammation should be noted. Inspection and palpation should be utilized to search for neoplastic lesions in these areas. The nasopharynx should be inspected for signs of infection, chronic inflammation, and mass lesions.

The neck should be inspected and palpated. Special attention should be directed to the laryngeal cartilages, thyroid gland, and deep jugular chain of lymph nodes.

The extent of a general physical examination required for the patient with a laryngeal complaint will vary with the patient's individual circumstances.

An indirect laryngoscopy should include a careful inspection of the inferior oropharynx, hypopharynx, and larynx. The indirect laryngoscopy is of major importance in the diagnosis of laryngeal disease.

Indirect Laryngoscopy

Historical Review. The origin of indirect laryngoscopy is obscure. Morell Mackenzie[2] credited M. Levret, a French surgeon, with having described the use of a polished metal instrument to examine the lower portions of the pharynx by reflected light and reflected imagery in 1743. Some historians[3] have questioned the accuracy of Mackenzie's interpretation of Levret's work. Bozzini's[4] "light conductor" was described in 1804, and there is general agreement that it was used for viewing the larynx (Fig. 4–1). Senn (1829) attempted indirect laryngoscopy by means of a mirror, but apparently failed to recognize the importance of an external source of illumination. Babington[5] exhibited his "glottiscope" in 1829. This instrument combined a laryngeal mirror with a tongue depressor (Fig. 4–2). Bennati (1832) is said to have used a "double-tubed speculum" to view the larynx. This instrument was designed and fabricated by Selligue, a patient of his who suffered from a laryngeal disorder. Baumès exhibited a laryngeal mirror of his own design at the Medical Society of Lyons in 1838. Liston described the use of a dental mirror to examine the larynx in 1840. Warden (1844) employed prisms in attempts to view the larynx. Avery (1844) designed a head mirror and candle holder combination, together with a speculum and laryngeal mirror combination, in an unsuccessful attempt to make indirect laryngoscopy practical (Fig. 4–3).

Manuel Garcia,[6] a singing teacher of Spanish descent, French birth, and English residence,

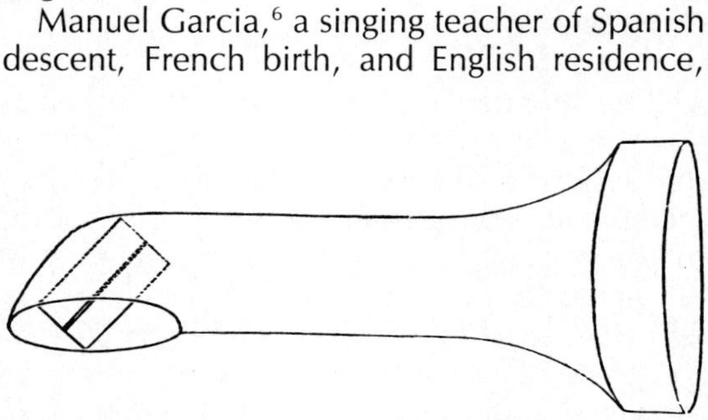

Figure 4–1. Bozzin's "Light Conductor." (From Mackenzie M: The Use of the Laryngoscope. Philadelphia, Lindsay and Blakiston, 1865.)

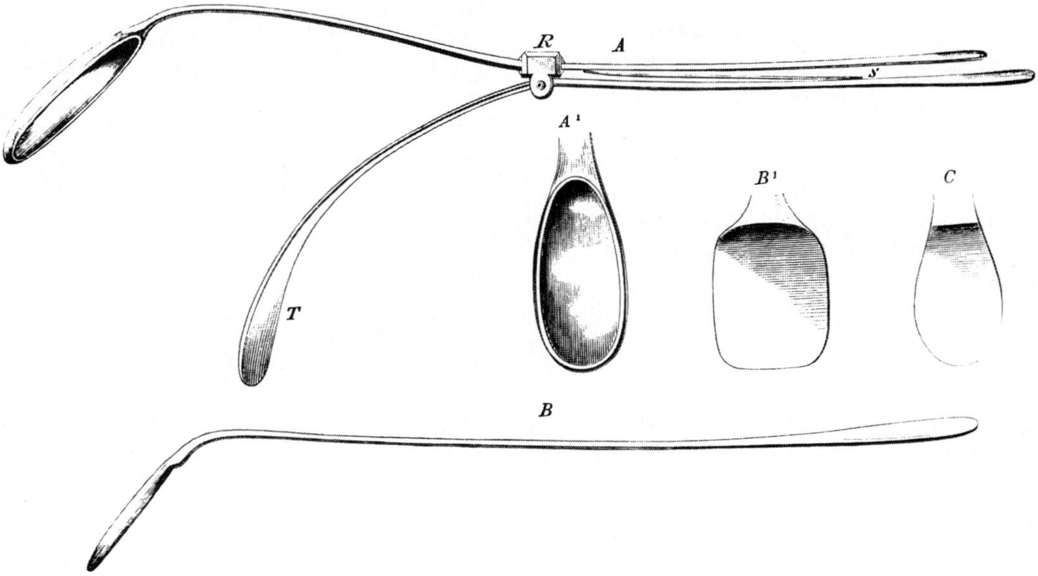

Figure 4–2. Babington's Glottiscope. (From Mackenzie M: The Use of the Laryngoscope. Philadelphia, Lindsay and Blakiston, 1865.)

viewed his own larynx in September 1854. He used a hand mirror both to reflect the sun rays to and receive his larynx's image from a dental mirror held in his oropharynx. He made detailed studies of his larynx in the dynamic state and contributed much to the early understanding of laryngeal physiology.

Basic Techniques. Proper positioning of the patient facilitates indirect laryngoscopy. The patient should be in the sitting position, leaning forward slightly. The neck should be flexed on the chest and the head extended on the neck. The mouth is open with the tongue maximally extended.

The examiner's position will vary with his personal preference and the conditions under which the patient is to be examined. The right-handed laryngologist will usually perform an

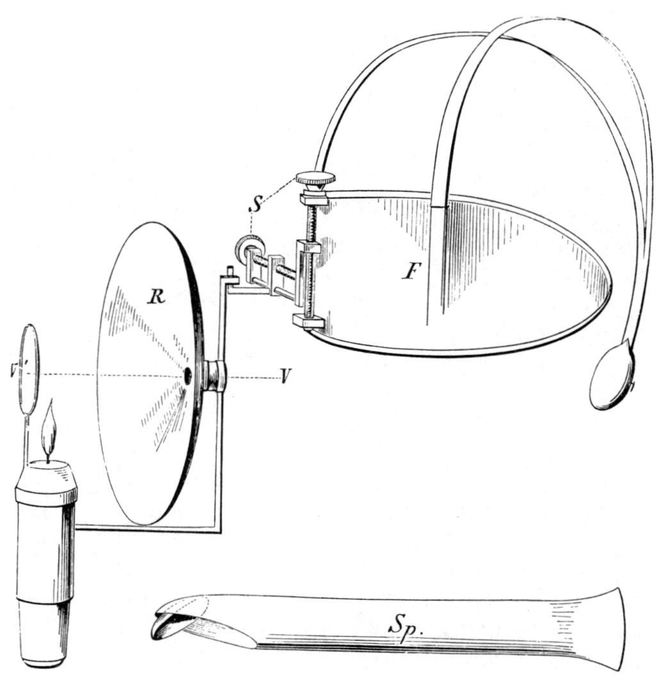

Figure 4–3. Avery's devices for indirect laryngoscopy. (From Mackenzie M: The Use of the Laryngoscope. Philadelphia, Lindsay and Blakiston, 1865.)

indirect laryngoscopy from directly in front of the patient or from the patient's right side. The examination may be accomplished from the sitting or the standing position.

Reflected light from a head mirror is the classic source of illumination for this examination. Headlights of various designs may be substituted for the head mirror and may facilitate examinations at locations other than the physician's office.

The right-handed laryngologist usually places the head mirror over his left eye and uses a light source from the patient's right side. Skillful use of a head mirror requires experience. Some basic rules for head mirror use are as follows: (1) use a high-quality mirror that focuses reflected light at a convenient working distance, (2) place the mirrror as close to the eye or spectacles as possible, (3) adjust the angle of the mirror to cast the light where you are looking, and (4) make minor adjustments in the patient's head position to take best advantage of the reflected light as the examination progresses.

A 2-inch square or 4-inch square gauze sponge (without cotton or other filler material) is wrapped about the tip of the patient's tongue and used to hold the tongue between the left thumb and middle finger. The forefinger of the left hand may be used to retract the patient's upper lip. A laryngeal mirror (size 5 or 6 for an adult) is held in the right hand and treated to prevent fogging. This may be accomplished by warming the mirror over the flame of an alcohol lamp, by dipping it into a glass bead sterilizer (a device used in dentistry to sterilize root canal instruments), or by applying an antifog solution (a detergent solution developed to keep dental mirrors from fogging). If a heat method is employed, the laryngologist is obligated to test the temperature of the back of the mirror on his skin before placing it in the patient's mouth. The skin of the left hand is a convenient place for this testing.

The laryngeal mirror is placed into the patient's mouth and carefully carried to the posterior oral cavity, keeping the plane of the mirror more or less parallel to the floor. The shaft of the mirror rests against the left commissure of the mouth, while the fingers of the right hand are braced against the cheek. The angle of the mirror is then changed to about 45 degrees, and the mirror is used to retract the soft palate posteriorly and superiorly. The left hand may exert gentle force on the patient's face to improve positioning while the angle of the mirror is changed to give a panoramic view. After focusing on the oropharynx, the hypopharynx should be inspected. Finally, attention is directed to the larynx. The supraglottic structures are reviewed, the endolarynx inspected next, and the subglottic areas studied last. The patient is asked to phonate to allow evaluation of vocal cord function. In fact, phonatory efforts are often required to permit adequate visualization of the endolarynx. Both "A-a-a-a" and "E-e-e-e" sounds should be tried. The "A-a-a-a" sound will often permit an optimal view of the hypopharynx, while the "E-e-e-e" or "H-e-e-e" sound will often afford the best view of the endolarynx. Having the patient laugh will sometimes improve the view of the endolarynx. The subglottis will often be revealed to its best advantage during pauses between vocalizations. The inexperienced laryngologist will usually have to perform the above series of examinations in several stages, giving the patient short breaks between efforts. The experienced endoscopist may be able to accomplish the entire examination with one mirror insertion. When an abnormality is discovered, a series of examinations will permit a more careful study.

When superior laryngeal nerve function is in question, the supraglottic larynx may be palpated with appropriate instruments to test sensation. A malleable calcium alginate swab (Calgiswab) is convenient for this purpose.

About one patient in twenty will have such an active gag reflex that even the most experienced laryngologist will be unable to perform an adequate indirect laryngoscopy without the aid of a pharmacologic agent.

Topical Anesthetics. The mucous membranes of the mouth, oropharynx, and hypopharynx may be anesthetized with a topically active local anesthetic. Agents such as lidocaine 4 per cent, dyclonine (Dyclone) ½ or 1 per cent, and combinations of benzocaine, butyl aminobenzoate, and tetracaine (Cetacaine) are quite effective in abating the gag reflex. Some precautions are in order prior to using topical anesthetics. The patient should be asked about possible allergies or intolerances to local anesthetics. The patient should be told that the agent will have an unpleasant taste and that the effects of the anesthetic agent will also be unpleasant. Most anesthetized patients feel as though their swallowing mechanism is impaired, and many experience an ill-defined sense of insecurity. Without adequate advance warning and reassurance, some patients will pass rapidly from insecurity into a state of panic. It is important to remember that topically applied local anesthetics are systemically absorbed across mucous membranes and that absorption may be very rapid in the presence of traumatized or inflamed tissues. Provisions for resuscitation and treatment of local anesthetic reactions should be immediately available before any of these agents is used.

Intravenous Diazepam. The gag reflex can be markedly reduced in the adult by the intravenous injection of 10 mg of diazepam (Valium). The effect is present within a few minutes and persists long enough to allow multiple endoscopic procedures. While it is not likely to be adopted as a routine substitute for topical anesthesia, intravenous diazepam may be used for the occasional patient who is allergic to local anesthetics or who requires both agents to allow an adequate examination.

There are several precautions regarding the intravenous use of diazepam. To reduce the possibility of venous thrombosis and phlebitis, the drug should be injected slowly (1 minute or more per each 5 mg) into a large vein. Also, diazepam should be used only with great caution in the elderly, very ill, or pulmonary-compromised patient because of the danger of precipitating apnea, cardiac arrest, or both. It is not recommended for use in children. Patients will experience sedation after intravenous diazepam, and proper provisions for their postexamination transportation and care must be made. As with local anesthetics, provisions for resuscitation should be made before use of this drug.

The Overhanging Epiglottis. A good view of the endolarynx is occasionally prevented by an overhanging epiglottis. Often the patient may be trained to move the epiglottis. This usually takes several examinations with reinforcement by the laryngologist when the patient performs an appropriate epiglottic movement. When this fails, a view can usually be obtained by mechanically retracting the epiglottis. This requires topical anesthesia and a cooperative patient. A Jackson cross-action forceps or a similarly shaped instrument may be guided by indirect visualization and the epiglottis held anteriorly. Use of a flexible endoscope to bypass the epiglottis is another satisfactory solution to this problem.

Office Endoscopy

Several instruments have been developed in recent years for indirect and direct examinations of the upper aerodigestive tract. These include right-angled telescopes and flexible fiberoptic endoscopes.

The major advantages of these instruments are that they (1) allow photographic or videotape records to be made for review at leisure, (2) allow observations to be made by more than one person at a time, and (3) are better tolerated by some patients than mirror examinations. Additionally, access problems may be overcome by the fiberoptic instruments that may be visually guided around obstructing anatomy or pathology.

Among rigid instruments for indirect laryngoscopy, those utilizing the Hopkins rod-lens system merit special mention. This unique lens system improves light transmission and magnification, while allowing miniaturization of the instruments. The improved image resolution and bright illumination provide the capability for endoscopic photography and video recordings of superb quality.[7]

Recorded Images

The value of recorded images of the larynx has long been recognized. Still photographs are helpful for documentation, teaching, and study; however, motion picture photography offers the major advantage of allowing study of the larynx in its dynamic state. Unfortunately, the cost and unwieldiness of equipment, as well as the delays associated with film processing, have kept laryngeal cinematography from gaining widespread use.

The ready availability of television video recording systems utilizing miniature color cameras, coupled with recent technologic advances in endoscopic instruments, has made video recording of endoscopic events a practical reality. Tape recordings are available for immediate playback, and much of the associated hardware has multiple uses.

RADIOGRAPHIC STUDIES AND SPECIAL STUDIES

The larynx may be studied with standard radiography, tomography, xeroradiography, contrast radiography, sonography and computerized tomography. These procedures are covered in detail in Chapter 5 of this volume, Radiologic Evaluation of the Larynx.

The larynx may be studied by stroboscopy, electroglottography, spectographic analysis, echoglottography, and electromyography. Each of these subjects is discussed in Chapter 28, Laryngeal Research.

Yumoto[8,9] has recently described a new method of objectively assessing hoarseness, utilizing the harmonics-to-noise ratio. A voice recording of a sustained vowel is processed by a computer to obtain the harmonics-to-noise ratio, expressed in decibels. The measurement is not affected by subjective influences of the examiner and is not beyond the capability of a microcomputer. Measurements such as this may soon be standard for pre- and post-treatment documentation, much as audiograms are used in otology.

Direct Laryngoscopy

Problems with the diagnosis of laryngeal disease in an historically prominent patient are thought by some historians to have contributed to conditions that led to World War I.[10]

The Case of Frederick the Noble.[3 11, 12] On June 15, 1888 Frederick III, Emperor of the German Empire and Prussia, died of laryngeal carcinoma. He had become symptomatic in January, 1887. In the spring of that year, his German physicians concluded that carcinoma was the probable diagnosis and recommended surgical excision via laryngofissure. However, British laryngologist Morell Mackenzie was called in for a second opinion. Sir Morell felt that the laryngeal lesion was probably benign but recommeded biopsy via indirect laryngoscopy to rule out malignancy. Several biopsies were obtained, but they were inadequate for diagnosis by renowned pathologist Rudolph Virchow. Mackenzie stood firm in recommending against surgical treatment, and a bitter controversy developed among those responsible for the Crown Prince's care.

By late November, 1887, all concerned agreed that the Crown Prince was suffering from an advanced laryngeal malignancy. At this point, the attending physicians offered their royal patient choice of palliative treatment or total laryngectomy. Frederick chose palliation. A tracheostomy was required in February, 1888, when airway obstruction became severe. In early March, Waldeyer was able to confirm the diagnosis of squamous cell carcinoma after examining soft tissue coughed from the tracheostomy tube. Frederick became Emperor on March 9, 1888, on the death of his father, William. The last several months of Frederick's life were complicated by mediastinal abscesses and pneumonia, while the lay press and medical jounals fed fuel to the raging controversy between Mackenzie and his German counterparts.

Frederick III was a political moderate and had hoped to lead Germany from the "Blood and Iron" policies of Bismarck and William I into a peaceful democracy. His ties to Great Britain were strong, largely through his wife Victoria, daughter of Queen Victoria. His son, William II, was quite the opposite, having matured under the influence of his grandfather, Kaiser Wilhelm I, and Bismarck. Under the leadership of William II, Germany pursued the nationalistic and imperialistic policies that led to World War I.[10]

The negative influences of several inflated egos were major factors in producing the bitterness among those who attended Frederick the Noble. The entire affair marked one of the low points in modern medical history. Had the direct laryngoscopy been an accepted procedure in the 1880s, world history might well have been altered.

Intraoperative Considerations. The technical details of direct laryngoscopy and endoscopic surgery of the larynx are well covered in Chapter 6 of this volume. In this chapter, we will be concerned only with the diagnostic considerations of direct laryngoscopy, especially as they relate to the evaluation of malignancies.

A careful examination of the oral cavity, oropharynx, and hypopharynx is important in the course of a diagnostic direct laryngoscopy. Digital palpation of these areas should precede the introduction of a laryngoscope.

The Jackson standard laryngoscope is an excellent instrument for the initial inspection of the upper aerodigestive tract. Its large lumen allows a panoramic view of the inferior oropharynx, the hypopharynx, and the larynx. Its wide blade fits nicely into the vallecula, allowing a stable, unencumbered view of the supraglottic structures. It is also useful for visualizing the pyriform sinuses and for lifting the larynx anteriorly to gain visualization of the postcricoid area and introitus oesophagi.

A narrow instrument, such as the Hollinger anterior commissure laryngoscope, may then be utilized to inspect the endolarynx and any other areas that were not well seen with the wider instrument. The ventricular folds, ventricles, vocal cords, and subglottis are inspected. When microscopic examination is deemed desirable, a Jako-Pilling or Dedo-Pilling laryngoscope of suitable size may be used (see Chapter 6).

When small or obviously benign lesions are discovered, they may be managed as outlined in Chapter 6. When a malignancy is suspected, great care must be taken not only to establish the correct diagnosis but also to determine the extent of tumor involvement accurately.

Several generous biopsies of the main body of the tumor should be obtained. If there is question about the extent of tumor involvement, biopsies may be used to aid in the mapping process. This is especially important when determining whether conservation surgery is applicable to a given lesion.

Pathologic confirmation of laryngeal malignancy will occasionally be a major problem. This is especially true when the tumor infiltrates and spreads submucosally, as is often the case with carcinomas arising within a ventricle. Deep, submucosal biopsies will usually provide the diagnosis in such lesions. When one or more such biopsies have failed to establish the diagnosis, the use of frozen-section techniques may be valuable. Serial biopsies are submitted for frozen section until the pathologist is able to declare a sample adequate for diagnosis.

At the termination of the operative portion of a direct laryngoscopy, it is wise to consider observing the larynx for vocal cord motion as the patient recovers from anesthesia. This is of the utmost importance in the occasional patient with a laryngeal complaint who cannot be adequately examined by indirect laryngoscopy.

When an apparent malignancy is discovered, the surgeon should accurately record the extent of tumor involvement on the patient's chart. Preprinted forms or rubber stamps with anatomic diagrams are convenient for this purpose.

Triple Endoscopy. A patient with squamous cell carcinoma of the upper aerodigestive tract has about a 20 per cent chance of developing

Table 4–2. CARCINOMA OF LARYNX—CLINICAL STAGING SYSTEM*

A. Tumor Size (T)
- 1. Supraglottis
  - Tis Carcinoma in situ
  - T1 Tumor confined to site of origin with normal mobility
  - T2 Tumor involves adjacent supraglottic site(s) or glottis without fixation
  - T3 Tumor limited to larynx with fixation or extension to involve postcricoid area, medial wall of pyriform sinus, or preepiglottic space
  - T4 Massive tumor extending beyond larynx to involve oropharynx, soft tissues of neck, or destruction of thyroid cartilage
- 2. Glottis
  - Tis Carcinoma in situ
  - T1 Tumor confined to vocal cord(s) with normal mobility (includes involvement of anterior or posterior commissures)
  - T2 Supraglottic or subglottic extension of tumor with normal or impaired cord mobility
  - T3 Tumor confined to the larynx with cord fixation
  - T4 Massive tumor with thyroid cartilage destruction or extension beyond the confines of the larynx, or both
- 3. Subglottis
  - Tis Carcinoma in situ
  - T1 Tumor confined to the subglottic region
  - T2 Tumor extension to vocal cords with normal or impaired cord mobility
  - T3 Tumor confined to larynx with cord fixation
  - T4 Massive tumor with cartilage destruction or extension beyond the confines of the larynx, or both

B. Nodal Involvement (N)
- NX Minimum requirements to assess the regional nodes cannot be met
- N0 No clinically positive nodes
- N1 Single clinically positive homolateral node, 3 cm diam. or less
- N2 Single clinically positive homolateral node, more than 3 but not more than 6 cm diam., or multiple clinically positive homolateral nodes, none more than 6 cm diam.
  - N2a Single clinically positive homolateral node more than 3 cm but not more than 6 cm diam.
  - N2b Multiple clinically positive homolateral nodes, none more than 6 cm diam.
- N3 Massive homolateral node(s), bilateral nodes, or contralateral node(s)
  - N3a Clinically positive homolateral node(s), one more than 6 cm diam.
  - N3b Bilateral clinically positive nodes (stage each side separately; e.g., N3b: right; N2a; left, N1)
  - N3c Contralateral clinically positive node(s) only

C. Distant Metastasis (M)
- MX Minimum requirements to assess the presence of distant metastasis cannot be met
- M0 No (known) distant metastasis
- M1 Distant metastasis present

D. Stage Grouping

Stage I	T1, N0, M0
Stage II	T2, N0, M0
Stage III	T3, N0, M0
	T1, T2, T3; N1, M0
Stage IV	T4, N0, N1; M0
	Any T, N2, N3; M0
	Any T, any N, M1

*From American Joint Committee on Cancer: Manual for Staging of Cancer, 2nd ed. Beahrs OH, Myers MH (eds). Philadelphia, JB Lippincott Company, 1983, pp. 41 and 42.

a second primary within five years.[13] Gluckman[14] reported having detected 15 synchronous second primaries when routinely performing triple endoscopies in 162 consecutive cases of carcinoma of the upper aerodigestive tract. Almost 50 per cent of these second primaries were unsuspected prior to endoscopy, and all fulfilled the strict criteria of Warren and Gates[15] (that is, each neoplasm clearly malignant; each geographically separate and distinct; possibility of one being metastasis from the other excluded).

Few would disagree with the rationale for performing examinations of the mouth, pharynx, larynx, esophagus, and tracheobronchial tree when a malignancy is discovered in the upper aerodigestive tract. An exception to this general rule would be nasopharyngeal carcinoma, a disease that does not seem to be etiologically related to other aerodigestive tract malignancies.

The triple endoscopy is ideally performed under the same anesthetic as the initial direct laryngoscopy. This is practical because the nature of a laryngeal malignancy is usually apparent preoperatively. When necessary, the additional endoscopic examinations may be performed at a second session, or even as a prelude to definitive laryngeal surgery.

Intraoperative Biopsies. During the course of definitive laryngeal surgery, it may be advantageous to obtain additional diagnostic information in the form of biopsies studied by the frozen-section technique. This is true when conservation surgery of the larynx is being performed and questions arise as to the extent of the lesion or the nature of adjacent epithelial changes.

Postoperative Examination of Excised Tissues. The laryngeal surgeon is well advised to examine the surgical specimen thoroughly after its removal. Taking precautions to insure against seeding tumors cells, the surgeon should thoroughly examine the laryngeal specimen. This will give feedback regarding the accuracy of preoperative and intraoperative assessments of tumor extent and may yield information that indicates the need for a change in the treatment plan.

Time taken to assist the pathologist in orientation of the fixed surgical specimen will yield rewards in the form of a more meaningful pathology report and a better working relationship with the pathologist. Review of the final histopathology section will be educational and may aid in therapeutic decision making.

CLASSIFICATION AND STAGING OF LARYNGEAL MALIGNANCIES

The current classification and staging system for tumors of the head and neck was updated and published by the AJCC in 1983. Table 4–2 presents those portions of this system applicable to the larynx.[16]

References

1. Brewer DW Sr: The early diagnostic signs and symptoms of laryngeal disease. Laryngoscope 85:499–515, 1975.
2. Mackenzie M: The Use of the Laryngoscope. Philadelphia, Lindsay and Blakiston, 1865.
3. Stevenson RS: Morell Mackenzie—The Story of a Victorian Tragedy. New York, Henry Schuman, 1947.
4. Bozzini P: Der Lichtleiter oder Beschreibung einer einfachen Vorrichtung, und ihrer Anwendung zur Erleuchtung innerer Höhlen und Zwischenräume des lebenden animalischen Körpers. Weimar, 1807.
5. Babington BG: Glottiscope. London Med Gazette 3:555, 1829.
6. Garcia M: Observations on the human voice. Philos Mag and J of Sci 10:218–226, 1855.
7. Ward PH et al.: Advances in endoscopic examination of the respiratory system. Ann Otol Rhinol Laryngol 83:754–760, 1974.
8. Yumoto E et al.: The harmonics-to-noise ratio as an index of the degree of hoarseness. J Acoust Soc Am 71:1544–1550, 1982.
9. Yumoto E: The quantitative evaluation of hoarseness. Arch Otolaryngol 109:48–52, 1983.
10. McInnis WD et al.: The management of carcinoma of the larynx in a prominent patient, *or* Did Morell Mackenzie really cause World War I? Am J Surg 132:515–522, 1976.
11. Schweig, H: Case of Emperor Frederick III. New York, Edgar S. Werner, 1888.
12. Mackenzie M: The Fatal Illness of Frederic the Noble. London, Sampson Lowe, 1888.
13. Gluckman JL et al.: Multicentric squamous-cell carcinoma of the upper aerodigestive tract. Head and Neck Surg 3:90–96, 1980.
14. Gluckman JL: Synchronous multiple primary lesions of the upper aerodigestive system. Arch Otolaryngol 105:597–598, 1979.
15. Warren S, Gates O: Multiple primary malignant tumors—A survey of the literature and a statistical study. Am J Cancer 51:1358–1414, 1932.
16. American Joint Committee on Cancer: Manual for Staging of Cancer, 2nd ed, Beahrs OH, Myers MH (eds). Philadelphia, JB Lippincott Company, 1983.

5

Radiologic Evaluation of the Larynx*

Arnold M. Noyek, M.D., Harry S. Shulman, M.D., Marvin I. Steinhardt, M.A., M.D., and Judah Zizmor, M.D.

The modern-day laryngologist is overwhelmed by the number of available laryngeal imaging modalities and their remarkable imaging potential; however, he perceives an increasing need for radiologic imaging to help him deal with clinically problematic areas. Equally, the modern-day laryngeal radiologist is amazed by the increasing array of treatment options open to his clinical colleagues. The imager may not understand the clinician's specific problem unless it is brought to his attention directly, but he fully understands that the imaging technology within his department can contribute in an exciting and significant way to improved patient management. The common meeting ground for these two laryngeal specialists is in the diagnostic imaging process, which has the potential of contributing so significantly to the contemporary management of the patient with laryngeal disease. It is the purpose of this chapter (1) to suggest a working role for diagnostic imaging in the most effective evaluation of the patient with laryngeal disease, (2) to discuss the current imaging modalities available and to define their roles by current need, and (3) to detail the specific applications of these various imaging modalities to a more precise process for differential diagnosis and treatment decision-making that is relevant to each major group of laryngeal disorders.

THE ROLE OF THE LARYNGOLOGIST

The laryngologist must place the patient's laryngeal disease in clinical context. He assesses his patient by history and physical examination, and by indirect, telescopic, and direct endoscopic examination. He attempts to place the patient's disease in a provisional or working diagnostic category, both in a qualitative or diagnostic sense and in a quantitative or size sense; however, this purely clinical process only approximates the real description of the disease. The laryngologist faces a variety of difficulties in diagnosis based upon the cooperation and habitus of the patient, the skill of the individual examiner in the particular situation, and the frequent problem of technical

*Supported by the Saul A. Silverman Family Foundation, Toronto, Ontario, Canada.

inaccessibility. These impede realistic and complete structural and functional analysis.

There are occult areas, at the mucosal, submucosal, and framework levels of the larynx, and disease is commonly underestimated to the detriment of the patient's health. It is here that the laryngologist must recognize his clinical limitations and turn to the laryngeal radiologist to supplement the diagnostic input and allow credible pretreatment disease staging—the basis for rational therapy. The laryngologist may not fully understand the technology of the imaging modalities, but he must make every effort to understand their clinical application.

There are a variety of imaging evaluations available, both roentgenographic and nonroentgenographic[1]. Many of these are now areas of subspecialization for the experienced radiologist. Certain disorders, such as laryngeal cancer (except for clearly small T1 lesions), fully deserve critical contemporary imaging as part of the diagnostic pretreatment work-up. There is no justification for a patient being denied the availability of such imaging; if he must attend a major center for optimum treatment, the same reason applies to the provision of a thorough and appropriate radiologic investigation. It must not be misconstrued, however, that all laryngeal disease requires extensive radiololgic work-up. Some disorders require only the critical clinical examination of an astute and interested laryngologist; other disorders may require the supplemental evaluation of only one lateral baseline x-ray (the soft tissue lateral radiograph). All these matters, from simple to complex, require sound clinical judgment.

The laryngologist is therefore the pivotal figure; he is the person to initiate a specific diagnostic evaluation and he forms the link to the radiologist. There is now such sophistication in imaging capability and such opportunity for improved patient care that never before has the need for meaningful clinician-imager dialogue been as great. The laryngologist has the responsibility for initiating this dialogue.

THE ROLE OF THE LARYNGEAL RADIOLOGIST

The radiologist recognizes that he participates in this dialogue; he is clearly something more than a technologist. He must be aware of modern technology and of its potential for application; above all, he must be interested and motivated in the possibilities of ever improving his diagnostic imaging yield. The sensitive radiologist, who takes pride in his work as a consultant and in his contribution to the patient's welfare, does himself much credit and the patient much gain.

After consultation, the radiologist must play an active role in the examination, regardless of the technique elected for radiologic evaluation. It is critical that the laryngologist familiarize the radiologist with the clinical problem at hand by means of a meaningful x-ray requisition supplemented when appropriate by a telephone call. An interested and enthusiastic radiologist can then respond by providing a diagnostic imaging solution of highest possible diagnostic return. A "routine" study done by a technologist is frequently inadequate or incomplete through no fault of the technologist but because the radiologist fails to understand the critical role of the diagnostic study that he is providing, usually because the clinician has not fulfilled his role.

The diagnostic imaging study should be reviewed by the radiologist while the patient is still in the radiology department to see whether or not the purpose of the radiologic examination has been fulfilled. If an advanced imaging study, such as CT, is required, the examination should be actively monitored by the radiologist and either the purpose of the examination achieved or its limitations recognized. The purposes range from rendering a specific diagnosis (such as laryngocele or fracture) to evaluating the three-dimensional extent of a laryngeal tumor and to determining whether certain regional boundaries (such as cartilage framework, neighboring luminal structures, or regional draining lymph nodes) have been transgressed or become involved.

The laryngeal radiologist has a further and final responsibility, not only to provide the best possible imaging study but to guarantee that this information is passed on to the clinician in a meaningful and direct way. Thus, through the two-way communication between clinician and imager, the entire process grows and becomes satisfying. Unfortunately, but importantly, much is learned from failure as well as from success; therefore, both the laryngologist and the laryngeal radiologist are obliged to review the hard-copy findings both before the fact and after patient treatment and to realistically assess the results, searching for constant improvement.

THE ROLE OF LARYNGEAL IMAGING

In these paragraphs we examine the need for laryngeal imaging; here, the question is "Why?" The later sections will answer "How?"

The larynx, a remarkable mucosa-lined complex organ comprising modified soft tissue sphincters supported by a unique cartilaginous framework, remains distant to the inspecting eye and the palpating hand. Mucous membranes can be examined directly by mirror, telescope, and endoscope, but areas such as the laryngeal ventricles and the subglottis often remain hidden from view. Beneath the mucous membrane, which offers visual assessment to greater or lesser degree, lie a series of muscular, ligamentous, and cartilaginous structures far more difficult to assess. Here, then, is the role of diagnostic radiologic imaging—it provides the possibility of a resting-state examination, free from encumbrances such as endoscopes and movement. By this examination the clinician may ultimately have a more definitive display of the true nature and extent of the pathology—or as close an approximation thereto as the imaging technology and circumstances will allow.

Radiologic evaluation can be both qualitative and quantitative. The qualitative diagnosis may be specific, or it may be only broadly specific as in indicating a group disorder (see below). An example of a specific qualitative diagnostic yield might be the recognition of a laryngocele. In clinical perspective, a large mass or bulge in the supraglottis, obscuring the bulk of the laryngeal airway and denying visual access to the vocal cords, may suggest a laryngocele or a large smooth supraglottic tumor. Here conventional radiology may rapidly indicate the qualitative diagnosis and conclude the diagnostic issue.

Occasionally a group disorder qualitative diagnosis is the radiologic yield. For example, the presence of calcific densities within an endolaryngeal mass may represent the multiple coarse calcifications of an osteochondroma; however, this finding is insufficiently specific to differentiate an osteochondroma from the similar appearance of an osteochondrosarcoma, which has a different biologic behavior. Coarse calcifications may suggest other calcific disease within the larynx such as the rare tracheopathia osteoplastica; spheroid phlebolithic calcifications may suggest a cavernous hemangioma. Though the astute laryngeal radiologist may be able to differentiate these lesions further by radiologic-pathologic correlations (for example, phleboliths are usually uniformly round), the radiologist serves his role best when he allows the evolution of a practical differential diagnosis through mutual clinician-imager consideration. The radiologist is not in competition with the pathologist to offer his own tissue specific diagnosis in advance of biopsy; his role should be to suggest diagnostic options to the clinician and to direct further studies if required. If a specific diagnosis comes forth, it is a bonus rather than the *raison d'être* for most radiologic examinations.

As for the more important quantitative diagnostic radiologic role, the radiologist is not in competition with the clinician to see who can define the smallest possible lesion.The laryngologist may need no diagnostic imaging whatever for a small T1 carcinoma of the vocal cord; however, a suspected larger lesion, which may have extension into the ventricle, becomes very much an opportunity for the radiologist to lend his expertise to the proper pretreatment staging of this cancer.

In quantitative diagnosis, the clinician in essence asks three groups of questions of the radiologist:

1. Can you demonstrate, through examinations in more than one plane, the full three-dimensional extent of the laryngeal lesion? Can you demonstrate extraregional extension that will alter my treatment approach?

2. Is the disease local or systemic? If it is local disease (here, cancer), does it extend subclinically to deep cervical nodes or beyond? (Can you help me place this patient's cancer in a working TNM category?) Could the laryngeal lesion be a local manifestation of a systemic disorder? (Could it be systemic arthropathy, relapsing perichondritis, or amyloidosis, for example?)

3. Can you demonstrate specific anatomic or physiologic deficits (for example, a fistula) that may alter my treatment approach?

In summary, the role of laryngeal imaging is to complement and supplement the entire diagnostic process. Radiologic evaluation is to be used selectively and wisely in order to direct further studies or give credibility to treatment options. A specific laryngeal study should solve a specific clinical problem; if it does not, it may give direction to a second study, perhaps different by mode and perhaps different by plane, which may answer the outstanding question. In essence, communication between the laryngologist and laryngeal radiologist may result in a shorter study or a longer study; above all, it should result in a meaningful study. The patient is the clear beneficiary.[2]

RADIOLOGIC MODALITIES IN LARYNGEAL IMAGING

Soft Tissue Lateral Radiography[3–9]

The soft tissue lateral radiograph is the mandatory preliminary film in the work-up of most laryngeal disease; it provides a baseline diagnostic study. It is inexpensive, easy to obtain, noninvasive, and permits an overview of the larynx that may be directive in initiating further diagnostic studies. The soft tissue lateral radiograph, within limits, can demonstrate findings related to both mucous membrane and the laryngeal cartilaginous framework (Figs. 5–1 and 5–2)

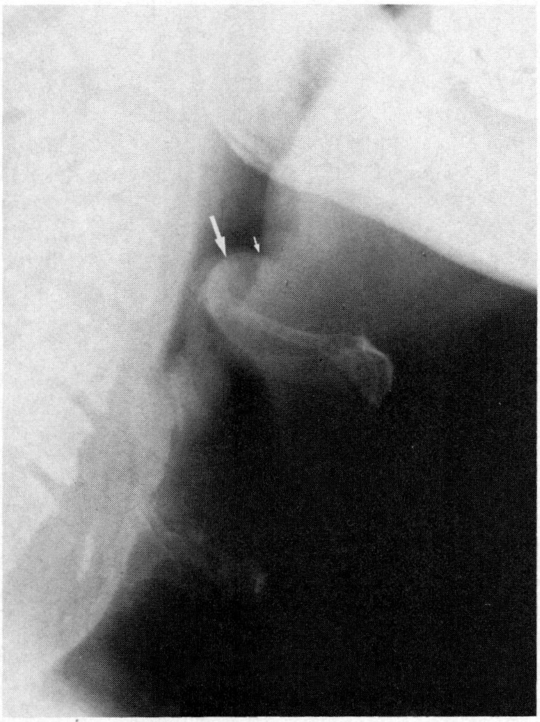

Figure 5–1. Acute epiglottitis. A lateral soft tissue radiograph of the larynx demonstrates the radiologic findings in acute epiglottitis in a 60-year-old male. The mucous membrane of the lingual and laryngeal surfaces of the epiglottis presents a smooth, rounded outline *(large white arrow)*. The valleculae are effaced, and the vallecular outline is elevated toward the base of the tongue *(small white arrow)*. The extent of compromise of the airway at this level is indicated by the air-containing lumen between the epiglottis and the posterior pharyngeal wall.

Acute epiglottitis is a potentially lethal disease, and initial treatment with establishment of an airway should not be withheld pending radiologic investigation. The radiograph indicates the findings in acute epiglottitis. It may be useful in following the course of the disease once treatment has been initiated, especially in the patient who is hard to examine. (From Zizmor J, Noyek AM: An Atlas of Otolaryngologic Radiology. Philadelphia, WB Saunders Company, 1978.)

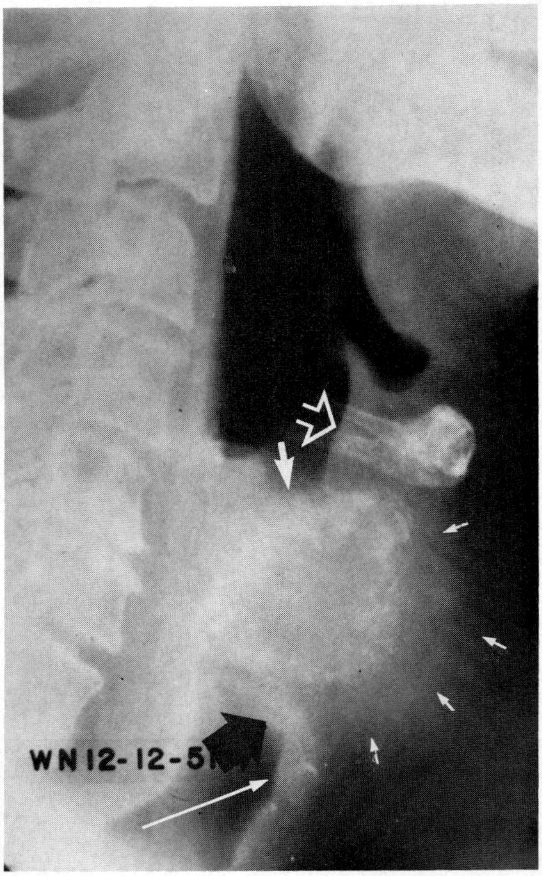

Figure 5–2. T4 carcinoma of the larynx, with cartilage destruction. A soft tissue lateral radiograph of the larynx demonstrates both soft tissue and framework imaging findings on a patient with an extensive transglottic carcinoma. The mucosal vertical dimension of disease appears, at first glance, to extend from the levels shown (*thick white arrow* above to the *very thick black arrow* below). However, critical examination of the x-ray film demonstrates posterior displacement of the smooth uninfiltrated surface of the epiglottis *(hollow white arrow)*. The retrodisplacement of this structure is undoubtedly caused by tumor infiltration superiorly into the preepiglottic space between the air column and the body of the hyoid bone. Further, the actual inferior extension of the tumor is seen anteriorly in the subglottis *(long thin white arrow)*.

Framework information is depicted as the overlapping thyroid cartilage alae are widely destroyed. Both thyroid alae are lytic in their central areas. Cartilage is fragmented anteriorly and obvious soft tissue thickening of tumor is noted within the soft tissue planes of the anterior neck itself *(four tiny marginating white arrows)*. This case demonstrates the significant diagnostic information that can be gleaned from one good quality radiograph. (From Zizmor J, Noyek AM: An Atlas of Otolaryngologic Radiology. Philadelphia, WB Saunders Company, 1978.)

The radiograph's major application lies in demonstrating the interface between mucous membrane and air in the sagittal plane, especially in the supraglottis. It permits a clear lateral profile of the base of the tongue, valleculae, epiglottis, aryepiglottic folds, and arytenoid eminences. The laryngeal surface of the epiglottis may be followed, in varying degree, inferiorly toward the level of its petiolus attachment above the vocal cords.

Though some glottic detail may be visualized (for example, the overlapping superior surfaces of the two vocal cords and the overlapping air shadows of the suprajacent ventricles), less subglottic detail is usually evident. This imaging limitation is largely caused by the density of the overlapping thyroid cartilages, which demonstrate calcification and ossification to varying degree beginning posteroinferiorly in the region of the inferior cornua. Detail is also obscured by the marked density of the cricoid signet below. Coincidentally, the prevertebral soft tissues are well seen on this technique, and the trachea is well profiled to the level of the thoracic inlet.

The soft tissue lateral radiograph is the diagnostic study of choice in evaluating mucosal epiglottic involvement in epiglottitis, tumor, tuberculosis, and so forth. The soft tissue lateral radiograph may also provide some information about the laryngeal framework, such as the possibility of thyroid cartilage destruction; however, the paired thyroid cartilages, which show overlapping images, are often irregularly calcified and ossified, and cartilage destruction can be quite difficult in interpretation. The lateralization of such cartilage destruction is not usually possible unless both alae are extensively destroyed. The apparent image of cartilage destruction should be confirmed or denied by a more sophisticated examination such as computed tomography (CT) or ultrasound (in skilled hands).

The major limitation in mucosal evaluation arises from the intrusion into the image of the overlying irregular calcifications of the overlapping paired thyroid alae. Additionally, this technique shows the anteroposterior (AP) relationship of structures but does not permit lateralization of lesions. Radiologic lateralization can only be achieved by a second planar study such as axial CT or coronal tomography. Further to lateralization of lesions, the AP soft tissue radiograph of the neck loses much of its laryngeal information because of the obscuring shadow of the cervical spine. AP information is therefore best sought by other techniques such as high kV selective filtration radiography, coronal tomography, AP laryngography, or AP xeroradiography. All of these are described later in this chapter.

The thyroid cartilage can be imaged by roentgenographic techniques once it becomes sufficiently calcified or ossified. Calcification may begin as early as eight years of age but is usually not recognized on x-ray until the adult years. Calcification or ossification of this cartilage commences posteroinferiorly, in the region of the inferior cornu of each thyroid ala. The calcification or ossification tends to advance both superiorly and anteriorly, decade by decade, and more actively in males than in females. The anterior plough-shaped attachment of the two thyroid alae provides a figure-eight lateral image of bicortical cartilage calcification by the middle adult years. The waist of this calcification corresponds to the region of vocal cord attachment. There is a notch above the prominence of the fused thyroid alae (the Adam's apple) that should not be confused with cartilage destruction on examination.

The thyroid cartilage not only calcifies but ossifies; this ossification follows the same pattern. Marrow-containing bone may be recognized within the thyroid cartilage by age 30. The cricoid cartilage calcifies and ossifies more uniformly than the thyroid cartilage. The arytenoid cartilages calcify variably but may present very dense radiographic images, especially in the elderly female.

There are several pitfalls in the interpretation of the soft tissue lateral radiograph. Soft tissue outline may fail to contrast sharply with the marginating air, and topographic detail may be so inadequate as to be overlooked. Cartilage destruction may be very difficult to evaluate, except in advanced lesions. Loss of any portion of the figure-eight configuration of the thyroid cartilage calcification anteriorly is usually presumptive evidence of cartilage destruction, most frequently by cancer invasion.

The soft tissue prevertebral shadow should not exceed, in sagittal dimension, the height of the body of the adjacent vertebra at that level of the larynx. Pediatric imaging may be made difficult or impossible because of respiratory or somatic movement. On expiration, the AP dimension of the trachea narrows; the trachea may buckle anteriorly with the larynx appearing to be pushed forward by a prevertebral soft tissue mass.[10] The larynx may rise during swallowing; air may unexpectedly be absent in the hypopharynx or be trapped within the cervical esophagus if the infant should swallow during the examination.

The soft tissue lateral radiograph is taken in

the upright position. Technical details vary from machine to machine, as will all other techniques. One suggested format is as follows: 1.0- to 1.6-mm focal spot, 70 to 75 kV, 5 mAs (milliampere-seconds), and 72-inch focal film distance; filtration is not needed and there is no need for a grid. Modern x-ray machines provide ultrafast exposure time, such as 1/60th of a second; this theoretically eliminates all possibility of motion artifact degrading the x-ray image. Unfortunately, good imaging results are not always obtainable.

For comparison of soft tissue radiography with other imaging modalities see Figures 5–11, 5–12, 5–14, 5–16, 5–19, 5–43, and 5–47 later in this chapter.

High kV Selective Filtration Radiography

This technique[11–13] is now discussed because of its simplicity and its natural screening relationship as the AP examination to complement the soft tissue lateral radiograph. It should be an important adjunct to the soft tissue lateral radiograph, but unfortunately it is little used because of lack of experience on the part of most laryngeal radiologists. Figures 5–3 and 5–4 demonstrate use of this technique.

High kV selective filtration radiography is an

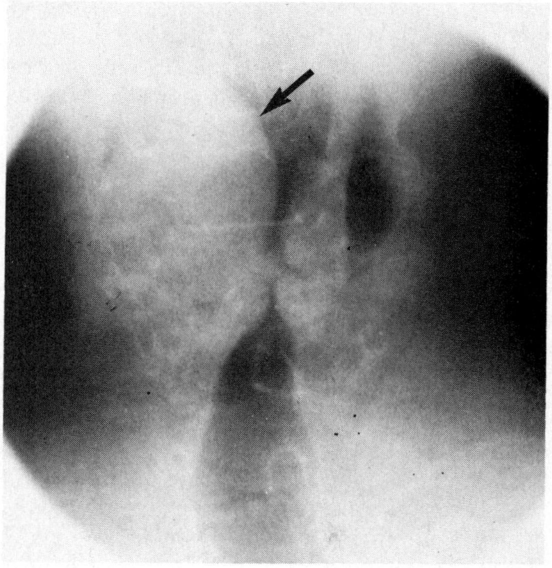

Figure 5–3. Laryngopyocele. An AP high-kilovoltage selective filtration radiograph of the larynx demonstrates a large, oval, cystic expansion, opacified by fluid, occupying the entire right aryepiglottic fold *(arrow)* and encroaching on the airway. The sharp delineation of the periphery of the lesion as well as the clear preservation of normal laryngeal structures at the cord level indicates the lesion to be a fluid-filled laryngocele, either infected or sterile. The right pyriform sinus is effaced by the lesion, as contrasted with the air-filled left pyriform sinus. The detail of this examination matches that of tomography, with less radiation exposure. (From Zizmor J, Noyek AM: An Atlas of Otolaryngologic Radiology. Philadelphia, WB Saunders Company, 1978.)

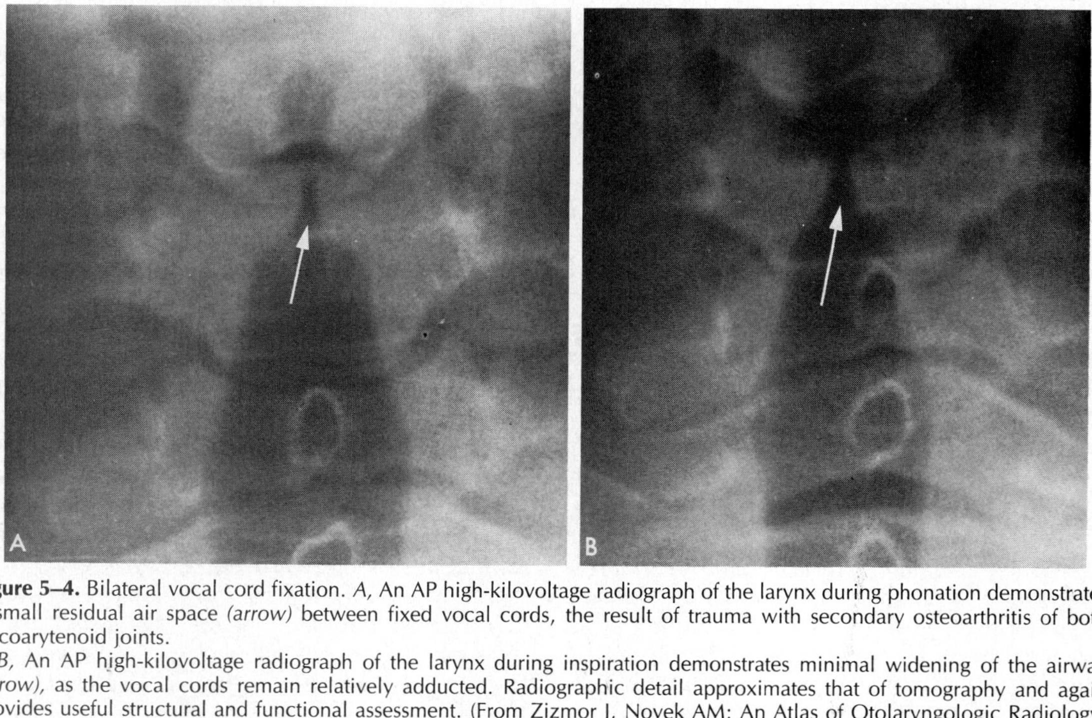

Figure 5–4. Bilateral vocal cord fixation. *A,* An AP high-kilovoltage radiograph of the larynx during phonation demonstrates a small residual air space *(arrow)* between fixed vocal cords, the result of trauma with secondary osteoarthritis of both cricoarytenoid joints.

B, An AP high-kilovoltage radiograph of the larynx during inspiration demonstrates minimal widening of the airway *(arrow),* as the vocal cords remain relatively adducted. Radiographic detail approximates that of tomography and again provides useful structural and functional assessment. (From Zizmor J, Noyek AM: An Atlas of Otolaryngologic Radiology. Philadelphia, WB Saunders Company, 1978.)

excellent screening technique for demonstrating glottic abnormalities without the shadow of the cervical spine, which usually obscures conventional radiographs. This simple screening study was first described by Maguire at McGill University in the mid-1960s. The high kV selective filtration radiograph can be combined with functional maneuvers such as inspiration, phonation, and a modified Valsalva maneuver for better mucosal display and for the detection of mobility defects and fixation. This examination actually approximates coronal tomographic imaging without the length of examination, expense, and radiation exposure that occurs with tomography.

This radiologic modality utilizes copper and aluminum filtration and as short an exposure time as possible; any technique requiring more than 0.1 s of exposure time runs the risk of poor detail due to movement artifact. The technique's usefulness lies in the obliteration of the shadow of the cervical spine while depicting clearly the laryngeal airway.

Technically, we currently favor 0.5-mm copper plus 0.5-mm aluminum filtration with 140 to 145 kV; a Bucky grid improves the detail. The central ray is centered at the thyroid notch at a distance of 100 cm (or 38 inches), utilizing a head unit; a short exposure time is essential (5 mAs). A single AP film during phonation is exposed. An additional inspiratory film may be obtained for the assessment of vocal cord paralysis or fixation, and any further selective physiologic maneuvers may also be recorded.

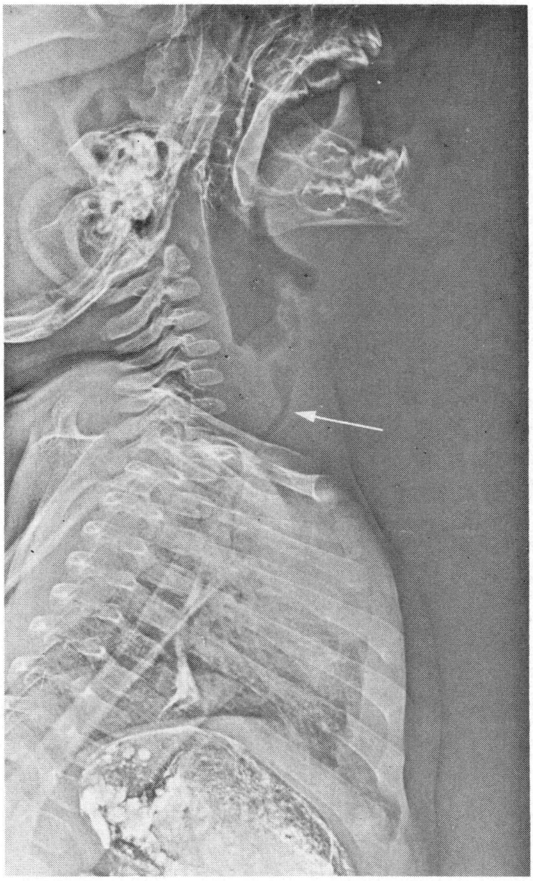

Figure 5–5. Extensive congenital subglottic and tracheal stenosis. A lateral xeroradiograph gives an excellent overview of the airway in this neonate who has an extensive subglottic and tracheal stenosis which extends to the level of the carina. The subglottic larynx narrows into a diminutive trachea *(white arrow)*. There is barium in the stomach, indicating patency of the esophagus as visualized by a previous barium esophagram. (From Noyek AM et al.: Otolaryngol Clin North Am 2(2):445–456, 1978.)

Xeroradiography

The simple technique of xeroradiography[13–20] logically follows the soft tissue lateral radiograph and the AP high kV screening examination. If a lateral radiologic study that yields more information is sought, the xeroradiograph is elected. Figures 5–5 to 5–10 are examples of this technique.

This technique, which uses a conventional x-ray source, suffers the disadvantage of a fourfold radiation dose; however, it owes its superior delineation of soft tissue and cartilage detail to the unique property of edge enhancement inherent in the xeroradiographic recording process. Any structure with a sharply defined edge is seen with particular clarity. Such structures include both the soft tissue elements bordering the air column and the cartilaginous structures supporting the soft tissue.

The lateral xeroradiograph provides excellent definition of laryngeal mucosa, especially in the supraglottic region. The lateral profile details of the valleculae, epiglottis, aryepiglottic folds, arytenoid eminences, and ventricles are all well demonstrated. Mucosal detail is excellent when air-profiled; however, for critical evaluation of mucosal surface contour, especially within the glottis or subglottis, other modalities (such as contrast laryngography and CT) remain superior. This deficiency is especially true in the AP examination, for which xeroradiography is sometimes elected. Occasionally, both for assessment of laryngeal function (vocal cord paralysis or fixation) and laryngeal structure (subglottic angle), AP xeroradiography may be combined with zonography to produce a satisfactory fixed-section

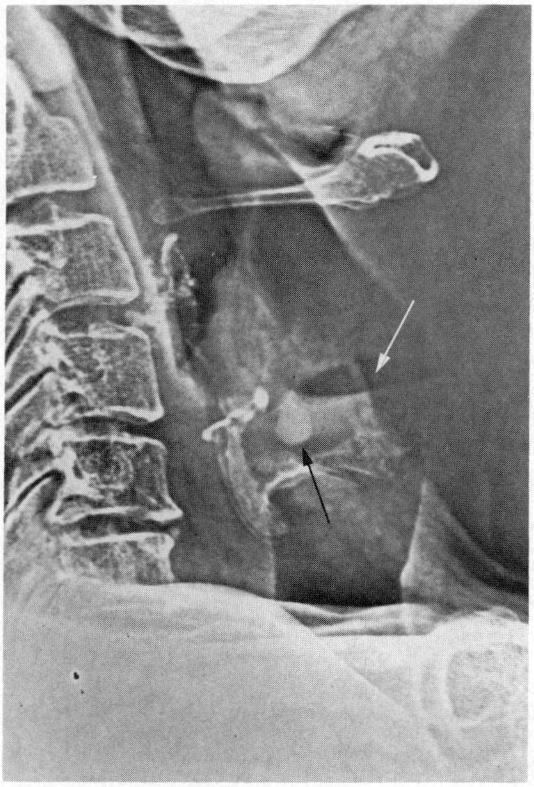

Figure 5–6. Contact granuloma, vocal process, arytenoid cartilage. A lateral xeroradiograph demonstrates the exquisite soft tissue detail by edge enhancement of a discrete polypoid contact granuloma *(black arrow)* as it hangs from its attachment to the vocal process of the arytenoid cartilage. Laterality is not determined. The overlapping air shadows of both ventricles are indicated *(white arrow)*. (From Noyek AM et al.: Otolaryngol Clin North Am 2(2):445–456, 1978.)

Figure 5–7. Leiomyosarcoma, trachea. A lateral xeroradiograph demonstrates a large soft tissue tumor mass, shaped like a kidney bean, virtually occluding the trachea beginning at the subglottic larynx. The point of anterior attachment to the trachea is clearly shown *(white arrow)*. (From Fredrickson J, MacDonald R: Toronto, private communication.)

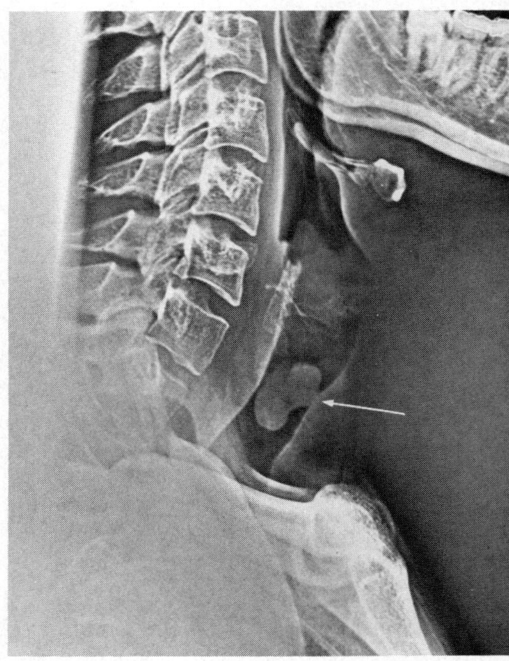

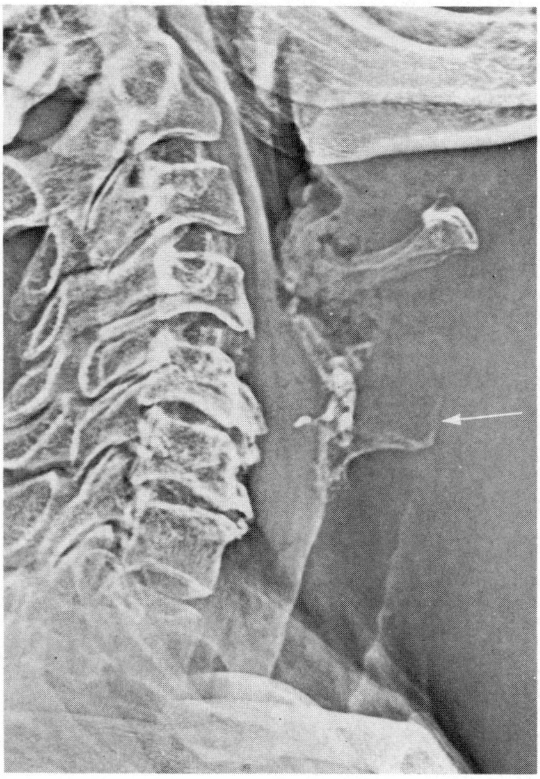

Figure 5–8. T4 carcinoma of supraglottis with cartilage destruction. A lateral xeroradiograph demonstrates a multinodular exophytic tumor bulging into the supraglottic airway and completely replacing the epiglottis. The thyroid cartilage image is completely demineralized and washed out. A small fragment of residual isolated cartilage remains anteriorly *(white arrow)* in the region where a clear figure eight should be visualized. This is unequivocal xeroradiographic evidence of cartilage destruction.

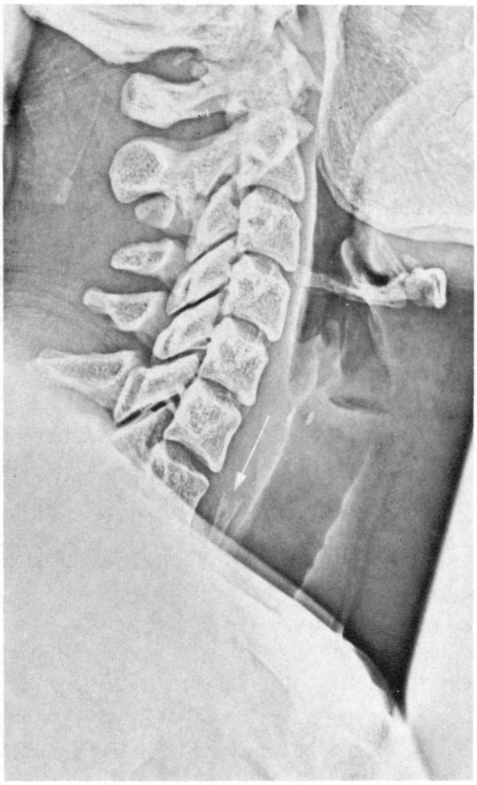

Figure 5–9. Chicken bone in esophagus. A lateral xeroradiograph demonstrates the spicular end of a calcified chicken bone *(white arrow)* as it lies within the upper cervical esophagus. The soft tissue detail of the larynx is well shown. The patient is a young female with minimal calcification within the larynx; however, the possibility of applying xeroradiography to distinguish between a calcified foreign body such as this bone and calcifications within the thyroid cartilage and cricoid cartilage is obvious. (From Noyek AM et al.: Otolaryngol Clin North Am 2(2):445–456, 1978.)

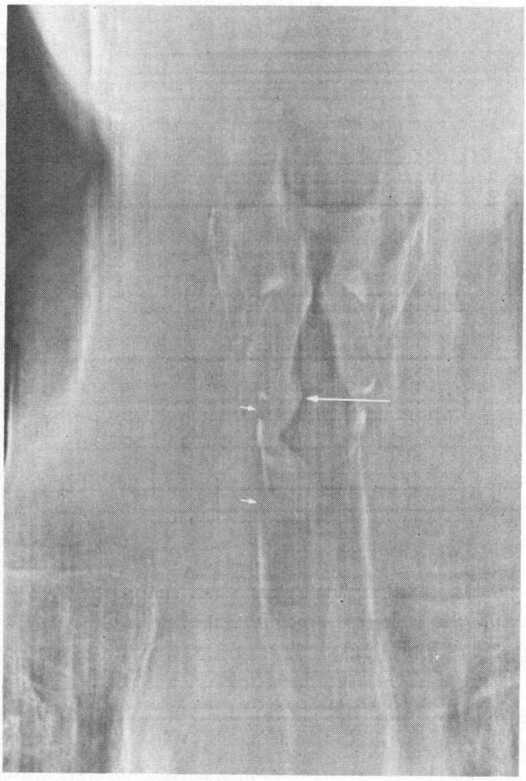

Figure 5–10. Anaplastic carcinoma, thyroid, with invasion of larynx and trachea. An AP xerotomogram (in which the image is reversed from the conventional AP tomogram) demonstrates the presence of a soft tissue mass in the left side of the root of the neck. This density has displaced the larynx and trachea from the midline to the left. This alteration is obvious at the level of the clavicular heads. Two areas of cartilage destruction by tumor are indicated *(tiny white arrows).* There are two large lobules of soft tissue tumor within the airway; the upper element, within the larynx, is indicated *(long white arrow).* One of the occasional uses of xerotomography is the detection of airway and mediastinal extension of known cancer in this region.

examination. This is carried out when AP examination is of paramount importance and especially when malignancy is evaluated as possibly extending into the trachea or even into the mediastinum. This examination is therefore restricted to the adult patient with known cancer.

Though the lateral xeroradiograph gives good delineation of cartilage structure, just as on the soft tissue lateral radiograph, cartilage destruction is still often difficult to interpret, unless it is extensive. It therefore remains the role of other modalities (especially CT and ultrasound) to confirm or deny the xeroradiographic findings suggestive of cartilage destruction.

The indications for xeroradiography are identical with those for the soft tissue lateral radiograph. Aside from the definition of mucous membrane and cartilage, particularly in the pretreatment evaluation of laryngeal cancer, xeroradiography has several special areas of application. It is useful in foreign body examination, for even the most faintly calcified foreign body can be differentiated from the normal calcification within the supporting laryngeal cartilaginous framework.

Traumatic lesions can be imaged by xeroradiography, but only by their secondary signs (for example, fracture or disruption of mucous membrane is inferred by the presence of air in the soft tissues of the neck) rather than by the demonstration of a specific fracture line. Mass lesions, especially with prolapse into the subglottic region, are very well demonstrated by this method. Postintubation granuloma is an example of such, and xeroradiography is especially useful where the inferior extent of some of the larger lesions cannot be determined by mirror or telescopic examination. Stenosis, stricture, and other lesions of the subglottic larynx and upper trachea may occasion xeroradiographic examination. Mucosal displacement by extrinsic lesions (granuloma, papilloma) or extrinsic elevations or compressions (tumor, vascular ring) are also well seen.

Special mention should be made of the role of xeroradiography in the study of the pediatric patient[20] with laryngeal and associated tracheal disease. Xeroradiography has value in providing a correlative overview of congenital or acquired laryngeal and tracheal stenosis, and is especially useful in the follow-up examination of these pediatric patients. Here it may obviate the need for repeated endoscopic procedures under general anesthesia or the use of tomography with its higher radiation dose over the entire tomographic series.

Though xeroradiography has some excellent applications and some obvious deficiencies, it is now not widely available because of the high cost of leasing arrangements that have allowed its use since 1971.

Coronal (AP) Tomography

The most accessible radiographic examination for general and detailed display of laryngeal anatomy remains coronal tomography.[21–25] Coronal (AP) tomography permits radiographic visualization of the entire larynx, free from the superimposition of the image of the cervical spine. It provides an overview of the larynx in the vertical dimension, seen best in natural relationship at mid-cord level. Coronal tomography is a primary imaging modality for assessing the structure of the epiglottis, the aryepiglottic folds, the false and true vocal cords with intervening ventricles, and the subglottic angles. Delineation of the laryngeal ventricles and pyriform sinuses may be inconsistent, but with effective radiologic monitoring of the procedure and patient cooperation, these areas can usually be satisfactorily assessed. Structures that cross the tomographic plane obliquely (such as the aryepiglottic folds) or that may be of unusual configuration (for example, the pyriform sinuses are cone-shaped) may or may not be well seen, depending upon the level of tomographic section and the presence or absence of distension. Equally, the epiglottis may lie in a plane well posterior to the section that best defines the glottis; thus a critical eye is required for meaningful radiologic interpretation. Figures 5–11 to 5–22 show the uses and limitations of this technique.

It is important to recognize that the major value of the technique lies in the demonstration of structures that are depicted at right angles to the tomographic (coronal) plane. Thus the glottis and the subglottic space are most favorably imaged; the subglottic angle, which usually lies between 90 and 120 degrees, is very well demonstrated by this technique. This is of critical importance in cancer evaluation.

Coronal tomography, however, is insensitive to small lesions and does not differentiate between edema and tumor. A lesion must be 3 to 4 mm in size for radiologic visualization on tomography, assuming a 0.5 cm survey examination technique as described below.

Functional assessment is favorably combined with structural assessment in this examination. The patient can perform a series of physiologic maneuvers (phonation, reverse phonation, Valsalva, modified Valsalva, inspiration), all of which give specific dynamic evaluation in terms of cord mobility and the presence or absence of laryngeal paralysis or fixation.

Though mucosal definition by AP tomography is inferior to that of laryngography in general and AP laryngography in particular, the technique is particularly acceptable because of

Text continued on page 69

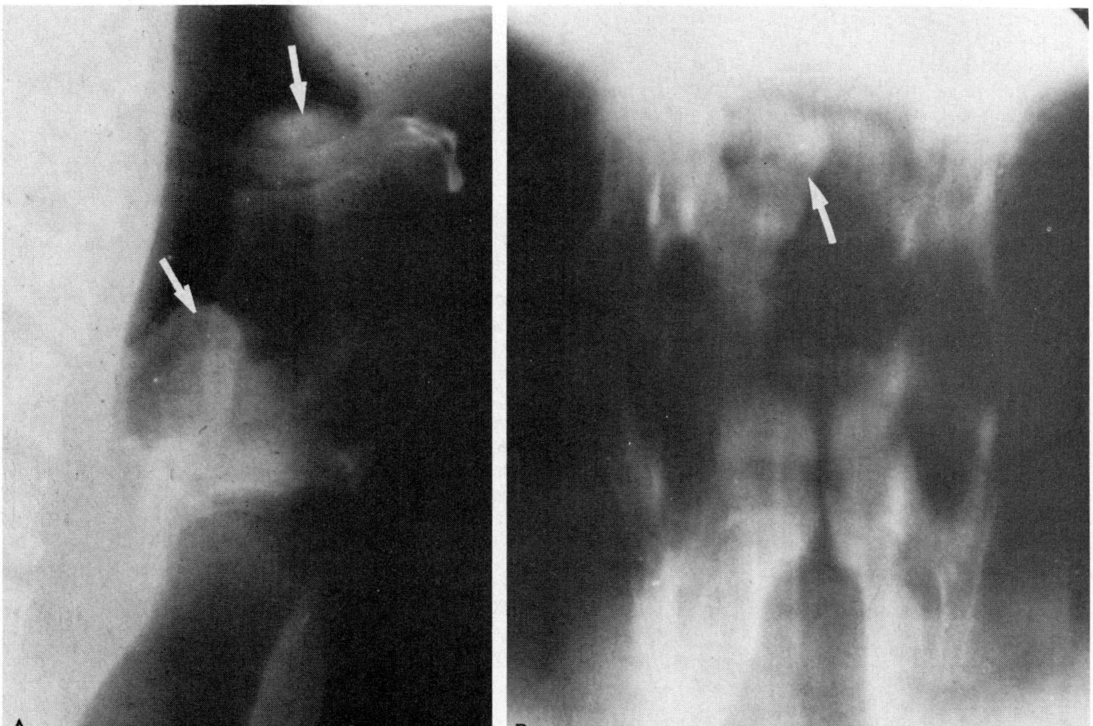

Figure 5–11. Laryngeal tuberculosis. The patient was a 40-year-old male with active cavitary pulmonary tuberculosis and positive sputum on bacteriologic examination.

A, A lateral radiograph demonstrates the findings in classic tuberculosis with involvement of supraglottic structures, especially the epiglottis. *Upper arrow,* thickened nodular epiglottis; *lower arrow,* enlargement of the arytenoid eminences.

B, An AP tomogram demonstrates the nodular thickening of the epiglottis *(arrow),* producing the turban deformity seen clinically. The ventricular outline is effaced bilaterally, in large measure. (From Zizmor J, Noyek AM: Semin Roentgenol 9(4):311–322, 1974.)

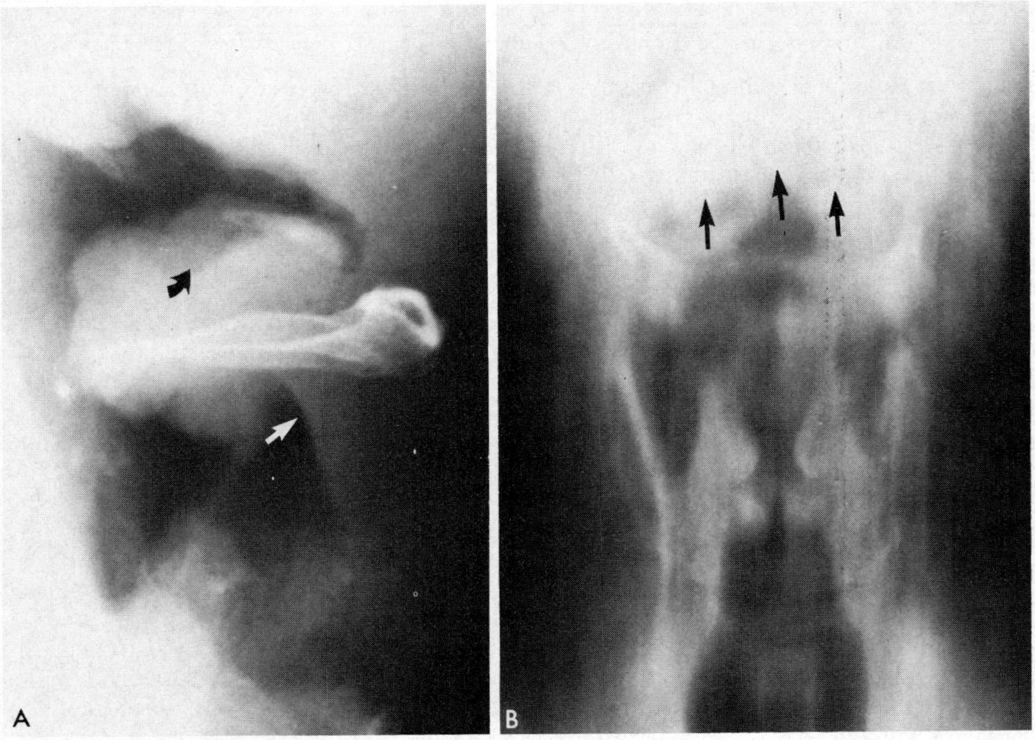

Figure 5–12. Carcinoma, epiglottis. The patient is a 75-year-old male.

A, A lateral radiograph demonstrates a bulky carcinoma involving the lingual and laryngeal surfaces of the epiglottis as well as its free margin. It overhangs the vestibule, obstructing the laryngeal airway in large measure. *Curved black arrow,* an area of ulceration involving the superior surface of the tumor. The tumor's relationship to the depth of the vallecula, as it involves the base of tongue, is well demonstrated. Note the infrahyoid laryngeal surface of the epiglottis; it is free of tumor *(white arrow).*

B, A coronal tomogram demonstrates the bulk of the squamous cell carcinoma to involve the suprahyoid epiglottis *(arrows).* However, this AP tomographic cut is designed to show vocal cord morphology in optimal relationship; the bulk of the epiglottic tumor itself is posterior to this plane, as can be best appreciated from the lateral soft tissue radiograph. This demonstrates one of the limitations of the AP tomogram. (From Zizmor J, Noyek AM: An Atlas of Otolaryngologic Radiology. Philadelphia, WB Saunders Company, 1978.)

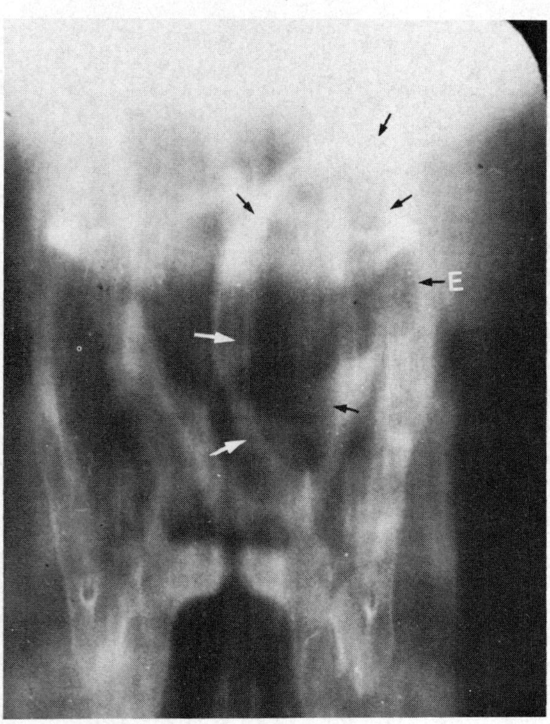

Figure 5–13. Internal laryngocele. A coronal tomogram demonstrates a large air sac *(arrows)* displacing the left aryepiglottic fold medially and encroaching on the supraglottic airway. A small external component to the laryngocele is noted in the region of the thyrohyoid membrane (E). The smooth, uniform displacement of mucous membrane in this region demonstrates the classic radiographic appearance of an internal laryngocele. In this instance, it is air filled. If the neck of the sac becomes obstructed, the laryngocele may become a fluid-filled cyst, in which case a similar radiographic appearance is seen without air content. If the fluid content becomes infected, it is termed a pyocele but retains the same radiographic appearance as a fluid-filled laryngocele. The patient is a 26-year-old male saxophone player. (From Zizmor J, Noyek AM: Semin Roentgenol 9(4):311–322, 1974.)

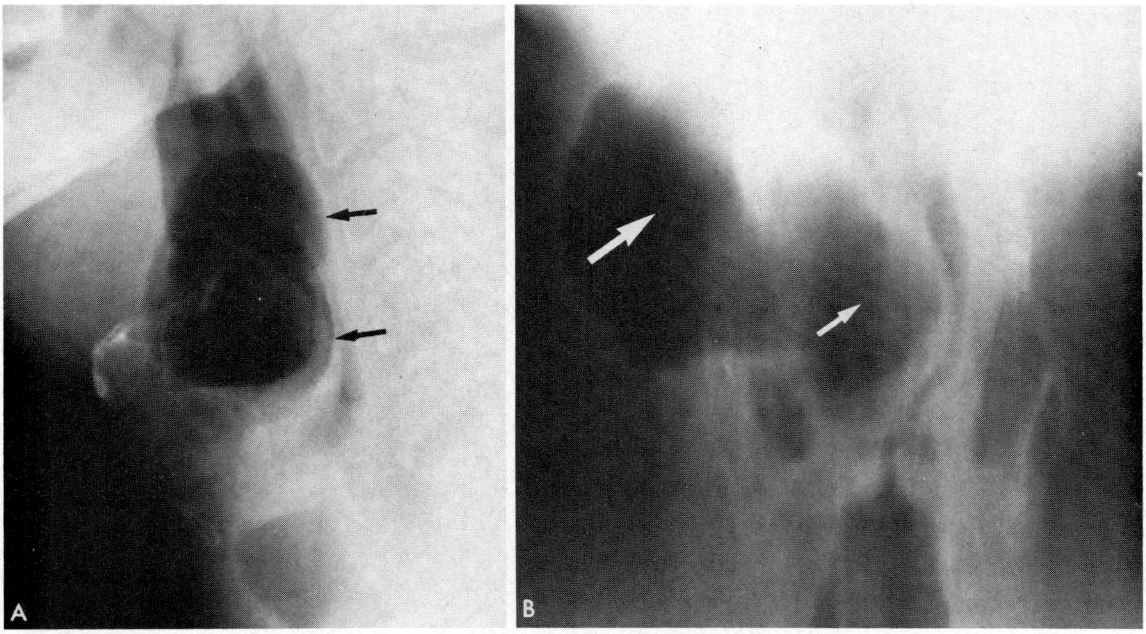

Figure 5–14. Mixed internal-external laryngocele. The patient is an 85-year-old female.

A, A soft tissue lateral radiograph demonstrates the classic "double bubble" sign of superimposed spheroid air shadows *(black arrows)* of the overlapping internal and external air-containing components of this mixed laryngocele.

B, An AP tomogram fully clarifies the diagnosis and the "double bubble" sign. *Small white arrow,* the internal component of the laryngocele, which bulges medially overlying the normal glottis and obscuring it from clinical evaluation. *Large white arrow,* extensive air-containing external component of laryngocele. The components communicate through a large channel through the thyrohyoid membrane.

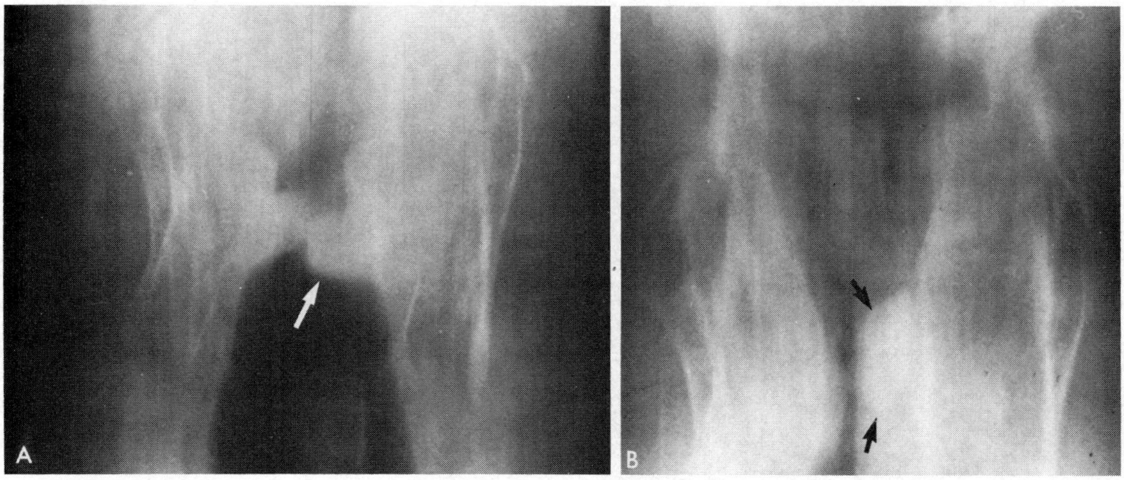

Figure 5–15. Laryngeal granuloma due to gastroesophageal reflux in a patient with recurrent hiatal hernia following two previous surgical repairs along with longstanding respiratory and laryngeal irritation symptoms.

A, A coronal tomogram of the larynx in phonation demonstrates a smoothly outlined granuloma arising from the free margin and subglottic surface of the left vocal cord *(arrow).* It is attached to the posterior two-thirds of the left vocal cord.

B, A coronal tomogram of the larynx during quiet breathing profiles the granuloma *(arrows)* as both vocal cords abduct. (From Goldberg M et al.: J Otolaryngol 7(3):196–202, 1978.)

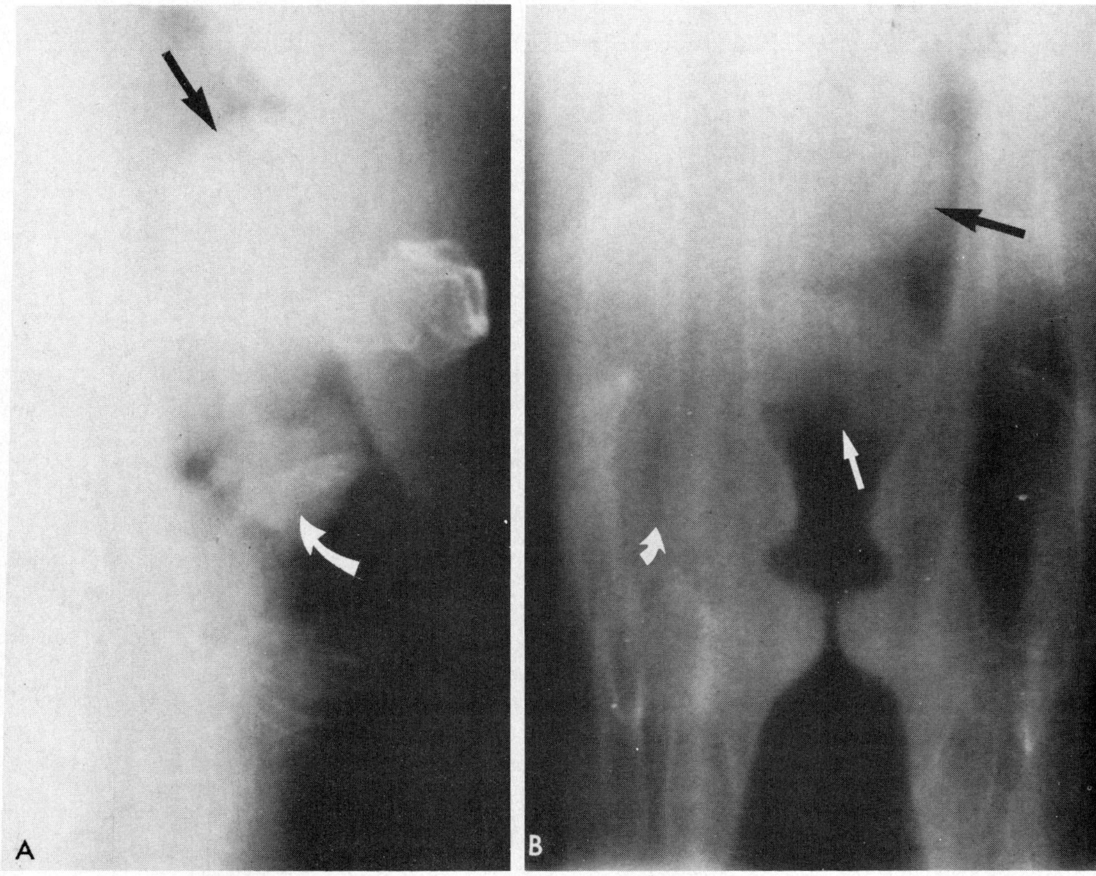

Figure 5–16. Carcinoma, epiglottis, with airway obstruction. The patient is a 52-year-old male.

A, Lateral radiograph of the larynx demonstrates a large, lobulated mass completely transforming the normal configuration of the epiglottis *(black arrow)*. The vallecula is obliterated, and a deep projection of the mass into the laryngeal vestibule *(curved white arrow)* almost completely obstructs the airway.

B, A coronal tomogram demonstrates the bulk of the lobulated squamous cell carcinoma of the epiglottis, which arises from the right side of the larynx and projects across the midline at the hyoid level *(black arrow)*. Another large lobulation is seen immediately above the level of the ventricular bands *(straight white arrow)*, virtually obstructing the airway. The right pyriform sinus is also obliterated *(curved white arrow)*. (From Zizmor J, Noyek AM: An Atlas of Otolaryngologic Radiology. Philadelphia, WB Saunders Company, 1978.)

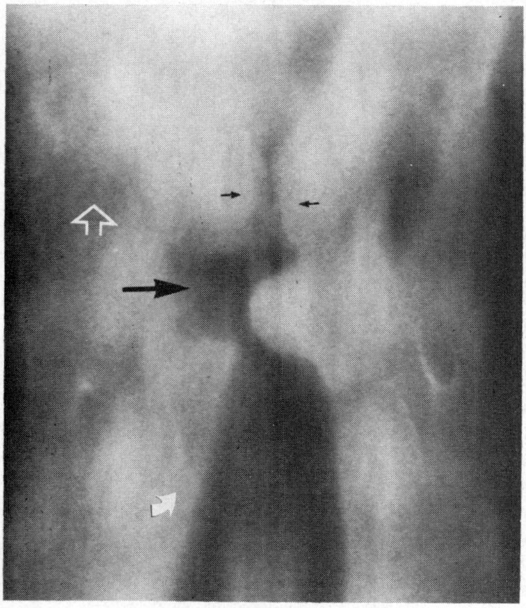

Figure 5–17. Ulcerative carcinoma, ventricle, with pyriform sinus extension. A coronal tomogram demonstrates a large, ulcerative, squamous cell carcinoma of the right ventricle. The carcinoma has extended deeply *(large black arrow)*. It has amputated the entire bulk of the right vocal cord, as contrasted with the left. Infraglottic extension is indicated *(curved white arrow)*. Both ventricular bands are somewhat thickened *(small black arrows)*. The carcinoma has extended into the right pyriform sinus *(hollow white arrow)*, which is obliterated by tumor and does not contain air. (From Zizmor J, Noyek AM: An Atlas of Otolaryngologic Radiology. Philadelphia, WB Saunders, 1978.)

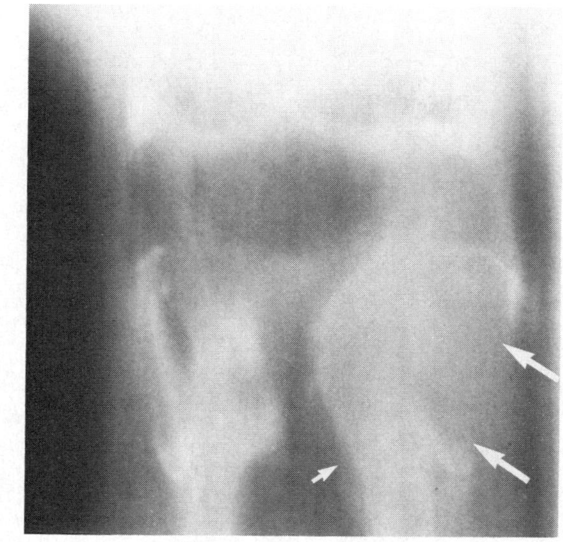

Figure 5–18. Transglottic carcinoma, larynx, with thyroid cartilage destruction. A coronal tomogram demonstrates an extensive squamous cell carcinoma, which involves the supraglottic, glottic, and subglottic regions of the larynx on the left side. The subglottic angle is effaced by tumor extension *(small arrow)*. Excellent cartilage definition is seen, and comparison of the involved left thyroid ala with the right clearly shows cartilage destruction (between the *two large arrows*). (From Noyek AM et al.: J Otolaryngol 6(5):368–373, 1977.)

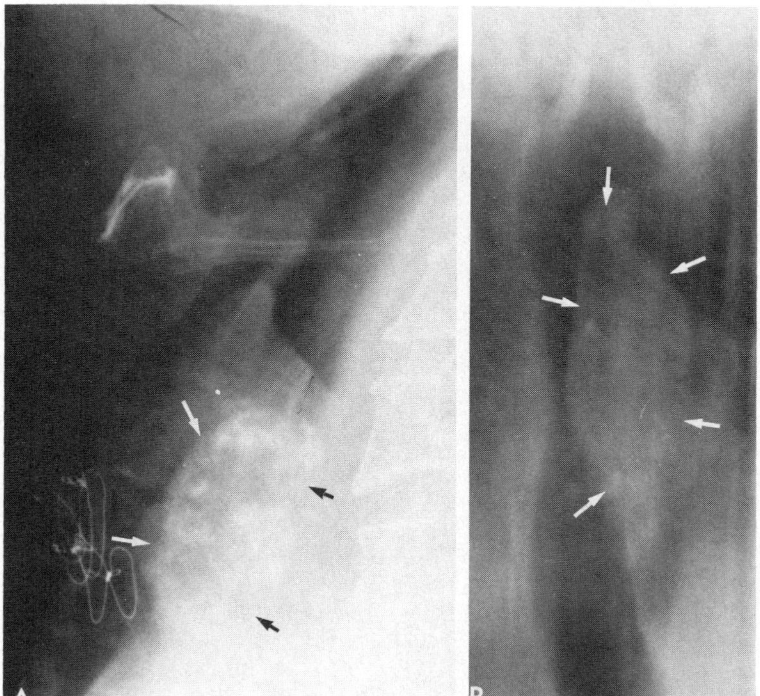

Figure 5–19. Chondrosarcoma, larynx.

A, A lateral radiograph demonstrates a low-grade chondrosarcoma arising from the internal surface of the posterior lamina of the cricoid cartilage *(arrows)*. It extends upward to the level of the arytenoid eminences, encroaching on the laryngeal airway, diminishing it by less than 50 per cent in anteroposterior diameter. Multiple foci of coarse calcification are present, a diagnostic feature.

B, A coronal tomogram demonstrates both the subglottic and the supraglottic extent of the lesion as well as coarse calcification in some areas. (From Zizmor J et al.: Arch Otolaryngol 101:232–234, 1975, and Briant TDR, private communication.)

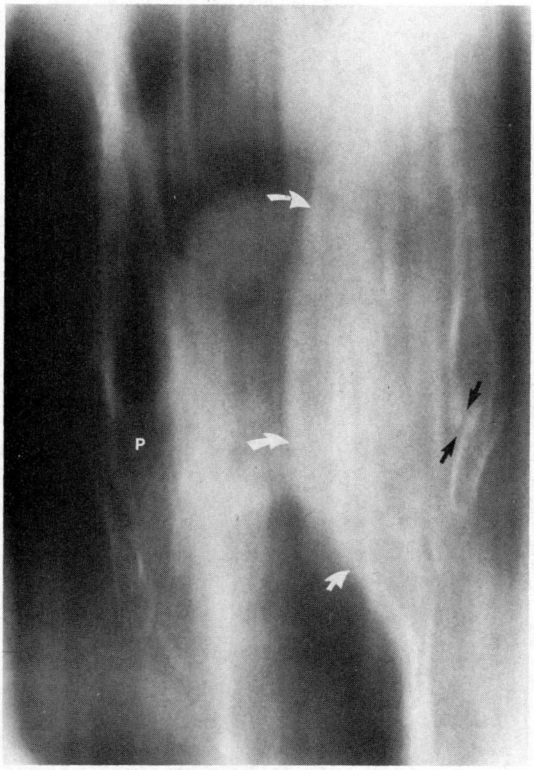

Figure 5–20. Laryngeal fracture, thyroid cartilage. A coronal tomogram demonstrates an overriding fracture line involving the inferior third of the left thyroid cartilage ala. *Black arrows,* the overriding of the internal calcified cortices on either side of the fracture line. The most common laryngeal fracture involves one of the thyroid alae, usually in a vertical direction. Fracture lines are uncommonly demonstrated unless, as in this instance, sufficient calcification or ossification has occurred to allow for radiographic visualization.

A massive hematoma involves the entire left lateral laryngeal wall from supraglottic to subglottic larynx *(white arrows).* The hematoma extends into the upper trachea, and the entire left lateral pharyngeal wall is effaced by hemorrhage as well. Note the obliteration of the left pyriform sinus (compare with right pyriform sinus, P). Radiographic examination of the larynx is of paramount importance not only for the study of possible fracture lines and displacement of cartilage but also for the assessment of airway adequacy. The cervical spine should also be carefully studied for coincident injury. Other signs of laryngeal fracture may include airway distortion and recognizable cartilage dislocation, usually in the arytenoid region.

The extensive vertical dimension of laryngeal hematoma can be best appreciated by this AP tomogram; however, the imaging methodology of choice for laryngeal trauma is CT, with the additional recognition of its capability in imaging the cervical spine in the at-risk patient, who remains safely in the supine position on the CT table. (From Zizmor J, Noyek AM: An Atlas of Otolaryngologic Radiology. Philadelphia, WB Saunders Company, 1978.)

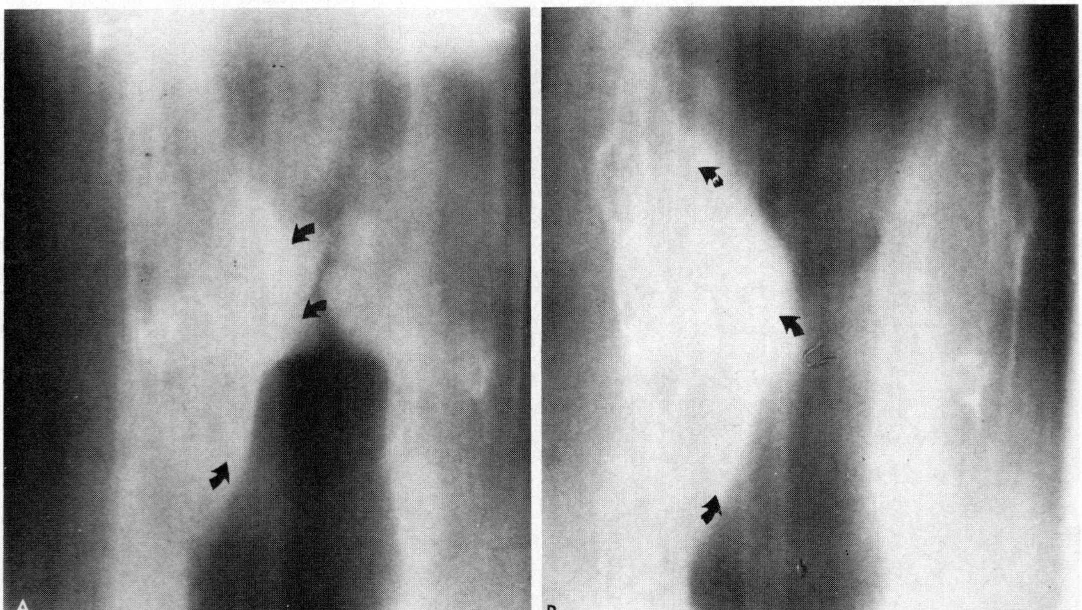

Figure 5–21. Carcinoma, ventricular band, with vocal cord fixation and subglottic extension.

A, A coronal tomogram, taken on phonation, demonstrates coalescent thickening of the right ventricular band and vocal cord along with loss of the right subglottic angle *(arrows).*

B, A coronal tomogram, taken on inspiration, demonstrates the relatively unchanged appearance of the confluent squamous cell carcinoma involving the right transglottic structures. The uninvolved left side of the larynx abducts during inspiration. This is a useful radiographic modality for the demonstration of vocal cord fixation. Right pyriform sinus extension is also demonstrated. (From Zizmor J, Noyek AM: An Atlas of Otolaryngologic Radiology. Philadelphia, WB Saunders Company, 1978.)

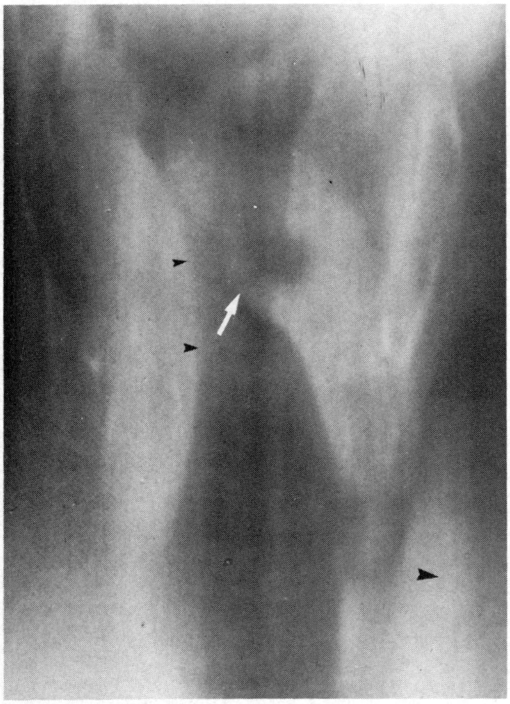

Figure 5–22. Left vocal cord paralysis caused by anaplastic carcinoma, left lobe of thyroid. An AP tomogram of the larynx during inspiration reveals an immobile left vocal cord *(white arrow)* remaining in median position. The left ventricle is well outlined above the immobile vocal cord. The normally mobile structures of the right hemilarynx are seen in abduction *(small black arrowheads)*. Increased tissue density involving the upper pole of the left lobe of the thyroid gland *(lowest black arrowhead)* indicates the site of an anaplastic carcinoma that has involved the left recurrent laryngeal nerve. (From Zizmor J, Noyek AM: An Atlas of Otolaryngologic Radiology. Philadelphia, WB Saunders Company, 1978.)

its noninvasiveness. The study is of maximal value in the patient who is fully able to cooperate in the functional display maneuvers previously mentioned. Thus tomography may clearly demonstrate vocal cord paralysis, loss of distensibility of the larynx, or tumor fixation. AP tomography is also useful in the demonstration of extralaryngeal tumor extension when carcinoma involves the marginal area (aryepiglottic fold or the pyriform sinus); here it demonstrates soft tissue extension by air profile. AP tomography is not the procedure of choice, however, for imaging extraregional extension; CT is mandatory to detect the posterior infiltrations of cancer into the postcricoid region or pyriform sinuses from glottic or marginal sources.

Small lesions of the true or false cord may be difficult to demonstrate, but these lesions are best assessed by clinical means. Radiologic studies are usually indicated only if ventricular extension is in question. Under optimal conditions, the ventricle is well outlined by modified Valsalva and reverse phonation maneuvers.

If the paired thyroid cartilages are sufficiently calcified or ossified, tumor destruction or fracture involving the internal and external cortices of either thyroid cartilage lamina may be shown.

The AP tomogram was formerly the standard pretreatment radiologic study contributing to the staging of laryngeal cancer (TNM classification) at the T level; it still provides the best correlative depiction of the vertical extension of laryngeal carcinoma[25] combined with functional display in a noninvasive procedure. Magnification factors have little importance in distorting the reliability of the study. Its major deficiency lies in the fact that the examination is often carried out in the AP plane best suited to demonstrate ventricular band, ventricle, and vocal cord morphology—that is, usually at midcord level—rather than toward the anterior commissure, where tumor pathology is more frequently maximal. Tomographic examination of the region of the anterior commissure, where the vocal cords approximate at their anterior tendinous insertions, is in fact poorly defined by this technique. Also, posterior extension of disease is poorly demonstrated. Both anterior and posterior commissures are best depicted in lateral oblique view by contrast laryngography or, more favorably yet, in axial display by the increasingly sophisticated use of CT.

The laryngologist who knows and understands the physical principles of tomography will have a better appreciation of its application and limitations. Tomographic equipment varies from institute to institute; our routine linear study is performed on the Polytome. The patient is positioned supine on the radiographic table with the neck hyperextended so the central x-ray beam enters the larynx parallel to the surface of the vocal cords. Correct positioning is critical. The central ray is centered on the thyroid notch and a four-cut screening examination, with cuts 0.5 cm apart, is initiated at 1.0 cm below skin level, the examination proceeding posteriorly. The patient is asked to phonate a continuous "EEE" during each x-ray exposure.

As a result of this survey, the appropriate level for further examination is chosen, and a single film is exposed during quiet inspiration, Valsalva maneuver, modified Valsalva maneuver, and arrested breathing after full inspiration. An additional exposure may be made during an inspiratory "EEE," which opens up the ventricles and allows for excellent display of their morphology and distensibility; a reverse Valsalva maneuver film may also be incorporated into the technique for improved assessment of the laryngeal ventricles and pyriform sinuses.

Utilizing the linear mode on the Polytome and a 20 (or 30) degree tube movement, the radiographic exposure factors suggested are as follows: 90 to 95 kV and 20 mAs; a grid is used but no filtration is required. We have attempted lateral tomography and find it of little value; thus, we do not include it on the routine examination.

For comparison of coronal (AP) tomography with other imaging modalities, see Figures 5–36, 5–37, 5–44 and 5–45 later in this chapter.

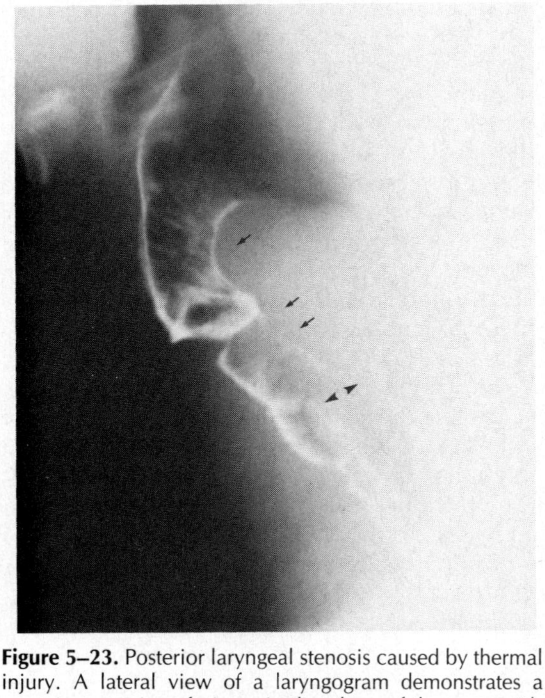

Figure 5–23. Posterior laryngeal stenosis caused by thermal injury. A lateral view of a laryngogram demonstrates a great increase in soft tissue in the plane of the arytenoids *(upper black arrow)* extending inferiorly into the subglottic larynx *(lower parallel black arrows).* Here, the posterior segment of the airway is narrowed by hypertrophic soft tissue response to a thermal injury of the larynx in a 23-year-old male who had been trapped in a house fire. *Paired black arrowheads,* upper limits of a Montgomery T-tube that had been positioned following tracheal resection for a segmental stenosis, the result of the same injury. It is anticipated that inhalation thermal injury would affect the larynx in the region of the posterior commissure, as happened in this instance. (From Zizmor J, Noyek AM: An Atlas of Otolaryngologic Radiology. Philadelphia, WB Saunders Company, 1978, and Cooper J, Toronto, private communication.)

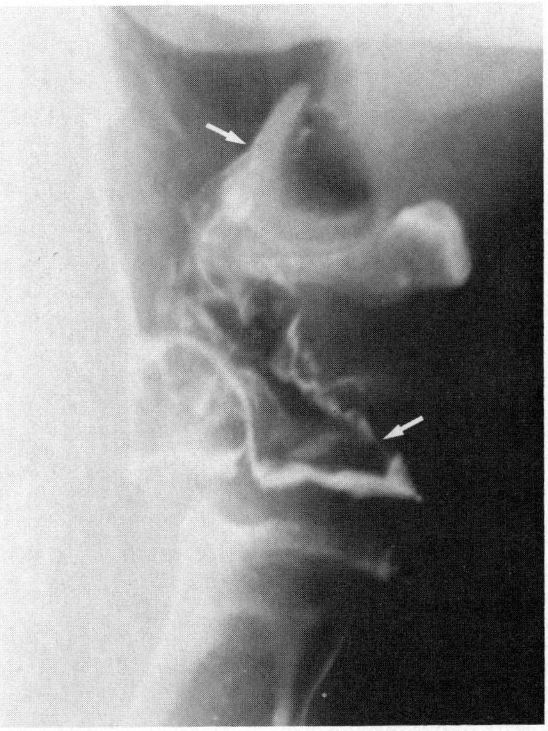

Figure 5–24. Carcinoma, laryngeal surface of epiglottis. A lateral view of a laryngogram demonstrates the irregular mucosal surface of an exophytic and ulcerative squamous cell carcinoma confined to the laryngeal surface of the epiglottis. Mucosal irregularity can be observed from immediately below the free margin of the top of the epiglottis *(upper white arrow)* to the lowest portion of the laryngeal surface of the epiglottis, immediately above its attachment above the anterior commissure *(lower white arrow).* (From Noyek AM et al.: J Otolaryngol 6(5):368–373, 1977.)

Laryngography

Historically, contrast laryngography[26–31] provided the most accurate means of assessment of laryngeal anatomy at the mucosal level. It also provided the most accurate assessment of laryngeal dynamics, especially if combined with cineradiography. Though its role has been largely superceded by the advent of CT, which competes not only at the mucosal level but has the added element of framework depiction, it has not been rendered entirely obsolete. Laryngography is now infrequently required, but it can still be of major value in critical mucosal imaging situations. Figures 5–23 to 5–26 show its capabilities.

Laryngography should not be undertaken or performed casually. This examination requires considerable skill—from the proper application of local anesthesia to the interpretation of films exposed in multiple projections. It remains the technique of choice for visualizing mucosal surface contours, especially in the definition of mucosal extension of cancer. Additionally, laryngography may contribute to the evaluation of the extent of malignancy by demonstrating functional as well as anatomic alterations caused by subtle changes such as tumor infiltration. It provides the best overview of the laryngotracheal airway when stenosis becomes a consideration following major trauma.

Its use is limited to the upright position in cooperative patients and is contraindicated in patients with stridor or respiratory insufficiency. Contrast laryngography is an invasive procedure. Careful consideration must be given to the use of premedication, topical anesthesia, and the contrast agent itself.

The patient is kept nil per os for six hours prior to the examination. The patient is premedicated with 60 mg of codeine and 0.4 mg of atropine 20 min prior to the examination; this dual premedication obtunds the cough reflex and dries out salivary secretion, which might interfere with contrast apposition against mucous membrane. Patients with glaucoma, asthma, and other contraindicating conditions should not receive atropine. History of possible sensitivity to the synthetic alkaloid anesthetic "-caine" derivatives, the iodinated contrast agent, or peanut oil should be elicited by questioning. Contrast laryngography is absolutely contraindicated if the laryngeal airway is compromised (stridor, bulky obstructive masses, and so forth). Contrast medium may be aspirated, and thus laryngography should be selected carefully if patients have significant pulmonary disease.

The pharynx is anesthetized with a lidocaine (Xylocaine) spray. The oropharynx and hypopharynx are swabbed topically with 1 per cent lidocaine. A soft rubber catheter coated with lidocaine jelly is introduced into the nose and positioned above the valleculae at the base of the tongue; its position is monitored briefly at fluoroscopy and 2 or 3 ml of 2 per cent lidocaine are dripped onto the vocal cords during inspiration.

Contrast laryngography practices vary. Some laryngeal radiologists utilize propyliodone (oily Dionosil) from which half of the supernatant oil has been removed and discarded. The residual oil and contrast medium is then warmed and thoroughly agitated prior to use. It is dripped into the larynx until adequate coating of all intrinsic and extrinsic structures is obtained. Other laryngeal radiologists prefer iopydol-iopydone (Hytrast), which is an aqueous preparation.

Frontal and lateral spot films are obtained in

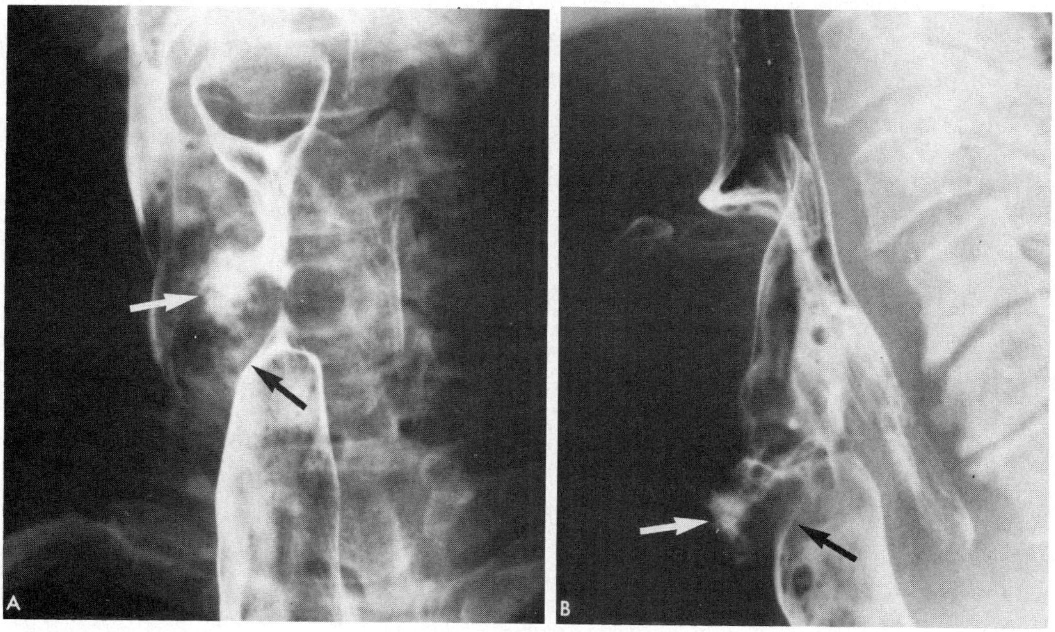

Figure 5–25. Carcinoma, laryngeal ventricle, with anterior commissure extension.

A, An anteroposterior view of a laryngogram demonstrates ulceration of a carcinoma of the right ventricle *(white arrow)*. The lesion has infiltrated inferiorly to efface the right subglottic angle, evidence of subglottic extension *(black arrow)*.

B, A lateral view of the laryngogram demonstrates quite clearly the anterior commissure extension of the ulcerative carcinoma involving the vocal cords and right ventricle *(white arrow)*. Subglottic extension is again evident in the anterior half of the subglottic larynx *(black arrow)*. (From Noyek AM et al.: J Otolaryngol 6(5):368–373, 1977.)

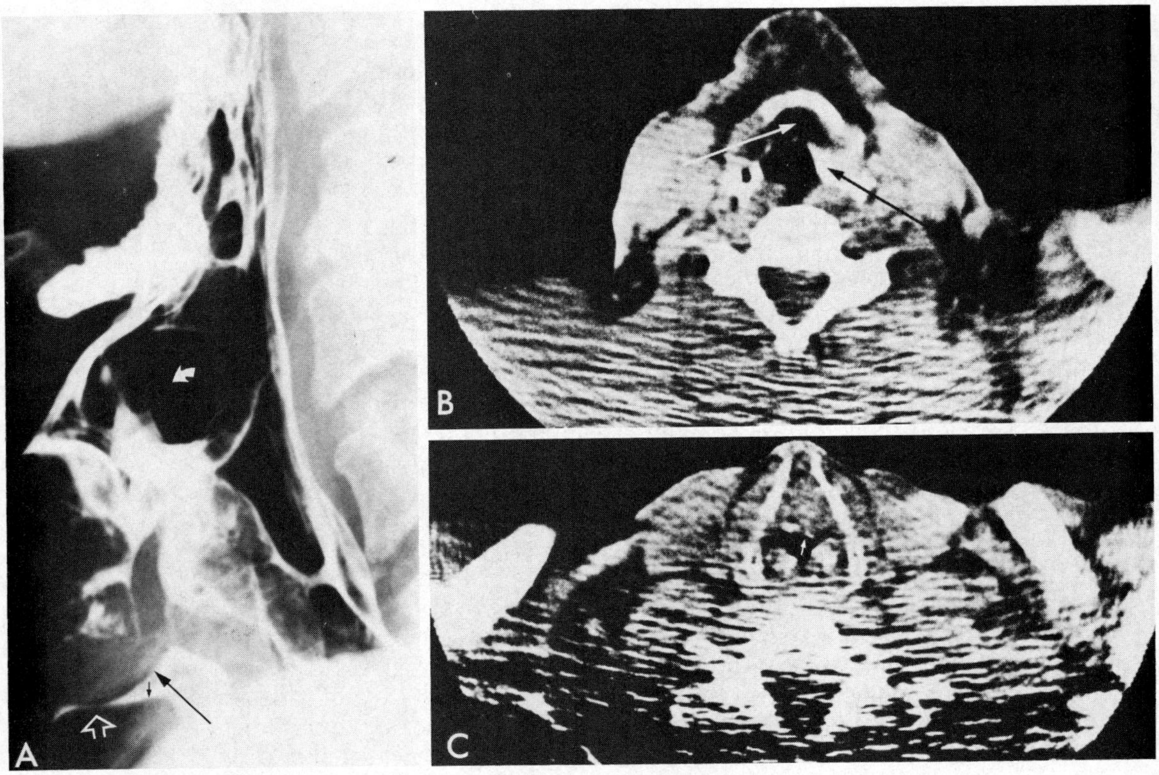

Figure 5–26. Lobulated supraglottic carcinoma, demonstrating critical application of laryngography.

A, A lateral view of a contrast laryngogram demonstrates a multilobular supraglottic tumor mass. *Curved white arrow,* a large segment of tumor at the level of the aryepiglottic fold, on the left. A large segment of tumor mass prolapses in globular fashion towards the vocal cords. The undersurface of this supraglottic tumor mass is indicated *(long black arrow).* The superior surface of the vocal cords is indicated posteriorly *(tiny black arrow).* The supraglottic mass is nearly in contact with the vocal cords *(hollow white arrow).* However, there is an obvious separation, critically demonstrated by the laryngogram, as the tumor arises from the supraglottis and maintains this regional relationship.

B, A higher supraglottic CT cut demonstrates the left aryepiglottic fold tumor mass *(black arrow)* and the uninvolved preepiglottic space, in the midline *(white arrow)* at the level of the hyoid bone.

C, An axial CT cut at the level of the arytenoid cartilages shows the presence of a soft tissue mass anteriorly within the larynx; it occupies the anterior three-quarters of the lumen. *Tiny white arrow* overlies the residual airway and indicates the posterior aspect of the mass. However, the axial morphologic display does not demonstrate the direction of tumor growth and its vertical relationship.

phonation, inspiration, Valsalva maneuver, modified Valsalva maneuver, and inspiratory phonation. Oblique films are also taken during the modified Valsalva maneuver to demonstrate the pyriform sinuses and aryepiglottic folds to best advantage. Cord movement is best demonstrated during quiet inspiration and phonation. The Valsalva maneuver provides improved demonstration of the subglottic angle. The modified Valsalva maneuver allows good distension of the hypopharynx and pyriform sinuses as well as of the ventricles; inspiratory phonation also improves visualization of these structures as well as the surface detail of the true and false vocal cords. These functional maneuvers of the larynx, particularly those of the vocal cords, can also be recorded by cineradiography or video tape and kept as a permanent record for repeated review.

One critical area of continued application of laryngography should be mentioned. Polypoid supraglottic carcinomas may prolapse and even abut the subjacent glottis and vocal cord surfaces. These cancers may not permit morphologic display as to site of origin independent from their prolapse against the vocal cords, even on axial CT, although it has such a critical mucosal imaging capability. In this instance, where the selection of patients for conservation laryngeal surgery is critical, only a sophisticated laryngographic examination will clarify the diagnostic situation. Figure 5–26 shows such a case.

The increasing availability and sophistication of CT, as well as an increasing dependence by both clinician and radiologist on CT, will no doubt contribute to contrast laryngography ultimately becoming a lost art. As less material becomes available for resident teaching, facility with the procedure will ultimately disappear.

For comparison of contrast laryngography with other imaging modalities, see Figures 5–28, 5–40, and 5–41 later in this chapter.

Computed Tomography (CT)

The neurosciences were immediately revolutionized by CT. Its impact on laryngeal radiology, while less dramatic in a temporal sense, has been no less definitive in its ultimate accomplishment.[32–41] It provides the possibility of the most exquisite soft tissue and framework imaging that can be sought. Further, it offers an axial dimension to laryngeal imaging that was never before obtainable; the uniqueness of this feature lies in its absolute correlation with the surgeon's axial approach to the structures of the head and neck.

While conventional radiographic techniques provide baseline data and even definitive laryngeal imaging, computed tomography has assumed an absolutely dominant role, particularly in the pretreatment staging and posttreatment evaluation of the patient with laryngeal cancer. Equally, it has altered the diagnostic approach to the patient with laryngeal trauma and offers a variety of singularly effective imaging options in many difficult diagnostic situations. For example, no other imaging modality will distinguish solid from cystic disease, as is done by CT number. With the advent of CT, the natural anatomic definition of tissue planes within the larynx has been recognized; it allows the recognition of normal fat planes (the preepiglottic space and the paralaryngeal spaces) and permits detection of altered density within these planes due to pathologic infiltration of malignancy. Further, the use of intravenous contrast enhancement, often as a rapid infusion technique, has special application to the study of laryngeal cancer in the regional first order lymph nodes.

We prefer 5-mm-thick contiguous slices, which permit a full laryngeal axial display; we find the study should be carefully preview-positioned. The scout preliminary digital radiograph can be utilized in lateral display to judge the level of the superior surfaces of the true vocal cords or in AP display to judge the same structures, the ventricles, or the ventricular bands. This allows for more precise slice localization and permits more critical transition judgments, particularly from supraglottis to glottis. Some laryngeal imagers record images of contiguous slices 3 to 4 mm in thickness. Regardless, all images should begin well above the anticipated site of lesion, in the supraglottis, and should be carried into the subglottis. As a general rule, the images provide very accurate correlation with the pathologic alterations. Invariably, the CT images indicate the presence of much more extensive disease than has been suspected on clinical grounds.

Current thinking now suggests that the rapid intravenous infusion of 60 per cent iodine-containing contrast agent (e.g., 150 cc over 3 min) provides an additional crucial element of soft tissue display. This enables the visualization of mucosal stain for delineation of soft tissues. Though squamous cell carcinoma is hypovascular, the rapid infusion technique differentially stains the normal adjacent mucosa from the advancing soft tissue infiltration of the carcinoma.

Scans must therefore be performed during the time of maximal flow. This also enables differential staining of the vascular structures adjacent to the regional first-order lymph node drainage sites. This is of critical importance in differentiating the vascular structures of the carotid sheath from the deep cervical lymph nodes, especially in the key area of the site of entry of the common facial vein into the internal jugular vein, because supraglottic cancer follows the lymphatics about the superior thyroid vasculature centrally.

CT will permit consistently the detection of lymph nodes with dimensions greater than 2 cm. These nodes are virtually always tumor-bearing. Lymph nodes between 1.5 and 2 cm in size can be detected, but they may represent either tumor or reactive hyperplasia.

As CT is a relatively new imaging modality, the normal CT anatomy of the larynx is depicted (Figs. 5–27 and 5–28) and discussed. The concept of reconstructed images (better termed reformations) is shown in Figure 5–29, which demonstrates the possibilities of coronal and sagittal display. Thyroid cartilage variations, not previously well appreciated, are shown in Figure 5–30. Figures 5–31 to 5–34 show the larynx after injury, while Figures 5–35 to 5–42 show disease processes in the larynx.

In the normal larynx, the supraglottic structures can be defined with precision. At and below the level of the hyoid bone, the space between the laryngeal surface of the epiglottis and the hyoid bone contains largely fat. It is, therefore, of reduced density with CT number below zero. This preepiglottic space is bounded periorly by the valleculae, posteriorly by the

Text continued on page 88

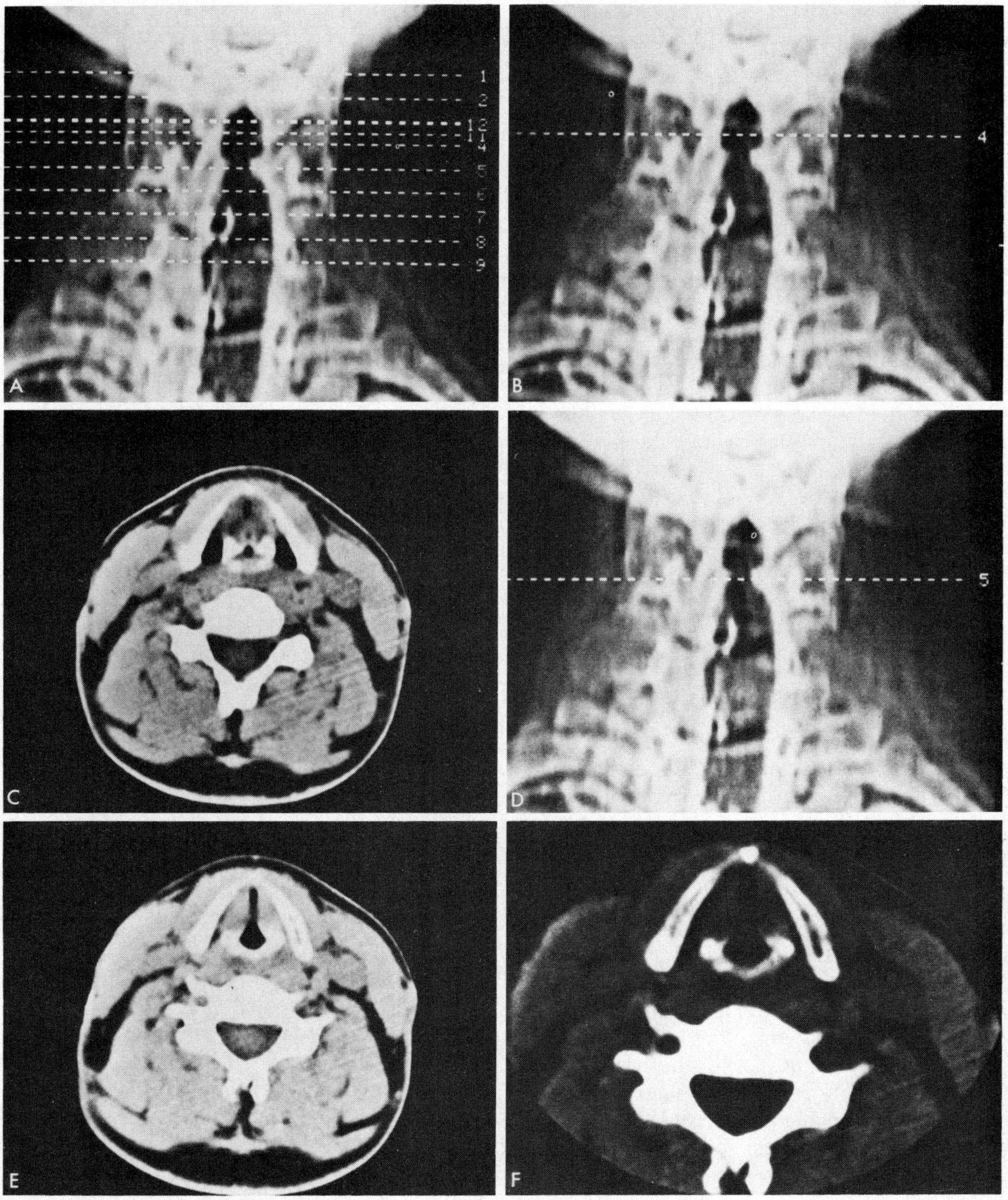

Figure 5–27. Normal CT larynx at false and true cord levels, with preliminary digital (scout) radiograph. All CT slices in this series were 5-mm thick and contiguous.

A, This AP scout view outlines all the slices obtained during the examination. After the initial nine slices were obtained, an additional three views were obtained in the supraglottic region, accounting for the crowding in this area. If a lateral scout view is obtained prior to the examination, the slices can be outlined on this view as well. Additionally, the scout view can be used to preselect a slice at a specific level. This allows clear definition of the transition from false cord to true cord.

B, Horizontal dotted line, location of CT slice 4 illustrated in *C.* If the scout view is obtained with the patient phonating, the precise location of the true cords may be facilitated.

C, The axial anatomy at the level of the false cords corresponding to the level indicated in *B* is clearly demonstrated. The upper portion of the arytenoids is visualized, confirming that the cut is at the level of the false cords. The false cords themselves are seen in adduction; they appear less dense than the muscular true cords (shown in *E*) because they contain fat and minor salivary glands.

D, The scout view demonstrates that CT slice 5 is taken at the level of the true cords.

E, CT slice 5 corresponds to the AP scout film illustrated in *D.* Note the superb delineation of the arytenoids, vocal processes, posterior arch of the cricoid cartilage, true cords, and glottis. Note the glottic shape; there is no anterior soft tissue seen in the midline at the anterior commissure.

F, The same slice shown in *E.* The window setting and level have been altered to highlight the cartilaginous structures.

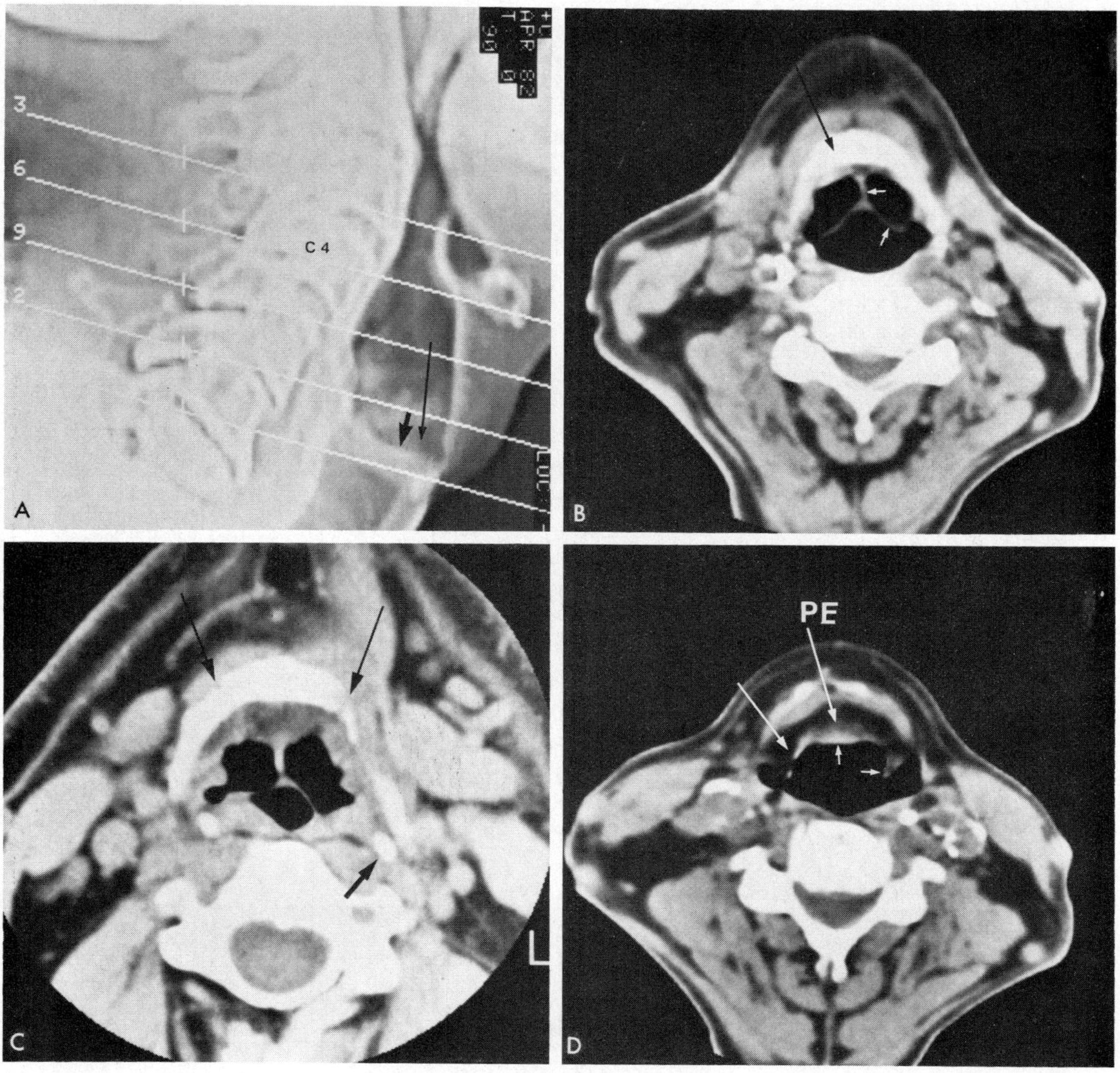

Figure 5–28. Normal CT larynx (supraglottic, glottic, and subglottic levels) with a lateral preliminary digital (scout) radiograph.

A, The lateral scout film demonstrates CT slices selected parallel to the true vocal cords. Fourth cervical vertebra (C4). *Heavy black arrow,* the superior surface of both vocal cords. Note the CT cuts have been positioned to lie parallel to this plane. *Long black arrow,* the overlapping air shadows of the ventricles.

B, A high supraglottic CT cut at the level of the hyoid bone. *Horizontal white arrow,* median glossoepiglottic ligament. *Oblique white arrow,* left lateral margin of the epiglottis extending laterally to the pharyngoepiglottic fold. *Black arrow,* hyoid bone. Note the air in the paired valleculae.

C, A CT cut at the same level as *B,* in a different patient, shows some base-of-tongue soft tissue anterior to the median glossoepiglottic ligament. This demonstrates the variation in soft tissue imaging at this level in the normal situation. The tripartite nature of the hyoid bone is recognized *(two long black arrows). Short black arrow,* superior cornu, left thyroid cartilage.

D, An axial section just at the inferior aspect of the hyoid bone demonstrates the imaging of the preepiglottic space (PE). The preepiglottic space is marginated anteriorly by the infrahyoid strap muscles and the thyrohyoid ligament. Posteriorly, this fat density is bounded by the epiglottis *(tiny vertical arrow). Horizontal tiny arrow,* upper portion of the left aryepiglottic fold. *Long oblique arrow,* the fat density of the right paralaryngeal space as it communicates anteriorly with the fatty preepiglottic space. This is a natural route for cancer extension.

Illustration continued on following page

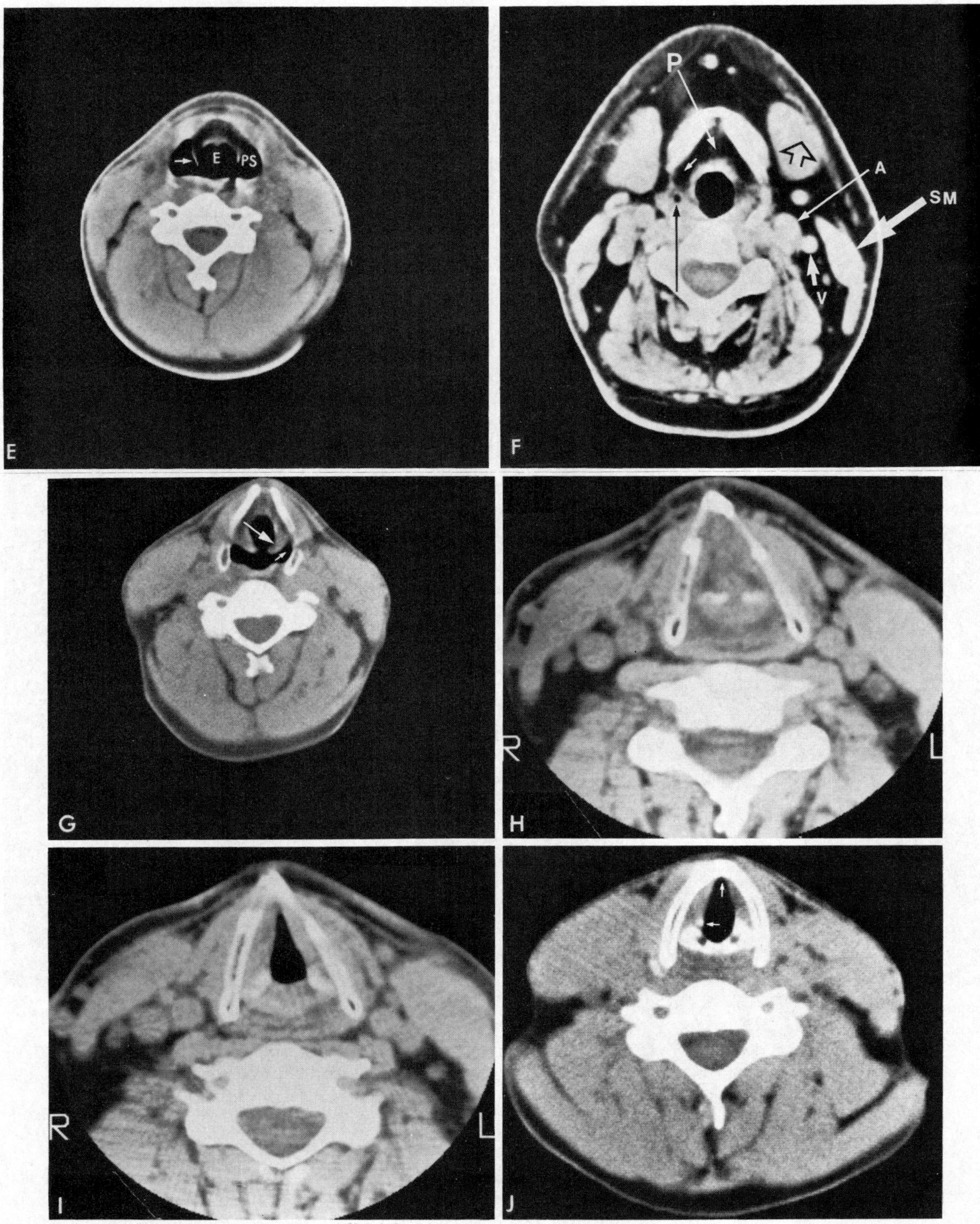

Figure 5–28 *Continued. E,* A supraglottic section lower than *D.* Epiglottis (E); right aryepiglottic fold (*arrow*); left pyriform sinus (PS).

F, A supraglottic section at the level of the thyroid notch. Both thyroid alae are well defined, with their overlying strap muscles; the thyroid cartilage is V-shaped. Preepiglottic space with its characteristic fat density (P). *Tiny white arrow,* continuity of the preepiglottic space with right lateral paralaryngeal space. In this section the infrahyoid strap muscles virtually merge with the thyroid cartilage. The pyriform sinuses are almost collapsed. *Long black arrow,* a tiny amount of air identifying the right pyriform sinus. *Hollow black arrow,* left submandibular gland. Deep to the left sternocleidomastoid muscle (SM) note the left internal jugular vein (V) and the left common carotid artery (A).

G, In a different patient, at approximately the same supraglottic level as *F,* the thyroid notch is shown. The patient has less fat and a longer gray scale setting. Here the pyriform sinuses are distended. *Tiny arrow,* left pyriform sinus. *Large arrow,* left aryepiglottic fold separating the pyriform sinus from the laryngeal vestibule. Note the symmetric near-homogeneous calcification of the thyroid cartilage.

Illustration continued on opposite page

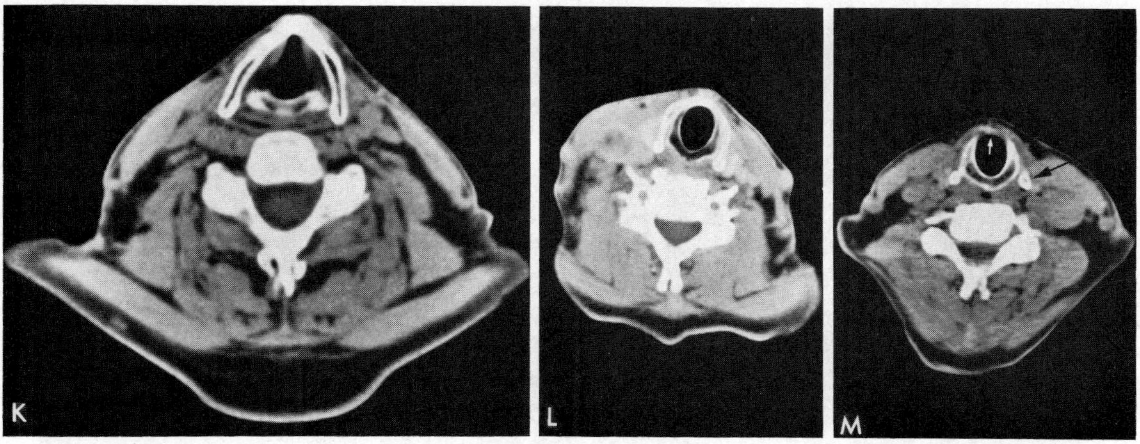

Figure 5–28 *Continued. H,* CT cut at upper false cord level with respiration suspended. There is no airway visible. The level of the false cords is recognized by the presence of the upper portion of the arytenoid cartilages. The minimal internal margination of both thyroid alae by the fat density of the paralaryngeal space is evident. Note the detail of the internal thyroid cartilage cortex.

I, A CT cut just below *H,* of same patient with quiet breathing. Note typical pear-shaped airway. The minor anterior soft tissue thickening in the midline indicates insertion of the thyroepiglottic ligament.

J, A CT cut at true cord level. The vocal cords are muscular and of the same soft tissue density as the other cervical muscles. The airway is now ovoid in quiet respiration. One can see the lower portions of the arytenoid cartilages and the posterior cricoid lamina, confirming the true cord level of the axial section. There is no anterior soft tissue mass marginating the inner surface of the thyroid cartilage in the midline *(vertical arrow).* The thyroid cartilage is becoming U-shaped. *Horizontal arrow,* the right vocal process of the arytenoid cartilage. The paralaryngeal space terminates at this level.

K, At the undersurface of the vocal cords, the anterior commissure is well seen. The level is identified by the cricoid arch posteriorly.

L, Subglottic larynx with the lower portion of the thyroid cartilage now U-shaped. The marrow-containing cricoid ring is well seen and an excellent demonstration of the airway at this level is shown.

M, A subglottic cut, lower than *L,* at the level of the cricothyroid articulations. *Black arrow,* left inferior thyroid cornu. This CT cut demonstrates the cricothyroid membrane anteriorly *(white arrow)* above the attachment to the forward-and-down sloping cricoid cartilage whose high-rising posterior signet is evident on this image. (*A, B, D, E, F, G, I, K, L,* and *M* from Shulman HS et al.: J Otolaryngol 11(6):395–406, 1982.)

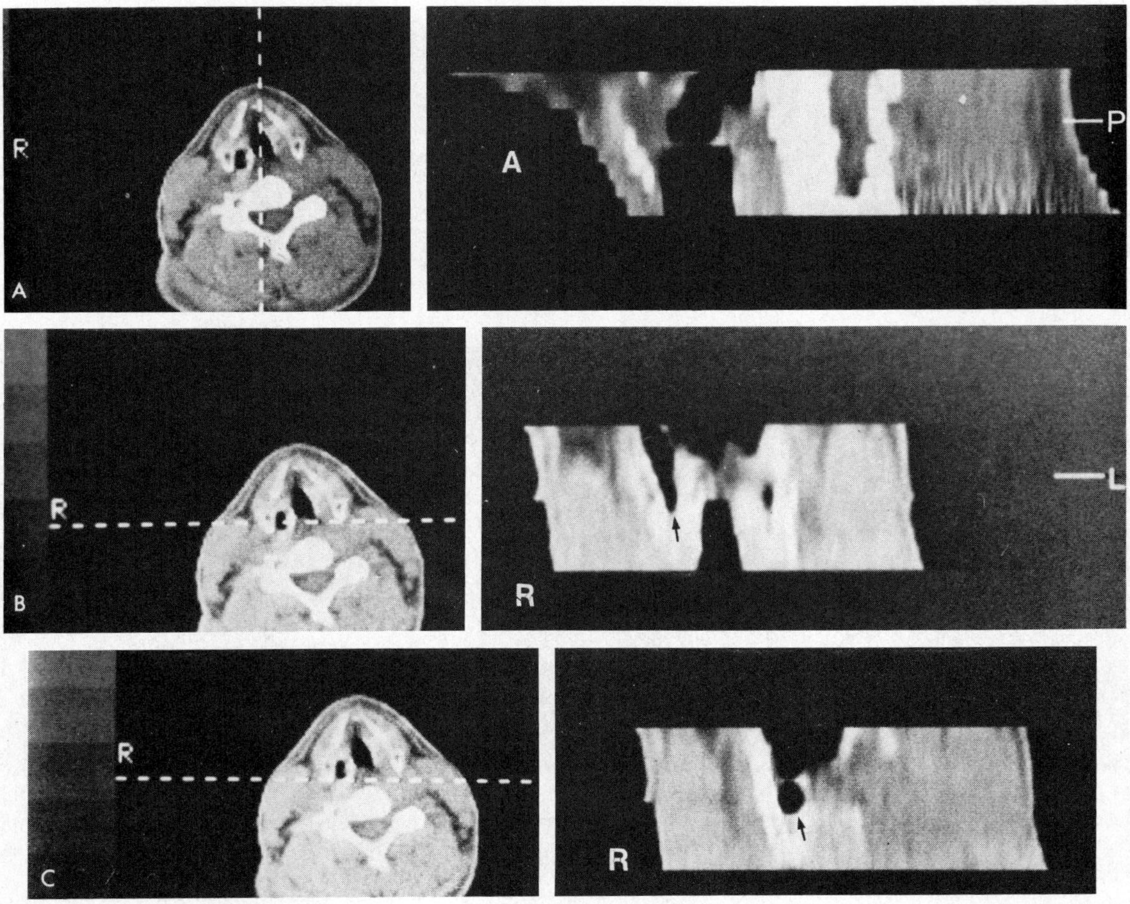

Figure 5–29. CT of normal larynx with sagittal and coronal reconstruction (reformation). A 29-year-old male presented with mucosal hemorrhage in both vocal cords following an injury to the lateral neck region with a deflected hockey puck. Clinical examination was otherwise unremarkable, as were other radiologic studies. CT scan was considered to be normal.

A, A sagittal reconstruction of the axial CT scan at the level indicated by the dashed line. Right (R); anterior (A); Posterior (P).

B and *C,* Coronal reconstructions at the levels indicated demonstrate the relationships of the right pyriform sinus *(arrow)* to the posterior aspect of the right thyroid ala.

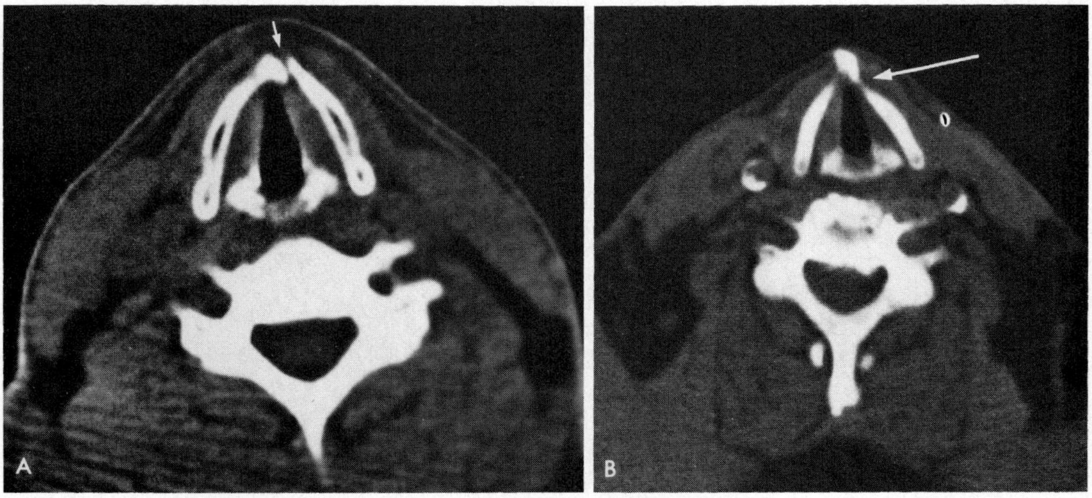

Figure 5–30. *See legend on opposite page*

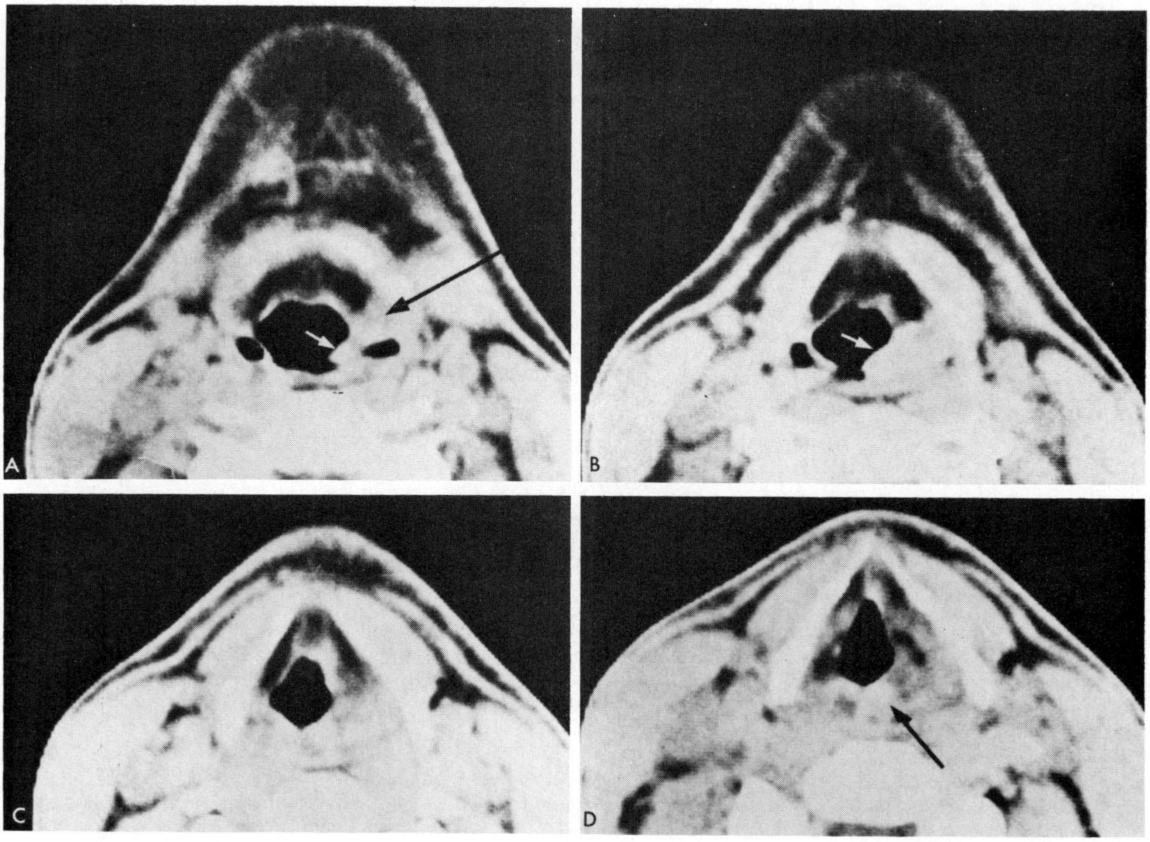

Figure 5–31. Laryngeal trauma with hematoma of aryepiglottic fold and displacement of arytenoid cartilage. CT imaging is carried out with 5-mm contiguous slices in a 26-year-old male who sustained a closed laryngeal injury.

A, The initial slice shows the asymmetry of the aryepiglottic fold. *White arrow,* the hematoma bulging into the lumen from the patient's left. The lateral extent of the hematoma anterior to the upper end of the pyriform fossa is indicated *(long black arrow).*

B, The involvement of the left aryepiglottic fold is more apparent on this examination *(white arrow).*

C, At the level of the false cord, thickening is evident on the left side of the larynx.

D, Inferior extension of the hematoma is indicated by the lateral thickening of the glottis at this level and the medial displacement of the arytenoid cartilage *(long black arrow).*

Figure 5–30. Normal CT of the larynx, demonstrating thyroid cartilage variations in two patients.

A, CT cut at the level of the vocal cords demonstrates the vocal processes of both arytenoid cartilages. The thyroid alae are well visualized. There is an area of probable fibrous union *(arrow)* joining the two normal thyroid alae. These appear to be abutting to the left of the midline. The appearance simulates a fracture, but the cartilage margins are smooth and round, and this probably represents a normal variation.

B, CT cut of a different normal larynx, again at vocal cord level, again shows an apparent thinning of both thyroid alae, in their most anterior portions; however, there appears to be a normal union of the two thyroid alae in the midline. Thinning is indicated on the left side *(arrow).* The authors can offer no explanation for this phenomenon, but it is thought to be a normal variation. This appearance may be due to incomplete calcification.

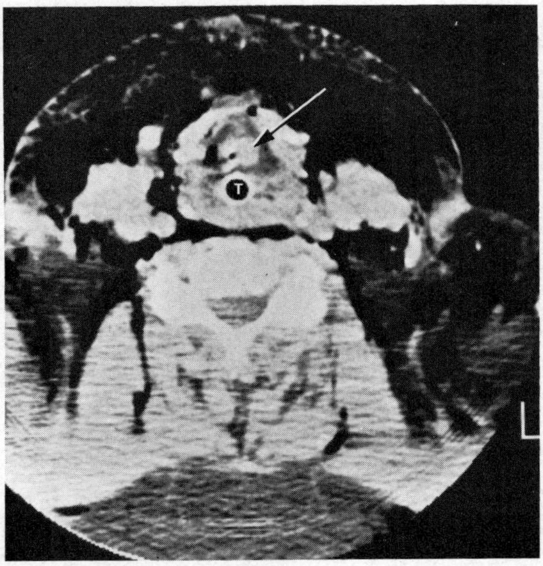

Figure 5–32

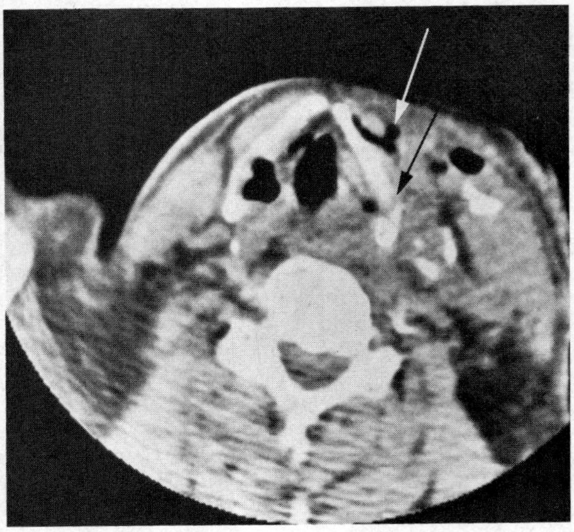

Figure 5–33

Figure 5–32. Laryngeal injury with thyroid cartilage fracture and dislocation of epiglottis. An axial CT cut demonstrates extensive subcutaneous emphysema. There is a vertical fracture of the thyroid cartilage, just to the left of the midline. The entire laryngeal airway is occluded by soft tissue density caused by hematoma. An endotracheal tube (T) is in position to secure an airway. The epiglottis is seen as a dense soft tissue structure *(arrow)* at this level; it is known to be dislocated because it should not be present in such configuration at this level. (From Shulman HS et al.: J Otolaryngol 11(6):395–406, 1982.)

Figure 5–33. Thyroid cartilage fracture. An axial CT cut demonstrates a vertical fracture of the left thyroid ala posteriorly *(black arrow).* There is considerable air within the soft tissues of the neck on the left *(white arrow).* Hematoma reduces the size of the left pyriform sinus. (From Shulman HS et al.: J Otolaryngol 11(6):395–406, 1982.)

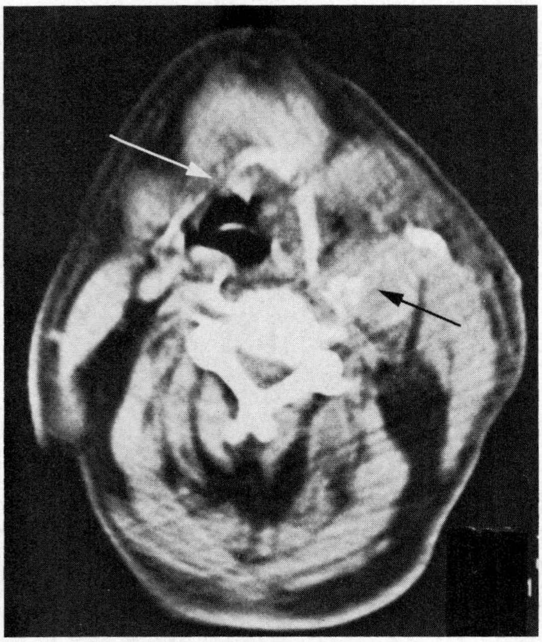

Figure 5–34

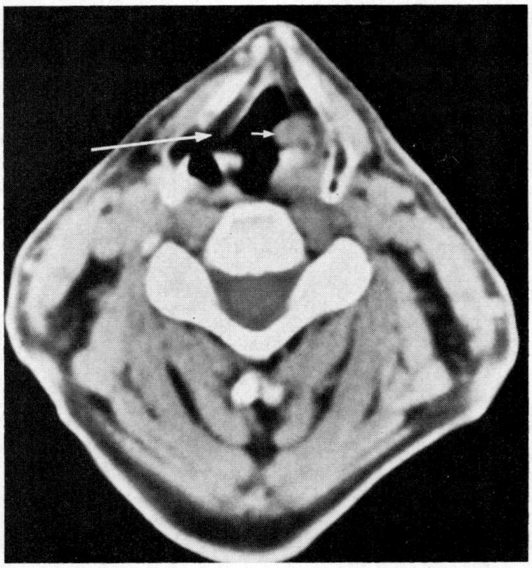

Figure 5–35

Figures 5–34 and 5–35. *See legends on opposite page*

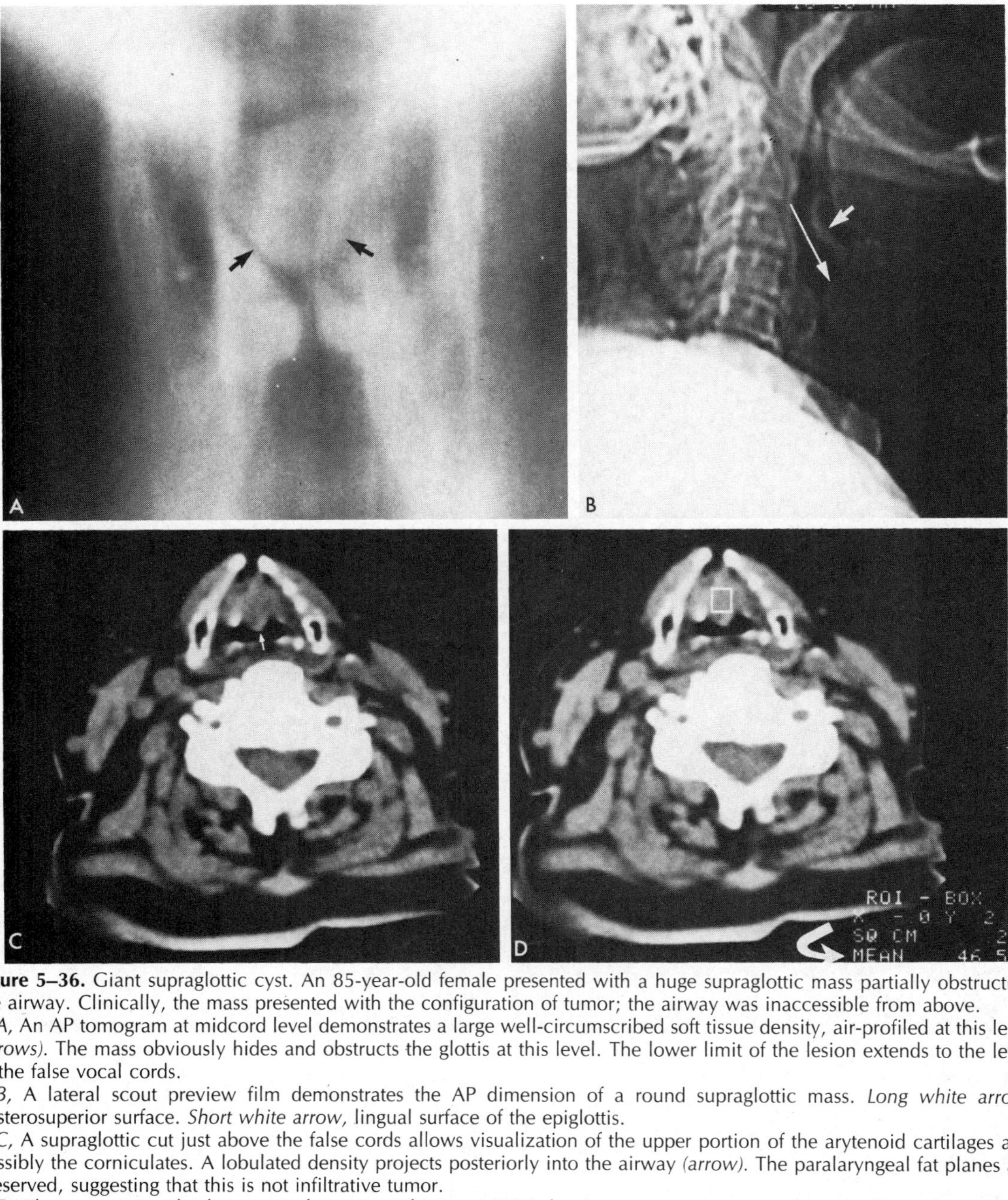

Figure 5–36. Giant supraglottic cyst. An 85-year-old female presented with a huge supraglottic mass partially obstructing the airway. Clinically, the mass presented with the configuration of tumor; the airway was inaccessible from above.

A, An AP tomogram at midcord level demonstrates a large well-circumscribed soft tissue density, air-profiled at this level *(arrows).* The mass obviously hides and obstructs the glottis at this level. The lower limit of the lesion extends to the level of the false vocal cords.

B, A lateral scout preview film demonstrates the AP dimension of a round supraglottic mass. *Long white arrow,* posterosuperior surface. *Short white arrow,* lingual surface of the epiglottis.

C, A supraglottic cut just above the false cords allows visualization of the upper portion of the arytenoid cartilages and possibly the corniculates. A lobulated density projects posteriorly into the airway *(arrow).* The paralaryngeal fat planes are preserved, suggesting that this is not infiltrative tumor.

D, The same cut with placement of a region of interest (ROI) density measurement cursor box. A CT number of 46.5 *(heavy curved arrow)* is indicated, suggesting inspissated fluid. This is greater than water density, and usually, but not always, less than solid tumor density. The findings were confirmed at surgery as a huge benign cyst.

Figure 5–34. Hyoid fracture with deep cervical hematoma. Axial CT cut demonstrates a shattering injury to the hyoid bone, the result of a direct blow. The *white arrow* indicates fracture of the hyoid arch. A bone fragment is displaced internally, partially encroaching on the preepiglottic space. The entire larynx is displaced to the right of the midline by a huge hematoma involving the soft tissue structures of the neck on the left *(black arrow).*

Figure 5–35. Small benign soft tissue mass, left false cord. *Tiny white arrow,* a discrete, small, soft tissue mass lying anteriorly to the left arytenoid cartilage attached to the left ventricular band. The benign nature of the lesion is suggested by the preserved fat density of the paralaryngeal space marginating the internal cortex of the left thyroid ala. The fat density of the right paralaryngeal space is well demonstrated *(long white arrow).* The lesion proved to be a mucous cyst on endoscopic removal; CT number does not always differentiate cysts from solid soft tissue masses. (From Shulman HS et al.: J Otolaryngol 11(6):395–406, 1982.)

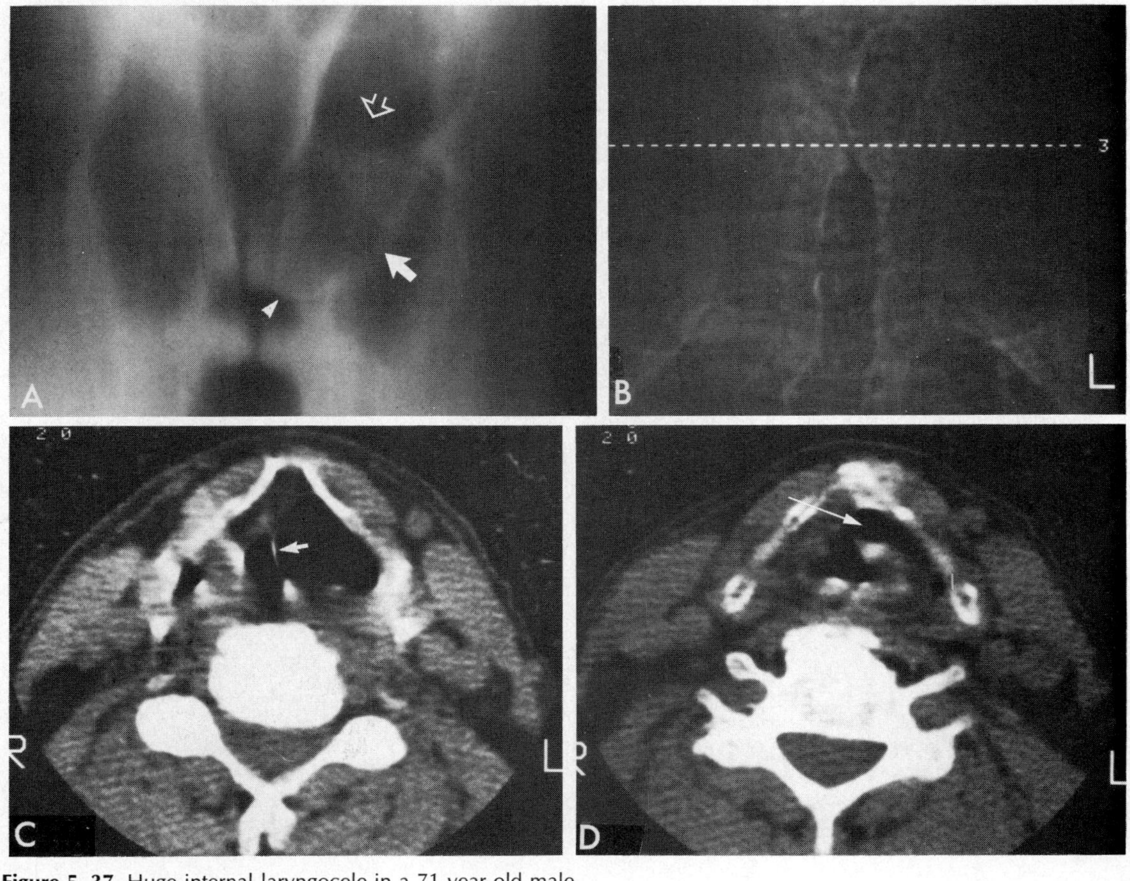

Figure 5–37. Huge internal laryngocele in a 71-year-old male.

A, An AP tomogram makes the diagnosis of a huge internal laryngocele *(hollow white arrow).* The laryngocele's origin in the roof of the laryngeal ventricle is indicated *(white arrowhead).* The lateral margin of the internal laryngocele, which marginates the left pyriform sinus, is indicated *(thick white arrow).*

B, An AP scout digital radiograph demonstrates the air-containing internal laryngocele sac. CT cut 3 is at the level of the neck of the laryngocele.

C, An axial CT cut through the bulk of the laryngocele defines its air-containing nature. *White arrow,* medial wall of the internal laryngocele.

D, A CT cut at the level of the neck of the laryngocele demonstrates the communication between the laryngocele and the laryngeal lumen *(white arrow).* CT has a major role in detection of the fluid-filled laryngocele and its differentiation from soft tissue tumor. Air-containing laryngocele is usually obvious on conventional radiographic examination.

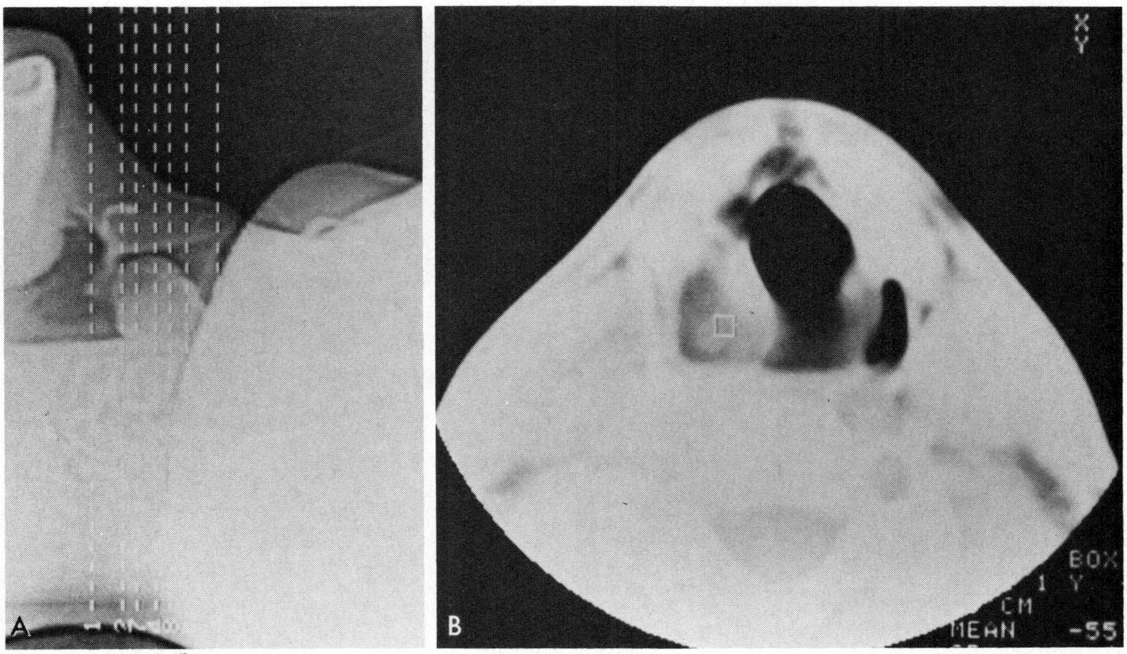

Figure 5–38. Lipoma, pyriform sinus. A 40-year-old male presented with stridor and airway obstruction caused by a mass lesion within the right pyriform sinus encroaching on the laryngeal airway by involvement of the right aryepiglottic fold and related structures. The diagnosis of lipoma was confirmed at surgery.

A, A lateral view of the preview feature film, prior to axial CT, indicates the direction and selection of CT slices. An obvious soft tissue mass, roughly spherical in nature, encroaches on or overlaps the supraglottic airway at the level of the epiglottis. The lateral placement of the lesion is not demonstrated.

B, CT cut 4 indicated on the preview lateral film. The section is at approximately midlevel of the mass, and reveals it to involve the right pyriform sinus. The left pyriform sinus is clear. The dimension of residual laryngeal airway is well shown. A cursor *(white square marker)* has been positioned over the pyriform sinus mass to take a density reading. The window level is −60, and the mean density of the mass is indicated as −55. This established the diagnosis of lipoma, as fat is the only imageable soft tissue with a density less than water (zero density) that can be imaged.

(From Nedzelski J, Toronto, private communication.)

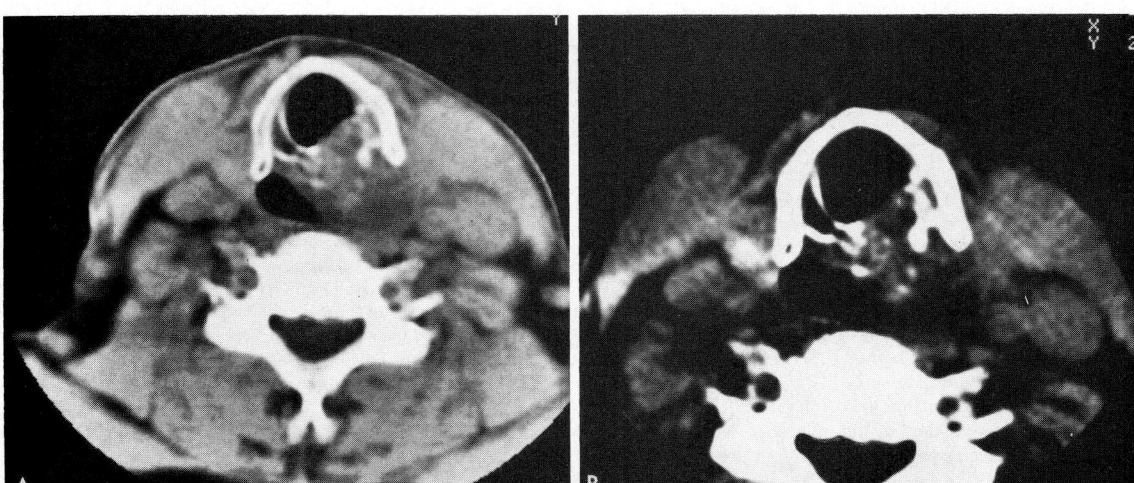

Figure 5–39. Chondroma, cricoid cartilage. A diagnosis of chondroma was confirmed at surgery.

A, A destructive tumor mass arises from the cricoid cartilage on the left and extends posteriorly and laterally, compressing or invading the hypopharynx and the left pyriform sinus.

B, At a lower window setting, extensive calcification can be seen within the mass. This is indicative of a cartilaginous tumor.

(From Nedzelski J, Toronto, private communication, and Shulman HS et al.: J Otolaryngol 11(6):395–406, 1982.)

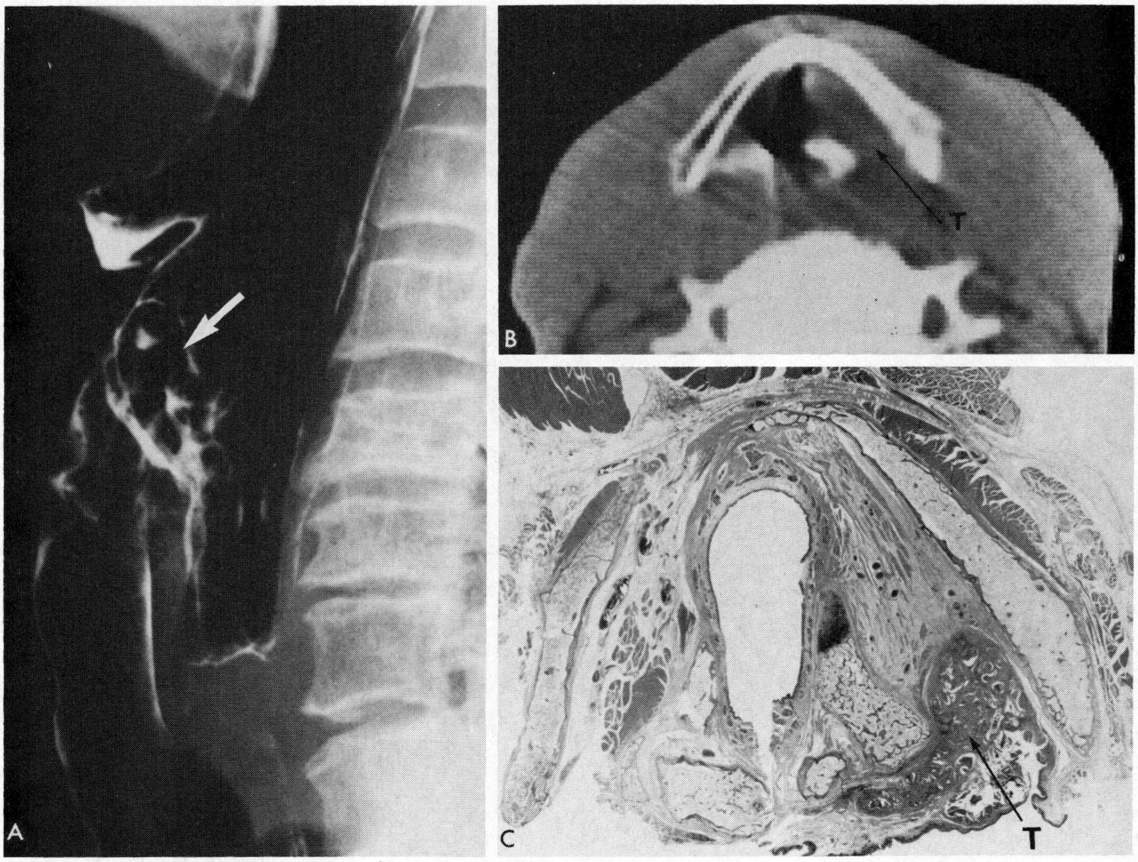

Figure 5–40. Carcinoma of aryepiglottic fold with infiltration of vocalis muscle and arytenoid cartilage displacement. Correlation of CT and pathology is shown. A 56-year-old male presented with a lobulated mass of the left aryepiglottic fold.

A, A lateral view of a laryngogram indicates the position of the mass *(arrow).*

B, A CT cut at the level of the vocal cords demonstrates infiltration of the left vocalis muscle by tumor (T). The arytenoid cartilage is displaced medially.

C, A photomicrograph demonstrates the squamous cell carcinoma (T) infiltrating the vocalis muscle between the thyroid ala and the displaced arytenoid cartilage. The histologic section exactly matches the CT scan. (From Van Nostrand P, Keene M, and Birt BD, Toronto, private communications.)

Figure 5–41. Supraglottic carcinoma with extension into base of tongue and adjacent deep cervical lymph nodes; no glottic involvement. A 65-year-old male presented with a large carcinoma apparently confined to the epiglottis. There was a suggestion of lymph node enlargement of the right side of the neck, but this was unclear.

A, A lateral view of a laryngogram defines the lobulated bulky epiglottic mass. The mass appears to be well clear of the vocal cord level inferiorly.

B, CT cuts of 5 mm thickness taken contiguously begin at the level of the base of the tongue. *Arrow,* the markedly thickened superior aspect of the epiglottis. Note the narrowing of the vallecular air space just anterior to the epiglottis.

C, The thickened epiglottis is still well seen. *Short horizontal arrow,* extension of the tumor into the upper end of the left aryepiglottic fold. *Long oblique arrow,* an ill-defined soft tissue density not seen on the patient's left side and presumably representing tumor extension either into the soft tissues of the neck or into draining lymph nodes.

D, The preepiglottic space is seen here as a more homogeneous soft tissue density than usual. Loss of the streaky fat density usually seen is strongly suggestive of anterior tumor extension into this space.

E, Note the posterior extent of this tumor, which results in narrowing of the airway. *Long white arrow,* the soft tissue density seen just posterior and inferior to the hyoid bone, indicative of tumor extension into the preepiglottic space.

F, This slice is taken at the level of the false cords. The arytenoid cartilages can be visualized. The airway is pear-shaped. There is no inferior tumor extension to this level.

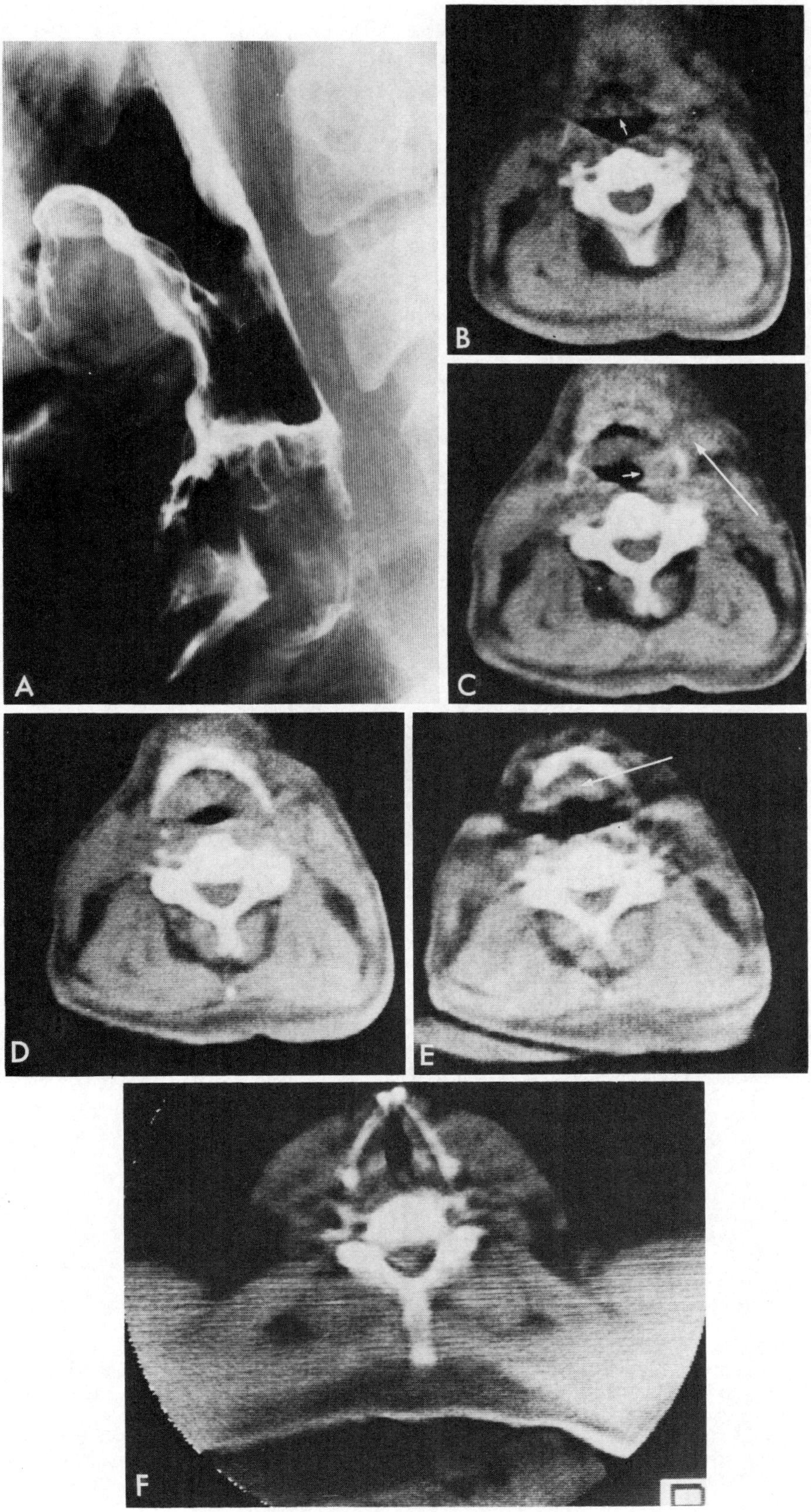

Figure 5–41. *See legend on opposite page*

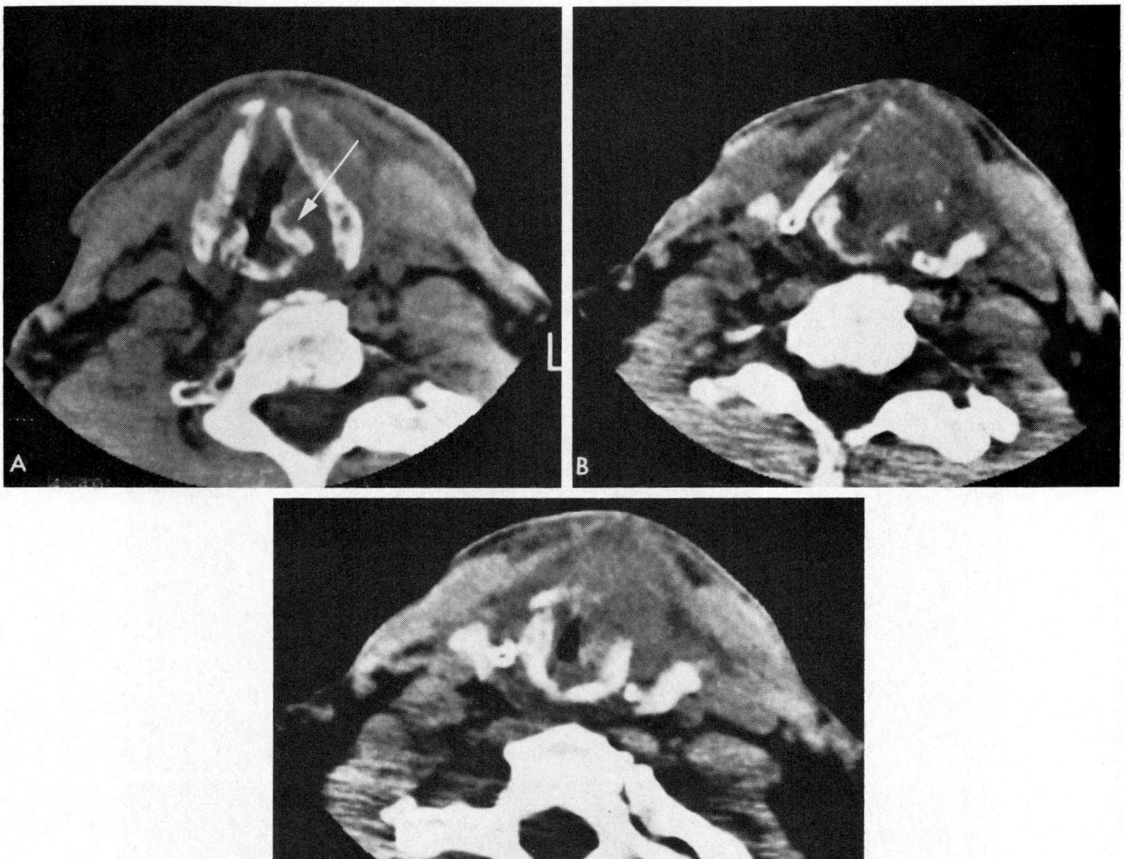

Figure 5–42. Transglottic carcinoma, T4, with cartilage invasion.

A, A large transglottic carcinoma displaces the left arytenoid cartilage medially *(white arrow),* as it infiltrates between the arytenoid cartilage and the thyroid cartilage on this side. There is considerable airway encroachment by tumor. There is marked soft tissue thickening anteriorly indicating anterior commissure extension.

B, The airway is virtually obliterated by soft tissue tumor mass, which has destroyed the entire left thyroid ala and the anterior half of the right thyroid cartilage. Displaced fragments of cartilage are pushed posteriorly.

C, A subglottic cut demonstrates the extensive subglottic extension of tumor as well as the continued presence of tumor beyond the larynx anteriorly and laterally. This detection of cancer extension beyond the confines of the larynx was never possible prior to the axial display of CT.

(From Shulman HS et al.: J Otolaryngol 11(6):395–406, 1982.)

Figure 5–43. Adenoid cystic carcinoma of trachea, with extension to subglottic larynx. The patient is a 21-year-old female presenting with episodes of stridor and fainting attacks. The lesion proved to be an adenoid cystic carcinoma; it was treated by debulking surgical procedure and radiation therapy.

A, A lateral radiograph demonstrates a dome-shaped, relatively smooth mass arising from the posterior wall of the trachea. The anterior limit of the trachea is defined *(two white arrows).* The tumor is an adenoid cystic carcinoma arising from minor salivary glands within the party wall between the trachea and the esophagus. The tumor encroaches on the inferior aspect of the cricoid signet posteriorly, but this is not well shown.

B, A barium esophagram demonstrates the thickening of the party wall *(arrow)* due to adenoid cystic carcinoma arising in glandular elements. The barium outlines the slightly retrodisplaced esophagus. The dome shape of the soft tissue mass contrasted against tracheal air is better seen here than in *A.*

C, A CT scan at the level of the bulk of the intratracheal tumor mass demonstrates the axial encroachment on the airway *(arrow).*

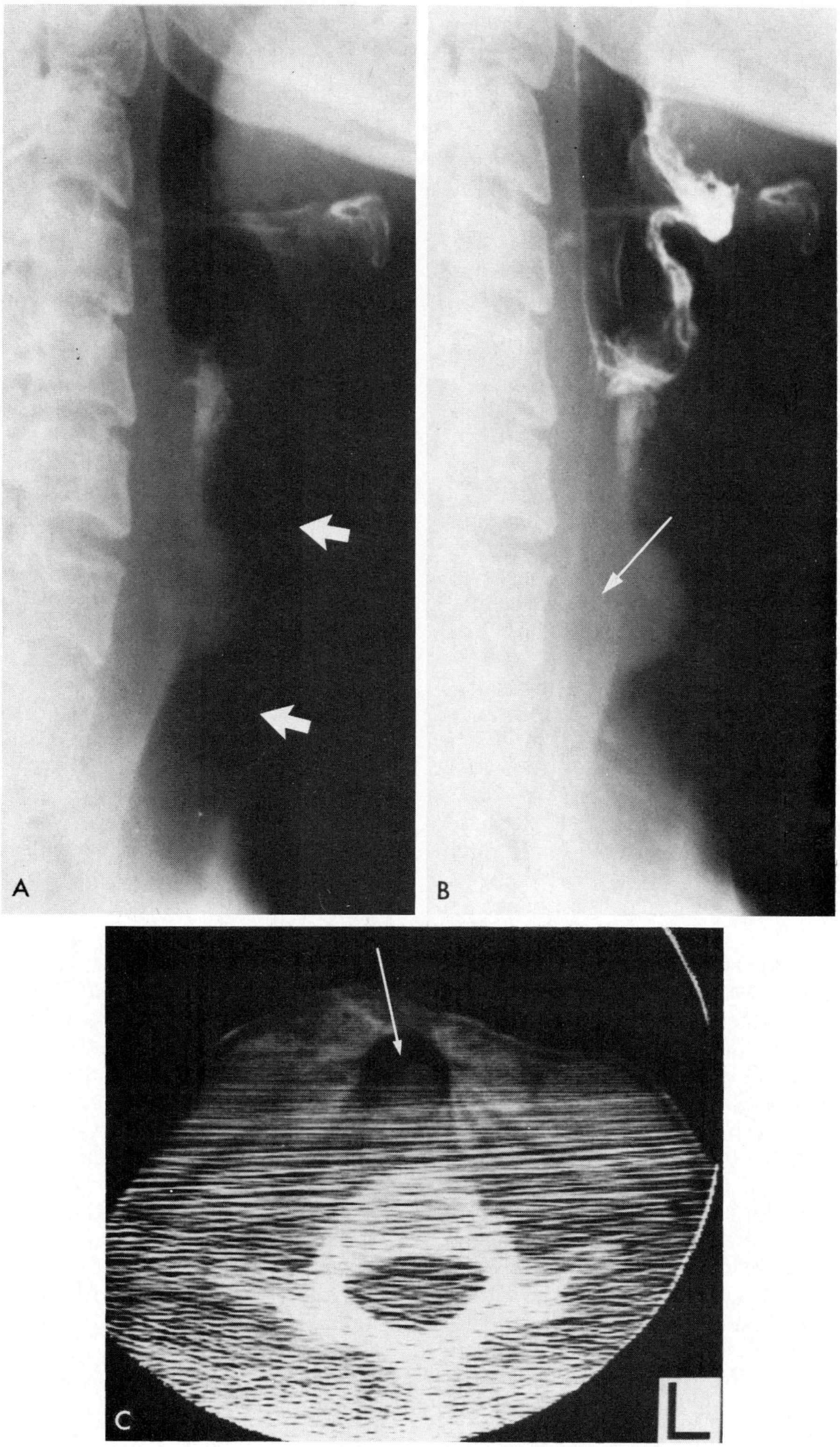

Figure 5–43. *See legend on opposite page*

epiglottis, and anteriorly by the thyrohyoid membrane. It is roughly triangular in shape, with the base of the triangle (above) just below the valleculae and the apex (below) just above the anterior commissure. Laterally, the edges of this inverted triangle merge with the paralaryngeal space.

The paralaryngeal spaces are the fat planes that marginate the internal cortices of the thyroid cartilage on each side. These paralaryngeal, low density fatty regions are an inferior extension of the preepiglottic space. Violation of their integrity indicates tumor infiltration. The paralaryngeal spaces gradually diminish and terminate inferiorly at the level of the vocal cords.

At the level of the ventricular bands, the airway is pear-shaped: the soft tissues of the ventricular bands are relatively less dense on CT than are the true vocal cords; they contain both fat and minor salivary gland structures. The level of this examination can always be determined by virtue of the shape of the airway and the fact that the arytenoid cartilages, in their upper portions, are noted in the axial image.

When the transition is made to the glottis, the airway assumes a more ovoid appearance. No soft tissue should be detectable in the midline anteriorly, a critical observation. The tendinous insertion of each vocal cord should be clearly seen as it attaches to the anterior commissure region of the larynx, immediately subjacent to the point of fusion of the paired thyroid alae. The paralaryngeal fat defines this tendinous insertion still better. Minor soft tissue thickening in this area always indicates the extension of disease into the anterior commissure. The airway at the level of the vocal cord examination can be recognized by its ovoid shape; the arytenoid cartilages and, possibly, the vocal processes are imaged in full display, as is the subjacent posterior lamina of the cricoid cartilage.

Additionally, the subglottis is extremely well imaged. It should be remembered that the cricoid cartilage, which has a signet ring shape, slopes inferiorly as it is followed anteriorly. The cricothyroid distance approximates 1.5 cm anteriorly, though the cricoid rises to the level of the vocal cords at the cricoarytenoid articulations posteriorly. This is again a critical transition point, because soft tissue cancer extension in the subglottis anteriorly does not produce cartilage involvement until it has made the full inferior infiltration to the level of the cricoid cartilage; however, posterior extension of glottic cancer has easy access to the high-rising cricoid signet, at which point cancer may exit the larynx posteriorly. Its route may lie either between the arytenoid and cricoid cartilages through their articulations, lateral to the arytenoid cartilage (between it and the thyroid cartilage), or more inferiorly amputating the upper portion of the cricoid cartilage itself either medially or laterally. In any event, cancer then gains access to the postcricoid region and the remainder of the hypopharynx. This posterior commissure extension and posterolateral exiting of cancer from the larynx could never be well appreciated prior to the introduction of CT. Even at endoscopy, this was always a difficult evaluation.

Cartilage destruction is precisely defined in the cricoid cartilage. Because this is a well calcified and ossified cartilage, transgression of its boundaries is clearly seen. The situation with the thyroid cartilage is less clear, though images are far more readily interpretable than those of conventional radiology. If the fat planes of the paralaryngeal space are encroached upon, this suggests tumor approaching and in contact with thyroid cartilage on its internal cortex. The calcification and ossification of thyroid cartilage may be irregular and even asymmetric, however; care must therefore be taken in evaluating thyroid cartilage integrity by CT. Ultrasound techniques, described later in this chapter, may assist in this evaluation.

It is possible to improve the display in certain areas, such as the pyriform sinuses, by having the patient maintain the Valsalva maneuver during the scan. Perhaps the best technique for evaluation of the glottis and ventricles by distension is to have the patient carry out a modified Valsalva maneuver during the scan. This can be undertaken by asking the patient to blow slowly and persistently into a partially crimped straw or other device. This allows the patient to maintain a position of comfort, without movement. Suspended respiration may have some additional selective advantage over standard imaging during quiet breathing, even with rapid scans.

As a final point at this junction, the CT study should not be done the same day as a laryngogram. Even a small amount of retained contrast medium may produce troublesome density artifacts.

For comparison of CT with other imaging modalities, see also Figures 5–43 to 5–45 and Figure 5–47 later in this chapter.

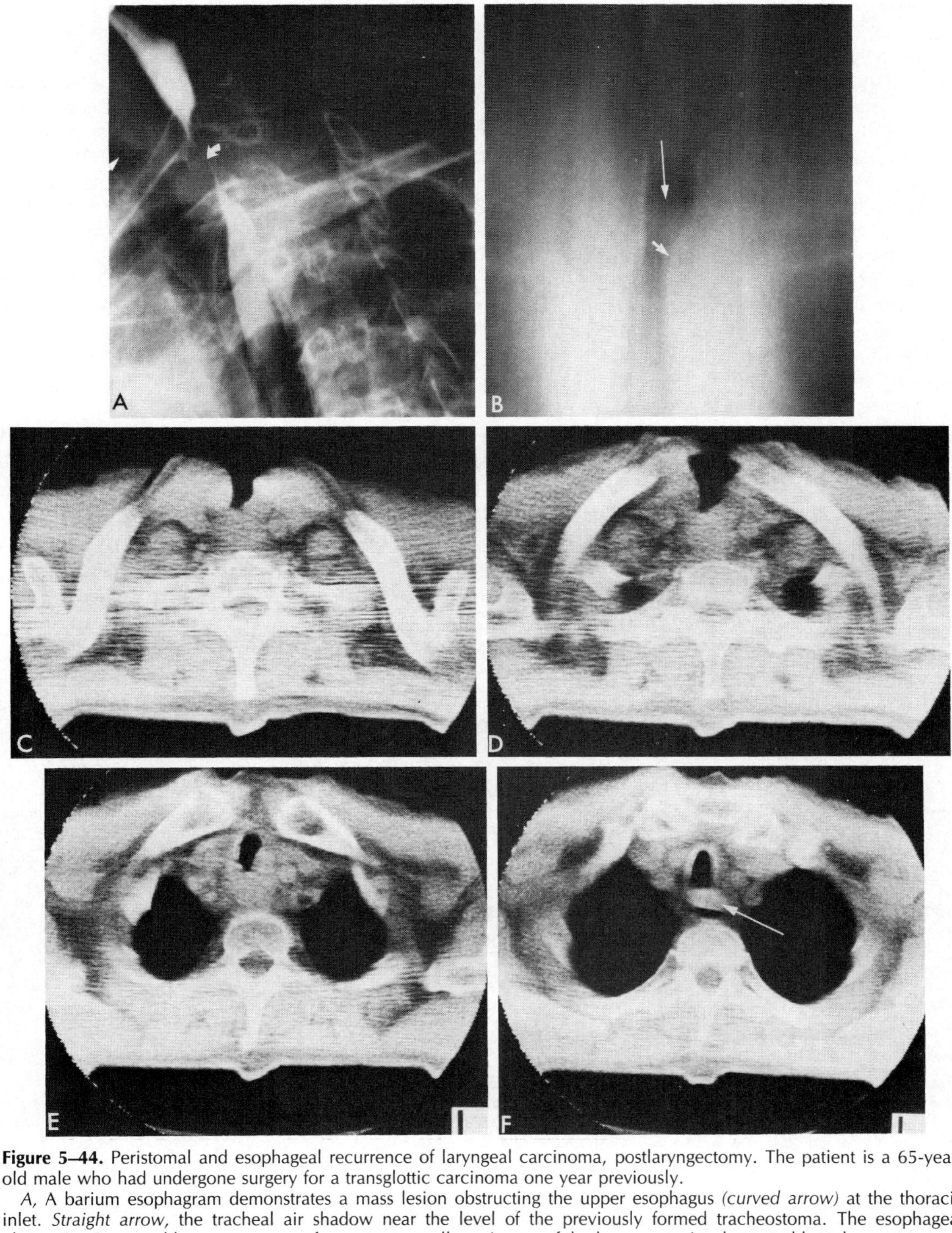

Figure 5–44. Peristomal and esophageal recurrence of laryngeal carcinoma, postlaryngectomy. The patient is a 65-year-old male who had undergone surgery for a transglottic carcinoma one year previously.

A, A barium esophagram demonstrates a mass lesion obstructing the upper esophagus *(curved arrow)* at the thoracic inlet. *Straight arrow,* the tracheal air shadow near the level of the previously formed tracheostoma. The esophageal obstruction is caused by a recurrence of a squamous cell carcinoma of the larynx, previously treated by a laryngectomy.

B, An AP tomogram at the level of the thoracic inlet demonstrates narrowing of the trachea by tumor, especially on its left lateral wall *(thick arrow).* The tracheostoma is indicated *(thin arrow).* The superior mediastinal tissues are infiltrated by tumor.

C, D, E, and *F,* A series of axial CT cuts, beginning at the level of the tracheostoma and descending inferiorly, show the extent of peristomal and superior mediastinal tumor involvment. *C* and *D,* The anteriorly placed tracheostoma and distortion of the tracheal walls by tumor are indicated. *E,* The superior mediastinal tumor is shown clearly, with narrowing of the trachea. *F,* The tumor extension into the common party wall between the trachea and esophagus is indicated *(arrow).*

Barium Swallow Examination

The barium swallow examination, which allows assessment of hypopharyngeal and esophageal structure and function, provides an important complementary study in laryngeal diagnosis (Figs. 5–43 and 5–44). Although not a routine examination, it is added to the laryngeal investigation of those patients with upper dysphagia in whom further evaluation of the hypopharynx, pyriform sinuses, postcricoid region, and cervical esophagus is mandatory. Contrast laryngography is insensitive to these latter areas, except for the pyriform sinuses. The barium swallow (actually barium sulfate) is also useful in the evaluation of possible laryngeal reflux from the hypopharynx or the esophagus.

During the pharyngeal phase of swallowing, the laryngeal introitus is closed as the aryepiglottic folds tend to constrict and the false and true vocal cord sphincters close. The larynx is elevated by the extrinsic strap muscles and the barium bolus pushes backwards and downwards and then flows over either side of the epiglottis, outlining the pyriform sinuses, the posterior pharyngeal wall, and the postcricoid region. The barium bolus enters the cervical esophagus at approximately the level of the sixth cervical vertebra.

The hypopharynx should be examined during its fully distended phase as well as during the time it is coated with the barium compound, both in frontal and lateral projections. Fluoroscopic spot films are made, and the distensibility and symmetry of the structures evaluated; the presence or absence of a mass lesion is recorded. Cineradiography or video recordings

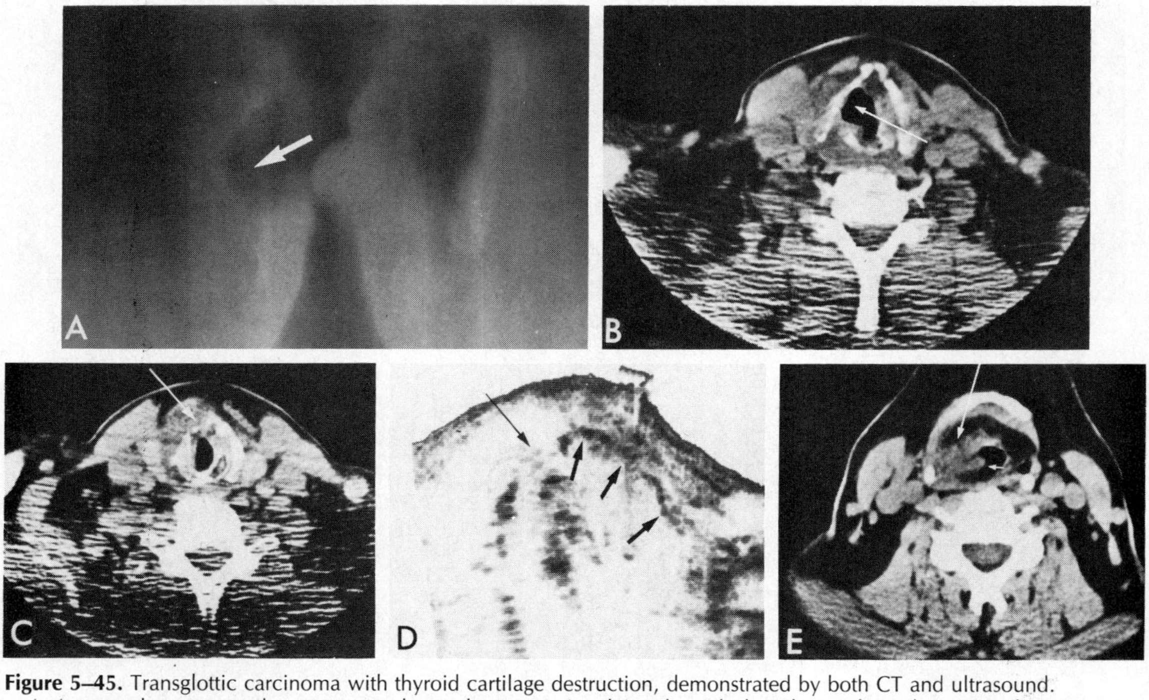

Figure 5–45. Transglottic carcinoma with thyroid cartilage destruction, demonstrated by both CT and ultrasound.

A, A coronal tomogram demonstrates a large ulcer crater involving the right hemilarynx from destruction by squamous cell carcinoma. This is a classic transglottic carcinoma, which has destroyed the entire right vocal cord and much of the right ventricular band. There is a rolled exophytic margin both above the destructive ulcer and below it, extending into the subglottic space. The left vocal cord is thickened by tumor infiltration across the midline. The left ventricle is obliterated. *White arrow,* the ulcer crater.

B, A CT scan through the midsection of the ulcer crater demonstrates the depth of its extension to the subjacent thyroid cartilage *(white arrow).* The thyroid cartilage appears intact at this level.

C, A CT scan at the lower level of the thyroid cartilage demonstrates destruction of the right thyroid ala anteriorly *(arrow)* as tumor extends from the glottis through the thyroid ala into the soft tissues of the neck. Subglottic tumor extension is obvious within the airway lumen.

D, A transverse contact B-mode ultrasound image at the same level as *C* demonstrates the intact left thyroid cartilage *(three short black arrows). Long black arrow,* the multiple echoes resulting from tumor destruction and infiltration through the right thyroid cartilage into the soft tissues of the neck. The image information is identical to that of the CT cut in *C.* (From Rothberg R, Toronto, private communication.)

E, A supraglottic cut shows lobulated tumor bulging into the airway *(tiny white arrow)* from the right aryepiglottic fold. It is above the ulcer crater seen in *C.* Tumor extension into the preepiglottic space is clearly shown *(long white arrow).*

are utilized for best dynamic evaluation. Cineradiography and video tape studies do not demonstrate anatomic detail as well as do spot films; however, cineradiography is a most important supplement to spot filming, especially during events of short duration or in the uncooperative patient.

At times, water soluble contrast examination of the hypopharynx and esophagus is deemed necessary. This is especially important where there is a chance of major fistulization of the digestive tract into the laryngotracheal airway, as in the neonate with tracheoesophageal fistula or the adult patient with malignant fistula.

Other Modalities

Certain radiologic studies, not usually considered as part of the ordinary laryngeal imaging armamentarium, may have selective diagnostic usefulness.[1] The innovative laryngologist and laryngeal radiologist may look to these other modalities to solve specific diagnostic problems or give direction to other studies.

Diagnostic Ultrasound Scans. Diagnostic ultrasound[1, 42] has the rapid, simple, relatively inexpensive, and highly sensitive capability of detecting whether or not the thyroid cartilage has lost its integrity (Fig. 5–45). It occasionally provides other cartilage information (arytenoid displacement, tracheal destruction). Ultrasound has two special features: (1) the ultrasonographer actively produces (and can reproduce) the transverse (axial) images by contact scanning and (2) the imaging information can be amplified by longitudinal contact scans that provide parasagittal information; for example, they can demonstrate cancer wrapping around the inferior margin of the thyroid cartilage from internal to external surface. Oblique views can also be provided.

Because ultrasound is an imaging phenomenon that lends itself best to detecting the difference in impedance characteristics between different tissue interfaces, it has the one highly specific application in cartilage assessment. We utilize it to confirm or deny cartilage destruction suspected on conventional lateral radiograph or in the face of an equivocal CT scan. These imaging studies may demonstrate areas of irregular calcification and ossification and the CT may fail to delineate the cortex margin. The B-mode ultrasound may yet define the integrity of the external cortex of the thyroid cartilage, independent of the degree of calcification or ossification within it.

Ultrasound is also useful in the detection of fractures and cartilage thickening due to perichondritis or tumor such as chondroma. Many apparent T3 laryngeal cancers are actually T4—both CT and ultrasound contribute to a better definition and evaluation of this problem. Ultrasound cannot, however, image the air column because of the high impedance of the air itself.

Radionuclide Bone and Gallium Scans. Diagnostic radionuclide scans have limited usefulness in laryngeal evaluation.[43, 44] The major role of bone scanning is in the detection of the reparative osteoblastic response to a destructive arthropathy, as in cricoarytenoid arthritis, in

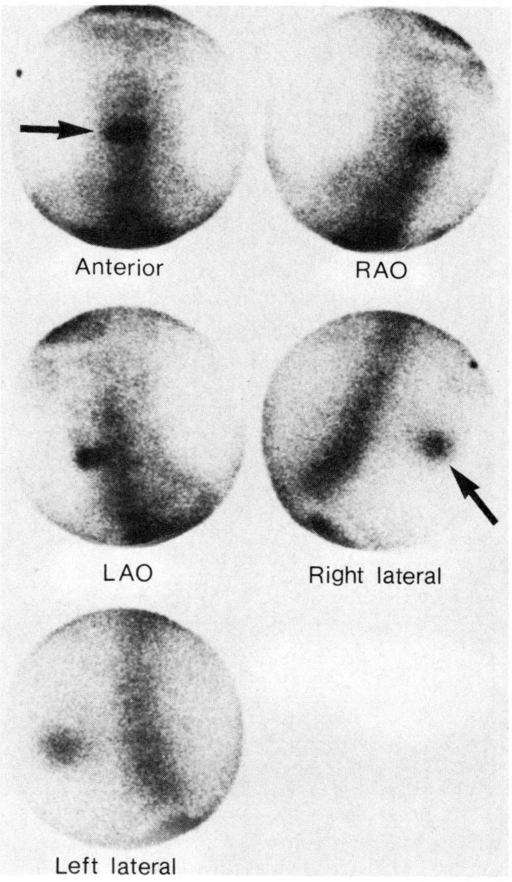

Figure 5–46. Cricoarytenoid arthropathy caused by gout; positive bone scan. The delayed phase of a ^{99m}Tc technetium methylene diphosphonate bone scan demonstrates the osteoblastic reparative response to a destructive arthropathy. The anterior view of the larynx *(horizontal arrow)* and the lateral view of the larynx *(oblique arrow)* allow for anatomic localization of this bone scan finding. The patient was confirmed as having gout by further laboratory investigations; his laryngeal complaints disappeared with effective treatment. (From Greyson ND, Noyek AM: Otolaryngol Clin North Am 2(2):541–560, 1978.)

delayed image. The bone scan, if "hot" on the pool phase soft tissue image, suggests whether there is a need for anti-inflammatory treatment as well. Further, a total body view will clarify whether this is a local arthropathy or merely a local manifestation of a systemic arthropathy. The bone scan (as with the liver-spleen scan) also contributes to the M staging of the TNM approach to laryngeal cancer. A positive bone scan after laryngeal injury has medicolegal usefulness rather than clinical value. Figures 5–46 and 5–47 show the use of radionuclides.

The gallium scan is of uncertain value. Gallium-67 citrate can detect certain inflammatory

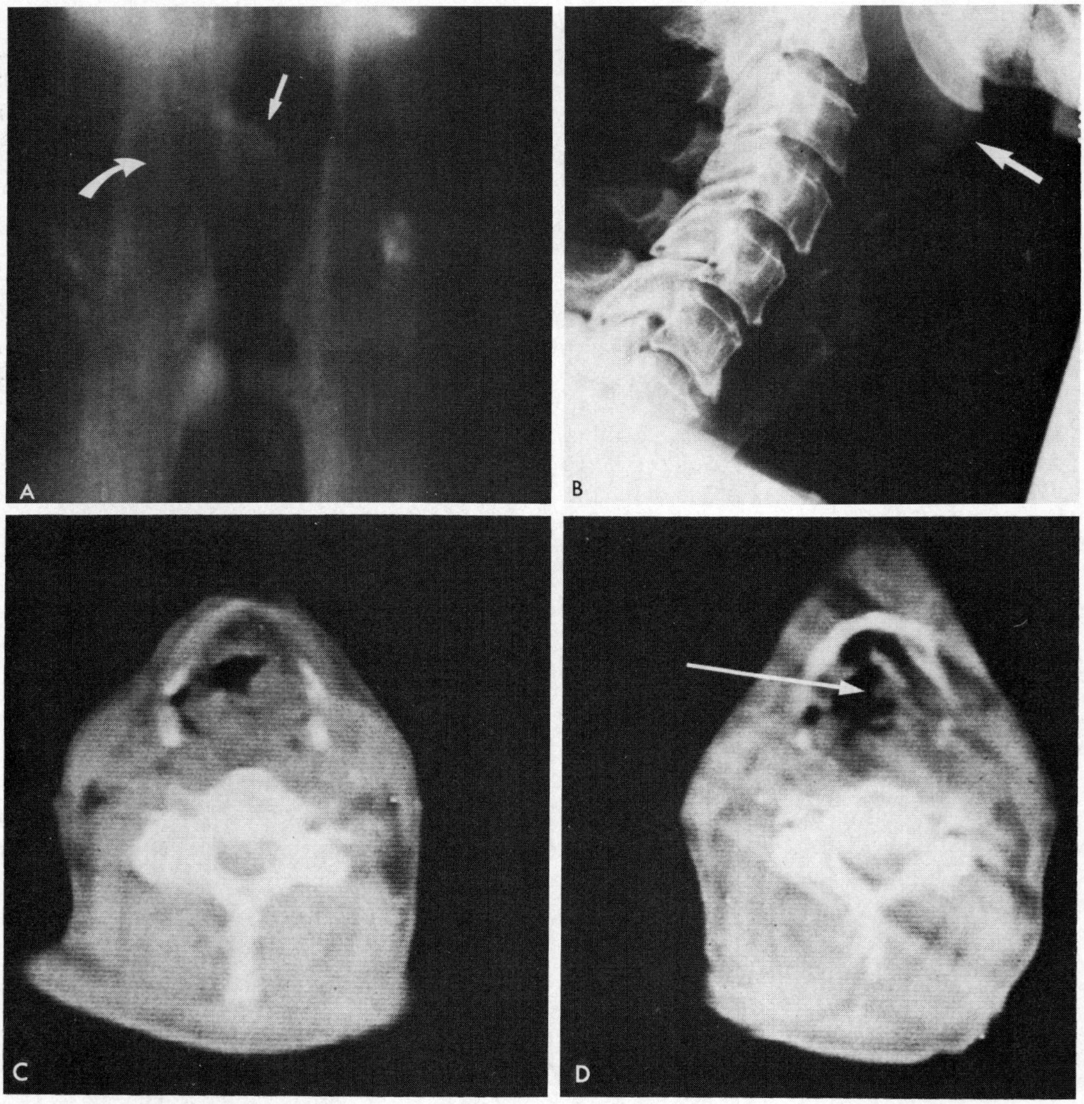

Figure 5–47. Massive carcinoma of the pyriform sinus, encircling the hypopharynx, involving the aryepiglottic fold, and infiltrating extensively superiorly in the posterior pharyngeal wall. Patient is a 50-year-old male, presenting with a one-year history of increasing dysphagia and right otalgia.

A, A coronal tomogram during phonation, which demonstrates thickening of the right aryepiglottic fold *(curved arrow)* from a poorly differentiated squamous cell carcinoma arising in the right pyriform sinus. The tumor encircles the larynx posteriorly. A large excrescence of tumor bulges from the right aryepiglottic fold into the airway *(straight arrow).* There is a submucosal infiltration of tumor at the level of the right ventricular band and cord.

B, A soft tissue lateral radiograph on admission demonstrates the massive extent of retropharyngeal tumor involvement *(arrow).*

C, D, E, and *F,* A series of CT cuts demonstrates the axial display of this tumor. The slices are 5 mm in thickness. The right of the figure (R) represents the patient's right side. *C,* Tumor display at the level of the inferior thyroid cornu. *D,* A cut slightly higher than *C,* demonstrating the aryepiglottic excrescence of tumor *(arrow)* as seen on the coronal tomogram. The paralaryngeal tissues are infiltrated.

Illustration continued on opposite page

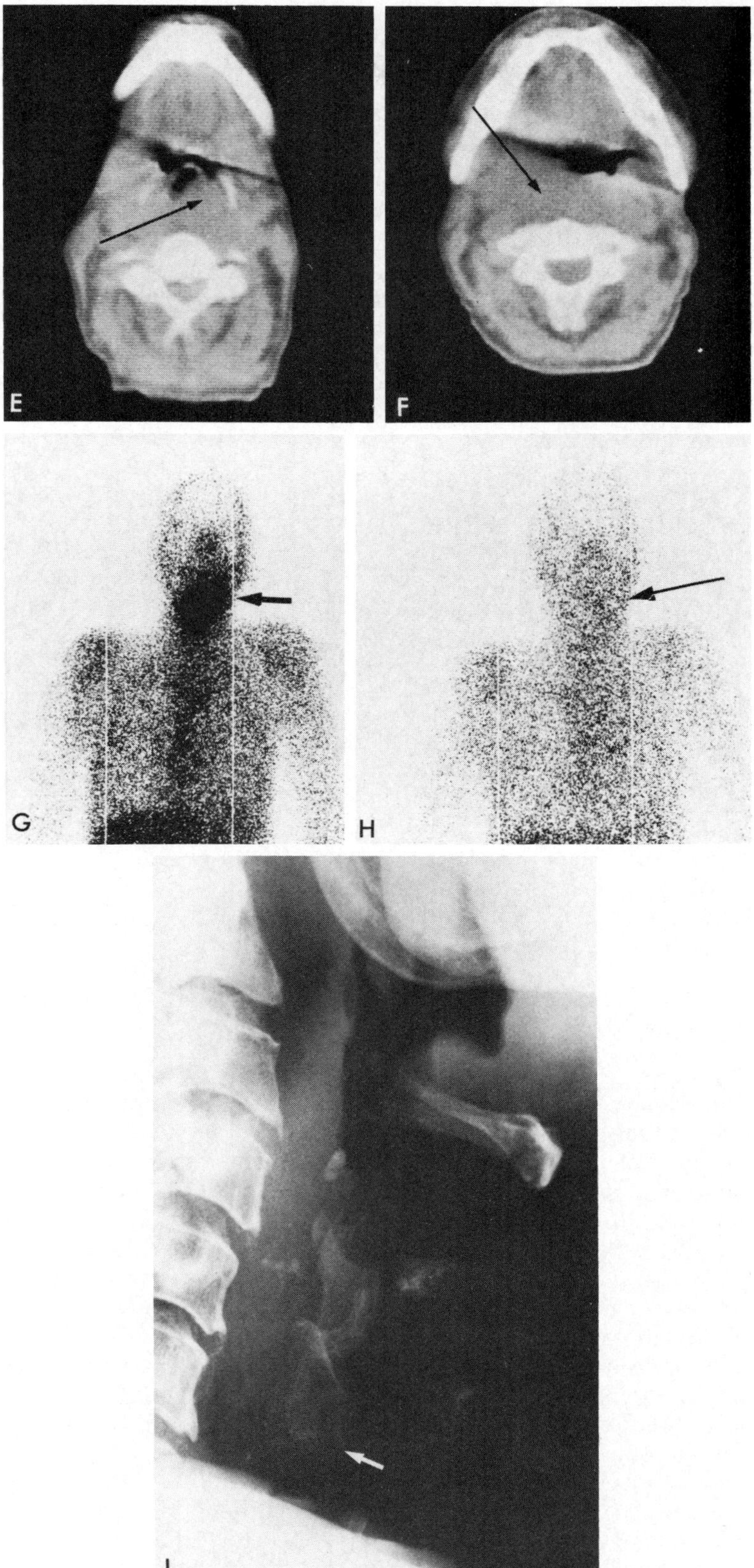

Figure 5–47 *Continued. E,* Encroachment of tumor on the epiglottis *(arrow).* The entire retropharynx is filled with tumor at this level. *F,* A cut considerably higher than *E,* showing the extension of the tumor in the retropharyngeal space *(arrow).*

G and *H,* Gallium-67 citrate scans before and after combination chemotherapy show the dramatic radionuclide response to tumor treatment. *G,* the gallium-positive scan prior to treatment *(arrow). H,* the radionuclide status two months after chemotherapy. The patient has experienced dramatic symptomatic improvement; the tumor has disappeared on gallium scan *(arrow).* (From Greyson ND, Toronto, private communication.)

I, Subsequently the patient's tumor recurred massively. A soft tissue radiograph demonstrates the lesser extent of tumor in the retropharynx, but an enormous mass is present in the hypopharynx and encroaches on the subglottic airway *(arrow).* The patient lived for six months after diagnosis.

diseases and tumors because of incorporation into actively reproducing cells. Its uptake in laryngeal carcinoma is inconsistent; it may image the primary carcinoma, its cervical lymph node metastases, neither, or both. It is useful, however, in the staging of the rare lymphoma or melanoma of the larynx; this is usually a postbiopsy diagnostic investigation.

Angiography. Superselective angiography[45–47] has application in the evaluation of major hemangiomas, other vascular tumors, and arteriovenous malformations involving the larynx. Here selective angiography may be combined with therapeutic intra-arterial embolization. Dynamic CT provides an effective imaging study for screening highly vascular lesions in the larynx and neck.

THE ROLE OF RADIOLOGIC EVALUATION IN THE DIFFERENTIAL DIAGNOSIS AND MANAGEMENT OF SPECIFIC LARYNGEAL DISORDERS

This section will attempt to correlate preferred radiologic imaging modalities with specific laryngeal disorders,[6, 40] with the purpose of allowing a realistic differential diagnosis and a rational basis for either further diagnostic studies or specific treatment options. These general correlations are amplified by a guide to laryngeal imaging, Table 5–1, which tabulates these concepts in detail.[40]

Congenital Disorders

In the area of congenital disorders, there are limited applications for radiologic evaluation.[48] Lateral soft tissue radiographs or xeroradiographs provide an overview of the airway; however, diagnostic imaging by these modes may be difficult because of the small size of the infant, especially if premature, and associated respiratory and somatic movement artifact. Radiographic images captured in expiration may appear to demonstrate more extensive airway collapse than is actually present. A water soluble contrast esophagram is mandatory if fistulas are considered or esophageal patency questioned. Major laryngeal abnormalities, such as laryngeal cleft, should be studied by CT; this may require a general anesthetic for appropriate examination.

Inflammatory Lesions

A variety of inflammatory lesions affect the larynx; radiodiagnostic imaging is useful both in primary diagnosis and in follow-up examination. Acute epiglottitis is usually a pediatric disorder; however, it can occur in the adult at any age and always produces a life-threatening situation. Massive edema displaces mucous membrane on both the lingual and laryngeal surfaces of the epiglottis, producing the radiologic image of an enlarged epiglottis. This correlates clinically with rapid but varying airway obstruction. As the inflammatory edema descends into the aryepiglottic folds and arytenoid region, airway compromise increases rapidly. The extent of airway compression can be evaluated on a soft tissue lateral radiograph or xeroradiograph by measuring the AP air space between the edematous epiglottis and the posterior pharyngeal wall; however, as acute epiglottitis is potentially a lethal disease, initial treatment with airway control should not be withheld pending radiologic investigation. Radiologic investigation is performed when the diagnosis is in doubt and foreign body or tumor remains a possibility. Soft tissue lateral radiography may also be useful in following the course of the disease, once treatment has been initiated, especially in the hard-to-examine patient. Acute supraglottic edema may appear as acute epiglottitis on soft tissue lateral radiographs. It occurs in the allergic patient as part of an acute hypersensitivity or anaphylactic reaction, or in the patient with angioneurotic edema.

Acute and chronic inflammatory disease of the laryngeal joints, especially the cricoarytenoid and cricothyroid articulations, can occur in rheumatoid arthritis and gout. Osteoarthritis usually presents with radiologic and clinical signs of fixation rather than inflammation. Conventional soft tissue lateral radiography may demonstrate edema confined to the region of the arytenoid eminences alone. This radiographic finding is not specific but is suggestive; however, especially in the acute phase of the disease, a positive delayed bone scan osteoblastic response should lead to the diagnosis of possible arthropathy, which should be clarified utilizing further appropriate additional laboratory methods.

Acute perichondritis usually complicates radiotherapy for laryngeal cancer. It can also occur following surgery or penetrating trauma. Most often, it indicates residual or recurrent

Table 5–1. GUIDE TO LARYNGEAL IMAGING*

Disorder	Soft Tissue Lateral	Xeroradio-graph	AP Tomo	High kV	Laryngogram	CT	Ultra-sound	Angio	Nuclear Medicine
Pediatric									
Subglottic and tracheal stenosis	G	G	E	E	C	G			
Laryngeal cleft	F	F				E			
Inflammation									
Epiglottitis	E	E	C	C	C	C			
Acute (e.g., diphtheria)	E	E		E	C				
Chronic (e.g., tuberculosis)	E	E			RIC	F			
Perichondritis and radionecrosis	G	G	G	G	C	E	G		G
Miscellaneous									
Foreign body	G	E	RIC			G			
Laryngocele	G	G	E	E		E	F		
Vocal cord paralysis			E	E	E				
Contact granuloma	G	E	G	F					
Arthropathy	F	F	F	F		F			G
Trauma									
Acute									
Airway	G	G	E	G	C	E			
Soft tissue	F	F	G	G	C	E			
Fracture	F	F	G		C	E	G		G
Sequelae									
Stenosis	G	G	E	G	E	RIC			
Fixation			E	E	E	RIC			
Benign tumors									
Multiple papillomatosis	G	G	G	G					
Hemangioma	G	G	E	E	C	E		RIC	G
Chondroma	G	E	E	G	F	E	E		
Lipoma		F	F		F	E			
Neurogenic	F	F	G	G	G	E		RIC	
Carcinoma site									
Supraglottic	E	E	G		E	E			
Glottic			E	F	E	RIC			
Subglottic	F	F	E	G	E	E			
Carcinoma extension									
Anterior commissure					E	E			
Opposite cord			G		G	G			
Preepiglottic space	F	F				E			
Subglottic space	F	F	E	E	E	E			
Cartilage/membrane	F	F	G			E	E		G
Laryngeal fixation			E	E	E	RIC			
Pyriform sinus			G		E	E			
Neck nodes						E	E		F

*Key: *E* = excellent; *G* = good; *F* = fair; *C* = contraindicated; *RIC* = requires intelligent communication between clinician and radiologist.
Adapted from Noyek AM et al.: J Otolaryngol. 11:178–185, 1982. Please see original article for particular footnotes and comments.

cancer in spite of radiation therapy (see the section on malignant tumors later in this chapter). In perichondritis, the laryngeal cartilage appears thickened, because of edema of the perichondrium itself. CT should detect this morphologic abnormality. Ultrasound may also demonstrate perichondrial thickening but is best utilized for the detection of focal abscess formation.

Relapsing perichondritis (or polychondritis) is a rare disorder in which there may be repetitive attacks of massive intralaryngeal edema caused by a sterile inflammatory reaction involving the perichondrium and adjacent soft tissues. This may be part of a systemic disorder affecting other cartilages (ear, nose, joint) and the cardiac valves. The blood pool phase of the bone scan will show marked hyperemia during the acute phase; this will clear dramatically with steroid therapy. The total body bone scan image should be reviewed critically.

Laryngeal tuberculosis is an occasional disorder. It usually occurs with active pulmonary tuberculosis and positive sputum. The nodular thickened turban epiglottis seen on mirror and telescopic examination produces a widened and deformed epiglottis on conventional soft tissue radiography and AP tomography. CT provides remarkable supraglottic detail, especially for both the destructive and proliferative signs of epiglottic involvement.

Other granulomas, whether from syphilis, fungus, or sarcoidosis, can also occur. The radiologic findings, regardless of modality utilized, usually suggest malignancy. Leprosy, for example, may present with a midline ulcer of the epiglottis. The pathologist, however, must provide the histologic diagnosis; the radiologist demonstrates only the extent of morphologic changes, which may also be important in post-treatment assessment.

Trauma and Its Complications

Laryngeal trauma[36, 50] comprises blunt and penetrating trauma, surgical trauma, endoscopic and postintubation trauma, and thermal and chemical injuries via the airway. Radiologic assessment[41, 42] is crucial for evaluation of the laryngeal airway, and CT is the critical definitive examination. Laryngeal trauma may be complex; it may involve mucosal integrity, soft tissue structures, and the cartilaginous framework. It may involve the airway at more than one level. It may affect vocal cord mobility either by primary neurogenic disruption or by the later onset of scarring, fixation, or cartilage displacements.

In acute trauma, compromise of the laryngeal airway at the supraglottic, glottic, and subglottic levels should be accurately and urgently assessed. Conventional radiology provides screening information and gives direction to CT studies. CT is a remarkable detector of laryngeal injury, at both the soft tissue and cartilage levels. Its use in laryngeal trauma is mandatory. CT detects hematomas, airway compromise, cartilage fractures, and cartilage fracture dislocations. It provides the critical assessment of the cervical spine at the same time in the patient who is at risk for cervical spine injury. This patient can be examined in a neck-stable position, while lying supine on the CT examining table. CT has thus superseded complex motion tomography in the evaluation of laryngeal trauma. Preliminary conventional films, however, give meaningful direction to CT studies.

Depending upon the nature and extent of the laryngeal trauma, and upon the success of initial treatment and healing capability, posttraumatic complications may ensue. Most complications result from extensive mucosal disruption with unfavorable healing, as well as significant cartilage displacement. Arytenoid dislocation is a common sequel and is easily imaged by CT.

Stenosis in one or more areas of the larynx requires careful diagnosis. Here, laryngography, in the uncompromised airway, gives an excellent overview of the vertical dimension of airway involvement at all levels. This is particularly important prior to surgical intervention or reconstruction. Individual areas of stenosis are very effectively imaged by CT but are best imaged when CT is given direction by other conventional studies. Thus xeroradiography, high kV selective filtration radiography, and even AP tomography have occasional application.

We must briefly acknowledge the continued role of laryngography in treatment of the posttraumatic stenotic larynx and trachea. When the airway is not grossly compromised, contrast laryngography still provides the best overview in the vertical dimension of the entire larynx and cervical trachea. It enables the surgeon to visualize, with clear measurements and reference points, those areas of the larynx and trachea that are so compromised as to require surgical intervention. Multiple CT slices, unless accurately preview-positioned, cannot provide the conceptual presurgical input that the laryngologist usually requires. While CT provides definitive axial information at a particular level, these localized images remain isolated in the mind's eye, and the overall architecture of the airway is thus more readily appreciated by utilization of a positive contrast study. Further, in order to study the entire laryngotracheal tree that might be at risk, an inordinate number of CT cuts would be required, each with its individual 2 rad radiation exposure. Additionally, if the possibility of stenosis exists at the level of the tracheal bifurcation, the role of the contrast laryngotracheogram is preeminent.

Extensive trauma may be followed not only by more than one area of stenosis but also by more than one type of complication. Vocal cord paralysis and vocal cord fixation are other important complications that should be evaluated by a laryngeal imaging functional study.

Laryngeal stenosis is not always a sequel of trauma; it can follow extensive scarring after inflammatory diseases such as tuberculosis or diphtheria. Inflammatory lesions such as these appear to produce delayed effects in the subglottic region with webs and stenosis. Acquired stenoses are usually eccentric, whereas congenital stenoses are uniform and centric.

Foreign Bodies

Foreign bodies in the larynx are relatively uncommon. When one is present, accurate radiologic assessment is crucial, especially if it is suspected in the subglottic area, which may be life-threatening. Foreign bodies may produce major airway obstruction and, as with acute epiglottitis, while radiologic examination may be of real value it should not precede the securing of an adequate airway if the patient's condition so warrants.

Conventional soft tissue radiographs may suffice for foreign body assessment, especially for radiopaque foreign bodies; however, when foreign bodies are only faintly calcified, xeroradiography may prove useful in distinguishing the calcified foreign body from the overlying or adjacent calcified or ossified laryngeal framework. As with stenoses, foreign bodies may be multiple.

In foreign body evaluation, a rare CT examination may be indicated when conventional studies are equivocal and suspicion of a small metallic foreign body remains exceedingly high. Here the image hopes for streaking density artifacts to help localize the elusive foreign body. CT has obvious value in the possible infective complications of foreign bodies and their operative manipulation.

When dysphagia is present in conjunction with a foreign body, conventional radiologic studies usually suffice. If, however, a foreign body within the upper digestive tract is not identifiable, a small amount of cotton soaked in barium sulfate should be utilized as a mini-esophagram.

Laryngocele

Laryngocele is a unique mechanical disorder of the larynx, arising from obstruction of the saccule of the laryngeal ventricle. The laryngocele may occasionally be fluid-filled, as a sterile noninfected lesion. Occasionally it may become a laryngopyocele from supervening infection. If air-containing, the internal laryngocele, the external laryngocele, and the mixed internal-external laryngocele should easily be recognized by conventional radiologic examination and by AP examination such as the high kV selective filtration radiograph or coronal tomogram. Though CT provides a definitive examination, it is often unnecessary. The critical role for CT lies in the differential diagnosis of the fluid-filled internal laryngocele from the solid supraglottic tumor mass.

Benign Tumors

A variety of benign tumors, most of which are rather rare, can affect the larynx.[6, 49–56] A small discrete lesion, confined to one region and clearly visualized clinically, requires no radiologic imaging. It is only when the extent of the lesion is uncertain or its nature is questioned that radiodiagnostic imaging is introduced.

Xeroradiography provides an excellent overview of the larynx and the trachea in disorders such as papillomatosis in the child, juvenile, or adult. The presence of diffuse or localized calcification in a submucosal mass, or even overt ossification, suggests a benign chondroma, osteochondroma, or tracheopathia osteoplastica. This latter lesion has a predilection for the cricolarynx.

Osteochondromas may arise from any of the laryngeal cartilages but have a predilection for origination from the inner aspect of the posterior portion of the cricoid arch; thus the tumor narrows the subglottic airway in AP dimension. This tumor is most effectively imaged by axial

CT; CT allows for diagnostic morphologic display and also detects the tumor's intraluminal and extralaryngeal extension. Even CT, however, does not differentiate between the benign osteochondroma and the malignant osteochondrosarcoma.

Other benign tumors do rarely occur. A lipoma may be identified on CT by its fat density and corresponding negative CT number. A cavernous hemangioma may be identified by its spheroid calcific phleboliths; its vascular physiologic nature may be detected by rapid sequential contrast-infusion CT scanning or dynamic scanning. The election of angiography more closely parallels treatment rather than diagnostic options.

Malignant Tumors

Of malignant tumors of the larynx[6, 32–35, 57–60] the most common is primary squamous cell carcinoma, which arises from the mucosal surface of the supraglottis or glottis. Rarely does it arise primarily in the subglottis. When extensive tumor involves both glottic and supraglottic regions, or when the tumor is transglottic, involving all three regions, determining an initial site of origin may be difficult. Other malignant tumors, though rare, may affect the larynx either primarily or secondarily. Tumors may be of minor salivary gland origin, as is the adenoid cystic carcinoma, or they may arise from the laryngeal framework, as do the sarcoma group of tumors.

The occasional lymphoma or sarcoma usually presents as a smooth mass lesion and, except for chondrosarcoma, presents little in the way of specific diagnostic roentgenographic signs. Leiomyosarcoma may present as a lobulated subglottic tracheal mass. Anaplastic carcinoma of the thyroid gland may invade the larynx, producing cartilage destruction and direct extension into the subglottic or tracheal airway. These changes should be detected by tomography, xeroradiography, or CT for proper treatment evaluation and follow-up. An occasional malignancy, such as hypernephroma, may metastasize to the larynx.

In all laryngeal malignancy, the role of radiology is to define both the site of malignancy and the extent of tumor. In squamous cell carcinoma of the larynx, the role is even more precise; it provides critical input for the TNM staging classification, particularly in terms of the T staging of the tumor and especially in the critical identification of the T3 and T4 laryngeal carcinoma. Hence it directs cancer management. The role of CT in this regard is paramount; prior to the advent of CT, approximately 50 per cent of T3 and T4 carcinomas were understaged. The contemporary role of laryngeal imaging involves both N stage diagnosis (especially in the search for occult neck node metastases) and M stage search for systemic metastases. The chest x-ray, the liver-spleen scan, and the total body bone scan provide the elements of this diagnostic search when occasioned. The correlation of laryngeal cancer with other primary malignancies of the lung and the rest of the upper aerodigestive tract is well established.

All laryngeal cancer treatment depends upon accurate staging and classification. Radiologic criteria often provide crucial input, particularly in the presence of bulky lesions that obscure underlying structures and are therefore inaccurately evaluated from the topographic point of view, even at direct endoscopy. The critical capability of radiologic imaging to localize most tumors by region and extension leads to effective informed decisions regarding conservation surgery. We still find a role for AP tomography, which gives an excellent overview evaluation, in vertical dimension, in the laryngeal cancer patient and directs the subsequent CT study: it may therefore result in a shorter CT study and a more directed and effective CT study. In either event, the multiplanar approach satisfies the need to understand the three-dimensional relationships of the tumor.

The initial baseline radiographic examination in suspected laryngeal cancer is the conventional soft tissue lateral radiograph. This usually permits adequate contrast of mucosal detail against the endolaryngeal air shadow, especially in supraglottic carcinoma. There is, of course, the additional possibility of detecting cartilage destruction. When supraglottic extension of squamous cell carcinoma into the base of the tongue is considered, the lateral conventional radiograph (or xeroradiograph) plays a role with CT. The role of xeroradiography in improving conventional lateral laryngeal imaging at both the mucosal and framework level has been noted earlier in this chapter. Similarly, the screening role of high kV selective filtration radiography has been placed in perspective for the laryngeal cancer patient.

If AP tomography is utilized for a vertical display overview in laryngeal cancer, it should always be combined with functional assessment. Subtle signs, such as loss of mucosal distensibility, are often indicants of subjacent tumor infiltration. Generally, AP tomography provides a good overview evaluation of the epiglottis, aryepiglottic folds, ventricles, false and true cords, and subglottic angles (which are normally 90 to 120 degrees). If cartilage destruction is demonstrated, it is usually a fortuitous finding in patients whose thyroid alae are sufficiently calcified or ossified to be imageable and where pathology can be recognized. Pyriform sinus evaluation may also be possible, depending upon the imaging plane. Functional assessment is important in the demonstration of vocal cord fixation caused either by neurogenic involvement of the recurrent laryngeal nerve or by direct tumor infiltration of the vocalis muscle.

Laryngography continues to have selective application, but its role has been diminished dramatically by CT; it now assumes a role complementary to CT in critical evaluation. As laryngography is an invasive technique, it must be elected with care. Its use is usually occasioned when a critical mucous membrane evaluation is still sought. Larger lesions, which prolapse into the glottis, might be better defined by laryngography. Ulcerative lesions in the region of the anterior commissure also lend themselves to laryngographic imaging.

In the radiologic evaluation of laryngeal cancer, the primary role now falls to computed tomography. Areas of application of CT will be discussed in detail after these comments on the use of ultrasound and radionuclide scans.

Ultrasound's sensitivity to thyroid cartilage destruction remains its only area of predictable value. It easily and inexpensively confirms or denies the suspicion of cartilage destruction seen on conventional or CT examinations. Vertical ultrasound demonstrates parasagittal anatomy in T4 cancer as well. Essentially, ultrasound defines the cortical surface of the thyroid cartilage independent of the degree of calcification.

Radionuclide techniques tend to have little application in the T stage radiologic diagnosis of laryngeal cancer. Positive bone scan changes reflect advanced and extensive cartilage destruction, which can usually be detected by other means; however, radionuclide scans do have value in M staging. Systemic bony metastases are detected by total body bone scan. Here physiologic changes in bone are detected in advance of the skeletal x-ray findings of the conventional metastatic survey. Of course, other studies such as liver-spleen scans and the conventional chest x-ray supplement the diagnostic process.

Gallium scanning has been referred to as a postbiopsy study, usually when an unexpected lymphoma is encountered within the larynx and systemic staging is sought. On the occasion when radionuclide gallium scanning does allow for squamous cell carcinoma imaging, it may be selectively useful in assessing the treatment response to chemotherapy and in the detection of recurrence.

The most dramatic addition to the armamentarium of the laryngologist and laryngeal radiologist in the evaluation of laryngeal cancer has been the advent of CT. It has a number of remarkable areas of application, and all should be enumerated here. Its role lies in the demonstration of mucosal extension, submucosal infiltration (whether of muscle or fat plane), and cartilage framework encroachment.

CT and Glottic Carcinoma. Localized lesions (T1), clearly recognized as such, require minimal if any imaging. When CT is performed, these early lesions may not be seen at all, or they may present as thickening (focal or diffuse) or merely as contour abnormalities. Because tumor and muscle are of the same CT density and characteristics, invasion of the true cord musculature is difficult to assess. For the same reason, edema related to tumor or to radiation treatment of tumor can mimic tumor extension itself. Tumor extending vertically in the paralaryngeal fat spaces or laterally into the neck can only be shown on CT.

With its inherent slice thickness, CT is occasionally unable to totally define the transition from glottis to supraglottis or from true to false cord. This is especially important in bulky supraglottic tumors and can lead to understaging of such tumors. While the true and false cords can be fairly accurately separated by morphologic CT characteristics based on size and shape of the airway, density, and recognition of surrounding structures (e.g., pyriform sinus), this is not entirely adequate for use as an absolute surgical guide. Glottic cancer assessment therefore remains the ultimate mandate of direct laryngoscopy or open surgery; however, recent CT work with infusion techniques shows promise of increased diagnostic contribution in this area, as subtle mucous membrane changes can be imaged. The major contribution of CT in glottic cancer, therefore, is in the evaluation of involvement of the anterior and posterior commissure, the cartilages, and the paralaryngeal space.

Anterior Commissure. As indicated previously, there is normally no anterior soft tissue thickness at the level of the anterior commissure. Any increase in thickness is therefore abnormal, but hemorrhage and edema will exhibit the same soft tissue density as tumor.

Posterior Commissure. Posteriorly, at this level, the space around the arytenoid and thyroid cartilages had never been satisfactorily visualized prior to CT. If the patient is properly centered, the arytenoids and their relationship to thyroid and cricoid cartilages are symmetric bilaterally. Tumor extension posteriorly may therefore be seen as an increase in thickness of the tissue between the arytenoid and the adjacent thyroid cartilage. Tumor extension may be accompanied by rotation or displacement of the arytenoid cartilage, or its inferior egress from the larynx posterolaterally may be noted.

Cartilage. Where cartilage is well mineralized, it is clearly depicted. Tumor involvement of cartilage may present as either a decreased density (because of destruction) or increased density (especially of the arytenoids, because of a primary osteoblastic response to the tumor itself). The difficulty in identifying cartilaginous involvement lies in the normal variability of the degree of mineralization, particularly when the pattern of calcification and ossification is not only nonhomogeneous but asymmetric. In the case of overt destruction of cartilage, there is little doubt on CT examination; subtle changes give cause for concern and suggest verification by other means (such as contact B-mode ultrasound).

Cartilage involvement may occasionally be inferred by distortion or bowing of the cartilage, without destruction. Such bowing is seen in anterior thyroid cartilage tumor extension. In addition to distortion of the cartilage contour, there may be collapse, displacement, or rotation due to tumor bulk. There may be loss of integrity of the connecting membranes (cricothyroid, thyrohyoid). This latter situation may result in the imaging of more of one cartilage than expected on a particular CT slice.

The Paralaryngeal Space. At the true cord level, this space may occasionally be seen as a fine line of reduced (fat) density lying just medial to the inner aspect of the thyroid cartilage. The absence of the paralaryngeal space, bilaterally, is not necessarily significant since this natural space terminates at the level of the glottis; however, if the line is visible on one side but absent on the side of the pathology, this is strongly suggestive of tumor invasion of the paralaryngeal space. At the false cord level, the widening of the paralaryngeal space makes invasion easier to detect. The paired paralaryngeal spaces communicate superiorly with the preepiglottic space; the paralaryngeal spaces provide easy access for vertical extension of laryngeal cancer.

CT and Supraglottic Carcinoma. Tumors above the false cords are mainly epiglottic and may be categorized as suprahyoid and infrahyoid, though this itself is descriptive rather than practical. Suprahyoid epiglottic lesions may vary in appearance from simple thickening of one of the margins of the epiglottis to a large bulky mass obscuring all normal landmarks. Extension can occur anteriorly to the valleculae and base of tongue, laterally along the pharyngoepiglottic folds, anteroinferiorly into the preepiglottic space, and posteroinferiorly along the aryepiglottic folds and into the marginal region. Access to the paralaryngeal space occurs in continuity with preepiglottic space involvement. Tumor spread into the preepiglottic space or paralaryngeal space is inferred by replacement of fat density by soft tissue density, keeping in mind that hemorrhage and edema are generally indistinguishable (by CT number) from tumor; equally, it should be kept in mind that these changes should always be considered tumor until proven otherwise.

CT and Subglottic Carcinoma. Extension below the cords posteriorly may result in medial displacement of the arytenoids. If the tumor mass extends below the glottis, the mass itself will be identifiable. At the level of the cricoid ring, any soft tissue thickness lining the airway is absolute evidence of subglottic tumor extension. Cricoid destruction, although not common, is critical information in the assessment of carcinoma for treatment. The constancy of calcification of this cartilage allows confident detection of destruction.

CT and Lymph Nodes. CT of the larynx with contrast enhancement allows the identification of normal and enlarged lymph nodes (the lymph nodes will have a soft tissue CT number while the contrast-enhanced vasculature will have a much higher number). Mancuso[38, 39] has developed criteria for assessing lymph nodes for malignant involvement and cautions that size alone may introduce false results. Small discrete nodes may or may not be involved with early tumor spread. Ill-defined nodes, particularly if enlarged (greater than 2 cm), are almost always involved with tumor.

CT and Postradiation Changes. Individual response to radiation therapy varies considerably. As tumor dose reaches 2,000 to 3,000 rads and above, edema of the mucosa and submucosa causes an increase in size of the soft tissues that is indistinguishable in density from tumor on CT. If the edema involves the cricoarytenoid joint, vocal cord mobility will be affected. Edema usually reaches its maximum two to five weeks after radiation therapy has terminated and slowly subsides over the ensuing four to six weeks.

Perichondritis, which may be visualized as an increase in cartilaginous density (especially of the arytenoids), may progress to chondronecrosis. The epiglottic cartilage is frequently involved. Involvement of the base of the epiglottis is manifested by thickening of the soft tissues just above the anterior commissure. Thyroid cartilage involvement is also common.

Postradiation recurrence of laryngeal cancer presents an especially difficult problem. The signs of residual or recurrent disease depend on comparative pretreatment and posttreatment radiologic studies. Until the 1980s, comparative coronal tomograms, with or without lateral xeroradiographs, were usually utilized to follow the postradiation larynx, supplemented by direct laryngoscopy and biopsy. CT has radically altered this imaging need, with postradiation baseline examinations being carried out at six to twelve weeks posttreatment and subsequently as required. Though CT (especially with rapid infusion mucosal staining) may suggest the presence of recurrent tumor, the differential problem of edema versus recurrent tumor largely remains. When a mass has not responded appropriately to radiotherapy, or when an enlarging soft tissue mass is noted following radiotherapy, recurrence is presumed and endoscopic biopsy is mandatory. The conventional radiographic signs[60] that suggest a recurrence or failure of therapy apply equally to CT examination. These signs are: (1) an increasing localized soft tissue mass on serial examination, (2) progressive loss of subglottic angle, (3) erosion or ulceration of mucosal structures within the larynx that were previously known to be intact, (4) vocal cord fixation or alteration in cord movement, as a new finding, (5) increase in cartilage demineralization or destruction, and (6) persistent mass three to four months after therapy.

Miscellaneous Disorders

As indicated previously, vocal cord paralysis or fixation can be primarily detected or confirmed by radiologic evaluation combined with functional studies. This has been dealt with earlier in this chapter.

The larynx is a unique structure within the airway. It can be affected by a variety of unusual conditions that the laryngologist should anticipate encountering, within the sphere of his practice, from time to time.[61] Unusual systemic diseases may present with laryngeal manifestations. Miscellaneous inflammatory disorders include fungal infections, infective granulomas such as syphilis and leprosy, sarcoidosis, and rhinoscleroma. Mechanical lesions such as large retention cysts or laryngeal tonsils may be encountered. Amyloidosis may occur within the airway; it has a predilection for deposits in relation to cartilage. Lethal midline granuloma can also affect the larynx and trachea. It is impossible to suggest the gamut of lesions that can affect the larynx; lesion localization and size evaluation may rest with the radiologist, but histologic diagnosis rests with the pathologist. For extensive coverage of such lesions, see Chapter 13 of this volume, Nonsurgical Conditions of the Larynx.

References

1. Noyek AM et al.: Sophisticated radiology in otolaryngology: II. Diagnostic imaging: Non-roentgenographic (non-x-ray) modalities. J Otolaryngol 6(Suppl. 3): 95–117, 1977.
2. Noyek AM: Some comments on the art of diagnosis. Otolaryngol Clin North Am 2(2):247–249, 1978.
3. Hickey PM: Radiography of normal larynx. Radiology 11:409–411, 1928.
4. Iglauer S: Value of roentgenography in the diagnosis of the larynx and the trachea. JAMA 63:1827–1881, 1914.
5. Noyek AM, Zizmor J: The evolution of diagnostic radiology of the larynx. J Otolaryngol 6(Suppl. 3): 12–16, 1977.
6. Zizmor J, Noyek AM: An Atlas of Otolaryngologic Radiology. Philadelphia, WB Saunders Company, 1978.
7. Gay BB Jr, Wilkins SA Jr: The fluoroscope with image amplifier in the study of the larynx and pharynx. Cancer 9:1253–1260, 1956.
8. Jackson C: Value of roentgenography of the neck. Trans Am Laryngol 58:112–131, 1936.
9. Coutard H: Note preliminaire sur la radiographie du larynx normal et du larynx cancereaux. J Belge Radiol 13:287, 1922.
10. Kushner DC, Harris GBC: Obstructing lesions of the larynx and trachea in infants and children. Radiol Clin North Am 16(2):181–194, 1978.
11. Maguire GH et al.: Selective filtration: Practical approach to high-kilovoltage radiography. Radiology 85:343–351, 1965.
12. Maguire GH: The larynx: Simplified radiological examination using heavy filtration and high voltage. Radiology 87:102–109, 1966.
13. Noyek AM et al.: Sophisticated radiology in otolaryngology: I. Diagnostic imaging: Roentgenographic (x-ray) modalities. J Otolaryngol 6(Suppl. 3):73–94, 1977.
14. Doust BD, Ting YM: Xeroradiography of the larynx. Radiology 110:727–730, 1974.

15. Hemmingsson A, Lofroth PO: Xeroradiography and conventional radiography in examination of the larynx. Acta Radiol [Diagn] (Stockh) 17:723–732, 1976.
16. Noyek AM et al.: Xeroradiography in otolaryngology. Otolaryngol Clin North Am. 2(2):445–456, 1978.
17. Holinger PH et al.: Xeroradiography of the larynx. Ann Otol Rhinol Laryngol 81:806–808, 1972.
18. Samuel E: Xerography or conventional radiography for laryngeal examination? Can J Otolaryngol 4(1):59–63, 1975.
19. Johns HE et al.: Electrostatic methods of imaging in diagnostic radiology. Can J Otolaryngol 4(1):102–110, 1975.
20. Noyek AM et al.: Xeroradiography in the assessment of the pediatric larynx and trachea. J Otolaryngol 5(6):468–474, 1976.
21. Canuyt G, Gunsett A: La tomographie ou planigraphie du larynx pathologique: Methode des coupes ou sections radiographiques. Ann d'Otolaryngol 987–994, 1937.
22. Leborgne FE: Tomography, Cancer Laryngotomographia. Montevideo, K. Garcia Morales, 1938.
23. Leborgne FE: Tomography and cancer of the larynx. Arch Otolaryngol 31:419–425, 1940.
24. Leborgne FE: Tomographic study of cancer of the larynx. Am J Roentgenol 43:493–499, 1940.
25. Olofsson J et al.: Radiologic-pathologic correlations in laryngeal carcinoma. Can J Otolaryngol 4(1):86–96, 1975.
26. Iglauer S: Use of injected iodized oil in roentgen ray diagnosis of laryngeal, tracheal, and bronchopulmonary conditions. JAMA 86:1879, 1926.
27. Farinas PL: Mucosagraphy of respiratory tract. Radiology 39:84–87, 1942.
28. Landman GHM: Laryngography cinelaryngography, and 70 mm intensifier fluorography in diagnosis of laryngeal cancer. Can J Otolaryngol 4(1):74–80, 1975.
29. Landman GHM: Laryngography and Cinelaryngography. Amsterdam, Excerpta Medica Foundation, 1970.
30. Ogura JH et al.: Laryngograms: Their value in the diagnosis and treatment of laryngeal lesions. Laryngoscope 70:780–809, 1960.
31. Powers WE et al.: Contrast examination of the larynx and pharynx. Radiology 68:169–177, 1957.
32. Mancuso AA et al.: The role of computed tomography in the management of cancer of the larynx. Radiology 124:243–244, 1977.
33. Mancuso AA et al.: Computed tomography of the larynx. Radiol Clin North Am 16(2):195–208, 1978.
34. Archer CR et al.: Computed tomography of the larynx. J Comput Assist Tomogr 2:404–441, 1978.
35. Mancuso AA, Hanafee WN: A comparative evaluation of computed tomography and laryngography. Radiology 133:131–138, 1979.
36. Mancuso AA, Hanafee WN: Computed tomography of the injured larynx. AJR 133:139–144, 1979.
37. Gamsu G et al.: CT in carcinoma of the larynx and pyriform sinus: Value of phonation scans. AJR 136:577–584, 1981.
38. Mancuso AA et al.: CT of cervical lymph node cancer. AJR 136:381–385, 1981.
39. Mancuso AA, Hanafee WN: Computed tomography of the head and neck. Baltimore, Williams and Wilkins, 1982.
40. Noyek AM et al.: Contemporary laryngeal radiology—A clinical perspective. J Otolaryngol 11(3): 178–185, 1982.
41. Shulman HS et al.: CT of the larnyx. J Otolaryngol 11(6):395–406, 1982.
42. Miskin M et al.: Diagnostic ultrasound in otolaryngology. J Otolaryngol 2(2):513–530, 1978.
43. Greyson ND, Noyek AM: Nuclear medicine in otolaryngological diagnosis. Otolaryngol Clin North Am 2(2):541–560, 1978.
44. Noyek AM: Bone scanning in otolaryngology. Laryngscope 89(Suppl. 18, No. 9, Part 2):1–87, 1979.
45. Freeland AP: Microfil angiography: A demonstration of the microvasculature of the larynx with reference to tumor spread. Can J Otolaryngol 4(1):111–127, 1975.
46. Holgate RC et al.: Angiography in otolaryngology: Anatomy, methodology, complications and contraindications. J Otolaryngol 2(2):457–475, 1978.
47. Holgate RC et al.: Angiogrpahy in otolaryngology: Indications and applications. J Otolaryngol 2(2):477–499, 1978.
48. Momose KJ, MacMillan AS Jr: Roentgenologic investigation of the larynx and trachea. Radiol Clin North Am 16(2):321–341, 1978.
49. Bachman AL: Benign, non-neoplastic conditions of the larynx and pharynx. Radiol Clin North Am 16(2):273–290, 1978.
50. Greene R, Stark P: Trauma of the larynx and trachea. Radiol Clin North Am 16(2):309–320, 1978.
51. Goldberg M et al.: Laryngeal granuloma secondary to gastroesophageal reflux. J Otolaryngol 7(3):196–202, 1978.
52. Cocke EW: Benign cartilaginous tumors of the larynx. Laryngoscope 72:1678–1730, 1962.
53. Ryan MD, Zizmor J: Chondroma of the larynx. Am J Roentgenol Radium Ther Nucl Med 62:715–717, 1949.
54. Zizmor J et al.: The radiologic diagnosis of chondroma and chondrosarcoma of the larynx. Arch Otolaryngol 101:232–234, 1975.
55. Weber AL et al.: Cartilaginous tumors of the larynx and trachea. Radiol Clin North Am 16(2):261–271, 1978.
56. Noyek AM et al.: Familial Warthin's tumor: 1. Its synchronous occurrence in mother and son, 2. Its association with cystic oncocytic metaplasia of the larynx. J Otolaryngol 9(1):90–96, 1980.
57. Noyek AM, et al.: The radiologic diagnosis of malignant tumors of the larynx. J Otolaryngol 6(5):368–373, 1977.
58. Jing B-S: Roentgen examination of laryngeal cancer: A critical evaluation. Can J Otolaryngol 4(1):64–73, 1975.
59. Jing B-S: Malignant tumors of the larynx. Radiol Clin North Am 16(2):247–260, 1978.
60. Rideout DF: Appearances of the larynx after radiation therapy. Can J Otolaryngol 4(1):98–101, 1975.
61. Zizmor J, Noyek AM: Some miscellaneous disorders of the larynx and pharynx. Semin Roentgenol 9(4):311–322, 1974.

PART II

SURGERY FOR BENIGN LESIONS OF THE LARYNX

6

Endoscopic Surgery of the Larynx

M. Stuart Strong, M.D.

Endoscopic examination and surgery of the larynx have come a long way since the advent of the early direct laryngoscopes used by Kirstein, Yankauer, and others at the turn of the century. Although it had become possible to obtain samples of tissue for biopsy by indirect laryngoscopy, it soon was recognized that the direct examination using a self-illuminated tube and cup forceps would allow more accurate sampling of the diseased tissue.

Direct laryngoscopy soon became firmly established as a diagnostic modality using inspection, palpation, and tissue biopsy. Treatment was limited to removal of polypoidal masses, applications of caustics, and dilatation. Operative laryngoscopy for localized cancers was successfully carried out and reported by Lynch[1] in 1920 and, thereafter, by New[2] and Lillie.[3]

Detailed inspection of the larynx and operation in other than the ideal candidate for laryngoscopy were difficult until the advent of the small bore, cuffed endotracheal tube.[4] This technological advance provided control of the airway so that examination and treatment could proceed in an orderly and unhurried fashion.

Laryngoscopy was limited by the use of narrow endoscopic tubes illuminated by incandescent bulbs. Jako and Kleinsasser spearheaded the development of wide bore laryngoscopes with fiberoptic illumination for use with the operating microscope. Microscopic laryngoscopy and microsurgery of the larynx came of age in 1970.[5]

Most recently, the carbon dioxide laser has been adapted to the surgical microscope, and extensive surgery can be performed endoscopically with minimal morbidity.[6]

INSTRUMENTS

Laryngoscopes. To meet the needs of the entire spectrum of patients with laryngeal disease, including the "difficult patient," a modest variety of laryngoscopes is needed (Fig. 6–1). The complete armamentarium is composed of four sizes of Jako-Pilling laryngoscopes, two sizes of Dedo-Pilling laryngoscopes, and one Lynch suspension laryngoscope.

The Jako-Pilling laryngoscopes are available either with large or small light cables; the large cables are needed for photography and television demonstration but are not necessary for routine surgery. The Dedo-Pilling instruments provide only incomplete binocular vision and limited illumination for teaching and photography. For getting the job done in the difficult patient, however, they are unsurpassed.

Adult Males. In the average male who does not present unusual difficulty factors,[7] the adult

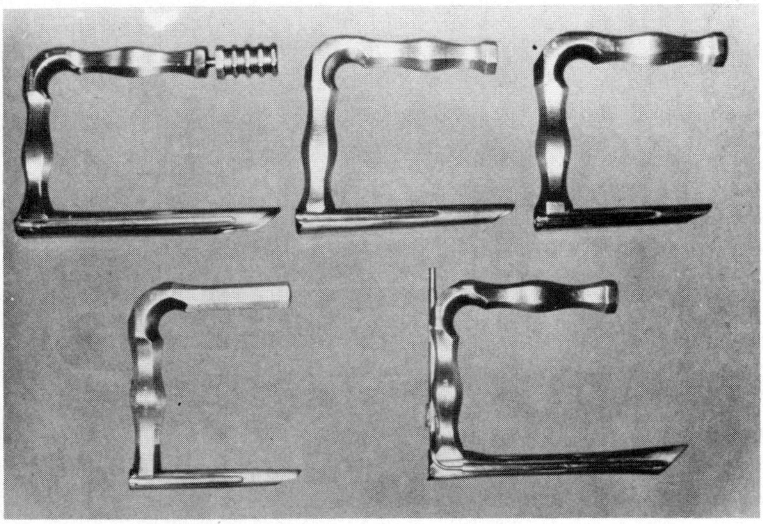

Figure 6–1. These laryngoscopes, four sizes of the Jako-Pilling instruments and the Dedo-Pilling laryngoscope, are needed to take care of males, females, children, infants, and the difficult adult. Note the detachable extension on the handle of the largest Jako-Pilling laryngoscope.

size Jako-Pilling laryngoscope with large fiberoptic bundles is ideal for inspection and microsurgery. In 10 per cent to 20 per cent of patients, however, this large bore laryngoscope cannot be used because of difficulty with lack of extension at the atlantooccipital joint, a narrow mandibular arch, or other commonly appreciated problems. In these patients, the Dedo-Pilling laryngoscope, which is modeled after the anterior commissure laryngoscope, can almost always be inserted to expose all areas of the larynx.

Adult Females. Usually the female size Jako-Pilling laryngoscope is suitable for microscopic examination and treatment of the adult female larynx. Occasionally the beak of the laryngoscope is too broad to fit into the anterior larynx between the false cords. In this case it is necessary to use the Dedo-Pilling laryngoscope to obtain a better view of the anterior commissure.

Children. The flexibility and mobility of the tissues and joints in children make it possible to use the Jako-Pilling child size laryngoscope in almost every instance. If the view of the anterior subglottic area is inadequate, the child size Dedo-Pilling should be used.

Infants. An excellent view of the infant larynx can be obtained with the infant size Jako-Pilling laryngoscope in almost every instance.

Special Procedures. In certain circumstances such as during endoscopic epiglottectomy or arytenoidectomy, it is difficult to work within the limited confines of a tubular laryngoscope. In most patients, increased access can be obtained with the Lynch suspension laryngoscope (Fig. 6–2). Depending on the procedure, it may

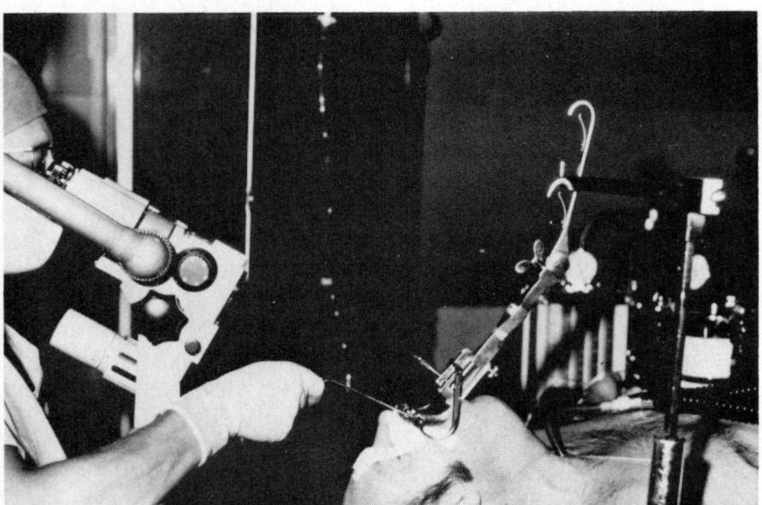

Figure 6–2. The Lynch suspension laryngoscope is seen here, suspended on the Killian gallows.

be necessary to augment the width of the tongue blade of the instrument to better support the base of the tongue.

Laryngoscope Suspension and Holder Devices. The adequacy of the exposure that can be obtained with a given laryngoscope depends in large measure both on the positioning of the patient and on the type of holding device that is used.

For all children and many easily examined adults (for example, edentulous patients), the standard Jackson type of laryngoscope handles can be fixed in position with the Lewy laryngoscope holder. This holder is light, easily attached and detached, and provides excellent stabilization of the laryngoscope within the larynx.

In the difficult patient, however, the Lewy holder does not allow proper positioning of the patient for endoscopy and is likely to exert unacceptable pressure on the maxillary teeth. For these patients, the Boston University–Pilling suspension gallows[7] provides ideal working conditions. The gallows allows proper positioning of the head and neck and minimizes pressure on the maxillary teeth while providing maximal exposure of the anterior commissure and stability for the laryngoscope. Use of the gallows does require the fitting of an inexpensive removable extension piece on the Jackson handle of the laryngoscope (Fig. 6–1). The gallows, of course, can also be used to suspend the Lynch suspension laryngoscope (Fig. 6–3).

Other Instruments. A standard operating microscope is necessary for precise examination and surgery of the larynx. To provide an adequate working distance and binocular vision, the microscope should be fitted with a 400-mm front lens. For surgeons of short stature, a 350-mm front lens may be used so that the surgeon may reach the operative site more comfortably while retaining nearly complete binocular vision.

Fine dissecting instruments are required for microsurgery of the larynx. The following should be available for routine use: suction tips (plain and insulated), cup forceps (upturned and straight), scissors (upturned and straight), probes (straight and right-angled), alligator forceps, scalpels, mirrors, sponge holder, and caliper (Fig. 6–4).

ANESTHESIA FOR ENDOSCOPIC SURGERY OF THE LARYNX

In order to carry out a thorough intralaryngeal examination and precise endoscopic surgery, ideal operating conditions must prevail. The patient must be completely relaxed at all times and the airway must be secure so that the procedure can be done in an orderly fashion without the need to hurry. These conditions are best provided through close collaboration between the surgeon and anesthesiologist. Thus, the anesthesiologist will understand the needs of the surgeon and can develop confidence in the surgeon so that he will not be concerned about losing control of the airway at any time during the procedure.

Details of the known pathological problems and the procedure must be discussed with the anesthesiologist prior to induction of the anesthesia. This is especially true if there are any

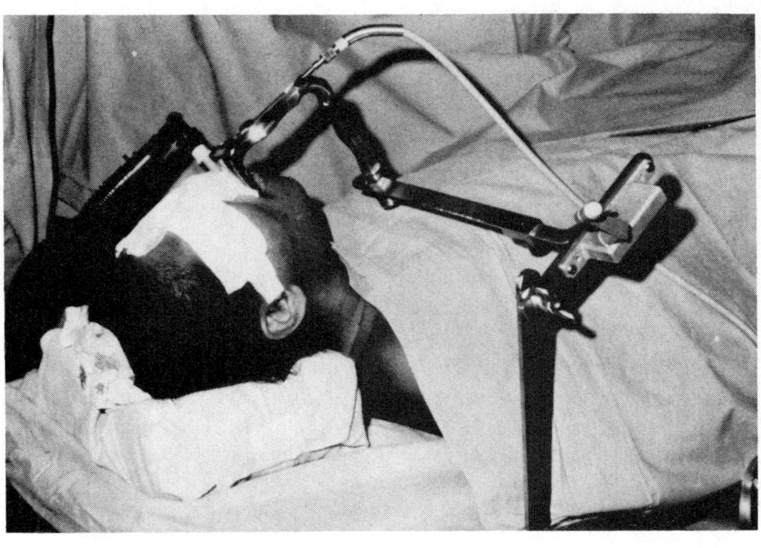

Figure 6–3. This patient is in the optimal endoscopic position. The laryngoscope is positioned within the larynx and is suspended by the detachable extension on the handle, on the Boston University–Pilling suspension gallows. The worm gear provides a lifting force that is always at right angles to the handle of the laryngoscope.

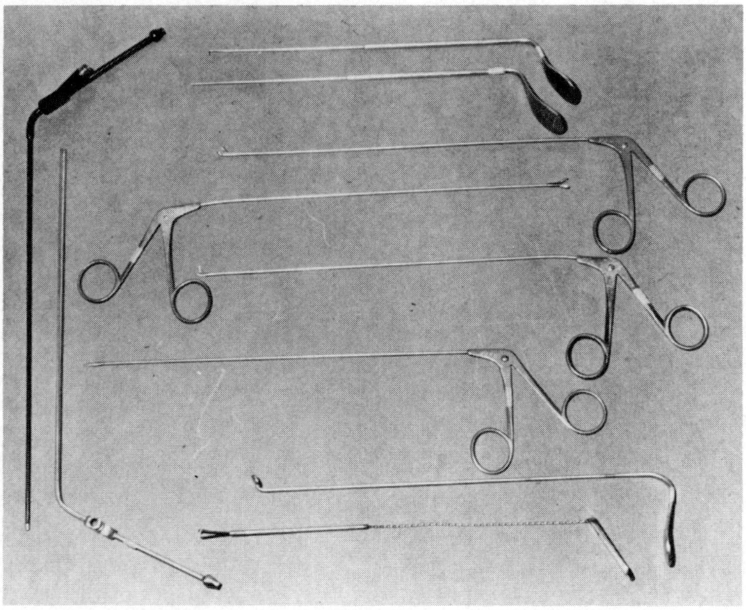

Figure 6–4. For routine endolaryngeal surgery, these instruments are usually sufficient.

gross abnormalities of the laryngeal inlet, for example, postirradiation edema, a partially obstructing mass, or paralysis. Foreknowledge of these problems will allow the anesthetist to plan ahead so that there will be no surprises during induction of anesthesia.

For all routine endoscopic surgery except augmentation of the paralyzed cord, the preferred technique is general anesthesia with a small bore, cuffed endotracheal tube. Most often, anesthesia is induced with thiopental sodium; the patient is paralyzed with succinylcholine chloride, oxygenated with a mask prior to intubation, and then intubated. Maintenance of anesthesia is commonly achieved with nitrous oxide, oxygen, and halothane or enthrane. This routine allows stabilization of the anesthesia and the airway before the endoscope is introduced; the laryngoscope can be introduced unhurriedly and exchanged for a more suitable instrument if necessary. The use of positive pressure ventilation through the small bore tube has been shown to provide adequate gas exchange for as long as one hour.[8]

All patients must have careful cardiac monitoring because of the known tendency for suspension laryngoscopy to precipitate cardiac arrhythmias, especially in patients with cardiac risk factors.[8] Surface anesthesia should be added at the time of intubation to reduce the incidence of postextubation laryngospasm. All areas of the larynx are accessible to inspection in the presence of a small bore endotracheal tube, but occasionally removal of the pathology (for example, papillomas situated below the interarytenoid space) is made easier by removing the tube and thereafter maintaining ventilation using the venturi injection needle attached to the barrel of the laryngoscope. It is the surgeon's responsibility to maintain proper alignment of the laryngoscope with the axis of the larynx and trachea and the position of the ventilation needle.

At the conclusion of the examination or surgery, the larynx should once again be sprayed with topical anesthetic solution and, while the laryngoscope is being withdrawn, all redundant secretions must be removed from the hypopharynx. Thereafter, the anesthesiologist will terminate the anesthesia by reintubation of the patient until reflexes and spontaneous breathing return. Alternatively, the anesthesiologist may elect to ventilate the patient using an oropharyngeal airway and mask.

Local anesthesia alone has limited application in endoscopic laryngeal surgery because of the patient's inability to tolerate fixation and suspension of the large bore laryngoscope in position. Because augmentation of the cord by injection usually requires cooperation of the patient during the procedure, local anesthesia is mandatory. Twenty minutes prior to the procedure, the supralaryngeal nerve should be blocked with 1 ml of 2 per cent lidocaine on each side, followed by surface application of 250 mg of 5 per cent cocaine solution to the mucous membranes of the oral cavity, pharynx, larynx, and upper trachea. This combination usually provides adequate anesthesia if the patient's anxiety can be alleviated by appropriate intravenous sedation.

Difficulties with general anesthesia do occasionally occur; they can usually be traced to a lack of understanding and cooperation between the anesthesiologist and the surgeon. It behooves the surgeon to cultivate the anesthesiologist, to gain his confidence, and to stimulate his enthusiasm for the job at hand.

TECHNIQUES OF ENDOSCOPY AND SURGERY

As soon as induction of anesthesia has been completed and the patient's condition has been stabilized, the patient's eyes must be taped shut or covered with wet eye pads. This precaution minimizes the risk of corneal abrasion during the insertion of the laryngoscope and performance of the procedure.

The patient's teeth should be inspected and a mental note made of the presence of crowns, caps, and bridges so that precautions can be taken to minimize the risk of injury to them. The absence of teeth should be noted with reference to positioning of the endotracheal tube and the laryngoscope.

Ordinarily, it is convenient for a right-handed team to position the endotracheal tube at the left corner of the mouth so that the tube passes behind the maxillary tuberosity; this removes the tube from the path of the laryngoscope through the right side of the oropharynx. The tube should be lightly taped at the left corner of the mouth so that it will not be forced too deeply into the trachea or inadvertently removed from the larynx. The anesthesiologist has freedom of movement and access to the patient at the patient's left shoulder and side.

If two or more adjacent teeth are absent, it is usually worthwhile to take advantage of this space by passing the laryngoscope through it, since it provides the most direct line to the larynx. The teeth adjacent to the space should be protected from abrasion by covering them with several layers of damp gauze or folded adhesive tape. A full set of teeth should be protected from abrasion by placing a plastic tooth guard over them (Fig. 6–5). The tooth guard does not, however, enable the surgeon to use the teeth as a fulcrum during exposure of the larynx in a difficult patient.

Correct position of the head is of the utmost importance in achieving successful laryngoscopy. In every case, the patient's head should be placed on a head support that raises the head 10 cm above the operating table; this flexes the neck on the chest and thereafter allows the head to be extended at the atlantooccipital joint to achieve the ideal endoscopic position.[7] This position, called the Boyce or sniffing position, always facilitates examination of the larynx in the easy patient and is mandatory in the difficult patient. It is this optimal endoscopic position that allows the operator to view the larynx while causing minimal pressure on the upper teeth or maxilla.

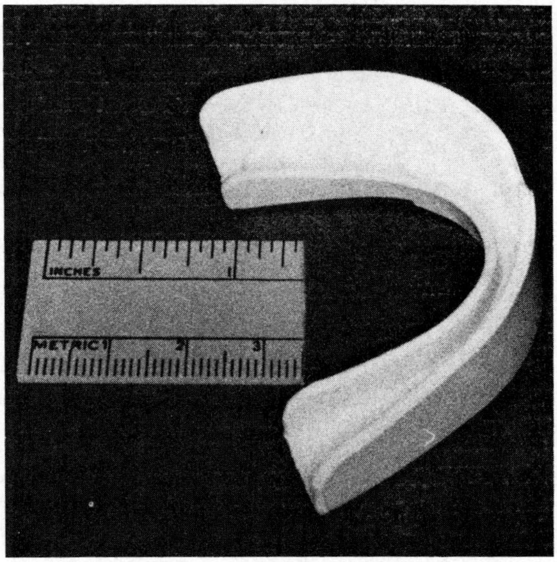

Figure 6–5. Plastic tooth guards are commercially available.

In selecting the best laryngoscope, consider which instrument will provide the best exposure and the best illumination of the larynx as a whole or of a particular area of the larynx. Usually the largest instrument that can be conveniently inserted to expose the anterior commissure region is the best choice—the adult size Jako-Pilling instrument with large light pipes, for example. The blunt distal end of this laryngoscope is specifically designed to push aside the false cords and give an improved view of the free edge and the upper surface of the vocal cords and the anterior commissure. In contrast, the distal end of the Dedo-Pilling laryngoscope is slim and is well suited for partial passage through the glottis to expose the immediate subglottic area. The surgeon may need to pass two or more laryngoscopes before deciding which instrument affords the best operating conditions. In general, it is preferable to use a smaller laryngoscope that is well aligned rather than a larger one that cannot be adequately aligned with the target area (for example, the anterior commissure).

For right-handed surgeons, it is most convenient to hold the laryngoscope by the vertical part of the handle (which is perpendicular to the endoscope tube) between the thumb and fingers of the right hand. In this way, the laryngoscope tube can be gently manipulated along the right side of the floor of the mouth past the right tonsil fossa towards the epiglottis. The tongue takes up a position to the left of the laryngoscope. Meanwhile, the left hand is used to keep the lips everted so that they do not get caught between the laryngoscope and the teeth.

Any secretions in the hypopharynx are removed with a velvet-eyed suction tip, so that the vallecula, the pyriform sinuses, and the postcricoid area can be carefully inspected. Thereafter, the tip of the laryngoscope is inserted under the epiglottis and in front of the endotracheal tube to expose the false cords and the true cords. At this juncture, the horizontal handle of the laryngoscope (which is parallel to the laryngoscope tube) is lifted forward and away from the patient's face by the upturned left hand; the lifting action must always be at right angles to the laryngoscope handle so that little or no pressure is exerted on the patient's teeth as the anterior commissure is brought into view.[7]

Usually the most direct path to the anterior commissure is over the right premolar area with the head rotated 5 to 10 degrees to the left; however, in patients with a narrow mandibular arch or with large medially rotated premolar and molar teeth, it may be best to pass the laryngoscope over the incisor area. Wide bore laryngoscopes with heavy light cables tend to impinge on the lower premolar area and to prevent a view of the anterior commissure. A slim laryngoscope will often slide forward and come to rest behind the lower incisor teeth, providing an adequate view of the anterior commissure with less lifting effort.

From time to time, it may be difficult to pass a wide bore laryngoscope (with a blunt end) under the epiglottis without infolding the epiglottis into the larynx. The infolding of the epiglottis can be prevented by exerting gentle pressure on the hyoid bone as the laryngoscope is advanced under the epiglottis or by withdrawing the patient's tongue with the left hand in order to lift the epiglottis forward and away from the endotracheal tube. The epiglottis rarely presents a problem when a slim laryngoscope is used.

For endoscopic surgery of the larynx, fixation of the laryngoscope is mandatory. This can be achieved by attaching the notched extension piece to the handle of the laryngoscope and suspending it on the cross bar of the Pilling suspension gallows. The angle at which the gallows lifts the laryngoscope is adjusted to ensure that the lifting force is always at right angles to the handle of the laryngoscope; in this way, exposure of the anterior commissure is achieved without risking damage to the maxillary teeth (Fig. 6–3).

Suspension of the laryngoscope on a gallows is mandatory in all but the easiest patients. In most edentulous patients and children, the laryngoscope may be fixed in position by the Lewy laryngoscope holder. The cross piece of the Lewy holder should be placed on a Mayo

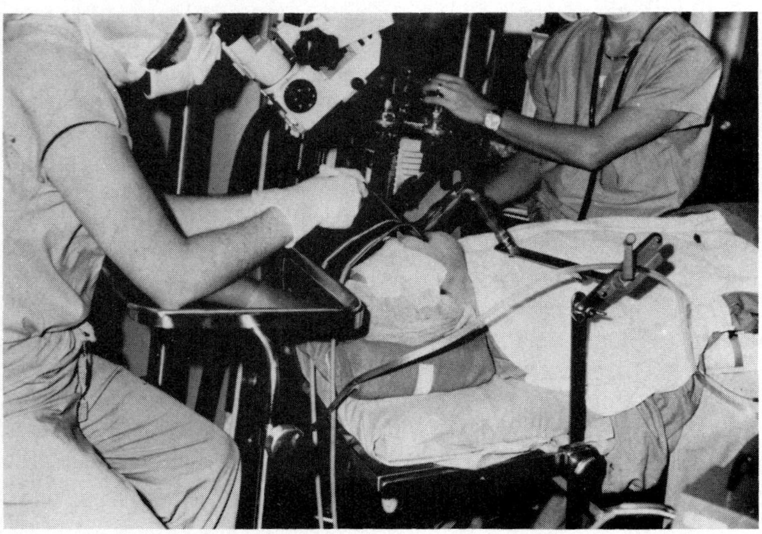

Figure 6–6. A view of the surgeon at work from behind the instrument table. Note the Mayo stand supporting the surgeon's elbows.

stand over the patient's chest. Under these circumstances, the laryngoscope does not cause unacceptable pressure on the alveolar ridge or teeth when the laryngoscope tube is rotated by the worm gear using the upper teeth as a fulcrum. The suspension gallows does make repositioning of the laryngoscope slightly more troublesome than when the Lewy holder is used, but the better exposure provided, with reduced threat to the patient's teeth, makes the effort worthwhile.

As soon as the laryngoscope is put on suspension, the cardiac monitor should be carefully observed in case cardiac arrhythmia develops secondary to the suspension. The surgical microscope, fitted with a front lens of 400 mm focal length, is placed to the left of the head of the operating room table. The back table with the instruments and light source can then be placed to the right of the patient's head (Fig. 6–6). The microscope head is swung into position and aligned with the barrel of the laryngoscope; then the vocal cords are brought into focus. If 20× eyepieces are on the microscope, a No. 10 power setting on the microscope turret is selected. This combination provides a magnification of 5 power, which is convenient for most endoscopic examinations and surgery. If 12.5× eyepieces are fitted on the microscope, a turret setting of 16 should be used to give the same magnification. With brilliant fiberoptic illumination provided by the laryngoscope, the microscope light should not be used; it adds little except glare from the barrel of the laryngoscope and the shafts of the instruments.

Evaluation of the pathology is carried out by inspection, using high power magnification when necessary. Occasionally, pressure on the cricothyroid area will give an improved view, particularly if the lesion arises in the ventricle or in the subglottis. The undersurface of the cords and the laryngeal surface of the epiglottis can be clearly viewed using a 00 laryngeal mirror (Fig. 6–7). The lesion can be further evaluated by palpation, using a suction tip or probe; the probe can be used to retract the false cords and the true cords to increase exposure beneath these structures.

If the lesion is situated in the interarytenoid space, the laryngoscope must be withdrawn and reinserted behind the endotracheal tube. After suspension of the laryngoscope in this position, the airway must be checked in case the tube has been partially collapsed and the airway reduced.

Differential staining with a nuclear stain, for example, toluidine blue, should always be done unless neoplasm has been confidently excluded from the differential diagnosis. This is most helpful in the presence of an unexplained localized area of redness (erythroplasia) or hyperkeratosis—carcinoma in situ and early nonkeratinizing carcinoma stain dark blue or black. This removes the element of guessing in selecting a site for biopsy when the malignant nature of the lesion is not obvious. All excess mucus must be removed before painting the entire glottic area with 2 per cent toluidine blue in water; the excess dye is irrigated away with saline after 15 to 30 sec. Biopsies taken from the stained area are the most likely to demonstrate the malignant nature of a lesion if cancer is present on the surface. Staining of the respiratory epithelium in the subglottis, on the ventricle, and on the false cords does not cause confusion.[9] Before biopsy or resection of the lesion is performed, an arm rest should be provided by placing a Mayo stand adjusted to a height comfortably below the surgeon's elbows; this allows improved control of the long-shafted, flexible instruments so that biopsy and resection can be done more deliberately (Fig. 6–6).

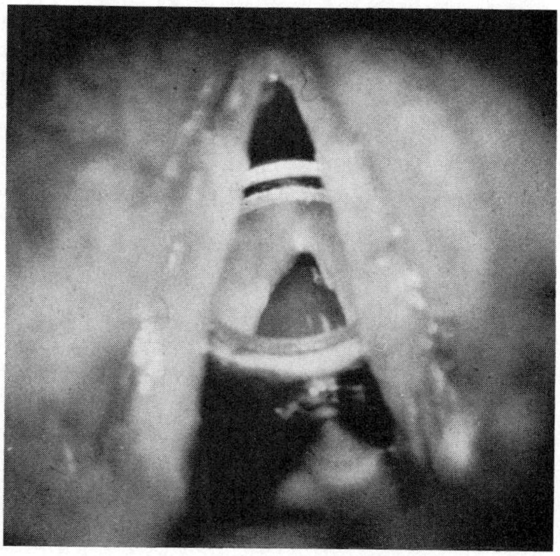

Figure 6–7. The undersurface of the cords can be seen in a 00 laryngeal mirror.

If the lesion is large (5 to 10 mm or more), a biopsy can be taken with standard 2-mm cup forceps; the fragment of tissue is merely avulsed from the mass. In the presence of a small mass (less than 5 mm), excisional biopsy is indicated. The mass is grasped in cup forceps held in the hand opposite to the side of the lesion, and the mass is excised with a scalpel or scissors held in the other hand. In this way, unnecessary stripping of adjacent mucosa is avoided.

During the removal of bilateral benign lesions (for example, vocal cord nodules or polyps), it is essential to incise the mucosa in front of the lesion first in order to avoid inadvertently removing the uninvolved mucosa up to the anterior commissure. If this occurs, only one side should be removed at a time. Bimanual dissection is carried out, with one hand providing retraction of and tension on the specimen to be removed and the other hand controlling excision of the lesion with a scissors or scalpel at the appropriate depth. Usually the plane of dissection is through Reinke's subepithelial space. No more mucosa should be excised than necessary so that the best possible vocal function can be preserved.

Cystic lesions (for example, those arising in the ventricle) should be aspirated and decompressed prior to excision as described above. When it is necessary to remove granulomas of the vocal process of the arytenoid area, they should be excised with great care to avoid further damage to the perichondrium and underlying cartilage. Hyperkeratotic verrucous lesions should be excised along with a layer of underlying muscle so that the presence or absence of verrucous carcinoma can be established. Hemostasis usually takes place spontaneously, but on occasion it may be necessary to control a persistent bleeding point by applying electrocoagulation via an insulated suction tip.

Prior to withdrawal of the laryngoscope, the laryngeal mucosa should once again be sprayed with a topical anesthetic agent that will reduce the incidence and severity of postextubation laryngospasm. The laryngoscope is removed from the suspension gallows and, while it is being withdrawn, any excess secretions or blood clots in the hypopharynx should be removed.

Usually the anesthesiologist will remove the endotracheal tube as soon as the patient has recovered his protective reflexes and is exchanging adequately without ventilatory assistance; delay in extubation until the patient begins to forceably strain on the tube is more likely to be followed by laryngospasm. As soon as the tube has been withdrawn, the anesthesiologist places an oropharyngeal airway and elevates the lower jaw to avoid airway obstruction at the level of the base of the tongue. If the patient shows signs of developing laryngospasm, the lower jaw should be subluxated anteriorly and then elevated. This maneuver will almost always reverse the developing laryngospasm and provide a smooth conclusion to the operation.

During the critical period of extubation, the surgeon should stand by and be ready to help the anesthesiologist if he requires the assistance of an additional pair of hands.

Inhalation of mist is most helpful in the recovery room and the immediate postoperative period, particularly if the patient tends to respond to the laryngeal irritation by coughing.

All patients over forty years of age and others with known cardiac risk factors should have an electrocardiogram in the recovery room and again on the following day, prior to discharge from the hospital. This must be done because of the known risk of silent myocardial infarction occurring after operative laryngoscopy.[8]

Most patients have little or no pain after endoscopic surgery and can tolerate their diets when fully recovered from the anesthesia. Postoperatively, patients are allowed to talk softly and should avoid whispering and vocal strain. The voice is likely to be hoarse, depending on the nature of the surgical intervention. If the air has low humidity, humidification of the environment (particularly of the bedroom) should be continued during the convalescent period.

COMPLICATIONS OF ENDOSCOPIC SURGERY

Contusions of the lips and tongue can occur unless great care is exercised during introduction of the laryngoscope. It should be possible to avoid these injuries.

Abrasion of the dental enamel or dislocation of dental crowns should occur rarely if the laryngoscope tube does not make contact with the teeth and if the laryngoscope is suspended with the patient in the optimal endoscopic position. Occasionally, a medially placed premolar tooth in the lower jaw can be damaged while a wide bore laryngoscope is being lifted away from the patient's upper jaw and placed on suspension. As the force of suspension is increased, the proximity of the laryngoscope to the lower premolar teeth should be monitored to avoid injury.

Interference with the airway can be caused by compression or kinking of the endotracheal tube. If the anesthesiologist has any difficulty with ventilation of the patient, the procedure must be discontinued until the cause of the obstruction has been identified and corrected.

During venturi ventilation, great care must be taken not to change the alignment of the laryngoscope with the larynx and trachea without observing the adequacy of ventilation. Partial reduction of the airway is likely to cause severe cardiac arrhythmias or worse.

A continuous watch must be kept for the development of cardiac arrhythmias, particularly premature ventricular contractions, bigeminy, or bradycardia. If they occur, the laryngoscope must be removed from the suspension and the patient hyperventilated with oxygen. Under these circumstances, these arrhythmias usually disappear promptly. Should the arrhythmia recur when suspension is resumed, it is unwise to proceed with the operation. In the presence of recurrent bigeminy, the incidence of occult postoperative myocardial infarction is 20 per cent. The procedure should be abandoned and rescheduled after appropriate cardiac consultation. On the next occasion, the deep receptors of the cardiodepressant reflex within the larynx should be blocked by preoperative infiltration of the superior laryngeal nerves with 2 per cent lidocaine, 20 min prior to induction. A similar blockade can be achieved by intravenous lidocaine administered intraoperatively. Surface anesthesia has no effect on this reflex.

There is no doubt that operative laryngoscopy poses a threat to the damaged myocardium. Unless appropriate monitoring and preventive measures are undertaken, the incidence of postoperative myocardial infarction will be unnecessarily elevated.

Swelling of the laryngeal mucosa, particularly in the subglottic area in children, must be avoided by gentleness of manipulation at all times. If extensive dissection is anticipated (for example, during the removal of multiple papillomas), posttraumatic swelling can be largely prevented by intraoperative, intravenous steroids. It is rare, except in infants, that postoperative swelling is so severe that the patient must be left intubated for a few hours in the recovery room.

Suspension of the laryngoscope often causes slight cyanosis of the tongue, which is of no consequence. If the cyanosis is severe and is allowed to continue for more than 5 min, the patient may develop severe edema of the tongue, floor of the mouth, submandibular area, and soft palate. Presumably this is caused by venous obstruction in the tongue. This type of swelling does not affect the larynx and is not responsive to intraoperative steroids. It does, however, interfere with ventilation after extubation unless a nasopharyngeal airway is introduced to bypass the obstruction. The swelling subsides spontaneously in 3 or 4 hours. It can be prevented by taking the laryngoscope off suspension every 5 min to allow the tongue to "breathe" and become pink again.

Postintubation laryngospasm is more likely to occur if extubation is delayed until the patient struggles and strains on the tube, even in the presence of surface anesthesia. The incidence is related to the amount of surgical interference and the presence of such predisposing causes as severe chronic mucositis of the larynx and tracheobronchial tree. It is essential to recognize laryngospasm as soon as it begins. Forward subluxation of the mandible will usually break the spasm and allow free ventilation.

SPECIAL PROCEDURES

Vocal Cord Augmentation. In patients with inadequate glottic closure because of vocal cord paralysis, the laterally placed cord can be augmented by intramuscular injection. Polytetrafluoroethylene (Teflon) paste is injected if permanent correction is desired, while glycerin or a paste of gelatin sponge (Gelfoam) is used if temporary augmentation is desired.

The injection can be carried out with the patient in the sitting position under local anesthesia, using indirect laryngoscopy if the patient has the ability to cooperate to such a high degree. Most often it is carried out using direct laryngoscopy after full local surface anesthesia has been induced with cocaine and supplemented by infiltration of the superior laryngeal nerves with lidocaine. The patient is then titrated against intravenous sedation until the proper degree of relaxation is achieved. The patient should be free of anxiety but able to respond to simple verbal instructions.

With the patient in the optimal endoscopic position, the larynx is exposed with a handheld small bore anterior commissure laryngoscope and the patient is asked to phonate. The degree of abduction of the paralyzed cord that must be corrected is then noted. A Bruening steel-barrelled syringe is loaded with the injection material and attached to the guarded laryngeal needle. Next, 0.3 to 0.5 ml of the material is injected, lateral to the tip of the vocal process of the arytenoid and deep into some musculature; 0.2 to 0.4 ml of material is placed lateral to the midpoint of the membranous portion of the cord, placing the point of the needle as far lateral as possible. After each injection, the patient is asked to phonate so that the degree of correction can be assessed. The use of Teflon requires slight over correction because of the eventual absorption of the glycerin component of the Teflon paste. It must be remembered, however, that it is safest to underestimate the amount of Teflon to be injected; more can be added later if necessary. This method is best suited for the occasional operator and makes it possible to avoid over augmentation fairly confidently.

Arytenoidectomy. Endoscopic arytenoidectomy for bilateral vocal cord paralysis can be performed through a large bore tubular laryngoscope, but the Lynch suspension laryngoscope provides better access. Most patients already have a tracheostomy in place when they first see the surgeon.

Anesthesia is administered through the tracheostomy tube so that the airway is under complete control. A tongue blade that will lift the epiglottis forward and give excellent exposure of the arytenoid area is selected for the Lynch laryngoscope. An incision is made in the mucosa over the anteromedial surface of the arytenoid cartilage to expose the cartilage. The cartilage is then grasped with cup forceps and put under tension. The surrounding muscles are dissected away by blunt dissection, leaving only the tip of the vocal process still attached to the vocal cord. A portion of the posterior end of the false cord may be excised to facilitate further abduction of the cord, or the aryepiglottic fold may be electrocoagulated submucously to induce scar formation and lateral retraction of the cord.

Endoscopic Placement of Keels and Stents. Anterior glottic webs can be divided with a laryngeal scissors, but, unless some unabsorbable material is placed between the raw surfaces, the web will probably re-form. After excision of the web, the straight Keith needle, attached to a cardiac pacemaker wire, is introduced percutaneously through one side of the thyroid cartilage immediately behind the new anterior commissure so that the tip of the needle can be seen in the lumen of the subglottis. A similar needle with the attached wire is introduced through the opposite side and made to enter the larynx immediately above the anterior commissure, so that only the tip of the needle protrudes into the larynx. A rectangular piece of reinforced Silastic sheeting (0.02 in thick) measuring 1.5 cm by 0.75 cm is then placed vertically in the anterior commissure and is transfixed by the two needles (Figs. 6–8 and 6–9). The pacemaker wires are then drawn through and tied over a button on each side of the neck, adjacent to the thyroid cartilage. While this could be carried out under general anesthesia with an endotracheal tube and without a tracheostomy, it is recommended that the patient be provided with a prophylactic tracheostomy. The keel can be removed in three to six weeks, depending on the extent of the denuded areas at the time of division of the web.

Cryosurgery. Cryosurgery, using the liquid nitrogen probe, is favored for the destruction of papillomas, small localized cord cancers, or small hemangiomas that do not lend themselves to excision.[10] After exposure of the larynx in the usual way, an iceball is created at the chosen location using a closed probe or an open microspray. The opposite cord must be protected from an inadvertent freeze by placing a small sheet of expanded polystyrene (Styrofoam) over the uninvolved cord.

Because the degree of postfreeze edema is unpredictable, it is important to administer intravenous steroids intraoperatively.

Surgery with the Carbon Dioxide Laser. The carbon dioxide laser, attached to the surgical microscope and controlled with the micromanipulator, is ideally suited for microsurgery of the larynx. After seven years of experience with the use of this laser in several thousand operations, the modality has become firmly en-

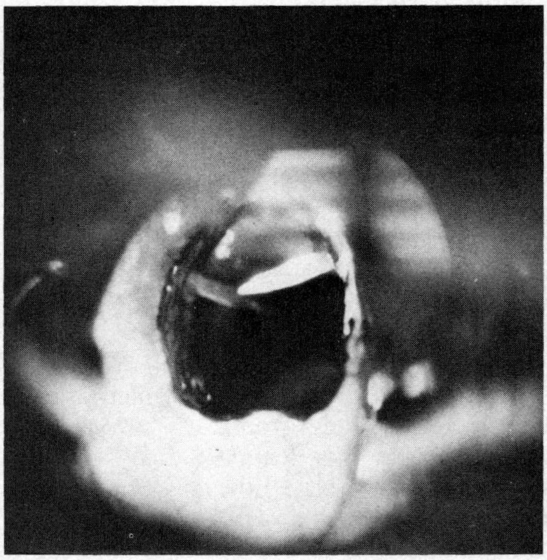

Figure 6–8. A dense subglottic scar has been removed. The two transfixion needles are seen entering the lumen of the larynx; prior to positioning the Silastic stent, the needles must be partially withdrawn until only the tips protrude into the lumen.

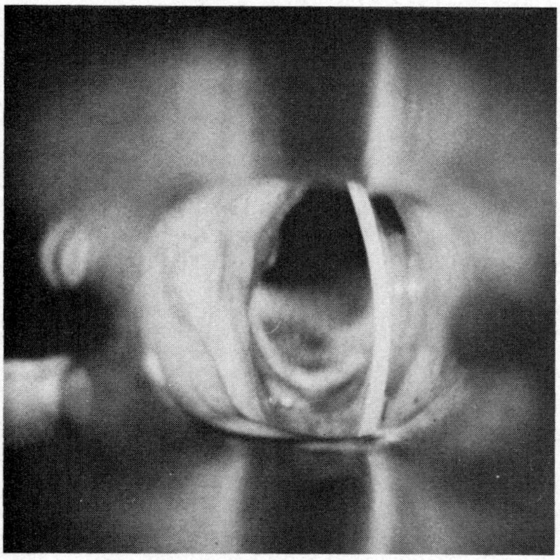

Figure 6–9. The upper edge of the Silastic stent is seen between the cords after transfixion with the suspension wires.

trenched in the armamentarium for laryngeal microsurgery.[6]

In addition to the usual precautions that must be taken during all microsurgical laryngeal procedures, a further precaution is peculiar to the laser—extreme caution must be used when using the laser in the immediate proximity of flammable materials in an oxygen-rich environment. Occasionally, moist neurosurgical cotton pads must be placed beneath the vocal cords to protect the anterior tracheal wall. Provided the pledgets of cotton are kept moist, there is no danger of ignition in the event of deliberate or inadvertent impact by the laser beam.

When operating with the laser within the larynx, the surgeon must prevent igniting the intratracheal tube by taking one of the following steps: (1) removing the tube and continuing ventilation by the venturi method, (2) protecting the tube by a covering of self-adhesive aluminum tape, or (3) replacing the tube with an all-metal flexible intratracheal tube.[11, 12] Unless one of these precautions is followed, there exists a real hazard of endotracheal tube ignition within the larynx. The consequences of such a fire would be very serious.

In microsurgery of the larynx, the laser can be utilized in two ways: it can be used to ablate by evaporation a previously biopsied lesion (for example, papilloma, leukoplakia, or a vocal cord nodule that is too small to biopsy), or it can be used for excision of tissue masses. The latter usage makes the instrument most versatile because the excised mass is available for histological evaluation.

Excisional biopsy by the carbon dioxide laser is carried out by grasping the lesion with cup forceps and placing the lesion under tension; the lesion is then excised at the desired level. Because of the absence of bleeding, the plane of dissection can be maintained exactly so that no more and no less surrounding tissue than necessary is included in the specimen. This technique is most suitable for the management of polyps, keratosis, cysts, granulomas, carcinoma in situ, early clearly localized T1 cord cancers, and lesions suspected of being verrucous carcinoma[13] (Fig. 6–10).

In a similar manner, the laser can be used to determine the extent of tumor for staging purposes. To determine whether an anterior commissure lesion is a T1 or T4 lesion, the tumor is removed until cartilage is encountered or until it is determined that the lesion has already penetrated the thyroid cartilage.

Occasionally, during the evaluation and staging of bulky cancers of the glottis and supraglottis, it is found that the airway has been so compromised that a tracheostomy needs to be done prior to extubation. Under these circumstances, the obstructive mass of tumor can be excised with the laser to temporarily restore an airway and thus avoid a tracheostomy prior to laryngectomy. More recently, it has been found

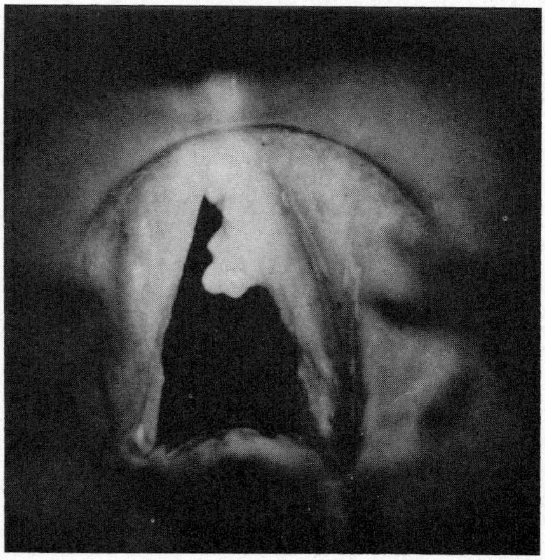

Figure 6–10. Keratotic lesions such as this should be removed in one piece so that the interface between the lesion and the underlying muscle can be evaluated histologically. This particular lesion demonstrated hyperkeratosis only, with no evidence of malignancy.

possible to do a partial supraglottic laryngectomy for T1 carcinoma of the epiglottis in suitable patients without the need for tracheostomy.[14]

During these major resections, intraoperative steroids are used intravenously to reduce the possibility of postoperative edema following surgical manipulation. The morbidity following laser resection is extremely low; pain and difficulty in swallowing are minimal and the patient can usually be discharged on the day after surgery.

Areas of stenosis, including subglottic stenosis and supraglottic hemangioma, can be vaporized with the laser to restore an airway in many cases. A lumen keeper may be needed to prevent restenosis if the area of resection is extensive. A roll of Silastic sheeting placed endoscopically and transfixed by stay wires, as already described, is most often used. The placement of the stent, of course, requires a tracheostomy.

SUMMARY

Endoscopic microsurgery of the larynx is now feasible because of advances in techniques of anesthesia and airway control, availability of prolonged operating time, adequate exposure of the operative site, and the availability of instruments for microsurgery, including the carbon dioxide laser. This is a desirable modality because of the ability to conserve or restore function, the low level of morbidity, and the cost effectiveness in managing larger lesions.

References

1. Lynch RC: Intrinsic carcinoma of the larynx with a second report of the cases operated upon by suspension and dissection. Trans Am Laryngol Assoc 42:119–126, 1920.
2. New G, Dorton HE: Suspension laryngoscopy in the treatment of malignant disease of the hypopharynx and larynx. Mayo Clinic Proc 16:411–416, 1941.
3. Lillie JC, DeSanto LW: Transoral surgery of early cordal carcinoma. Trans Am Acad Ophthalmol Otolaryngol 77:92–96, 1973.
4. Priest RE, Weselowski S: Direct laryngoscopy under general anesthesia. Trans Am Acad Ophthalmol Otolaryngol 64:639–648, 1960.
5. Strong MS: Microscopic laryngoscopy. Laryngoscope 80:1540–1552, 1970.
6. Strong MS et al.: The use of the CO_2 laser in otolaryngology: A progress report. Trans Am Acad Ophthalmol Otolaryngol 82:595–602, 1976.
7. Grundfast KM et al.: Suspension microlaryngoscopy in the Boyce position with a new suspension gallows. Ann Otol Rhinol Laryngol 87:560–566, 1978.
8. Strong MS et al.: Cardiac complications of microsurgery of the larynx: Etiology, incidence, and prevention. Laryngoscope 84:908–920, 1974.
9. Strong MS et al.: Toluidine blue in diagnosis of cancer of the larynx. Arch Otolaryngol 91:515–519, 1970.
10. Miller D: Cryosurgery as a modality in the treatment of carcinoma of the larynx. Laryngoscope 85:1281–1285, 1975.
11. Norton ML et al.: Endotracheal intubation and venturi (jet) ventilation for laser microsurgery of the larynx. Ann Otol Rhinol Laryngol 85:656–663, 1976.
12. Norton ML, DeVos P: New endotracheal tube for laser surgery of the larynx. Ann Otol Rhinol Laryngol 87:554–558, 1978.
13. Vaughan CW et al.: Laryngeal carcinoma: Transoral treatment utilizing the CO_2 laser. Am J Surg 136:490–493, Oct 1978.
14. Vaughan CW: Transoral laryngeal surgery using the CO_2 laser: Laboratory experiments and clinical experience. Laryngoscope 88:1399–1420, 1978.

7

Surgical Management of the Paralyzed Larynx

Howard L. Levine, M.D. and Harvey M. Tucker, M.D.

Laryngeal paralysis is a frequent problem. It may cause the patient little or no difficulty, or it can be life-threatening. It presents a variety of symptoms, some of which will be transient and others permanent. Successful management of laryngeal paralysis depends upon accurate diagnosis and command of a broad armamentarium of methods to treat the specific disorder. In this manner, problems of laryngeal paralysis can be individualized and the most appropriate management selected.

DIAGNOSIS

Position of the Vocal Cords. The position of the vocal cord or cords will usually correlate with the symptoms, narrow the range of possible diagnoses, and indicate appropriate treatment. Accurate inspection of the larynx and thorough understanding of laryngeal physiology and anatomy are, therefore, crucial. Vocal cord position will help the laryngologist to determine whether the problem is unilateral or bilateral and whether it is caused by injury to the superior laryngeal nerve or to the recurrent laryngeal nerve, or both.

Superior Laryngeal Nerve Paralysis. Injury to the external branch of the superior laryngeal nerve will result in paralysis of the cricothyroid muscle on the side of the injury. If the injury is unilateral, the opposite cricothyroid muscle acts unopposed. According to some authors, the anterior commissure will deviate to the side of the lesion,[1, 2] thus causing shortening and loss of tension in the affected vocal cord. More recent work[3] has shown that the posterior commissure is actually displaced, instead, but the ultimate effect is the same. Since the superior laryngeal nerve serves as both a tensor of the glottic musculature and a sensory nerve to the superior larynx, symptoms of its paralysis will include voice change because of loss of tension in the vocal cord and occasional aspiration. As a result of loss of tension in the vocal cord, the arytenoid cartilage on the side of the paralysis will prolapse inward. The vocal fold will appear to be at a lower level on inspiration and will be driven upward on expiration.

Recurrent Laryngeal Nerve Paralysis. Injury to the recurrent laryngeal nerve results in paralysis of all intrinsic muscles on that side. The vocal cord assumes a paramedian position, and there is no lateral motion on inspiration. The vocal cord may adduct during phonation because of the normal function of the ipsilateral superior laryngeal nerve, thus permitting the intact cricothyroid muscle to act by adduction when unopposed by abductor tonus.

Many theories have attempted to explain the

median or paramedian position that the vocal cord assumes in recurrent laryngeal nerve paralysis. In 1881, Sir Felix Semon[4] stated that abductor fibers of the recurrent laryngeal nerve are more susceptible to injury than the adductor. This theory has not really been disproved to the present time and may be an explanation for the position of the vocal cord in gradual paralysis, but it cannot be used to explain those cases where the recurrent laryngeal nerve has been sectioned. A more widely accepted explanation of the paramedian position of the vocal cord is the unopposed adductor function of the ipsilateral cricothyroid muscle, as noted above.

Of individuals with unilateral abductor paralysis caused by injury of the recurrent laryngeal nerve, 35 per cent may be asymptomatic and may have an essentially normal voice.[4] By the phenomenon of "compensation," glottic closure may be achieved by action of the ipsilateral superior laryngeal nerve or by the contralateral vocal cord, which, when sufficiently mobile, may cross the midline to reach the paralyzed cord. As a result, unilateral vocal cord paralysis caused by recurrent laryngeal nerve injury may go undetected.

If there is bilateral abductor paralysis, the voice may also be quite good because the vocal cords will come to rest close to the position of phonation. The airway, however, will be poor because of lack of abduction during inspiration. Although it is not a common occurrence, some patients with bilateral abductor paralysis have sufficient exercise tolerance that this condition may also go unrecognized. The vast majority will, of course, present with airway obstruction.

Complete Paralysis. Complete paralysis can occur with injury to the vagus nerve above the point of departure of the superior laryngeal nerve. There will be ipsilateral paralysis of the larynx with loss of sensation and muscular control in such cases. The vocal cord rests in a "cadaveric" or intermediate position just lateral to the paramedian position. This is because of loss of the slight adduction provided by the cricothyroid muscle seen in isolated recurrent nerve paralysis.

Adductor Paralysis. Since the vocal cords have bilateral innervation from the motor cortex, it is unusual for a central lesion to cause laryngeal paralysis. Nevertheless, it is possible to have an isolated adductor paralysis, which is usually caused by an injury within the central nervous system. In the past, patients who had such massive brain-stem lesions usually were not salvaged. Patients with adductor paralysis may be seen more frequently in the future because of better means of resuscitation following cerebral vascular accident. The vocal cords remain in a paramedian position on phonation but abduct on inspiration. The voice is extremely weak, breathy, and hoarse. While the airway will remain quite good, cough is inadequate because of inability to close the glottis, which may also result in significant problems with aspiration.

ETIOLOGY OF VOCAL CORD PARALYSIS

The recurrent laryngeal nerve may be paralyzed because of disease or injury anywhere along its course from the brain stem to the larynx. The left vocal cord is the more commonly paralyzed of the two, probably because its course is longer and more vulnerable than that of the right. Parnell and Brandenberg[5] studied 100 consecutive cases of vocal cord paralysis and classified them using the following etiologic categories: trauma; neoplasm; mechanical dysfunction; central nervous system dysfunction; toxic, idiopathic, and metabolic causes; and inflammation (Table 7–1).

While central vocal cord paralysis does occur, it is by no means as common as peripheral paralysis, comprising only 10 per cent of all cases. Central paralysis can occur with various bulbar disorders such as amyotrophic lateral sclerosis, poliomyelitis, multiple sclerosis, pseudobulbar palsy, syringomyelia, syphilis, cerebral vascular hemorrhage, thrombosis, Parkinson's disease, Guillain-Barré syndrome, and Charcot-Marie-Tooth syndrome.

While thyroid surgery remains a common cause of peripheral vocal cord paralysis, all surgery within the neck and thorax can result in vocal cord injury.[6] Vocal cord paralysis has been associated with influenza, diphtheria, typhoid fever, and lead and arsenic ingestion. Benign and malignant tumors (such as glomus jugulare, glomus vagale, and carotid body tumors) in and around the jugular foramen also are not infrequent causes.

Diseases within the mediastinum can produce vocal paralysis—aortic aneurysms, mediastinal involvement by carcinoma, cardiac enlargement, and scarring of the pulmonary apices by tuberculosis have all been implicated. Vocal cord paralysis may also be seen in the presence of benign thyroid disease, although this is not very common. About 4 per cent of patients with unilateral vocal cord paralysis will have disease within the thyroid gland. Approx-

Table 7–1. ETIOLOGY OF VOCAL CORD PARALYSIS—100 CASES*

Causes	Number of Cases	Total Cases
Trauma		34
Thyroidectomy	28	
Neck trauma	2	
Mediastinal and thoracic surgery	3	
Parathyroidectomy	1	
Neoplasm		32
Carcinoma of lung	15	
Carcinoma of thyroid	5	
Metastatic breast carcinoma	2	
Hodgkin's disease	2	
Adenocarcinoma	1	
Lymphoma	1	
Malignant melanoma	1	
Malignant thymoma	1	
Multiple myeloma	1	
Esophageal carcinoma	1	
Anaplastic carcinoma	1	
Mechanical dysfunction†		11
Cardiovascular pathology	6	
Pulmonary tuberculosis	2	
Leukemic hilar enlargement	1	
Hyperthyroidism	1	
Neurofibroma of parapharyngeal space	1	
Central nervous system dysfunction		7
Amyotrophic lateral sclerosis	2	
Bulbar poliomyelitis	1	
Cerebral vascular disease	1	
Severe head injury	1	
Multiple congenital anomalies	1	
Arnold-Chiari malformation	1	
Toxic and metabolic causes		5
Thyroiditis	2	
Toxic neuritis	2	
Bell's palsy	1	
Inflammation		1
Mediastinal abscess	1	
Idiopathic causes		10

*From Parnell FW, Brandenberg JH: Laryngoscope 80:1036, 1970

†Pressure by heart, great vessels, or organomegaly

imately 0.7 per cent of patients with benign thyroid disease will have recurrent nerve paralysis.[7] These figures suggest that these two conditions may not necessarily have a cause-and-effect relationship.

INDICATIONS FOR SURGICAL INTERVENTION FOR VOCAL CORD PARALYSIS

Unilateral Vocal Cord Paralysis. The patient with unilateral vocal cord paralysis will most commonly recover spontaneously or compensate. In either situation, no intervention will be required. When recovery or compensation does not occur, the patient will have major problems with voice and, to a lesser extent, problems with glottic competence. If the recurrent laryngeal nerve only is affected, there is breathiness, air wastage during phonation, and breathlessness after speaking only a few words, because of rapid air escape. The volume of the voice is diminished and the pitch lowered. If the ipsilateral superior laryngeal nerve is also involved, the adductive effect of the cricothyroid muscle will be lost and all of these symptoms will be more pronounced.

The glottic folds, base of tongue, and false vocal folds all play an integral part in preventing aspiration during swallowing. Competence of the true vocal cords is not, however, the major barrier to aspiration during deglutition. With unilateral paralysis that does not involve the sensory division of the superior laryngeal nerve, aspiration is uncommon. When the superior laryngeal nerve is involved, however, the patient is likely to have sudden minor coughing episodes or a need for throat clearing—not during swallowing of food or liquids but when swallowing saliva. In this situation, normal secretions and saliva tend to accumulate on the flaccid cord and spill over into the larynx unexpectedly.

On the other hand, the vocal cords play an extremely important role in the cough mechanism. During the first stage of the cough, the vocal cords are widely abducted as a large inspiratory effort is made. During the second stage, the vocal folds are tightly approximated and intrathoracic pressure is increased. Once intrathoracic pressure is raised sufficiently, the glottis is suddenly opened by the air forced upward by contraction of the abdominal and thoracic musculature. If there is paralysis of the vocal cord, adequate buildup of pressure within the larynx cannot be attained and the cough is often inadequate.

While these problems of voice and glottic competence can be quite significant, most cases of unilateral vocal cord paralysis can be expected to resolve spontaneously, depending upon the etiology. Indeed, unless the nerve is mechanically interrupted, recovery is the rule, rather than the exception. Most surgeons agree that recovery will take place within six months to a year of onset, or will not take place at all.

In most patients who do not recover recurrent nerve function, the contralateral vocal fold will compensate by moving across the midline to achieve satisfactory glottic closure. This restores a reasonable voice and glottic competence, preventing aspiration and producing an adequate cough; however, even when there is compensation of the opposite vocal fold and the voice is satisfactory for day-to-day communication, the professional voice user may find that phonation is still inadequate, especially with regard to pitch control. If the cause of the paralysis is known and is of the type from which one would not expect complete or adequate recovery, intervention earlier than six months may be considered. For the professional voice user, it might be wise to consider such earlier intervention to allow the patient a quick return to employment.

Bilateral Vocal Cord Paralysis. Most patients with bilateral paralysis will manifest upper airway problems varying from near total obstruction to slight problems with exercise tolerance. In some instances, patients whose exercise and daily activity is limited may be nearly asymptomatic, but this state of affairs is unusual. The majority of patients with bilateral vocal cord paralysis need something done, often as an emergency, to provide an adequate airway. Volume flow loop studies may be used to determine an individual's upper airway resistance and also as an objective measure of the degree of success of many of the laryngeal procedures that have been used for bilateral vocal cord paralysis. The decision as to which of several procedures may be undertaken to provide an adequate airway should be determined by the patient's individual needs and preference. There are those patients who will want to maintain a permanent tracheotomy and a normal voice. There are others who will prefer decannulation at the expense of voice. Still a third group might like to maintain adequate voice and airway.

TREATMENT OF BILATERAL VOCAL CORD PARALYSIS

Tracheotomy. The initial step in the management of bilateral abductor paralysis is to overcome potentially life-threatening airway obstruction. This can be accomplished most quickly and directly by a tracheotomy. Once the airway itself is stabilized, consideration can be given to further management of bilateral vocal cord paralysis, if indicated. In the past, and for some patients today, a tracheostomy was all that was necessary. The voice remains fairly good because the vocal cords are in the paramedian position. The obstruction is safely bypassed through the tracheotomy. Tracheotomy will be at least a temporary measure in the management of most patients with bilateral vocal cord paralysis.

Table 7–2. LATERALIZATION PROCEDURES FOR BILATERAL VOCAL CORD PARALYSIS—STATIC PROCEDURES

Investigator	Procedure
Kelley (1941)	Arytenoidectomy
Woodman (1946)	Arytenoidectomy, lateral laryngeal
Thornell (1949)	Arytenoidectomy, translaryngeal
Downey and Keenan (1968)	Arytenoidectomy, laryngofissure
Montgomery (1961)	Arytenoidopexy

Lateralization Procedures (Table 7–2). In an attempt to give the patient an adequate airway, various operative procedures have been developed with the common aim of permanently lateralizing at least one vocal cord, thus permitting decannulation. Some of the early procedures performed to this end involved removing the vocal cord itself. Cordectomy and submucous resection of the vocal cord can, indeed, improve the airway but at considerable expense to voice quality. Various surgical procedures have been employed to fix the arytenoid cartilage laterally in an attempt to gain an adequate airway but again at the expense of good voice.

An arytenoidectomy was performed by Kelley[8] in 1941, through a window in the thyroid cartilage. His results, while successful in early attempts, were not consistent.

In 1946, Woodman[9] used a lateral laryngeal approach to perform an arytenoidectomy. He removed the body of the arytenoid and fixed the vocal process of the arytenoid laterally to the thyroid cartilage. This produced a satisfactory airway when the posterior commissure was between 4 mm and 6 mm, but when it was greater than 6 mm, a poor voice resulted. The Woodman arytenoidectomy remains one of the most popular procedures for managing bilateral vocal cord paralysis (Fig. 7–1).

Thornell[10] described translaryngeal arytenoidectomy by a submucous resection of the arytenoid cartilage. The deep tissues were cauterized with the intention of causing retraction of the vocal cord laterally. This approach, with recent modifications, remains quite popular[11] (Fig. 7–2).

In 1968, Downey and Keenan[12] suggested laryngofissure as an approach through which arytenoidectomy could be performed. Mont-

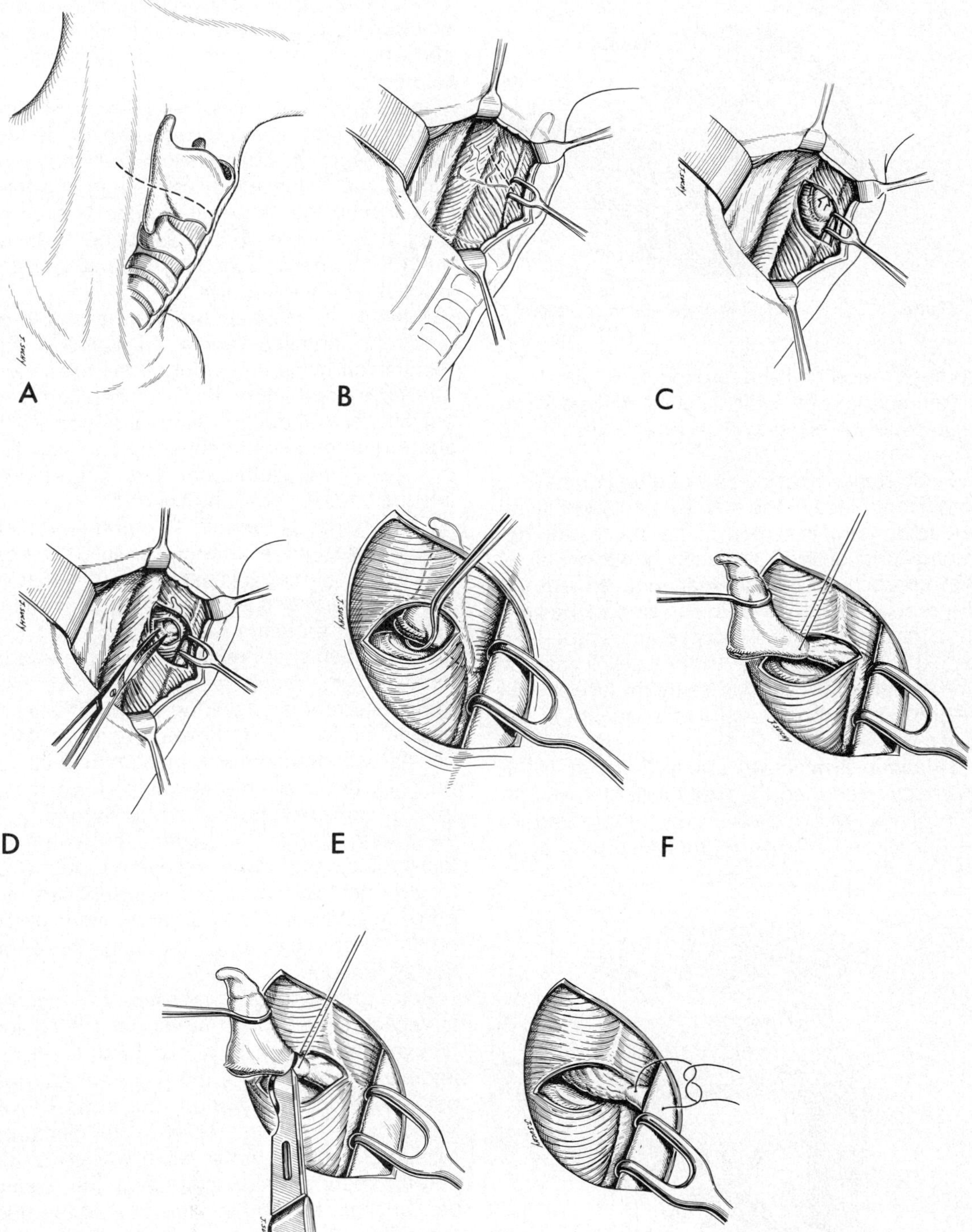

Figure 7–1. Woodman arytenoidectomy. *A*, Skin incisions. *B*, Hook on posterior ala of thyroid cartilage, rotation of larynx, and incisions in inferior constrictor muscle. *C*, Superior displacement of pyriform sinus. *D*, Exposure of cricoarytenoid joint. *E*, Hook used to mobilize arytenoid cartilage from joint space. *F*, Suture placed in vocal process of arytenoid to assist in dissection. *G*, Severing of arytenoid cartilage from its vocal process. *H*, Tying vocal process to thyroid ala to complete lateralization of arytenoid.

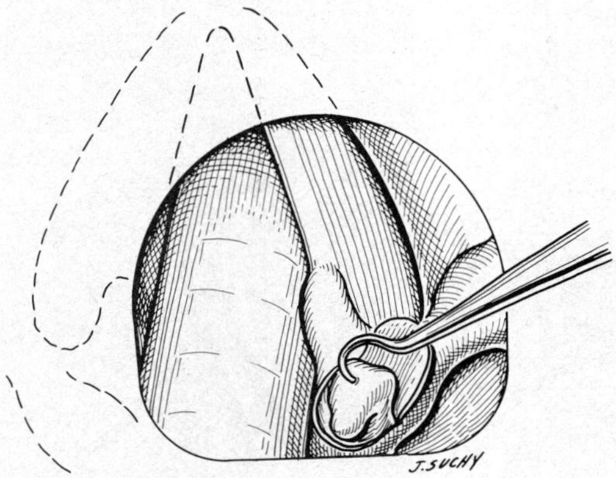

Figure 7–2. Thornell translaryngeal arytenoidectomy.

gomery[13] modified this procedure to allow an arytenoidopexy in which the lateralized cartilage could be fixed with a pin to the cricoid (Fig. 7–3).

Such static procedures continue to have a significant place in the management of bilateral abductor paralysis, permitting successful decannulation of most patients; however, all of these procedures are done at some expense to the remaining voice. Some degree of breathiness, hoarseness, or excessive air escape is to be expected in virtually every case. It may be said, in general, that the resultant airway will be inversely proportional to the quality of the voice remaining.

Dynamic Procedures (Table 7–3). In 1909, Horseley[14] reported the first successful restoration of vocal cord mobility by simple end-to-end anastomosis of an injured recurrent laryngeal nerve. Since that time, investigators have tried to reinnervate the paralyzed larynx using various techniques. If successful, reinnervation would restore a dynamic larynx, allowing both abduction for airway and adduction sufficient to preserve a good voice.

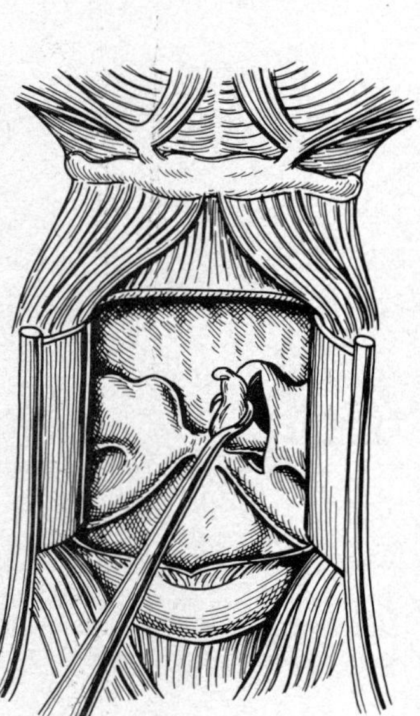

Figure 7–3. Laryngofissure arytenoidectomy.

In 1924, Fraser[15] achieved partial restoration of function by anastomosing the descendens hypoglossi to the cut recurrent laryngeal nerve. Barnes and Balance[16] performed an anastomosis between the recurrent laryngeal nerve and the phrenic nerve. There was good adduction but only partial abduction, resulting in a good voice but only a fair airway.

Lahey[17], in 1928, performed an end-to-end recurrent laryngeal nerve anastomosis eight months following injury during thyroid surgery. This gave good adduction with excellent voice but only fair abduction, with the glottis being about one-third of the normal glottic space. In this case, the glottic chink was considered adequate for exercise, however.

Doyle[18] also performed an end-to-end recurrent laryngeal nerve anastomosis after the nerve was injured during thyroid surgery. He felt that success was only partial, with adduction being better than abduction, as observed by Lahey. Of ten patients, six received end-to-end anastomosis of the recurrent laryngeal nerve to the same recurrent laryngeal nerve shortly after the original injury. Five showed recovery, while one had no improvement. In the remaining four patients, the anastomosis was performed from three months to two years following injury. Of these four, all had good adduction with excellent voice, but none recovered abduction. Doyle concluded that if a recurrent laryngeal nerve anastomosis is to be performed, it must be done early after injury for adequate restoration of function.

Boles and Fritzell[19] crushed the recurrent laryngeal nerve in dogs and demonstrated good recovery of motion in six to eight weeks. In another group of dogs, the recurrent laryngeal nerve was cut and grafted, but none showed recovery of motion. There was electromyographic recovery, however. It was concluded that the recurrent laryngeal nerve will regenerate, but that there is misdirection of the fibers that results in poor return of motion.

Miehlke[20] described an approach in which the vagal laryngeal trunk was anastomosed to the posterior ramus of the recurrent laryngeal nerve. He did this to exclude the remaining recurrent laryngeal nerve fibers in an attempt to achieve abductor function only with simultaneous denervation of the antagonistic mus-

Table 7–3. MANAGEMENT OF BILATERAL VOCAL CORD PARALYSIS—DYNAMIC PROCEDURES

Investigator	Procedure
Horseley (1909)	Anastomosis—recurrent laryngeal nerve to recurrent laryngeal nerve
Fraser (1924)	Anastomosis—descendens hypoglossi to recurrent laryngeal nerve
Barnes and Balance (1927)	Anastomosis—phrenic nerve to recurrent laryngeal nerve
Lahey (1928)	Anastomosis—recurrent laryngeal nerve to recurrent laryngeal nerve
Doyle (1964)	Anastomosis—recurrent laryngeal nerve to recurrent laryngeal nerve
Miehlke (1974)	Anastomosis—vagal laryngeal nerve trunk to recurrent laryngeal nerve
Iwamura (1974)	Anastomosis—split vagus nerve to adductor recurrent laryngeal nerve
	Anastomosis—phrenic nerve to abductor recurrent laryngeal nerve
Moreledge (1973)	Implanted phrenic nerve into posterior cricoarytenoid muscle
Miglets (1974)	Implanted recurrent laryngeal nerve into posterior cricoarytenoid muscle
Tucker (1971)	Nerve-muscle pedicle technique

cles. He found that he could achieve synchronous vocal cord abduction during inspiration on both the reinnervated and unoperated sides in dogs. In 1972, he performed the same procedure on a patient who had suffered an iatrogenic lesion of both recurrent laryngeal nerves four months prior to referral. Lateral motion of the vocal cord could be seen ten weeks following surgery; however, six months after surgery, medial motion of the reinnervated vocal cord could no longer be observed during phonation, and the vocal cord was found in an intermediate position comparable to that observed in successful lateral fixation.

In 1974, Iwamura,[21] working intralaryngeally in dogs, anastomosed a portion of split vagus nerve to the adductor division of the recurrent laryngeal nerve. Simultaneously, he anastomosed the phrenic nerve to the abductor division of the recurrent laryngeal nerve extralaryngeally. All experimental animals regained normal and symmetrical electromyographic function postoperatively. Voluntary synchronous adduction measuring from 50 per cent to 100 per cent of normal and spontaneous synchronous adduction ranging from 10 per cent to 60 per cent of normal were noted.

While these investigators were working on methods of reinnervation using neurorrhaphy, other researchers attacked the problems in a different manner by performing direct nerve implantation into the abductor group of muscles. Moreledge[22] implanted the phrenic nerve into the posterior cricoarytenoid muscle in 12 adult dogs. He found that when implantation was performed less than six months after denervation, some abduction could be achieved. Abduction ranged from 25 per cent to 70 per cent, with an average of about 40 per cent as compared to controls. When reimplantation was delayed more than six months, however, no abduction could be observed.

Miglets[23] reported reimplantation of the recurrent laryngeal nerve into the posterior cricoarytenoid muscle following traumatic laryngeal tracheal separation with avulsion of both recurrent laryngeal nerves. One year following surgery, the patient had good abduction and adduction of the vocal cords on one side. Miglets felt that the adduction resulted from intact cricothyroid function but that the abduction was a result of reimplantation.

Laryngeal Reinnervation—The Nerve-Muscle Pedicle Technique. Neurorrhaphy techniques requiring anastomosis between the recurrent laryngeal nerve and any other source of nerve fiber regrowth have failed to gain popularity because of inconsistent results. Implantation of the recurrent laryngeal nerve into the posterior cricoarytenoid muscle is not often possible clinically. Until recently, therefore, vocal cord lateralization has been essentially the only means of restoring an adequate airway in bilateral vocal cord paralysis, short of permanent tracheotomy. The patient has always been faced with a choice between preservation of voice or having an adequate airway without the need for tracheotomy.

Characteristic of all neurorrhaphy techniques are problems with (1) technical difficulty, (2) prolonged delay in reinnervation, (3) loss of nerve fiber population, (4) neuroma formation, and (5) inappropriate reinnervation. Inappropriate reinnervation is expected even in successful neurorrhaphies because adductor fibers are present in the recurrent nerve at a ratio of 3:1 over abductor fibers.[23]

The nerve-muscle pedicle technique described by H. M. Tucker et al.[24, 25] was originally intended to be used as a means for reinnervating the transplanted larynx. It has since been modified[26, 27] and is now used successfully in reinnervation of bilaterally paralyzed vocal cords in human beings.[28–30] This approach avoids all of the problems listed above for neurorrhaphy procedures.

The rapidity with which reinnervation can be achieved by this technique has been thought a result of the need to wait only for healing between the nerve-muscle pedicle and the recipient muscle into which it is implanted. Once this has been achieved, incoming nerve impulses in the intact nerve fibers can cause depolarization of motor units in the pedicle and, apparently by "spillover," also of the muscle fibers in the recipient muscle. The problem of inappropriate reinnervation or misdirection of fibers is avoided by selective reinnervation of the abductor muscles only. Phonation is preserved because of the tendency of the vocal cord to return to the paramedian position when not actively abducted.

Technique.[29, 30] The patient is examined with an anterior commissure laryngoscope. A suction tip or spatula is used to palpate the arytenoids to be certain that at least one of them is passively mobile while the patient is completely paralyzed. If the patient has a previous tracheotomy, such evaluation will be simplifed, but it can also be performed without intubation under apneic technique with paralysis. If both arytenoids are limited in motion or fixed in addition to being paralyzed, reinnervation surgery will not be successful and an arytenoidectomy should then be performed (with permission from the patient). If at least one arytenoid is mobile, a tracheotomy is performed if the patient does not already have one. This is advisable because the patient whose glottis has been barely adequate may have significant upper airway obstruction postoperatively.

An incision is then made transversely in a natural skin crease at about the lower border of the thyroid cartilage, just lateral to the midline, to a point posterior to the anterior border of the sternocleidomastoid muscle. The skin, platysma, and subcutaneous fat are carefully traversed, maintaining good hemostasis so that the various tissue planes can be identified. The sternocleidomastoid muscle is identified at its anterior border and mobilized posteriorly. The anterior belly of the omohyoid muscle and the jugular vein are identified. The ansa hypoglossi can usually be seen lying upon or crossing the internal jugular vein (Fig. 7–4A). The fascia overlying the ansa hypoglossi is carefully incised, and the nerve is traced proximally and distally to the first major branch, which is usually the one to the anterior belly of the omohyoid. If there is difficulty in identifying the ansa, the superior border of the anterior belly of the omohyoid muscle may be followed posteriorly from its insertion into the thyroid cartilage until the nerve is identified entering the muscle on its undersurface, usually in company with a small artery. A nerve tester is used to demonstrate that the branch in question causes contraction of the omohyoid muscle when stimulated. The muscle bundles of the omohyoid muscle are gently separated so that the actual point of entry of the nerve into the muscle is observed (Fig. 7–4B). A 2-mm to 3-mm square block of muscle, just large enough to include the point of entry and arborization of the nerve, is dissected from the omohyoid muscle using a sharp scissors or razor knife. The nerve-muscle pedicle is then isolated for a sufficient length to reach the larynx.

The retrolaryngeal prevertebral space is entered posterior to the thyroid cartilage by blunt and sharp dissection. In this fashion, the larynx can be rotated away from the operator to expose the posterior aspect. The inferior constrictor fibers can be seen passing diagonally from a posterosuperior point to an anteromedial position, and these may be gently separated with blunt dissection (Fig. 7–4C). This is continued until either the pyriform sinus is encountered and displaced superiorly, or the posterior cricoarytenoid muscle is observed (Fig. 7–4, D and E). This muscle is identified by observing that its fibers pass at right angles to those of the inferior constrictor. Two or three 5-0 nylon sutures are placed in the posterior cricoarytenoid muscle and then sutured to the block of muscle that is part of the nerve-muscle pedicle (Fig. 7–4F).

The larynx is allowed to rotate back into position. The nerve-muscle pedicle will rest in contact with the posterior cricoarytenoid muscle under little or no tension, in normal anatomic position. The wound is closed in the usual fashion after the insertion of a small Penrose drain. Postoperatively, the patient may

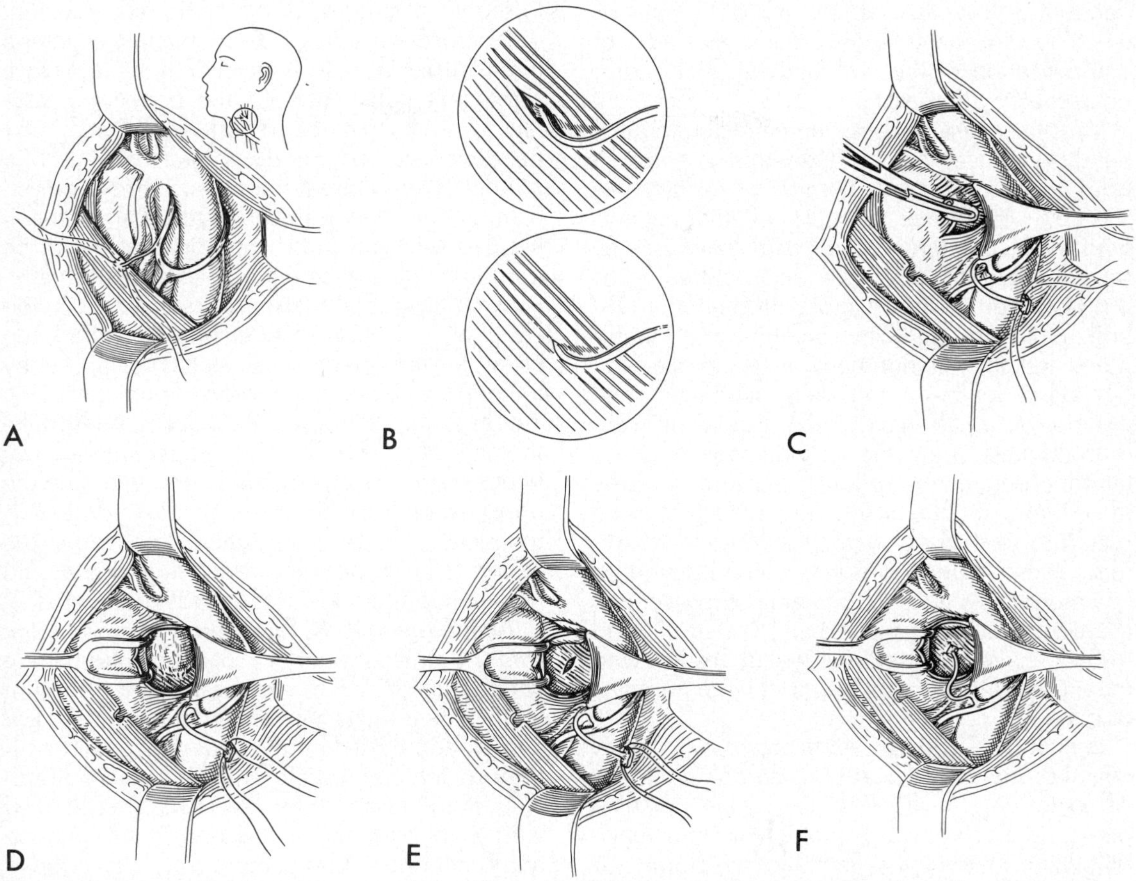

Figure 7–4. Laryngeal reinnervation. *A*, Isolation of branch of ansa hypoglossi to the omohyoid muscle. *B*, Dissection of ansa hypoglossi terminating fibers into the omohyoid muscle. *C*, Separation of inferior constrictor muscle fibers and exposure of the pyriform sinus. *D*, Identification of pyriform sinus and superior reflection to gain exposure to the posterior cricoarytenoid muscle. *E*, Incision into the posterior cricoarytenoid muscle. *F*, Insertion of ansa hypoglossi–omohyoid nerve-muscle pedicle into posterior cricoarytenoid muscle.

be fed the next morning and no antibiotics are necessary.

To date, more than 150 patients have undergone selective laryngeal reinnervation using the ansa hypoglossi and omohyoid muscle as the nerve-muscle pedicle. The short-term and long-term success rate to date has been 90 per cent. Success is judged by observation of appropriate vocal cord abduction or by sufficient improvement in airway for adequate day-to-day activity. Of the thirteen failures, three have been successfully managed by nerve-muscle reinnervation on the opposite side, resulting in satisfactory improvement in the airway and permitting decannulation. Two patients in the group underwent attempted reinnervation of the contralateral side, which also failed. These patients subsequently required a Woodman arytenoidectomy, which resulted in adequate airway.

The length of time between onset of paralysis and reinnervation does not seem to be critical; several of the patients in this series had paralysis for many years prior to successful reinnervation.[27, 28]

TREATMENT OF UNILATERAL VOCAL CORD PARALYSIS

Vocal Cord Injection. Unilateral vocal cord paralysis does not present the life-threatening problem of airway limitation that occurs with bilateral vocal cord paralysis. The patient with unilateral paralysis usually is hoarse but has no real respiratory distress. He may occasionally have minor problems with aspiration of saliva but not usually of food or drink. Depending on the etiology of the unilateral vocal cord paralysis, spontaneous recovery can often occur. If not, frequently there is compensation by the opposite vocal cord, which moves across the midline to reach the paralyzed cord and produces a satisfactory voice. In those patients who do not have spontaneous recovery or compensation of the contralateral vocal cord, hoarseness will persist.

Various materials have been injected into the paralyzed vocal cord in attempts to move it from a paramedian to a midline position. In 1911, Bruning[31] successfully treated patients who had unilateral vocal cord paralysis by injecting paraffin. This gave good initial results but lasted only a short time. Problems of embolization, drifting of the paraffin, and paraffinoma led to abandonment of this procedure. Glycerin, tantalum powder, cartilage, and ground bone all have been used but were discontinued since the introduction of polytetrafluoroethylene (Teflon) paste and silicone injections. Silicone, while initially a promising material, sets up no local reaction and, therefore, does not remain where placed beyond a few months. As a result, the initial improvement in voice quality is lost. Lewy,[32] Dedo,[33] and Rubin[34] have reported successful results with intracordal injection of Teflon in large numbers of patients.

Injection of Teflon is indicated for (1) unrecovered unilateral vocal cord paralysis, (2) vocal cord volume defects, (3) congenital dysplastic dysphonia, (4) glottic incompetence following cordectomy, hemilaryngectomy, or blunt laryngeal trauma, and (5) glottic incompetence following arytenoidectomy[33] (Table 7–4). Teflon is contraindicated in myasthenia laryngis and hypogenesis vocalis. This is because the tonal clarity present prior to injection may be replaced by huskiness that is more objectionable to the patient than the high pitch and thin quality of the voice produced by these conditions.[35]

Teflon can be injected into the middle third of the true vocal cord, but care must be taken to place the material as far laterally as possible. If Teflon is placed near the edge of the vocal cord, it may be rejected and it will change the mass vibratory characteristics of the cord with less than satisfactory voice results. Because of the tight adherence of the mucous membrane to the vocal process of the arytenoid, injection in the posterior third of the cord must be lateral to this structure. It is, therefore, difficult to close significant gaps between the arytenoid cartilages. In 135 patients reported by Dedo,[33] 81 per cent regained a fairly normal voice and 96 per cent were at least improved. Other complications from Teflon injection also can occur. If there is over-injection, the vocal cord can be immobilized and will not oscillate normally. Airway obstruction also may occur with too large an injection. Placement of Teflon too close to the margin, as stated above, may interfere with good vibratory function. If the Teflon is injected too superficially, it will take the path of least resistance and accumulate just beneath the mucous membrane, ballooning the upper surface of the cord. An injection that is too deep, on the other hand, can cause the Teflon to be displaced through the cricothyroid membrane and appear as a mass in the neck.[35]

Table 7–4. INDICATIONS FOR TEFLON INJECTION—UNILATERAL VOCAL CORD PARALYSIS

Unrecovered unilateral vocal cord paralysis
Vocal cord volume defects
Congenital dysplastic dysphonia
Glottic incompetence following cordectomy, hemilaryngectomy, or blunt laryngeal trauma
Glottic incompetence following arytenoidectomy

Technique of PTFE Injection. The ambulatory surgical unit is used for patients undergoing Teflon injection. The anesthesiologist is present in the operating room to monitor the patient and to administer intravenous diazepam (Valium) or fentanyl citrate with droperidol (Innovar), if necessary. The larynx is anesthetized with 5 ml to 8 ml of 0.5 per cent tetracaine hydrochloride (Pontocaine), which is dripped onto the upper surface of the true vocal cords until the cough reflex is abolished. A 2-ml Bruning syringe is filled with Teflon. The anterior commissure laryngoscope is used to identify the true vocal cords, and the Bruning syringe is used to inject the Teflon paste (Fig. 7–5A). The first injection is made in the posterolateral aspect of the middle third of the true vocal cord, just anterior to the vocal process, until the area of the vocal cord swells toward the midline (Fig. 7–5, B to F). The patient is then asked to phonate, and the vocal cords are observed. The voice will often change from a husky, breathy quality to a clear voice. If necessary, a second injection is made in the anterolateral aspect of the middle third of the true vocal cord. At the conclusion of Teflon injection, the true vocal cord that received the injection should appear straight and should meet the contralateral vocal cord. Antibiotics or corticosteroids are not needed. Some edema may develop within the true vocal cord several minutes after the injection, and this may make the final endpoint rather difficult to determine if one does not work quickly. The patient may have a husky voice for several days following the injection because of residual edema.

When there is a poor cough, aspiration, or a

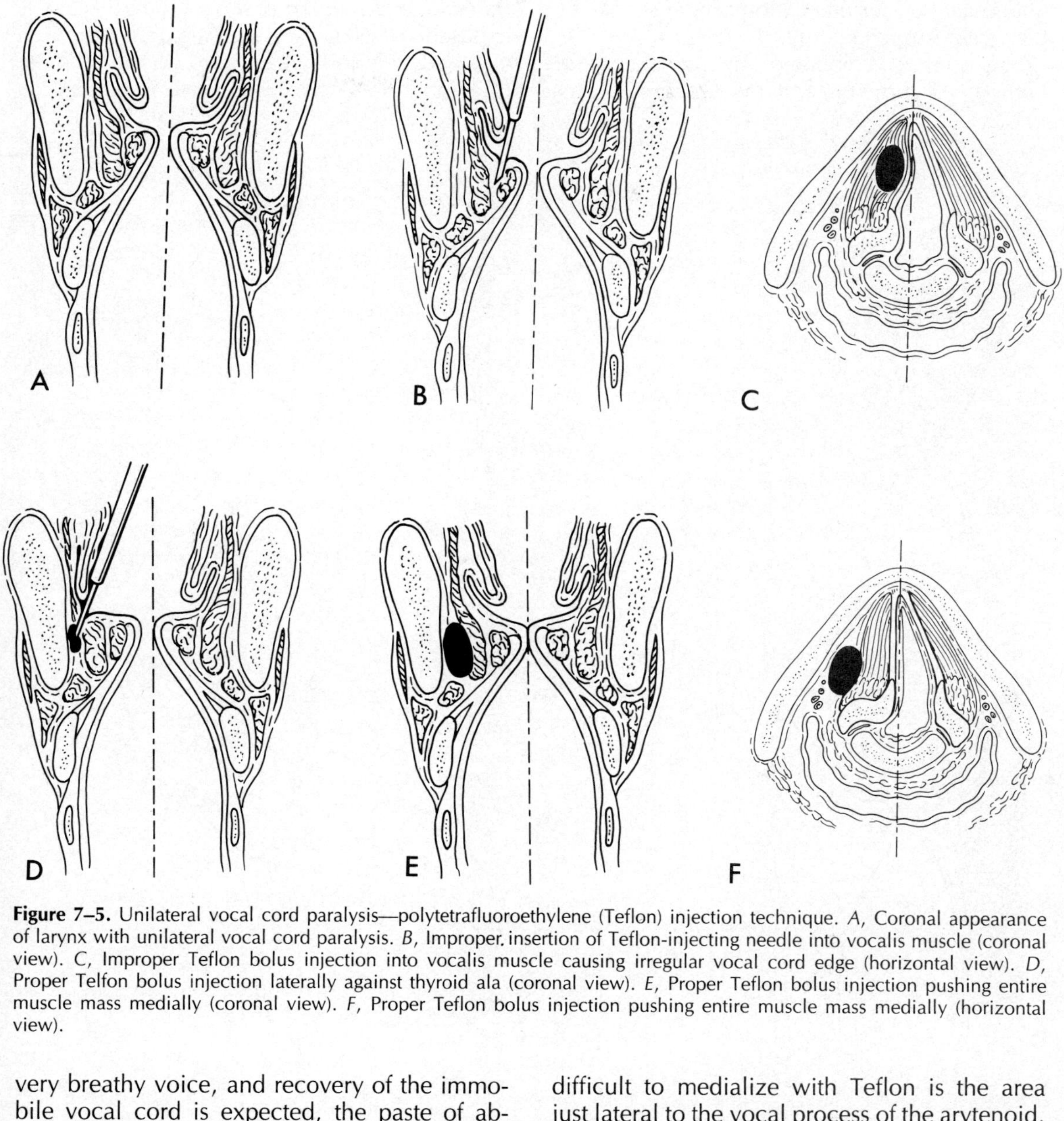

Figure 7–5. Unilateral vocal cord paralysis—polytetrafluoroethylene (Teflon) injection technique. *A*, Coronal appearance of larynx with unilateral vocal cord paralysis. *B*, Improper insertion of Teflon-injecting needle into vocalis muscle (coronal view). *C*, Improper Teflon bolus injection into vocalis muscle causing irregular vocal cord edge (horizontal view). *D*, Proper Telfon bolus injection laterally against thyroid ala (coronal view). *E*, Proper Teflon bolus injection pushing entire muscle mass medially (coronal view). *F*, Proper Teflon bolus injection pushing entire muscle mass medially (horizontal view).

very breathy voice, and recovery of the immobile vocal cord is expected, the paste of absorbable gelatin sponge (Gelfoam) can be injected into the vocal cord using the same technique as for Teflon. This gives relief for several weeks until the Gelfoam is absorbed.[36]

Vocal Cord Medialization. In those cases where satisfactory glottic competence cannot be achieved with Teflon alone, surgical medialization may be considered. In the patient who has both recurrent and superior laryngeal nerve paralysis, the vocal cord will be farther from the midline. In addition, paralysis of the cricothyroid muscle will result in total flaccidity. It is difficult to place a sufficient amount of Teflon into such a vocal cord to give adequate voice and prevent aspiration. The area most difficult to medialize with Teflon is the area just lateral to the vocal process of the arytenoid. In 1952, Meurmann[37] reported the insertion of autogenous costochondral cartilage through a median incision between the thyroid cartilage and its inner perichondrium. He reported successful restoration of voice in nine of fifteen cases. One patient required an emergency tracheotomy because of airway obstruction, and, in another patient, the graft spontaneously extruded because of infection.

Opheim[38] also medialized the vocal cord with cartilage, but he obtained the cartilage from the superior aspect of the thyroid ala and placed it medial to the inner perichondrium of the thyroid cartilage, where he felt he had more control in placement. Because of intralaryngeal manipulation, resultant glottic edema usually necessitates tracheotomy.

Sawashima[39] combined the advantages of both the Meurmann and the Opheim procedures. The upper part of the thyroid cartilage is exposed and is excised with the perichondrium attached anteriorly (Fig. 7–6, A and B). The thyroid ala is then excised vertically along the

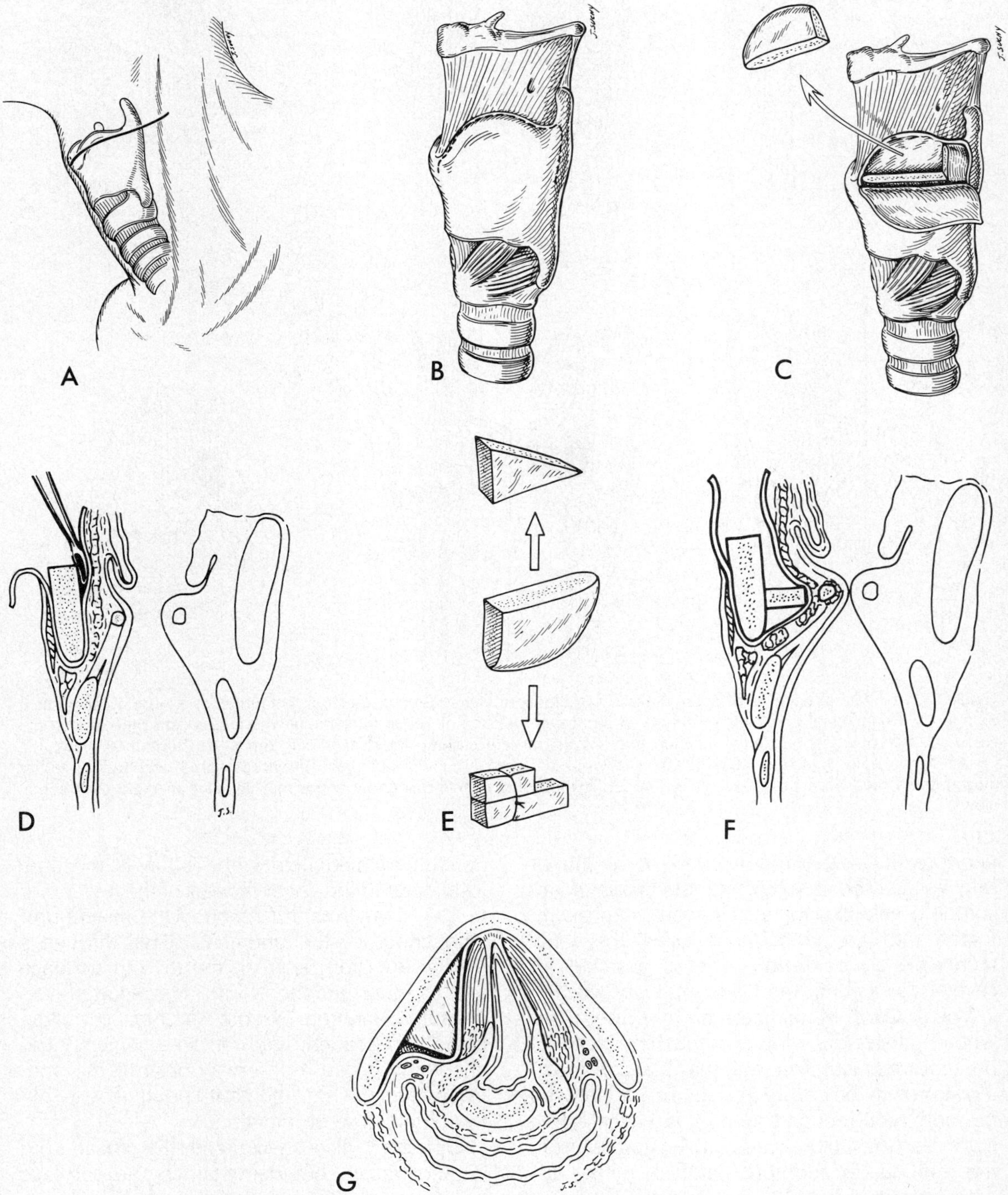

Figure 7–6. Vocal cord medialization. *A*, Skin incision for cartilagenous vocal cord medialization. *B*, Perichondrial incision for cartilaginous vocal cord medialization. *C*, Excision of superior one-third of thyroid cartilage ala for graft. *D*, Internal thyroid cartilage perichondrial elevation to create pocket for cartilage graft. *E*, Fashioning cartilage graft. *F*, Insertion of cartilage graft for medialization (coronal view). *G*, Cartilage graft in position achieving medialization.

midline, care being taken not to enter the inner perichondrium (Fig. 7–6C). The thyroid ala is elevated at the level of the vocal cord, and the cartilage is inserted (Fig. 7–6, D to G). Sawashima reported 20 cases with good, subjective patient improvement in 18. One patient from the two unsuccessful cases was operated on again with good results.

Reinnervation of the Unilaterally Paralyzed Vocal Cord. Although the majority of patients suffering from unilateral vocal cord paralysis regain motion spontaneously or achieve compensation of the contralateral vocal cord, there remain some patients who experience persistent glottic insufficiency causing hoarseness or aspiration. It is generally agreed that the treatment of choice in patients with unilateral vocal cord paralysis is Teflon injection. While Teflon or surgical medialization, or both, can restore glottic competence, these procedures do not provide dynamic motion or tensing ability to the paralyzed vocal cord. In addition, it is possible that the presence of the bolus of Teflon in the vocal cord may alter the mass characteristics of the cord and, therefore, affect its passive vibratory qualities.

Many surgeons find it difficult to alter the posterior third of the glottis to the extent necessary to correct glottic insufficiency in this region with Teflon alone. The most difficult cases to correct are those in which both superior and recurrent laryngeal nerve paralysis are present. The "professional voice," such as the actor, singer, minister, salesman, or lawyer, may require vocal quality superior to that which can be achieved with either Teflon or surgical medialization. For these reasons, investigations designed to correct glottic insufficiency and restore motion and tensing ability to the unilaterally paralyzed cord have been undertaken by H. M. Tucker.[40–42]

Technique for Unilateral Vocal Cord Reinnervation. The incision and preparation for unilateral vocal cord reinnervation is identical to that for bilateral vocal cord reinnervation with regard to design of the nerve-muscle pedicle from the ansa hypoglossi and omohyoid muscle (Fig. 7–7A). The strap muscles are then retracted on the side of the larynx to be reinnervated and mobilized to expose the lower 50 per cent of the thyroid cartilage, in an approach similar to that for a hemilaryngectomy. A posteriorly based perichondrial flap is created by making an incision through the perichondrium of the thyroid cartilage at the midline and carrying it posteriorly along the lower border of the thyroid cartilage and superiorly along a point approximately midway between the superior and inferior borders of the thyroid cartilage (Fig. 7–7B). A block of cartilage is removed with the Stryker saw from the lower 50 per cent of the thyroid ala so that an intact posterior and inferior strut of cartilage is left (Fig. 7–7C). If this is done carefully, the inner layer of the perichondrium on the thyroid cartilage remains intact. This can then be incised to expose the fibers of the lateral thyroarytenoid muscle, the major adductor and tensor of the larynx (Fig. 7–7C). The nerve-muscle pedicle is approximated to this muscle and sutured in place with two or three 5-0 nylon sutures (Fig. 7–7D). The wound is closed in a fashion similar to that for bilateral reinnervation (Fig. 7–7E).

Results (Table 7–5). In the nine cases originally reported by Tucker,[40] the cause of the paralysis was surgical sectioning of the vagus nerve high in the neck in the course of removal of a neoplasm. In all 31 cases to date (1982), there has been some observable degree of spontaneous return of adductor function seen in the reinnervated cord approximately two to eighteen weeks postoperatively.[41] In 12 cases, there was appropriate synchronous adduction and tensing of the reinnervated vocal cord with each phonatory effort. Normal or near-normal sound of voice, as well as good pitch control, was observed in each of these cases. In 15 cases, the reinnervated vocal cord became more or less continuously adducted to the midline but tensed with phonation, again resulting in a good voice. Four cases exhibited partial adduction with some tensing but without the ability to bring the vocal cord all the way to the midline. In these, while there was improvement, it was not to a satisfactory degree, and three of these patients had subsequent small Teflon injections to bring the voice to the desired level. All patients regained an effective cough with cessation of aspiration.

This modification of the nerve-muscle pedicle technique for the unilaterally paralyzed larynx is possible because the omohyoid mus-

Table 7–5. UNILATERAL LARYNGEAL REINNERVATION BY NERVE-MUSCLE PEDICLE TECHNIQUE—17 CASES

Outcome	Number of Cases
Synchronous adduction with each phonatory effect	8
Continuous adduction, tension with phonation	4
Partial adduction, Teflon needed	5

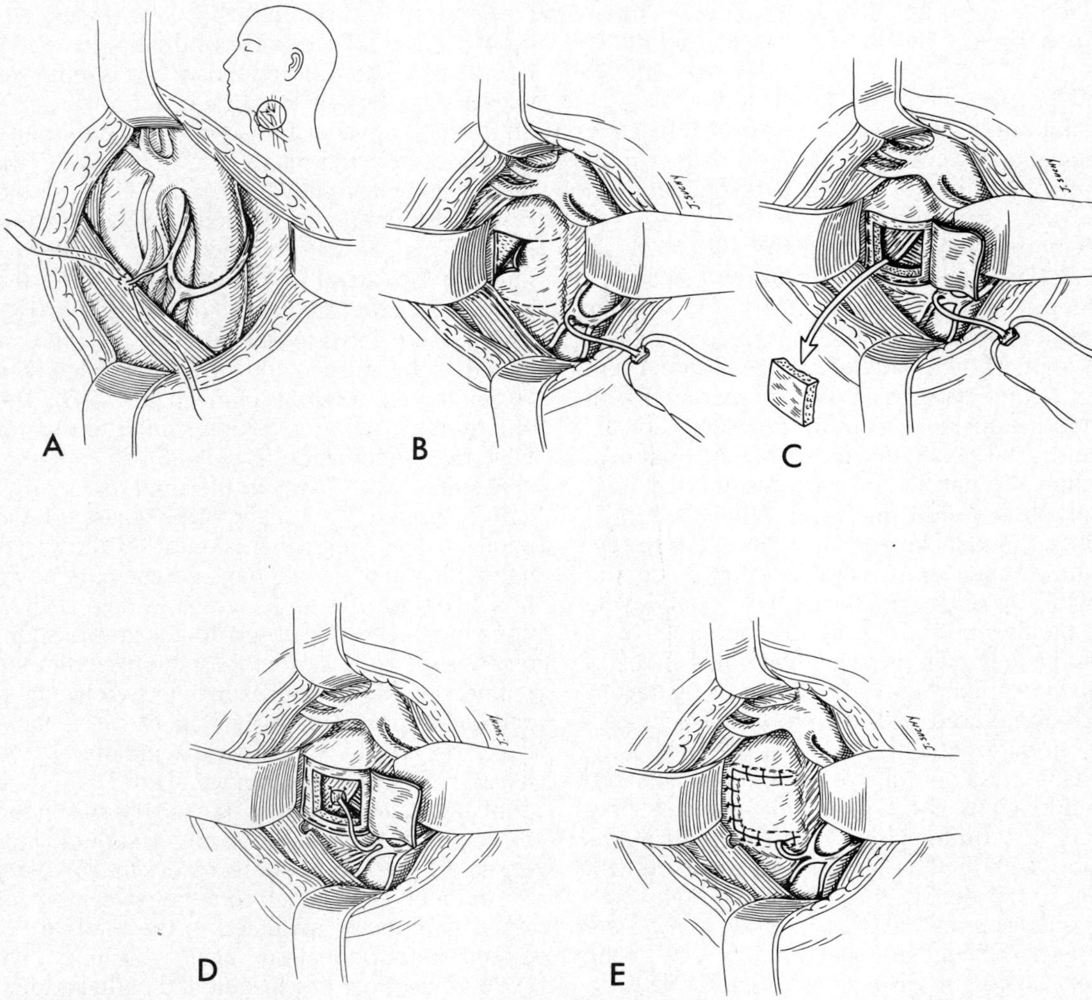

Figure 7–7. Unilateral reinnervation. *A*, Creation of nerve-muscle pedicle. *B*, Posteriorly based thyroid cartilage perichondrial graft. *C*, Removal of block of thyroid cartilage to expose adductors of larynx. *D*, Insertion of ansa hypoglossi–omohyoid nerve-muscle pedicle into adductors of larynx. *E*, Closure of thyroid cartilage perichondrium.

cle and other strap muscles of the neck are accessory muscles of phonation and respiration. There is voluntary tensing of these muscles during attempts at high pitch and loudness. Motor activity during such efforts, when rerouted to the lateral thyroarytenoid muscle, results in appropriate adduction and tensing of the vocal cords.

VOCAL CORD PARALYSIS AND SURGERY FOR CHRONIC ASPIRATION

The larynx plays an important role in avoiding aspiration of food, saliva, and other secretions, even though aspiration is mainly prevented by the action of the base of the tongue and epiglottis during swallowing. The approximation of the true vocal cords and other sphincteric actions of the larynx are also essential for adequate cough because they permit the buildup of subglottic pressure. When adequate airway protection is lacking, the result may be aspiration, pneumonia, eventual lung abscess, and subsequent death.

Although a cuffed tracheotomy tube may be an effective temporary protection against aspiration, it is not a suitable long-term solution because of complications of tracheotomy. The laryngologist is, therefore, faced with the problem of controlling aspiration in patients whose laryngeal difficulties may or may not be expected to recover eventually. Total laryngectomy is a possible means of eliminating aspiration and must be considered in those cases where other methods have failed. Such an approach, while effective, remains distasteful in dealing with nonmalignant disease. Several other approaches may be useful.

Vocal Cord Injection for Aspiration. While Teflon has been used for the most part in the improvement of voice in patients with unilateral vocal cord paralysis, it also can have an important role in the treatment of acute and chronic aspiration. Teflon injection can be rather easily performed under local anesthesia and, therefore, may be used in the debilitated patient with long-standing aspiration. Injection of Teflon into the paralyzed vocal cord can improve glottic competency, thus limiting further aspiration, and also improve cough to better clear secretions from the tracheobronchial tree. Either glycerin or Teflon paste can be used, depending upon the etiology and expected recovery of the vocal cord paralysis. Rontal et al.[43] reported the use of such an approach in the treatment of acute and chronic aspiration. Teflon in the true vocal cord increased the ability of his patients to maintain maximum peak intraluminal air pressure with a mean increase of 174 per cent above preinjection level.

Vocal Cord Fusion. Montgomery[44] has described a surgical technique for vocal cord fusion to prevent aspiration. This is performed through a midline thyrotomy. The glottis is denuded of epithelium circumferentially along its entire length, resecting a strip of mucous membrane between two parallel incisions. A 3-0 polyethylene suture is passed through the anterior aspect of each true vocal cord and out through the vocal process of the arytenoid. This allows fusion of the two true vocal cords to each other after healing has occurred (Fig. 7–8). In 12 patients, vocal cord fusion eliminated aspiration and restored deglutition. Three patients were able to communicate after vocal cord fusion by using an electronic larynx.

The Arytenoid-Epiglottic Flap. The arytenoid-epiglottic flap has been used successfully to close off the aditus laryngis by folding the epiglottis posteriorly, suturing it to the arytenoid cartilages, and thus preventing aspiration. Hable and Murray[45] reported on seven cases, all with good results. Four of these patients did extremely well with the arytenoid-epiglottic flap. One patient, who had failure with this flap, had undergone previous radiation to the larynx. A second patient continued to aspirate but showed definite clinical improvement. A third patient had subsequent revision of the flap with resulting normal upper airway and normal speech.

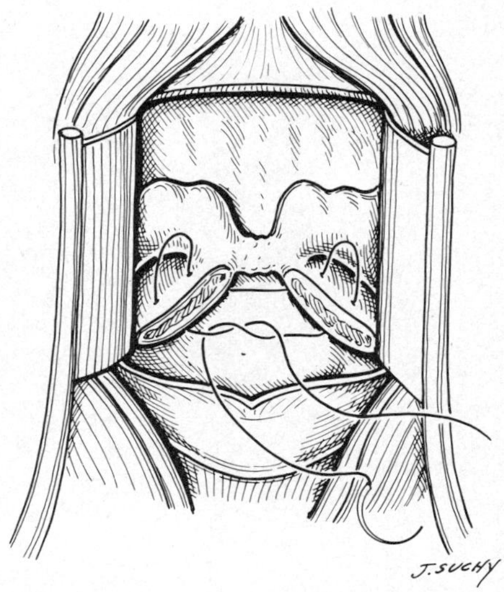

Figure 7–8. Vocal cord fusion achieved through laryngofissure.

Laryngeal Diversion Procedures. Secretions can be prevented from traveling into the tracheobronchial tree by diverting the larynx into the esophagus. Lindeman[46] reported tracheoesophageal dissociation with the larynx completely diverted from the trachea. After success was demonstrated in six dogs, the procedure was applied clinically. The proximal end of the trachea was diverted into the esophagus and the distal end brought out as a permanent tracheostoma (Fig. 7–9). Lindeman felt that tracheoesophageal diversion could be well tolerated by patients with lower cranial nerve deficits and severe chronic aspiration. The patient is followed clinically and if aspiration through the larynx decreases satisfactorily, it becomes possible to reconstruct the trachea.

Cricopharyngeal Myotomy in Management of Vocal Cord Paralysis and Chronic Aspiration. Cricopharyngeal myotomy has been employed to facilitate effective swallowing after partial laryngeal surgery. Without it, the patients may have significant aspiration and dysphagia. Cricopharyngeal myotomy has also been used to achieve improved swallowing and to discourage recurrence following excision of Zenker's diverticulum. Individuals who have multiple cranial nerve paralyses as a result of a stroke or intracranial surgery may exhibit dyssynergia of the inferior constrictor or of the cricopharyngeal muscles, or both, in addition to varying degrees of laryngeal paralysis. Such a situation is not compatible with normal swal-

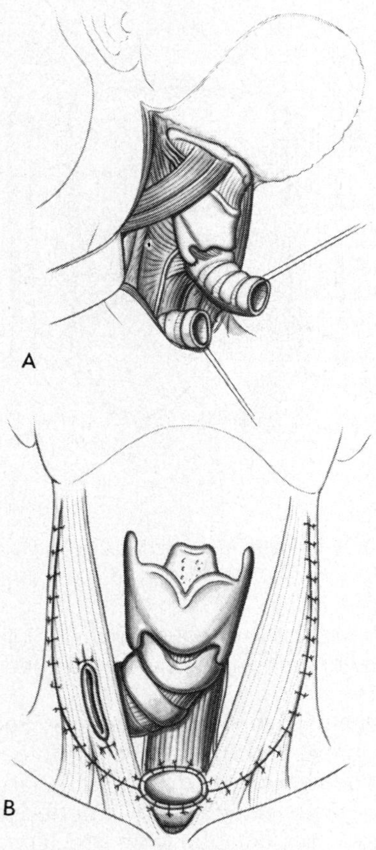

Figure 7–9. Tracheal transection and laryngeal diversion.

lowing. For this reason, cricopharyngeal myotomy should be considered as part of the surgical management of these patients. Although something can be done to create a more competent glottis, aspiration will usually persist unless appropriate relaxation of the cricopharyngeal muscle is achieved. This can be best accomplished through a cricopharyngeal myotomy.

Technique. The procedure can be performed under local or general anesthesia through a transverse incision at the level of the cricoid (Fig. 7–10A). A dissection is carried anterior to the sternocleidomastoid muscle and carotid sheath into the retropharyngeal space (Fig. 7–10B). The larynx is rotated, the cricopharyngeal muscle identified, and the fibers sectioned in the midline (Fig. 7–10C). By an approach from above and in the midline, the recurrent laryngeal nerve can be avoided completely; thus, further injury to it may be prevented (Fig. 7–10, D and E).

Cricopharyngeal myotomy should be considered before more aggressive, irreversible procedures, such as laryngectomy, are undertaken. It may also serve in place of laryngeal closure or diversion procedures, since it is an operation readily performed with little morbidity.

THE CHILD WITH VOCAL CORD PARALYSIS

Of 389 cases of partial or complete bilateral abductor paralysis, 149 were infants and children under the age of 12.[47] Fifty-five per cent of the patients had a congenital cause for paralysis, while 40 per cent had acquired laryngeal nerve paralysis (Table 7–6).[48]

Appropriate management of vocal cord paralysis in children is similar to that for adults. Tracheotomy is often indicated because of the problem of airway obstruction. This solves the initial life-threatening problem. In those patients with congenital paralysis, correction of the congenital lesion may result in resolution of the paralysis. Children with idiopathic vocal cord paralysis may recover within one year. For these reasons, it is wise to avoid irreversible

Table 7–6. ETIOLOGY OF VOCAL CORD PARALYSIS IN THE PEDIATRIC PATIENT—149 CASES*

Cause	Number of Cases	Total Cases
Congenital		
Without associated anomalies	39	39
With associated anomalies		
Neurologic	21	
Laryngeal	10	
Cardiac	8	
Other	4	
		43
Total congenital		82 (55%)
Acquired		
Secondary to congenital anomalies		
Meningomyelocele, A-CM, hydrocephalus	24	
Hydrocephalus unrelated to A-CM	6	
Postoperative for congenital lesion	11	
		41
Secondary to acquired conditions		
Infectious	7	
Neoplasm	7	
Birth trauma	2	
Guillain-Barré syndrome	2	
		18
Total acquired		59 (40%)
Undetermined	8	8 (5%)
Total cases		149 (100%)

*From Holinger LD et al.: Ann Otol Rhinol Laryngol 85:428, 1976.

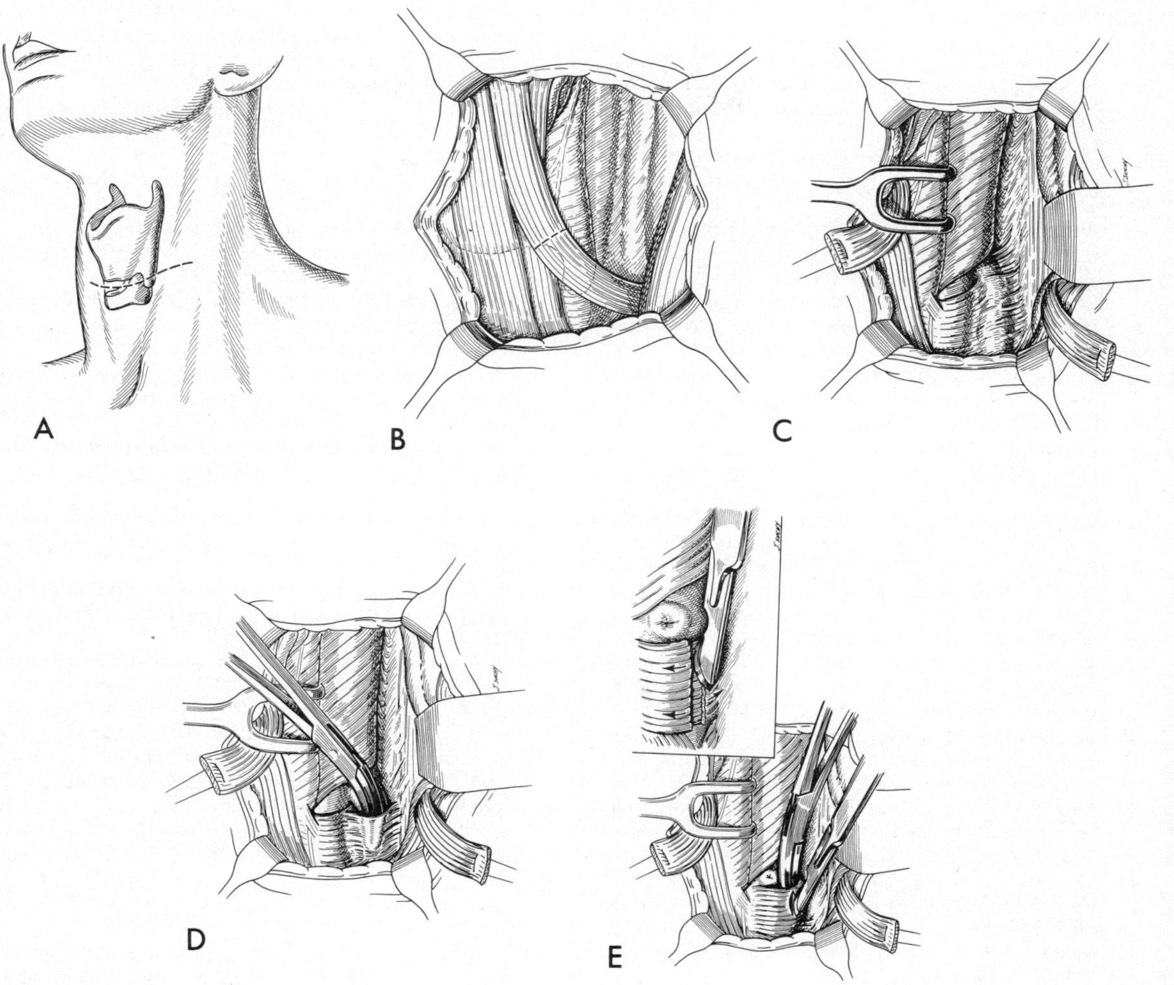

Figure 7–10. Cricopharyngeal myotomy. *A*, Skin incision. *B*, Division of omohyoid muscle to gain exposure of posterior edge of thyroid ala. *C*, Hook inserted on posterior edge of thyroid ala, rotation of larynx, and exposure of inferior constrictor muscle and cricopharyngeal muscle. *D*, Insertion of clamp under cricopharyngeal muscle fibers to aid in myotomy. *E*, Cutting cricopharyngeal fibers to achieve myotomy.

or dangerous procedures since the possibility exists that the vocal cord paralysis will resolve itself. When resolution of vocal cord paralysis can no longer be expected, a definitive approach such as vocal cord reinnervation using the nerve-muscle pedicle technique should be attempted. Arytenoidectomy should generally be avoided, at least until the child starts school, because it is irreversible and more difficult to perform satisfactorily in infant larynges. While arytenoidectomy is an uncommon operation in children, 11 cases were reported by Cohen.[48] He advocated waiting two or three years after vocal cord paralysis before proceeding with this definitive surgical procedure, trying to accomplish it before the child entered school. He employed a Woodman type of external arytenoidectomy in all cases except one in which a midline thyrotomy was employed. He found that the procedure was well tolerated with little postoperative morbidity, and decannulation was successful in all children. He reported preservation of satisfactory vocal quality in all cases. Nevertheless, stridor was noted on exertion in almost all of his cases.

The nerve-muscle pedicle technique is particularly attractive in children. It has resulted in successful decannulation in 14 of 16 children under the age of 12 operated on by H. M. Tucker. It has the advantage, in addition to preservation of voice, that it does not interfere with either the recurrent nerve or the arytenoid as arytenoidectomy techniques might. Therefore, if there is even a slight chance of spontaneous recovery, that chance will remain after such an attempt.

References

1. Thornell WC: Vocal cord paralysis. *In* Paparella MM, Shumrick DA (eds): Otolaryngology Vol. 3: Head and Neck. Philadelphia, WB Saunders Company, 1973, pp 650–651.
2. Faaborg-Anderson K, Munk-Jensen A: Unilateral paralysis of the superior laryngeal nerve. Acta Otolaryngol 57:155, 1964.
3. Abelson TI, Tucker HM: Laryngeal findings in superior laryngeal nerve paralysis: A controversy. Otolaryngol Head Neck Surg 89:463–470 (May–June) 1981.
4. Semon F: Clinical remarks on the proclivity of abductor fibers of the recurrent laryngeal nerve to become affected sooner than the adductor fibers, or even exclusively in cases of undoubted central or peripheral injury or disease of the roots or trunks of the pneumogastric, spinal accessory, or recurrent nerves. Arch Otolaryngol 2:197, 1881.
5. Parnell FW, Brandenberg JH: Vocal cord paralysis: A review of 100 cases. Laryngoscope 80:1036, 1970.
6. Tucker HM: Vocal cord paralysis—1979: Etiology and management. Laryngoscope 90:585–590, 1980.
7. Rueger RG: Benign disease of the thyroid gland and vocal cord paralysis. Laryngoscope 84:897, 1974.
8. Kelley JD: Surgical treatment of bilateral paralysis of abductor muscles. Arch Otolaryngol 33:293, 1941.
9. Woodman DG: A modification of the extralaryngeal approach to arytenoidectomy for bilateral abductor paralysis. Arch Otolaryngol 43:63, 1946.
10. Thornell WC: Intralaryngeal approach in arytenoidectomy in bilateral abductor vocal cord paralysis. Trans Am Acad Ophthalmol and Otolaryngol 53:631, 1949.
11. Kirchner FR: Endoscopic rehabilitation of the airway in laryngeal paralysis. Trans Am Laryngol Assoc 103:46–47, 1982.
12. Downey WL, Keenan WG Jr: Laryngofissure approach for bilateral abductor paralysis. Arch Otolaryngol 88:513, 1968.
13. Montgomery W: Cricoarytenoid arthrodesis. Ann Otol Rhinol Laryngol 70:451, 1961.
14. Horseley JS: Suture of the recurrent laryngeal nerve with report of a case. Trans South Surg and Gynecol Assoc 22:161, 1909.
15. Fraser CH: The treatment of paralysis of the recurrent nerve by nerve anastomosis. Ann Surg 79:161, 1924.
16. Barnes EB, Balance C: Anastomosis of recurrent laryngeal to phrenic nerves: Some recovery of function. Br Med J 2:158, 1927.
17. Lahey FH: Suture of the recurrent laryngeal nerve for bilateral abductor paralysis. Ann Surg 87:481, 1928.
18. Doyle PJ: Bilateral laryngeal nerve repair. *In* Gurria, AB, Salmon LFW (eds): Proceedings of the IX International Congress of Oto-Rhino-Laryngology in Mexico City, 1969. Amsterdam, Excerpta Medica, 1970, p 297.
19. Boles R, Fritzell B: Injury and repair of the recurrent laryngeal nerves in dogs. Laryngoscope 79:1405, 1969.
20. Miehlke A.: Rehabilitation of vocal cord paralysis. Arch Otolaryngol 100:431, 1974.
21. Iwamura S: Functioning remobilization of the paralyzed vocal cord in dogs. Arch Otolaryngol 100:122, 1974.
22. Moreledge DR et al.: Delayed reinnervation of paralyzed larynx. Arch Otolaryngol 97:291, 1973.
23. Miglets AW: Functional laryngeal abduction following reimplantation of the recurrent laryngeal nerves. Laryngoscope 84:1966, 1974.
24. Tucker HM et al.: Vocal cord remobilization in the canine larynx. Arch Otolaryngol 92:530, 1970.
25. Tucker HM: Laryngeal transplantation: Current status 1974. Laryngoscope 85:787, 1975.
26. Lyons RM, Tucker HM: Delayed restoration of abduction in the paralyzed canine larynx. Arch Otolaryngol 100:176, 1974.
27. Tucker HM: Human laryngeal reinnervation. Laryngoscope 86:769, 1976.
28. Tucker HM: Human laryngeal reinnervation: Long-term experience with the nerve-muscle pedicle technique. Laryngoscope 88:598, 1978.
29. Tucker HM: Laryngeal paralysis: Etiology and management. *In* English GM (ed): Otolaryngology Vol 3. Hagerstown, MD, Harper and Row, 1981.
30. Tucker HM: Nerve-muscle pedicle reinnervation of the larynx: Avoiding pitfalls and complications. Trans Am Laryngol Assoc 103:104–108, 1982.
31. Bruning W: Uber eine neue Behandlungsmethode der Rekurrenslahmung. Ver Deutsch Laryngol 18:23, 1911.
32. Lewy RB: Glottic rehabilitation with Teflon injection: The return of voice, cough, and laughter. Acta Otolaryngol 58:214, 1964.
33. Dedo HH et al.: Intracordal injection of Teflon in the treatment of 135 patients with dysphonia. Ann Otol Rhinol Laryngol 82:661, 1973.
34. Rubin HJ: Intracordal injection of silicone in selected dysphonias. Arch Otolaryngol 81:604, 1965.
35. Rubin HJ: Misadventures with injectable polytef (Teflon). Arch Otolaryngol 101:114, 1975.
36. Schramm VL et al.: Gelfoam paste injection for vocal cord paralysis: Temporary rehabilitation of glottic competence. Laryngoscope 88:1268, 1978.
37. Meurmann Y: Operative mediofixation of the vocal cord in complete unilateral paralysis. Arch Otolaryngol 55:554, 1952.
38. Opheim O: Unilateral paralysis of the vocal cord. Acta Otolaryngol 45:226, 1955.
39. Sawashima M et al.: Surgery for hoarseness due to unilateral vocal cord paralysis. Arch Otolaryngol 87:87, 1968.
40. Tucker HM: Reinnervation of the unilaterally paralyzed larynx. Ann Otol Rhinol Laryngol 86:789, 1977.
41. Tucker HM: Laryngeal reinnervation for unilateral vocal cord paralysis: Long-term results. Ann Otol Rhinol Laryngol 90:457–459, 1981.
42. Tucker HM: Preservation and restoration of voice after laryngeal paralysis. *In* Surgery for Phonatory Disorders. New York, Churchill Livingstone, 1981.
43. Rontal E et al.: Vocal cord injection in the treatment of acute and chronic aspiration. Laryngoscope 86:625, 1976.
44. Montgomery W: Surgery to Prevent Aspiration. Arch Otolaryngol 101:679, 1975.
45. Hable MB, Murray JE: Surgical treatment of life endangering chronic aspiration pneumonia. Plast and Reconstr Surg 49:305, 1972.
46. Lindeman RC: Diverting the paralyzed larynx: A reversible procedure for intractable aspiration. Laryngoscope 85:157, 1975.
47. Holinger LD et al.: Etiology of bilateral abductor vocal cord paralysis. Ann Otol Rhinol Laryngol 85:428, 1976.
48. Cohen SR: Arytenoidectomy in children. Laryngoscope 83:1293, 1973.

8

Update of Laryngeal Reinnervation Concepts and Options

Roger L. Crumley, M.D.

Since Horsley's initial report in 1909, surgeons have attempted many techniques to achieve functional reinnervation of the paralyzed larynx.[1] Like Horsley, some investigators have described initial success with a particular operative procedure, only to be forced to recant after clinical experience proved otherwise. Others have simply not written follow-up reports and their techniques have been presumed failures. Others, most notably Tucker, have described continued clinical success following initial animal studies.

This chapter will discuss the theoretical problems inherent in muscle reinnervation as it relates to the larynx. Previously described techniques will be enumerated and their limitations noted. Since laryngeal reinnervation remains a controversial field at the time of this writing, it is hoped that this chapter can simplify some of the concepts that fuel the controversy.

BASIC CONCEPTS IN MUSCLE REINNERVATION

The first concept to be considered is that when the motor nerve to a muscle is severed, both muscle and nerve undergo profound changes. Transection of the nerve triggers biochemical reactions in the muscle, making it more receptive to reinnervation. Substances called *neurocletin,*[2] *nerve-growth-factorlike substance,*[3] and others have been found in the vicinity of the motor end plates in denervated muscle. These substances are thought to arise from the muscle fiber near the motor end plate, the motor end plate itself, or the distal nerve fiber (axon) near it; they are known to promote axon sprouting (Figs. 8–1 and 8–2).

Another substance, known as *axon-sprouting inhibitor factor,* is normally found in innervated muscle near the motor end plate and disappears following denervation, allowing adjacent fibers to sprout axons toward the denervated motor end plate and muscle fiber (Fig. 8–1). The biologic interplay of these chemical substances results in a highly favorable situation for regenerating nerve fibers to innervate the degenerated muscle fiber, whether they come from the original innervating motor nerve or from a different (foreign) nerve supplied by a surgical nerve transfer procedure.[4, 5]

A second important concept regarding muscle reinnervation pertains to the ablity of muscle

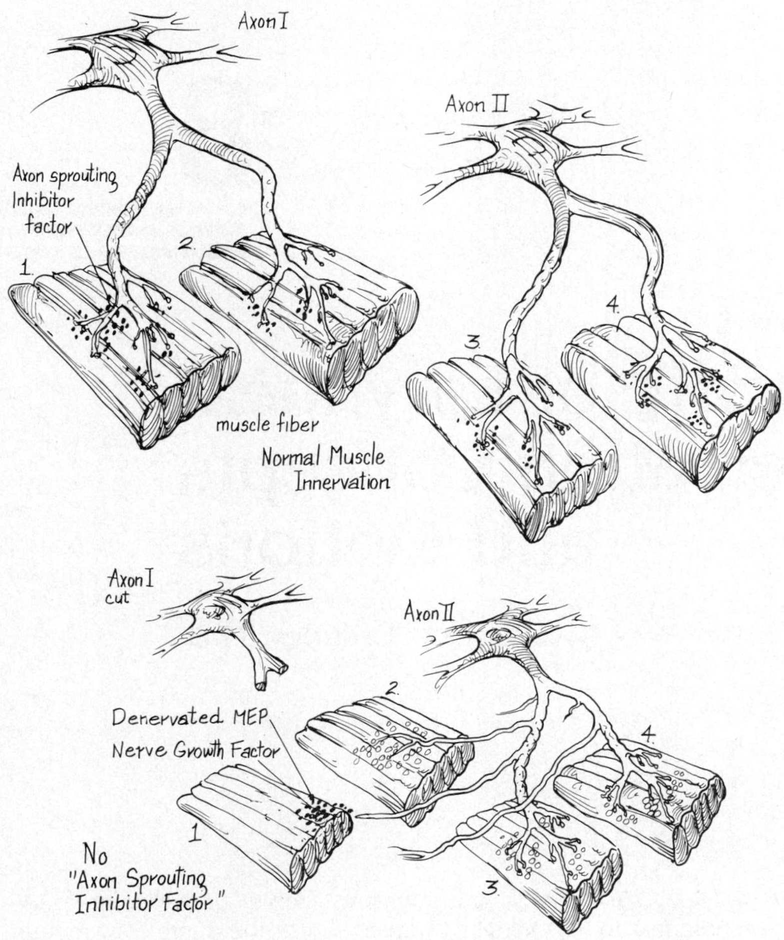

Figure 8–1. *Top,* Normal innervation. Axon I innervates muscle fibers 1 and 2; Axon II innervates muscle fibers 3 and 4. Axon-sprouting inhibitor factor *(see fiber 1)* suppresses axon sprouting and stabilizes the status quo. *Bottom,* After Axon I is cut, there is no longer any axon-sprouting inhibitor factor near the motor end plate (MEP) of fiber 1 and axon sprouting from Axon II begins. Note that nerve growth factor *(near fiber 1)* acts as a chemotactic force to attract the sprouting axons.

to accept new innervation from transplanted foreign nerves. Exner (1885), Steindler (1916), and Elsberg (1917) were among early surgical pioneers who demonstrated that denervated muscles could be reinnervated by nerve transfers.[6–8] Exner's report describing innervation of the cricothyroid muscle in the rabbit establishes this investigator as the father of laryngeal reinnervation. These early reports and many since have confirmed the feasibility of muscle reinnervation by nerve transfer.

Elsberg's work defined some of the limits of reinnervation. He showed that a normal muscle would not accept any additional reinnervation (hyperneurotization) by a nerve implant. Guth, however, demonstrated that an innervated muscle could be induced to accept additional innervation from an implanted nerve if the original nerve were injured at the time of nerve transfer. This results in the phenomenon called *dual innervation.*[9]

Perhaps the most significant factor controlling acceptance in clinical muscle reinnervation is the status of the motor end plates in the paralyzed muscle. Motor nerve fibers are well known to ramify and undergo axon sprouting among denervated muscle fibers. Avon sprouting results in characteristic electromyographic (EMG) patterns known as polyphasic potentials and giant motor units. It is seen histologically as type-grouping in biopsies of reinnervated muscle.

Axon sprouting also increases the number of muscle fibers innervated by a single nerve fiber. (One nerve fiber, or axon, and its innervated muscle fibers constitute a *motor unit.*) This expansion in the size of motor units enables fewer than normal nerve fibers to innervate the entire muscle. Hence, a small number of regenerating nerve fibers can sprout and "tie up," or occupy, all the motor end plates in the muscle. This apparently restricts subsequent reinnervation surgery, because the existing motor end plates are innervated by nerve fibers even though the number is too small to produce muscle contraction. Because these innervated

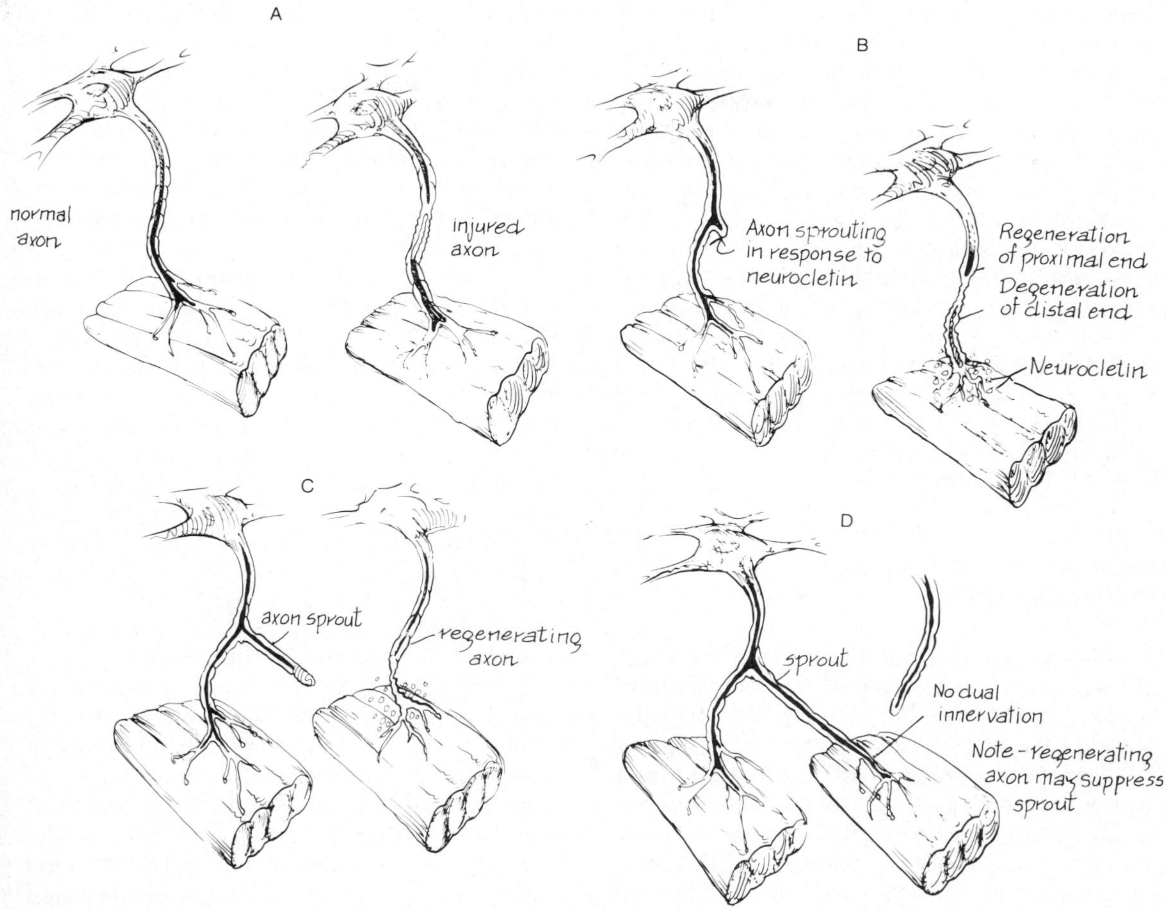

Figure 8–2. *A*, Normal and injured axons near motor end plate. *B*, Injured axon undergoing Wallerian degeneration. Intact axon begins to sprout in response to neurocletin. Neurocletin may be similar or identical to nerve growth factor. *C* and *D*, Axon sprout reaches denervated muscle fiber before the original axon has regenerated. The regenerating axon may subsequently suppress the sprout, but these mechanisms are still poorly understood.

motor end plates cannot accept new innervation or undergo hyperneurotization, any reinnervation attempt will fail unless the surgeon transects, or otherwise injures, the existing subclinical innervation.

A third important concept is that muscle reinnervation by nerve implantation always results in the reinnervated muscle assuming the contraction and biochemical characteristics of the implanted nerve. Hence, anastomosis of the hypoglossal and facial nerves results in facial muscle contraction only when lingual movements are attempted, whether they are involuntary or voluntary. Similarly, the phrenic nerve's cyclic inspiratory firing pattern can be transferred to other muscles. Lurje described how brachial plexus injuries could result in the innervation of upper arm muscles by regenerating phrenic fibers, and Hardy reported transfer of the phrenic's respiratory pattern to the muscles of facial expression with phrenicofacial anastomosis.[10, 11]

The fourth important concept regarding muscle reinnervation is that of *denervation atrophy,* which is thought to render muscle incapable of undergoing reinnervation following a period of denervation. The time from nerve injury to onset of atrophy is unclear, probably varying from species to species, among individuals within a certain species, and among different muscles of the same subject.[12] Evidence indicates that the laryngeal muscles are among the least hardy in regard to length of survival without innervation.[13] The best evidence in human beings, however, suggests that muscular cytoarchitecture and survivability are retained for at least three years following denervation.[14]

The earlier that reinnervation occurs, the greater the chance that functional muscle contractions will be regained. In the larynx, this is most important because cricoarytenoid joint fixation may impair vocal cord abduction and adduction if reinnervation is delayed.

The best indicator of muscle survival after

denervation is the demonstration of fibrillation potentials by EMG.[15] Such potentials require the presence of an intact muscle fiber without an innervating axon and indicate the most favorable situation for muscular reinnervation. Unfortunately, EMG of the posterior cricoarytenoid muscle is quite difficult to perform in the clinical setting. Because the denervated posterior cricoarytenoid muscle is extremely thin and delicate, needle electrodes placed percutaneously or during direct laryngoscopy are likely to record muscle action potentials from the adjacent pharyngeal constrictor muscles or from the inferior constrictor muscle.[16–18] As a result, candidates for laryngeal reinnervation are best identified at this time by history and physical findings alone.

HISTORY OF LARYNGEAL REINNERVATION

Although we have described Exner as the first investigator to describe laryngeal reinnervation (1885), it was not until 1909 that Horsley reported the first successful repair of the recurrent laryngeal nerve.[1, 6] He simply performed neurorraphy in a 40-year-old woman whose recurrent laryngeal nerve had been severed by a bullet from a pistol. Nineteen years later, Lahey reported a similar case, but he admitted in a subsequent manuscript that he had failed to demonstrate vocal cord function.[19, 20]

Frazier, Colledge, and Ballance all reported repairs to the recurrent laryngeal nerve in the 1920s.[21–23] In 1927, Colledge and Ballance first noted the problem of paradoxical movements—expiratory abduction and inspiratory adduction—following simple suture anastomosis of this nerve.[24] With this observation, they set the stage for subsequent laryngologists to introduce selective reinnervation techniques.

Other surgeons felt that neural techniques were not worthwhile; consequently, most patients were treated with arytenoidectomy or tracheotomy, or both. Baker (1916), Jackson (1922), and Hoover (1932) removed parts of one vocal cord to enlarge the glottis, but their procedures left the arytenoid intact.[25–27] Meanwhile, Loré, Woodman, Kelly, King and others advocated various arytenoidectomy and arytenoidopexy procedures.[28–31] Introduction and refinement of EMG allowed an improved understanding of experimental reinnervation techniques. Siribodhi's report in 1963 yielded evidence of laryngeal synkinesis, which had first been described clinically in 1927.[15] This proof that adductor muscles become reinnervated by abductor nerve fibers, and vice versa, confirmed the futility of recurrent laryngeal nerve repair and correlated with clinical findings of medial bulging of the vocal cord during inspiration. This reinnervation results in muscular competition for control of the arytenoid by adductors and the abductor in both inspiration and expiration.

The clinical result of anastomosis of the recurrent laryngeal nerve is a vocal cord that neither abducts nor adducts and that bulges medially during inspiration. Obviously, if both vocal cords are so afflicted, airway compromise results. If only one cord is paralyzed and is reinnervated randomly as above, as with recurrent laryngeal nerve neurorraphy, the airway is usually satisfactory because of the abduction of the normal cord, and the voice may be better than it would be if the cord were left paralyzed. This has been debated for years.[32 33]

Salassa has described partial airway obstruction resulting from medial bulging of a unilateral reinnervated vocal cord (following recurrent laryngeal nerve section for spastic dysphonia).[34] This obstruction may represent one of the major deterrents to anastomosis of this nerve as a means of providing vocal cord tone for phonation following unilateral paralysis. At present, treatment for unilateral vocal cord paralysis rarely involves any reinnervation technique.

The foregoing discussion explains why reinnervation of the larynx with bilateral vocal cord paralysis must be selective. Doyle, who appreciated this problem, pioneered the selective reinnervation of the larynx. He implanted the posterior cricoarytenoid muscle with the recurrent laryngeal nerve in dogs and in human beings, thereby achieving selective reinnervation in the sense that he implanted one nerve into one muscle; however, it was unselective in the sense that the implanted nerve contained both abductor and adductor fibers.[35–37] Although both Doyle and Miglets described this technique of nerve implantation into the paralyzed posterior cricoarytenoid muscle in human beings, it has not gained subsequent clinical acceptance, probably because it requires that the recurrent laryngeal nerve be intact and viable near the larynx, a situation not commonly found in paralyzed larynges.[37, 38]

Doyle and Miehlke independently reported implanting the posterior cricoarytenoid muscle with the vagus nerve with good results.[37, 39] This procedure also has not gained clinical acceptance because of its unselective nature in that

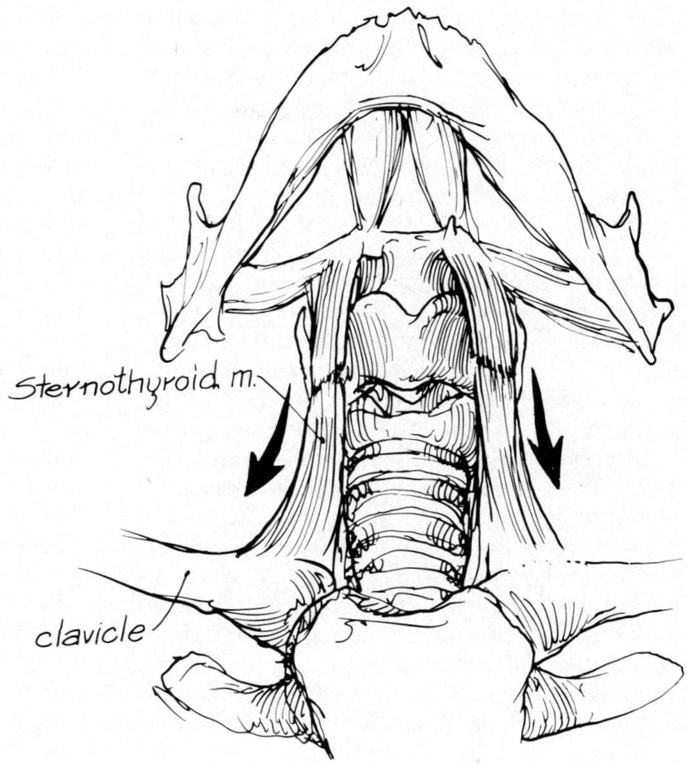

Figure 8–3. Sternothyroid muscle contraction produces divergence and downward displacement of the thyroid cartilage laminae.

the muscle is implanted with both abductor and adductor fibers.

The ansa hypoglossi, which innervates the strap muscles, was first proposed as a neural source for laryngeal reinnervation in 1924 by Frazier et al.[40] The ansa has been shown to fire during partial airway obstruction and hypoxia but not during quiet respiration.[41] The strap muscles situated below the larynx act as accessory muscles of inspiration, while the thyrohyoid muscle is accessory to phonation and other adductive functions (Fig. 8–3). Fink's excellent

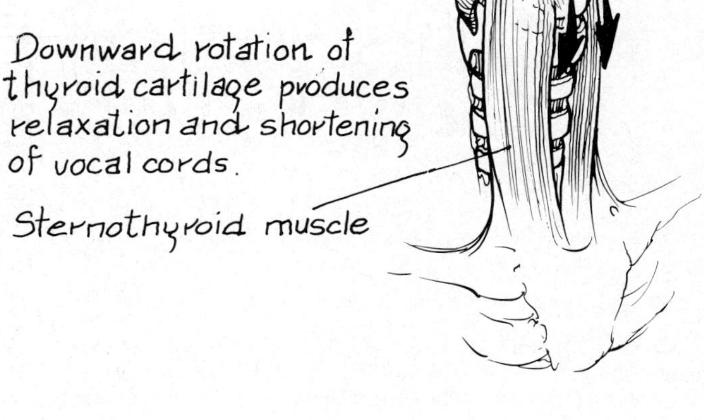

Figure 8–4. Sternothyroid muscle contraction causes relaxation and shortening of the vocal cords, if neither cricothyroid nor thyrohyoid muscles contract simultaneously.

work outlines clearly the role of sternothyroid muscle contraction (during labored respirations) and how it results in lateralization of the vocal cord, whether it is paralyzed, normal, or reinnervated (Fig. 8–4).[42] Conversely, the thyrohyoid muscle, by drawing the thyroid cartilage superiorly, results in a medial positioning of the cord (Fig. 8–5). In both situations, this cord positioning is effected by lateral or medial movement of the entire thyroid lamina, with the vocal cord inside the larynx following passively (Fig. 8–3). The opposing respiratory functions of the two muscles make their respective nerve supplies excellent candidates for selective adductor (thyrohyoid) and abductor (sternothyroid) nerve implants. Tucker utilized this principle in his neuromuscular pedicle procedure, although he considered the omohyoid muscle as physiologic a source of inspiratory stimulation as the sternothyroid.[43–45] Indeed, Evoy reported transfer of the sternothyroid muscle to the posterior cricoarytenoid tendon but did not pursue this procedure after initial successes in animals.[46] King's arytenoidopexy operation utilized this principle in transferring the omohyoid muscle to the muscular process of the arytenoid cartilage.[31]

The inspiratory nature of the phrenic nerve makes it an ideal implant for the denervated posterior cricoarytenoid muscle. EMG has shown the phrenic nerve to fire only 40 to 100 milliseconds later in inspiration than the abductor fibers to the posterior cricoarytenoid muscle.[47] Other biologic similarities exist between this muscle's motor nerve and the phrenic nerve. Hypoxia and hypercarbia cause an increased firing rate in both nerves, while decreasing muscular activity in the adductors.[48] In addition, the phrenic nerve resembles the nerve to the posterior cricoarytenoid in that it undergoes inhibition during coughing and phonation. The diaphragm and posterior cricoarytenoid muscle are so similar that some investigators have suggested the two muscles are innervated by the same collection of neurons in the brain stem.[49, 50]

Although the phrenic nerve is the main motor nerve to the diaphragm, transection of the phrenic nerve is remarkably well tolerated by human beings.[51] Fackler et al. studied 14 pa-

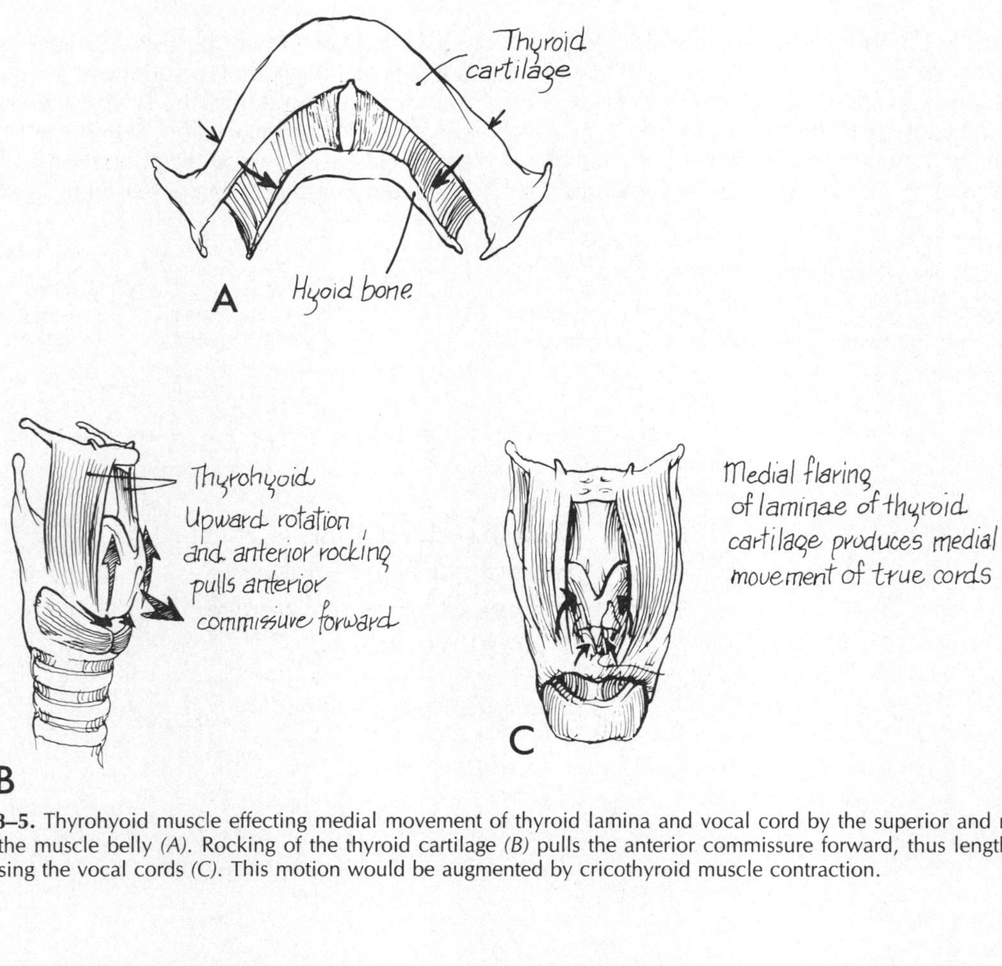

Figure 8–5. Thyrohyoid muscle effecting medial movement of thyroid lamina and vocal cord by the superior and medial pull of the muscle belly *(A)*. Rocking of the thyroid cartilage *(B)* pulls the anterior commissure forward, thus lengthening and tensing the vocal cords *(C)*. This motion would be augmented by cricothyroid muscle contraction.

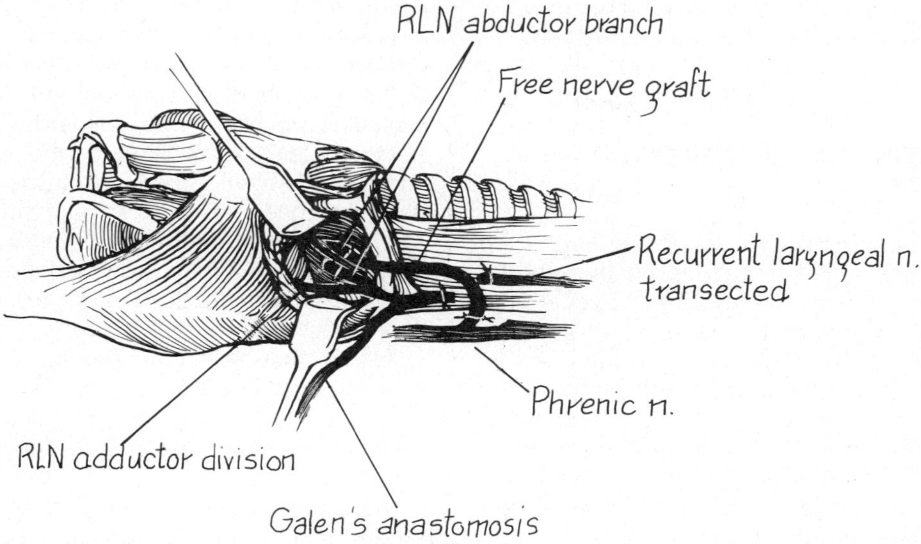

Figure 8–6. Phrenic nerve graft procedure described by this author. Phrenic nerve fibers, firing on inspiration, pass through a free nerve graft to the distal abductor branch, which directs them to the posterior cricoarytenoid muscle. (RLN, recurrent laryngeal nerve.)

tients who had phrenic nerve transection for phrenicofacial anastomosis; they found that all 14 had recovered normal vital capacity and maximal breathing capacity six months later.[52] This probably arises from reinnervation of the diaphragm by accessory phrenic nerves or lower thoracic nerves, or both. Thus, the phrenic nerve can be used as a donor for laryngeal reinnervation with minimal physiologic insult.

Transfer of the phrenic nerve's inspiratory pattern to other muscles is well known.[11] Lurje suggested the phrenic as a nerve graft donor for Erb's palsy, while Swift et al. showed that brachial plexus injuries could result in phrenic nerve misdirected regeneration, producing inspiratory muscular activity in the upper arm muscles, a phenomenon he termed *arm-diaphragm synkinesis*.[10, 53]

These features have made the phrenic nerve an obvious candidate for surgical transfer to the paralyzed larynx. Ballance described anastomosis of the phrenic nerve to the recurrent laryngeal nerve in 1924.[54] This, of course, resulted in inspiratory motion of the vocal cord, but motion that was synkinetic. Subsequent investigators were aware of the necessity for direct routing of the transferred nerve to the paralyzed posterior cricoarytenoid muscle. Fex implanted the distal stump of the phrenic nerve into the muscle in 23 cats. Eight animals developed abduction of the vocal cord in inspiration after nine months. Fifteen of the animals had no reinnervation because of avulsion of the nerve graft from the muscle.[55] Morledge and Taggart et al. described successful phrenic nerve reinnervation of the posterior cricoarytenoid muscle in animals and also reported that avulsion of the nerve graft prevented successful reinnervation in some instances.[56, 57] Crumley et al. succeeded in reinnervating the muscle with phrenic nerve fibers that were split into a free nerve graft, thereby retaining diaphragmatic innervation (Fig. 8–6).[58] We updated that initial study in 1982, describing a larger animal series in which posterior cricoarytenoid reinnervation was confirmed by muscle histology, EMG, nerve excitation, and nerve histologic studies.[59]

Rice similarly used the phrenic nerve to produce reinnervation of the posterior cricoarytenoid muscle in dogs.[60] His method, like ours, consisted of anastomosis of the phrenic nerve to the tiny abductor branch of the recurrent laryngeal nerve. Rice has one clinical case that appears to show reinnervated abduction, while our first four cases, reported in January 1983, did not result in visible cord abduction and were presented as failures.[61]

In addition to reinnervation techniques, other methods of reenergizing the paralyzed muscle have been investigated. Investigators have shown experimentally that electrical stimuli can trigger the laryngeal muscles. Zealear and Dedo described such a triggering device and Bergmann in Berlin reported further promising experimental results.[62, 63] Because clinical trials with such devices have been limited by delays in developing satisfactory implantable devices, these techniques do not warrant further discussion.

EVALUATION OF CONTEMPORARY METHODS

As the ansa hypoglossi and the phrenic nerve are the two nerves most frequently used in laryngeal reinnervation for bilateral vocal cord paralysis, and we know that paralyzed muscle can be reinnervated by implanted motor nerves, clearly reinnervation of the paralyzed posterior cricoarytenoid muscle is possible with either nerve. Why then is this surgically important topic so controversial? The answer lies in the difficulty of documenting and confirming successful cases in human beings.

Tucker and others reporting clinical experiences with the neuromuscular pedicle technique describe successful cases in terms of subjective improvement, but they do not report the percentage of tracheotomized patients able to undergo decannulation, change in vital capacity and pulmonary flow-volume loops, or visual documentation in the form of endoscopic movie footage or videotape.[64, 65] Ward showed movies of such a patient at the American Laryngological Association's annual meeting in 1982, but he admitted that the visual evidence of reinnervated abduction was unclear, at best. Applebaum and May independently reported clinical successes but used none of the above parameters in confirming actual reinnervation.[66, 67]

Proof of reinnervation would require either EMG discharge synchronous with ansa firing or direct observation of muscle contraction produced by electrical stimulation of the neuromuscular pedicle. Both are, of course, extremely difficult to accomplish at this time.

Compounding the difficulty of proving success (of any posterior cricoarytenoid reinnervation technique) is the fact that vocal cord positioning is affected by the strap muscles, the cricothyroid muscle, and the respiratory movements of the trachea and larynx (Figs. 8–3 to 8–6). In our experimental study, apparent abduction was seen in all dogs undergoing the ansa hypoglossi neuromuscular pedicle procedure; however, what we thought to be vocal cord abduction proved to be lateral vocal cord positioning by the strap muscles. Furthermore, the lateral positioning of the vocal cord was abolished by paralyzing the cricothyroid and sternothyroid muscles. None of the neuromuscular pedicles could be electrically stimulated. Histologic sections of the apparently reinnervated larynges showed dense scar tissue lateral to the posterior cricoarytenoid muscle and the muscular process of the arytenoid. Faced with evidence that denervation of the muscle induced nerve fiber sprouting towards the posterior cricoarytenoid muscle (from small nerves passing through the inferior constrictor), we could not explain why axon sprouting from the neuromuscular pedicle did not result in reinnervation.[59] After further research, I have come to believe that the seemingly ingenious step of preserving a muscle block with the motor end plates and the transferred ansa nerve instead presents a biologic obstacle to actual reinnervation.

The reason lies in the substances described earlier in the chapter (neurocletin, axon-sprouting inhibitor factor, and nerve-growth-factorlike substance). The interactions of these and other substances in denervated muscle promote axon sprouting. Axon sprouting is the critical neurophysiologic step in actual reinnervation in that it allows the nerve fibers from an implanted nerve to reach and mate with the denervated muscle's motor end plates. Since the ansa's fibers are still in contact with, and are transferred with, their respective motor end plates, there is no metabolic stimulus for the fibers to sprout toward the denervated muscle. Hence the transferred muscle block remains innervated but fails to interact with (sprout within) the posterior cricoarytenoid muscle (Fig. 8–7).

What about the effects of the axon-sprouting substances elaborated by the denervated muscle? We simply do not have answers to these questions at this time, but data from our studies imply that scarring in the interface between the muscle block and posterior cricoarytenoid muscle, or in the muscle block itself (due to ischemic necrosis of the muscle), acts as a strong deterrent to axon sprouting.

What might allow axons to sprout from a transplanted muscle block with an intact nerve supply? If the muscle block were quite small, perhaps a millimeter or two in diameter, two effects, both conducive to reinnervation, might occur:

1. This smaller volume of muscle would more easily survive on the delicate blood supply of the vasa nervorum accompanying the ansa hypoglossi.

2. Transection of the nerve fibers proximal to their motor end plates (yet within the muscle) would cause the transected axons to sprout in search of denervated motor end plates.

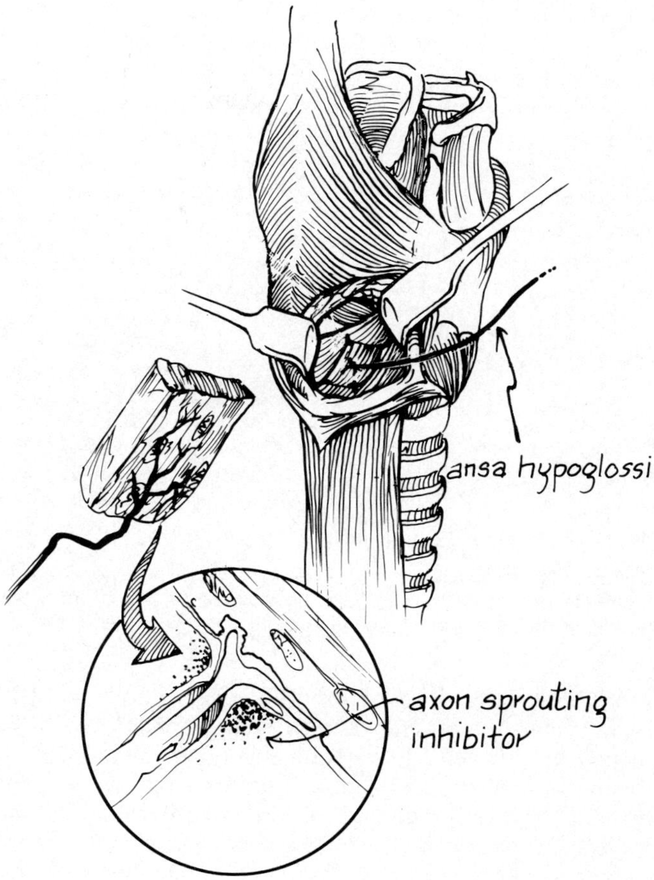

Figure 8–7. Neuromuscular pedicle. Retained continuity of nerve fibers and their motor end plates as described by Tucker. Since terminal axons remain intact, axon-sprouting inhibitor factor is present (*inset*). This substance is a powerful deterrent to axon sprouting.

Creation of such a small muscle block would not preserve motor end plates, as advised by Tucker, and would result in transection of the distal nerve branches between their muscle entry and the motor end plates. This would then allow axon sprouting and reinnervation to occur.

Why go to the trouble of creating such a muscle block when it acts as an impediment to axon sprouting? The ansa hypoglossi can just as well be transected, transferred, and sutured to the abductor branch of the recurrent laryngeal nerve or implanted into the posterior cricoarytenoid muscle, as recently reported by Rice.[68] Direct nerve implantation appears to be a much more physiologic approach to reinnervation with the ansa and deserves careful investigation, both basic and clinical.

One last point should be made regarding the ansa hypoglossi neuromuscular pedicle. No question exists that apparent abduction is seen during hyperpnea in some canine and human subjects that have had the procedure. That this observation was mistaken for posterior cricoarytenoid reinnervation is understandable, but at this time the mechanisms of vocal cord positioning must be clarified. These positioning factors seem to be responsible for the apparent abduction produced by the neuromuscular pedicle procedure.

Glottic enlargement during inspiration occurs by several mechanisms in intact larynges:

1. Lateral arytenoid rotation by posterior cricoarytenoid contraction.
2. Arytenoid stabilization and rocking by posterior cricoarytenoid contraction and lateral cricoarytenoid contraction.
3. Lateral positioning of the vocal cord by sternothyroid muscle contraction (lateralization of the lamina of the thyroid cartilage).
4. Lengthening of the vocal cord by cricothyroid muscle contraction.

Horiuchi and Sasaki have shown how the cricothyroid muscle pulls the anterior commisure anterior relative to the arytenoid and posterior commissure. The cricoarytenoid muscles act to stabilize the arytenoid and resist this force, which tends to pull the arytenoid ante-

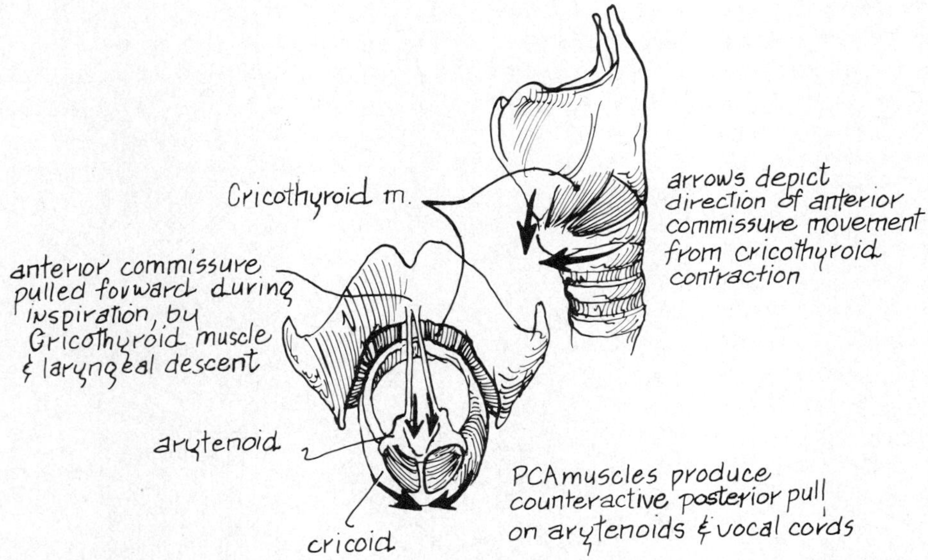

Figure 8–8. Effects of simultaneous cricothyroid and posterior cricoarytenoid contraction. Cricothyroid muscle pulls anterior commissure, vocal cord, and consequently the arytenoid anteriorly, while the posterior cricoarytenoid muscle (PCA) stabilizes the arytenoid by providing a counteractive posterior pull on the arytenoid.

riorly (Fig. 8–8).[42, 69] Recurrent laryngeal nerve paralysis results in loss of the first two mechanisms. In addition, loss of the second mechanism (arytenoid stabilization) produces partial loss of the fourth mechanism. The cricothyroid muscle's anterior pull on the anterior commissure and vocal cord now causes the arytenoid to be pulled medially and anteriorly, further compromising the glottic airway.

In this situation, surgery in and around the posterior cricoarytenoid muscle, regardless of whether reinnervation is achieved or not, produces the following effects:

1. Scar tethering of the arytenoid laterally to the thyroid cartilage.
2. Some degree of arytenoid stabilization.
3. This fixation allows the sternothyroid's pull on the thyroid cartilage to become transferred to the arytenoid, thereby enhancing the sternothyroid's effect on glottic enlargement.
4. Arytenoid stabilization provides the cricothyroid with a more physiologic fulcrum and allows it to once again produce vocal cord lengthening.[59]

In my opinion, these appear to be the methods by which the neuromuscular pedicle technique produces airway improvement. Certainly any reinnervation of the posterior cricoarytenoid that might be achieved would be additionally beneficial. Any procedure that yields hematoma with resultant scarring lateral to that muscle, however, should result in some benefit to the airway by any or all of the latter four effects.

CURRENT STATUS OF PHRENIC NERVE METHODS

Certainly no technique for laryngeal reinnervation has been used as widely as the neuromuscular pedicle technique. Clinical utilization of phrenic nerve transfers is limited to a handful of cases at this time. Our first four cases, reported in 1983, yielded only one patient with airway improvement documented by pulmonary function studies and, in that patient, no visible inspiratory vocal cord abduction was seen.[60]

Knowing that muscles can be innervated by foreign nerves and that the phrenic nerve and the posterior cricoarytenoid's nerve are so physiologically similar, we still find the phrenic transfer the most physiologic approach to reinnervation. That visible clinical success has not been seen does not mean that the concept is not valid; rather, techniques have not been perfected for effecting satisfactory reinnervation.

Our procedure, successful in less than one-half of animal tests, has physiologic disadvantages in that it requires regenerating nerve fibers to cross two neural suture lines and it requires a lengthy free nerve graft. We know nerve regeneration is much stronger in dogs than in human beings. On the other hand, the graft required in human beings (from phrenic split site to the posterior cricoarytenoid muscle) is much shorter than it is in dogs. Nevertheless, the sum of these two factors may preclude effective reinnervation by the split phrenic technique.

A different neurorraphy technique may be clinically successful. Iwamura's procedure of anastomosis of phrenic nerve to recurrent laryngeal nerve has appeal in that the adductors are denervated, thereby nullifying any opposition to posterior cricoarytenoid contraction.[70] The regenerating phrenic fibers must cross only one suture line and traverse an existing vascularized nerve segment (the recurrent laryngeal nerve), not a free nerve graft.[71] The adductor division is ligated to prevent axon regeneration and escape of regenerating phrenic fibers into the adductor muscles. Our group is working in this direction at present.

REINNERVATION FOR UNILATERAL VOCAL CORD PARALYSIS

Injection of polytetrafluoroethylene (Teflon) remains the treatment of choice for most patients with recurrent laryngeal nerve paralysis. The technique usually results in cessation of diplophonia and aspiration and in a markedly improved phonatory quality, although rarely a normal voice. Large series have shown the technique to be a safe, well-tolerated, inexpensive, easily performed, and expeditious treatment.

Nonetheless, several investigators have described operative procedures designed to reinnervate the paralyzed laryngeal muscles rather than relying on the replacement of muscle bulk with Teflon.[72, 73] Indeed, the phonatory function of the vocal cords is best served by two vocal cords with equal muscle tension and mass and with symmetric position. High-speed glottic motion pictures reveal that normal vocal cords beat and undulate symmetrically and synchronously; a paralyzed cord injected with a bolus of Teflon is not capable of this behavior. Consequently, to the end of improving voices in patients with unilateral vocal cord paralysis, reinnervation techniques are worth pursuing.

Tucker has described unilateral reinnervation using the neuromuscular pedicle technique, placing the muscle block into the adductor musculature through a window cut in the lamina of the thyroid cartilage.[73] Japanese investigators have also used this technique. These authors report an improved voice and resolution of aspiration in some cases.[72]

Although technically feasible, recurrent laryngeal nerve neurorraphy has not proved to be a workable option. Misdirected regeneration results in vocal cord spasm and medial inspiratory bulging. The vocal cord does not regain normal phonatory capabilities, despite reinnervation.

Nerve transfers have been reported since the 1920s. The author has one patient in whom ansa hypoglossi anastomosis to the recurrent laryngeal nerve and contralateral ansa hypoglossi implantation into the cricothyroid muscle resulted in an excellent voice, normal to several experienced listeners, and with near-normal voiceprint oscilloscopic analysis.

Such reinnervation for unilateral paralysis has appeal in that the vocal cord's intrinsic musculature can regain its normal mass. Since vibration of the two vocal cords is a passive event, the equal mass of the two cords is as important to vocal quality as is vocal cord position, provided that the two cords can approximate. Reinnervation of the posterior cricoarytenoid muscle, along with the adductors, results in arytenoid stabilization and assists the cricothyroid muscle in vocal cord elongation and tensing. Denervation of the sternothyroid muscle results in medial vocal cord positioning and allows the cords to approximate more easily.[74]

Patients with both superior laryngeal nerve and recurrent laryngeal nerve paralysis often have poorer voices following Teflon injection than do patients with paralysis of the recurrent nerve alone. This is presumably caused by the large posterior glottic chink seen in such cases and is thought to result from lack of the cricothyroid's tensing motion. Reinnervation of the cricothyroid muscle may serve as an adjunct to Teflon injection in these patients.

Such procedures for unilateral paralysis are to a certain degree experimental and should be performed by clinicians experienced in treating laryngeal paralysis. At this time, nerve transfers in such cases should be left to experienced investigators and the time-tested technique of Teflon injection used for the routine management of symptomatic, persistent, unilateral vocal cord paralysis.

References

1. Horsley JA: Suture of the recurrent laryngeal nerve with report of a case. Trans South Surg Gynecol Assoc 22:161, 1909.
2. Hoffman H: Local re-innervation in partially denervated muscle: A histo-physiological study. Aust J Exp Biol Med Sci 28:383, 1950.
3. Spiro RG: Nature of the glycoprotein components of basement membranes. Ann NY Acad Sci 312:106, 1978.

4. Dogliotti AM: Etudes experimentales et premiere application clinique d'une nouvelle operation destinee a augmenter et a equilibrer la fonction neuro-musculaire dans la paralysie des nerfs. J Chir (Paris) 45:30, 1930.
5. Hines HM et al.: Functional changes in nerve and muscle after partial denervation. Am J Physiol 145:48, 1945.
6. Exner S: Notiz zu der Frage von der Faservertheilung mehrerer Nerven in einem Muskel. Pflugers Arch Ges Physiol 36:572, 1885.
7. Steindler A: Direct neurotization of paralyzed muscles: Further study of the question of direction nerve implantation. Am J Orthopedic Surg 14:707, 1916.
8. Elsberg CA: Experiments on motor nerve regeneration and direct neurotization of paralyzed muscles by their own and foreign nerves. Science 45:318, 1917.
9. Guth, L: Neuromuscular function after regeneration of interrupted nerve fibers into partially denervated muscle. Exp Neurol 6:129, 1962.
10. Lurje A: Concerning surgical treatment of traumatic injury of the upper division of the brachial plexus. Ann Surg 127:317, 1948.
11. Hardy R et al.: Phrenicofacial anastomosis for facial paralysis. J Neurosurg 14:400, 1957.
12. Sunderland S: Nerve and Nerve Injuries. New York, Churchill-Livingstone, 1978, pp 303–305.
13. Gutmann E, Young JZ: The reinnervation of muscle after various periods of atrophy. J Anat 78:15, 1944.
14. Bowden REM, Gutmann E: Denervation and reinnervation of human voluntary muscle. Brain 67:20, 1944.
15. Siribodhi C et al.: Electromyographic studies of laryngeal paralysis and regeneration of laryngeal motor nerve in dogs. Laryngoscope 73:148, 1963.
16. Hiroto I et al.: Electromyographic investigations of human vocal cord paralysis. Ann Otol Rhinol Laryngol 77:296, 1968.
17. English DI, Blevins CE: Motor units of laryngeal muscles. Arch Otolaryngol 89:778, 1969.
18. Nakamura F et al.: Electromyographic study of respiratory movements of the intrinsic laryngeal muscles. Laryngoscope 68:109, 1958.
19. Lahey FH: Suture of the recurrent laryngeal nerve for bilateral abductory paralysis. Ann Surg 87:481, 1928.
20. Lahey FH, Hoover WB: Injuries to the recurrent laryngeal nerve and thyroid operations. Ann Surg 108:545, 1938.
21. Frazier CH, Mosser WB: Treatment of recurrent laryngeal nerve injury. Surg Gynecol Obstet 43:134, 1926.
22. Colledge L: On the possibility of restoring movements to a paralyzed vocal cord by nerve anastomosis. Br Med J 2:547, 1925.
23. Ballance C: Some experiments on nerve anastomosis. Mayo Clin Proc 3:317, 1928.
24. Colledge L, Ballance C: The first surgical treatment of paralysis and the diaphragm. Br Med J 1:553, 1927.
25. Baker CH: Report of a case of abductor paralysis with removal of one vocal cord. J Mich Med Soc 15:485, 1916.
26. Jackson C: Ventriculocordectomy: A new operation for the cure of goitrous paralytic laryngeal stenosis. Arch Surg 4:247, 1922.
27. Hoover WB: Functions of the diaphragm and their diagnostic importance. Arch Otolaryngol 15:339, 1932.
28. Loré JM: Symposium on the larynx. I. Practical anatomical considerations of the larynx. Laryngoscope 43:693, 1933.
29. Woodman DeG: Bilateral abductor paralysis: Survey of 521 cases of arytenoidectomy via open approach as reported by 90 surgeons. Arch Otolaryngol 58:150, 1953.
30. Kelly JD: Surgical treatment of bilateral paralysis of the abductor muscles. Arch Otolaryngol 33:293, 1941.
31. King BT, Gregg RL: An anatomical reason for the various behaviors of paralyzed vocal cords. Ann Otol Rhinol Laryngol 57:925, 1948.
32. Gordon JH, McCabe BF: The effect of accurate neurorrhaphy on reinnervation and return of laryngeal function. Laryngoscope 78:236, 1968.
33. Sato F, Ogura JH: Neurorrhaphy of the recurrent laryngeal nerve. Laryngoscope 88:1034, 1978.
34. Salassa JR et al.: Respiratory distress after recurrent laryngeal nerve sectioning for adductor spastic dysphonia. Laryngoscope 92:240, 1982.
35. Doyle PJ: Surgical treatment of bilateral adductor laryngeal paralysis. Proc Can Otol Soc 18, 1964.
36. Doyle PJ et al.: Results of surgical section and repair of the recurrent laryngeal nerve. Laryngoscope 77:1245, 1967.
37. Doyle PJ et al.: Treatment of recurrent laryngeal injury. Arch Surg 96:517, 1968.
38. Miglets AW: Functional laryngeal abduction following reimplantation of the recurrent laryngeal nerves. Laryngoscope 84:1996, 1974.
39. Miehlke A: Zur Indikation und Technik der Recurrensz:neurolyse. Z Laryngol Rhinol Otol 37:44, 1958.
40. Frazier CH: Anastomosis of the recurrent laryngeal nerve with the descendens noni. JAMA 83:1637, 1924.
41. Ellenbogen BG et al.: Accessory muscle activity and respiration. Otolaryngol Head Neck Surg 89:370, 1981.
42. Fink B: Folding mechanism of the human larynx. Acta Otolaryngol (Stockh) 78:124, 1974.
43. Hengerer AS, Tucker HM: Restoration of abduction in the paralyzed canine vocal cord. Arch Otolaryngol 97:247, 1973.
44. Lyons RH, Tucker HM: Delayed restoration of abduction in the paralyzed canine larynx. Arch Otolaryngol 100:176, 1974.
45. Tucker H: Human laryngeal reinnervation. Laryngoscope 86:769, 1976.
46. Evoy M: Experimental activation of paralyzed vocal cords. Arch Otolaryngol 87:155, 1968.
47. Iwamura S: Functioning remobilization of the paralyzed vocal cord in dogs. Arch Otolaryngol 100:122, 1974.
48. Suzuki M, Kirchner JA: The posterior cricoarytenoid as an inspiratory muscle. Ann Otol Rhinol Laryngol 78:848, 1969.
49. Wyke BD: Effects of anaesthesia upon intrinsic laryngeal reflexes. J Laryngol 82:603, 1968.
50. Brewer DW, Dana ST: Investigations in laryngeal physiology: The canine larynx. Ann Otol Rhinol Laryngol 72:1060, 1963.
51. Kelley WD: Phrenic nerve paralysis: Special consideration of the accessory phrenic nerve. J Thorac Surg 19:923, 1950.
52. Fackler CD et al.: Effect of unilateral phrenic nerve section on lung function. J Appl Physiol 23:923, 1967.
53. Swift TR et al.: Arm-diaphragm synkinesis: Electrodiagnostic studies on aberrant regeneration of phrenic motor neurons. Neurology 30:339, 1980.
54. Ballance C: Results obtained in some experiments in which the facial and recurrent laryngeal nerves were anastomosed with other nerves. Br Med J 2:349, 1924.

55. Fex S: Functioning remobilization of vocal cords in cats with permanent recurrent laryngeal nerve paralysis. Acta Otolaryngol (Stockh) 69:294, 1970.
56. Taggart JP: Laryngeal reinnervation by phrenic nerve implantation in dogs. Laryngoscope 81:1330, 1971.
57. Morledge D et al.: Delayed reinnervation of the paralyzed larynx. Arch Otolaryngl 96:291, 1973.
58. Crumley R et al.: Laryngeal reinnervation using the split-phrenic nerve graft procedure. Otolaryngol Head Neck Surg 88:159, 1980.
59. Crumley RL: Experiments in laryngeal reinnervation. Laryngoscope 92 [suppl 30]:1, 1982.
60. Rice D: Personal communication.
61. Crumley RL: Nerve transfer for clinical vocal cord paralysis. Laryngoscope (in press).
62. Zealear DL, Dedo HH: Control of paralyzed axial muscles by electrical stimulation. Acta Otolaryngol (Stockh) 83:514, 1977.
63. Bergmann K: Personal communication, 1982.
64. Tucker HM: Human laryngeal reinnervation: Long-term experience with the nerve-muscle pedicle technique. Laryngoscope 88:598, 1978.
65. Tucker HM: Reinnervation of the paralyzed larynx: A review. Head Neck Surg 1:235, 1979.
66. Applebaum EL et al.: Human laryngeal reinnervation: The Northwestern experience with laryngeal reinnervation. Laryngoscope 89:1784, 1979.
67. May M et al.: Rehabilitation of the crippled larynx. Laryngoscope 90:1, 1980.
68. Rice DH, Colman M: Repair of subglottic stenosis with a free perichondrial graft. Arch Otolaryngol 108:25, 1982.
69. Horiuchi M, Sasaki C: Cricothyroid muscle in respiration. Ann Otol Rhinol Laryngol 87:386, 1978.
70. Iwamura S: Functioning remobilization of the paralyzed vocal cord in dogs. Arch Otolaryngol 100:122, 1974.
71. Rice D: Laryngeal reinnervation. Laryngoscope 92:1049, 1982.
72. Takenouchi S, Okamoto Y: Vocal cord reconstruction using pedicle muscle graft. Jpn J Logopedics Phoniat 14:39, 1973.
73. Tucker H: Reinnervation of the unilaterally paralyzed larynx. Ann Otol Rhinol Laryngol 86:789, 1977.
74. Fink B, Demarest R: Laryngeal Biomechanics. Cambridge MA, Harvard University Press, 1978, pp 15–44.

9

Management of Acute Laryngeal Trauma

Hugh F. Biller, M.D.
and William Lawson, M.D., D.D.S.

Traumatic injuries of the larynx may be classified according to three criteria: (1) type of wound—blunt or closed versus penetrating or open; (2) point of application of the wounding force—external or internal; and (3) anatomic site of the injury—supraglottic, glottic, subglottic, or combined.[1, 2]

The penetrating wound of the airway is obvious and surgical exploration is usually performed immediately. Blunt trauma creates a different situation, however, because the extent of injury may not be appreciated so that the patient fails to receive prompt treatment. This can result in death from sudden airway obstruction. More commonly, the injury results in loss of the phonatory function or in laryngeal stenosis with its significant morbidity from reduced respiratory function.

Internal airway injuries may result from endotracheal intubation, laryngoscopy, bronchoscopy, or a foreign body. External injuries usually occur secondary to motor vehicle accidents, in which a blow to the anterior neck compresses the larynx against the rigid vertebral column, thereby fracturing the cartilages and contusing or lacerating the mucosal lining.

In any injury in which trauma occurs against the extended anterior neck, laryngeal fracture must be suspected and ruled out. The relatively lower observed incidence of laryngeal fractures in children may reflect the resilience of the young elastic cartilages.[3]

DIAGNOSIS OF ACUTE LARYNGEAL TRAUMA

The signs and symptoms of acute laryngeal trauma are airway obstruction, subcutaneous emphysema, hoarseness or aphonia, hemoptysis, odynophagia, and loss of the normal external contour of the larynx. Injuries to the esophagus, cervical spine, and spinal cord should always be considered in a patient who has sustained a laryngeal injury. If initial examination reveals an unobstructed airway, then the routine evaluation to determine whether laryngeal trauma has occurred may proceed. If, on the other hand, the airway is compromised, the patient should have a tracheotomy performed in the emergency room to prevent precipitous airway obstruction. Peroral intubation can be performed occasionally, provided that indirect laryngoscopy indicates the obstruction is secondary to mucosal swelling or hematoma. Blind intubation should be avoided.[4] If indirect laryngoscopy cannot be performed or the larynx cannot be visualized, intubation should not be performed; a tracheotomy should be the procedure to obtain an airway.

A tracheotomy below the second tracheal ring may be performed under local anesthesia. The operating surgeon should be aware that there may be tracheal separation and that palpation of the cartilaginous rings of the trachea may not be possible. In these cases, the distal trachea may be retracted into the upper mediastinum and the operating surgeon must explore the area, find the avulsed trachea, and retract it into the neck wound. It is also important to recognize perforating injuries of the lower respiratory tract as administration of a general anesthetic with positive pressure may result in massive subcutaneous emphysema, pneumomediastinum, or tension pneumothorax.[5]

Mirror laryngoscopy should be performed if possible to assess vocal cord mobility, the presence of mucosal edema, ecchymosis, mucosal tears, exposed cartilage, or evidence of dislocation of the arytenoid cartilage. Mirror laryngoscopy usually permits accurate assessment of the injury. Sometimes mirror laryngoscopy cannot be performed adequately or the extent of injury cannot be assessed accurately, requiring a direct laryngoscopy. The information obtained from the indirect and the direct laryngoscopy will dictate whether exploration is indicated. Those patients with cervical spine injury may need fiberoptic laryngoscopy for assessment. Radiologic studies are performed only when the airway is secure.[6] The radiographs obtained are usually not important determinants of whether an open operation is indicated. Fractures visualized on radiographs may or may not indicate the need for a surgical procedure. In most cases, the clinical assessment determines whether a surgical procedure is indicated. Radiographic contrast studies assume more importance in chronic than in acute cases.[7]

Computed tomography (CT) is a valuable diagnostic tool for assessing acute laryngeal injury.[8] CT provides information of high specificity and is particularly useful in patients with moderately severe injury, when the indications for surgery may be in doubt. In cases of severe injury, this study can give detailed information that is valuable for preoperative counseling if the surgical management is likely to involve extensive tissue resection, such as supraglottic partial laryngectomy.

ACUTE INTERNAL TRAUMA FROM INTUBATION

A traumatic endotracheal intubation may result in diffuse edema, laceration, perforation, or vocal cord paralysis. Early manifestations of these postoperative complications are usually pain, hoarseness, airway obstruction, or subcutaneous emphysema. Treatment of the internal injury depends upon its severity. Indirect laryngoscopy (and at times direct laryngoscopy) should be performed to establish the type and degree of injury. Edema of the laryngeal mucosa is treated expectantly with humidification or, if severe, with steroids. Lacerations are usually minor and require no therapy. Perforations may be associated with subcutaneous emphysema. If the emphysema is progressive, tracheotomy is indicated. The perforations tend to be small and generally do not require drainage. A unilateral or bilateral vocal cord paralysis probably develops secondary to recurrent laryngeal nerve injury resulting from the endotracheal tube balloon pressure at the glottis or subglottic level. The paralysis usually subsides spontaneously but may require six to nine months for resolution. Consequently, temporary tracheotomy is generally necessary in patients with bilateral vocal cord paralysis.

Trauma from direct laryngoscopy and vocal cord surgical procedures may result in anterior webbing or cord notching, which will result in hoarseness. Subglottic ulceration that may result in subglottic stenosis is not frequently seen in the acute state. In those cases when it is noted soon after extubation, the clinician may observe ulceration or granulation tissue in the subglottic area. In these patients, antibiotics and steroids may prevent the subsequent complication of stenosis. At present, we have no surgical procedure that will prevent this complication.

EXTERNAL TRAUMA

Laryngeal injuries with an open wound are rarely misdiagnosed by the examining physician. Airway obstruction, if present, frequently is relieved by intubation through the laceration. The presence of a laceration dictates surgical exploration of the larynx and neck.

Closed injuries where the overlying skin is intact, with or without contusion, present the clinician with the problem of whether to perform a surgical exploration. In these closed cases of laryngeal trauma, the decision against exploration may result in subsequent laryngeal stenosis. Early exploration decreases the incidence of stenosis.

The most important issue in acute closed laryngeal trauma is deciding when to surgically explore the larynx. This decision can be made only after adequate examination of the larynx utilizing indirect and at times direct laryngoscopy. A tracheotomy should be performed if needed for safe, adequate direct laryngoscopy. Generally, conservative management with voice rest, bed rest, and humidification is employed with those cases having only mucosal ecchymosis or small lacerations without airway obstruction.[9] Absolute indications for exploring the larynx include (1) airway obstruction requiring tracheotomy, (2) progressive subcutaneous emphysema, (3) extensive mucosal lacerations, (4) exposure of the cricoid cartilage, and (5) bilateral paralysis of the vocal cords. Some exceptions may arise, but if the patient's condition permits, surgical exploration is generally indicated to avoid or diminish the incidence of laryngeal stenosis. Olson[7] found that the presence of early airway obstruction, bare cartilage in the laryngeal lumen, or cricoid collapse requires early and aggressive treatment. Once the decision is made to explore the larynx, the clinician should determine whether the injury is glottic, supraglottic, subglottic, or a combination of these.

ACUTE SUPRAGLOTTIC INJURY

Acute supraglottic injuries are usually associated with fracture of the thyroid cartilage and hyoid bone. The thyroid cartilage fracture is generally horizontal, producing loss of prominence of the thyroid notch with the epiglottis being displaced posteriorly and superiorly.[10] This may result in inspiratory stridor and airway obstruction. With disruption of the thyrohyoid membrane and thyroepiglottic ligament, a laryngeal fistula may be created through the false cords into the anterior neck, producing subcutaneous emphysema. Dysphagia and aspiration may be prominent features. Indirect laryngoscopy may show only the posterior aspect of the vocal cords, with the anterior portion obscured by the dislocated epiglottis. Vocal cord mobility must be determined. Direct laryngoscopy will show the petiole to be displaced posteriorly, but elevation of the petiole will reveal a normal anterior commissure, anteroposterior extent of the vocal cords, and normal motion. At times, the severity of injury will not be appreciated because the anterior lip of the laryngoscope will correct the posterior displacement of the epiglottis during direct laryngoscopy. Therefore, remember that supraglottic injury frequently is better assessed by indirect laryngoscopy. There may be edema of the arytenoids, aryepiglottic folds, and false cords. When an arytenoid is dislocated, it is generally displaced posteriorly.

In pure cases of supraglottic injury, the larynx is approached through an anterior pharyngotomy followed by a supraglottic resection. The fractured thyroid lamina and false cords are usually removed along with the epiglottis. Closure is the same as after resection for neoplasm. In those patients with limited injury, resection of the epiglottis only may be possible.

If the vocal cords do not move or if there is an associated glottic injury, supraglottic resection should not be performed.[11, 12] In these cases, an approach by a midline thyrotomy is preferred, with a submucosal resection of the petiole of the epiglottis followed by suturing of the mucosa anterior to the infrahyoid area.

ACUTE GLOTTIC INJURY

Glottic injuries usually accompany fractures of the thyroid cartilage that are vertical, transverse, or cruciate. The voice is poor, and airway obstruction is produced by vocal cord edema. Direct laryngoscopy may reveal lacerations or distortion of the true vocal cords, disruption of the anterior commissure, foreshortening of the anteroposterior diameter of the larynx, or impaired cord mobility. Frequently, extensive lacerations are present within the ventricle bilaterally. The lacerations in this area cannot be appreciated by indirect laryngoscopy. Therefore, direct laryngoscopy should be done if extensive lacerations are seen on indirect examination. The clues for extensive lacerations include hemoptysis, evidence of bleeding at the ventricular level on indirect examination, and edema of the false cords. Because of the minimal findings of indirect examination related to airway obstruction, these patients frequently are not explored and, indeed, may well go on to form circumferential scarring and laryngeal stenosis. Therefore, in these cases, direct laryngoscopy should be performed to assess the nature of the lacerations; if the lacerations are significant and bilateral, an open procedure is indicated.

Surgical exploration is by midline thyrotomy.

The perichondrium should be elevated minimally from the fracture sites. Fractured pieces of cartilage are removed or reapproximated with 3-0 chromic catgut sutures. Free cartilage fragments devoid of perichondrium are sacrificed. Mucosal lacerations are repaired with interrupted 4-0 chromic catgut sutures. If the thyroarytenoid muscle is ruptured, it is similarly repaired. An ophthalmologic needle holder is helpful for precise suture placement. Areas that are devoid of mucosa and cannot be covered by local advancement flaps from the aryepiglottic fold, epiglottis, or postcricoid area are covered by buccal mucosal grafts, dermal grafts, or split-thickness skin grafts. Unilateral arytenoid displacement is corrected by repositioning the cartilage. Bilateral arytenoid dislocation will require an arytenoidectomy and cordal lateralization on one side. Stents are used to maintain the position of free grafts or to provide support for cartilage fractures that are unstable. Stents are removed ten to fourteen days later. The stent should be soft and may be fashioned from a sterile fingercot filled with plastic foam or a silicone rubber (Silastic) tube oversewn at its upper end to prevent aspiration. Severe injuries may require the surgeon to perform a hemilaryngectomy because of the inability to reposition segments of the thyroid cartilage. Loss of thyroid cartilage, with resultant decrease in the anteroposterior diameter of the larynx, requires reconstruction. If the loss is minimal, the anteroposterior diameter may be maintained with the insertion of a silicone rubber or tantalum keel. With severe cartilage loss, the anteroposterior diameter may be regained by creating a laryngostoma after rotating the residual thyroid alae 90 degrees anteriorly and covering them with advanced cervical skin flaps. The laryngostoma is closed in approximately three weeks.

ACUTE SUBGLOTTIC INJURY

This type of laryngeal fracture involves the cricoid cartilage and it is often associated with injury to the cervical trachea. Clinically, there is loss of the prominence of the cricoid arch. As subglottic edema increases, airway obstruction rapidly appears. Hoarseness is not marked unless the recurrent laryngeal nerves have been injured. Direct laryngoscopy reveals a subglottic narrowing, often accompanied by bare cartilaginous fragments within the lumen. Once this diagnosis is entertained, intubation should not be performed. An elective tracheotomy should be performed. Surgical exploration may reveal depression of the anterior arch of the cricoid, comminution of the anterior aspect of the cricoid arch, or fracture and separation of the cricoid from the thyroid or tracheal cartilage. Anterior cricoid depression is approached through a thyrotomy. The depressed cricoid arch is elevated, and a stent is inserted for one week. Mucosal defects of more than 25 percent of the circumference of the subglottis require resurfacing with free mucosal or skin grafts. Occasionally, the anterior arch injury may be stabilized by fine wire sutures alone. Comminution and loss of the anterior arch is repaired by either a thyrotracheal anastomosis or interposition of a pedicled hyoid bone graft. Use of the latter method requires that a skin graft be placed to separate the bone graft from the tracheal lumen. A stent is inserted for two weeks.

Laryngotracheal Separation. A specialized type of subglottic injury, laryngotracheal separation, is generally produced by the shearing force of a restraining object, such as a cable, against the upper trachea. This injury is seen principally in motorcycle injuries and auto and sports accidents. For example, when a motorcycle rider makes forceful contact with the cable, this causes avulsion of the cricoid cartilage from the trachea with retraction of the larynx upward and the trachea downward. Avulsion of the strap muscles, recurrent laryngeal nerves, and even the anterior wall of the esophagus may occur.[13] Airway obstruction develops rapidly.

When separation is suspected, peroral intubation is contraindicated and an emergency tracheotomy is required. Palpation of the neck will reveal a loss of continuity between the larynx and trachea, as the trachea generally retracts substernally. Careful attention must be given to the chest because pneumothorax is often present, as reported by Alonso et al.[14] in four of seven cases.

After the airway is secure and there is no evidence of cervical spine injury, preliminary endoscopic examination under general anesthesia is followed by a surgical exploration. It is important to determine whether vocal cord mobility is intact because of the high incidence of avulsions of the recurrent laryngeal nerve with this type of injury. If found, a laceration of the esophagus is repaired and the strap muscles are interposed between the trachea and the esophagus to prevent fistula formation. The trachea is then mobilized upwards and a tracheal-cricoid anastomosis is performed with stainless steel sutures. To prevent granuloma formation, the sutures should not enter the lumen of the airway. If there is an injury to the inferior aspect of the posterior plate of the cricoid, it is smoothed and trimmed with a rotating bur. Bilateral vocal cord paralysis requires an arytenoidectomy because reanastomosis of the recurrent laryngeal nerve is rarely successful and return of function is delayed, necessitating prolonged tracheal cannulation. Alonso et al.[14] stressed the importance of the placement of a stent to reduce the incidence of subglottic stenosis. Failure to repair this type of injury immediately results in fibrosis and distortion of the airway that is extemely difficult to reconstruct later.

COMBINED INJURY

Supraglottic and Glottic. The exposure for correction of this type of injury is achieved by midline thyrotomy. A supraglottic resection cannot be performed unless normal mobility of the vocal cords is anticipated. If there is good cord mobility, a standard supraglottic resection is performed. With an acute combined injury in which cord mobility is uncertain, the supraglottic component is corrected by a submucosal resection of the petiole of the epiglottis. The mucosa is then sutured anteriorly to the infrahyoid structures with a 2-0 chromic catgut suture. The glottic injury is corrected as required. This may entail simple suturing of lacerations, reattaching an avulsed cord, or placing a keel anteriorly. The thyroid cartilage fractures are stabilized by stainless steel wires, an internal stent, or both.

Glottic and Subglottic. This type of injury is managed by correcting each component separately; however, a thyrotracheal anastomosis cannot be performed because of the instability of the thyroid cartilage. An internal stent is generally required after lacerations and avulsions are repaired and the cartilage fragments are repositioned.

Supraglottic, Glottic, and Subglottic. These injuries are the most difficult to repair and often require numerous secondary procedures to achieve a patent airway without aspiration and with an adequate voice. The surgical approach is through both an anterior pharyngotomy and midline thyrotomy. The principles of reconstruction are the same as those mentioned above; however, with severe combined injuries, exteriorization of the larynx by creation of a trough (laryngostoma) may increase the probability of ultimate success. Such direct observation of the larynx permits closure to be deferred until complete healing has occurred.

PRINCIPLES OF MANAGEMENT AND RESULTS

The neck may be entered for exploration and repair of laryngeal fractures through a vertical or horizontal incision. The latter incision is generally used since it produces a scar that is more cosmetically acceptable. The thyrotomy is performed with an oscillating saw in the midline and an incision is made in the cricothyroid membrane so that the larynx can be divided through the anterior commissure ligament to prevent disruption of the vocal cords and to achieve better speech postoperatively. If the arytenoid cartilage is found to be dislocated, it is repositioned; however, avulsion of the cartilage may require its removal. All exposed cartilaginous fragments should be provided with an epithelial covering. An endolaryngeal stent is placed to support unstable cartilaginous fragments and grafts. If a stent is used to maintain a lumen while healing occurs by secondary intention, perichondritis and laryngeal stenosis will often result. Consequently, all denuded areas must be covered by local flaps or grafts.[15] Split-thickness skin grafts sutured to the mucosa or wrapped around a stent have successfully covered such bare areas.[16] Soft stents seem more physiologic when we consider the constant motion of the larynx during respiration and deglutition.[17] The stent is stabilized by a wire or heavy nonabsorbable suture passed translaryngeally and suspended over buttons to prevent accidental dislodgement. It is removed endoscopically ten to fourteen days later, depending on the injury. Prolonged stenting beyond two weeks, even with grafting, should be avoided. Prophylactic antibiotics are generally administered after open reduction of laryngeal fractures.

The best results with laryngeal fractures are obtained in those cases managed acutely. As reported by Olson and Miles[18] (25 cases), Pennington[19] (22 cases), and Potter et al.[16] (27 cases), uniformly good results were obtained with treatment within the critical first week following the injury. Delayed repair showed a high incidence of failure of decannulation, aspiration, and poor speech. The use of steroids has been suggested to delay wound healing when immediate repair cannot be performed because of other injuries sustained.

Table 9–1. TREATMENT GROUPS—87 CASES*

Group	Retrospective 1965–1977	Prospective 1978–1982	Total
1	7	7	14
2	5	17	22
3	14	4	18
4	26†	7	33

*From Schaeffer SD: Ann Otol Rhinol Laryngol 91:400, 1982.
†Excludes one patient reported previously.

Primary closure of the laryngeal mucosa and surgical management within 24 hours of the injury are the two principles Schaeffer[20] emphasizes in his review of 87 patients with laryngeal injuries. He proposes using a classification system based on severity of the tissue trauma that defines four groups of injury. Table 9–1 shows the results of this management regimen.

Group 1. Minor Hematoma or Lacerations, Without Fracture

Conservative management is recommended.

Group 2. Edema, Hematoma, Lacerations Without Exposed Cartilage

Direct laryngoscopy and esophagoscopy are indicated with tracheotomy, if needed. Exploration of the larynx is deferred if CT shows nondisplaced fractures.

Groups 3 and 4. Massive Edema, Mucosal Tears, Exposed Cartilage, and Cord Immobility

Tracheotomy, laryngoscopy, esophagoscopy, and laryngeal exploration are recommended, with careful repair of all lacerations. Suture repair of anterior commissure disruption eliminates need for stent in many patients. Patients are classified (after surgery) in Group 3 if no stent was used and in Group 4 if stenting was necessary.

Leopold[21] evaluated the reported experience in managing laryngeal injuries from eight large treatment series and added data from the experience at Upstate Medical Center, Syracuse, New York. He noted that among those patients who required laryngeal exploration and repair, airway adequacy was independent of the use or method of stenting. Further analysis revealed that both vocal quality and airway are better when surgical intervention occurs within the first 24 hours.

There is no one surgical technique to reconstitute the traumatized larynx. The surgeon must have at his disposal many techniques and the ability to select the particular technique for the individual case. Precise surgical technique and knowledge of basic surgical principles will improve results.

References

1. Ogura JH: Management of traumatic injuries of the larynx and trachea including stenosis. J Laryngol 85:1259–1261, 1971.
2. Ogura JH, Biller HF: Reconstruction of the larynx following blunt trauma. Ann Otol Rhinol Laryngol 80:492–510, 1971.
3. Fitz-Hugh GS, Powell JB: Acute traumatic injuries of the oropharynx, laryngopharynx and cervical trachea in children. Otolaryngol Clin North Am 3:375–393, 1970.
4. Yarington CT: Trauma involving the air and food passages. Otolaryngol Clin North Am 12:321–327, 1979.
5. Herrin TJ et al.: Anesthetic management of neck trauma. South Med J 72:1102–1106, 1979.
6. Greene R, Stark, P: Trauma of the larynx and trachea. Radiol Clin North Am 16:309–320, 1978.
7. Olson NR: Surgical treatment of acute blunt laryngeal injuries. Ann Otol Rhinol Laryngol 87:716–721, 1978.
8. Maceri DR et al.: Value of computed axial tomography in severe laryngeal injury. Arch Otolaryngol 108:449–451, 1982.
9. Brandenburg JH: Management of acute blunt laryngeal injuries. Otolaryngol Clin North Am 12:741–751, 1979.
10. Bryce DP: The surgical management of laryngotracheal injury. J Laryngol 86:547–587, 1972.
11. Harris HH: IV. Management of injuries to the larynx and trachea. Laryngoscope 82:1924–1929, 1972.
12. Harris HH, Tobin HA: Acute injuries of the larynx and trachea in 49 patients. Laryngoscope 80:1376–1384, 1970.
13. LeJeune FE: Laryngotracheal separation. Laryngoscope 88:1956–1961, 1978.
14. Alonso WA et al.: Complications of laryngotracheal disruption. Laryngoscope 84:1276–1290, 1974.
15. Pratt LL: Laryngotracheal separation: Late complications. Trans Am Acad Ophthalmol Otolaryngol 80:452–453, 1975.
16. Potter CR et al.: Blunt laryngotracheal trauma. Trans Am Acad Ophthalmol Otolaryngol 86:909–923, 1978.
17. Harris HH, Ainsworth JZ: Immediate management of laryngeal and tracheal injuries. Laryngoscope 75:1105–1115, 1965.
18. Olson NR, Miles WK: Treatment of acute blunt laryngeal injuries. Ann Otol Rhinol Laryngol 80:704–709, 1971.
19. Pennington CL: External trauma of the larynx and trachea. Ann Otol Rhinol Laryngol 81:546–554, 1972.
20. Schaeffer SD: Primary management of laryngeal trauma. Ann Otol Rhinol Laryngol 91:399–402, 1982.
21. Leopold D: Laryngeal trauma. Arch Otolaryngol 109:106–111, 1982.

10

Management of Acquired Laryngeal Stenosis

William A. Alonso, M.D.

HISTORICAL BACKGROUND

In the beginning of the twentieth century, most cases of laryngeal stenosis of the acquired type were the residual of infectious diseases such as syphilis, laryngeal diphtheria, tuberculosis, and typhoid fever. Chevalier Jackson, in 1917, brought attention to an iatrogenic cause, involving the development of subglottic stenosis after a high tracheotomy. Infectious diseases and a high tracheotomy remained the principal causes of laryngeal stenosis until World War II. The conquest of infection almost totally eliminated infectious diseases as a cause for laryngeal stenosis. Enhanced educational efforts reduced the surgical error of the high tracheotomy. After World War II, the growing availability of motor vehicles and the practice of driving at greater speeds produced an alarming increase in serious automobile accidents. In the 1960s, blunt trauma to the neck after an automobile collision became known as the "padded dash syndrome." Inadequately treated acute laryngeal injuries commonly ended as severe laryngeal stenosis. In the 1970s, the emphasis on safety restraints such as seat belts, shoulder straps, and air bags greatly reduced the incidence of serious neck injuries. Concomitantly, a national speed limit of 55 mph was instituted, further reducing the incidence of serious automobile collisions.

Although advances in respiratory care over the last 20 years have produced many survivors of respiratory failure, the need for prolonged intubation and mechanical ventilation has caused an increase in cases of subglottic and tracheal stenosis. Today, this iatrogenic complication is the principal cause of laryngeal stenosis. Penetrating injuries of the larynx from high-velocity projectiles or sharp objects such as knives can also lead to laryngeal stenosis, depending on the extent of the damage and the method of management of the laryngeal injury.

The growing popularity of recreational vehicles such as minibikes, trail bikes, go-carts, and snowmobiles has also resulted in serious injuries to the larynx and trachea. In particular, laryngotracheal separation, commonly encountered in these injuries, can result in a subglottic stenosis even after early diagnosis and treatment.[1]

In the latter part of the nineteenth century, laryngologists began treating laryngeal stenosis. Initial treatment consisted of dilation with metal bolts and hard India rubber tubes.[2] Before these efforts at dilation, the condition had been considered incurable. Limited success was achieved with dilation, and that only in uncomplicated cases. Early in the twentieth century, some surgeons[3] advocated laryngostomy, an open exploration of the larynx with a tracheotomy. An indwelling stent was placed in the open wound and the size of the indwelling prosthesis was gradually increased over a period of months. This long, arduous procedure was very painful and had a high mortality rate.

Schmiegelow[4] is credited with being the first to advocate scar excision at the time of open exploration. After resection of the stricture, the lumen was enlarged as much as possible, and an indwelling stent was placed so that the indwelling prosthesis extended beyond the stenotic area but not into the pharynx. The wound was closed, and the stent was held in position with multiple stainless steel wire sutures through the skin, the subcutaneous tissue, the thyroid cartilage, and the prosthesis. This procedure was adapted for children and for adults. In children, a tracheotomy was left below the stent. In adults, the tracheotomy was commonly removed, since the prosthesis was hollow and adequate for respiration. The indwelling prosthesis was left in place for many months and often required repeated procedures. Removal of the internal stent was accomplished by the transoral route.

In the late 1920s, Arbuckle[5] modified Schmiegelow's method by placing a split-thickness skin graft around the indwelling prosthesis. Instead of Schmiegelow's India rubber tubes, a solid sea sponge was selected as the internal stent. Sometimes this method was supplemented with repeated dilations with electrically heated bougies.

In the late 1930s and the 1940s, Figi[6] and Negus[7] further refined Arbuckle's methods and laid the principles for skin grafting within the laryngeal lumen. Both these laryngologists emphasized the advantage of skin grafting raw areas rather than waiting for slow cicatrization and the importance of prolonged stenting to limit the tendency for contracture. Figi advocated using Jackson's core molds in increasing sizes to over-dilate the endolarynx and, thus, maintain the pliability and softness of the skin graft.

In the late 1940s and 1950s, a search for a less reactive substance for stent reconstruction was initiated. Initially, obturators composed of dental acrylic were advocated. These acrylic molds were customized through a laryngostomy and fashioned at the time of surgery in a rather tedious procedure. In the early 1950s, Woodward[8] modified the treatment of laryngeal stenosis by advocating extensive submucosal dissection of the cicatricial area and by preserving as much intraluminal mucosa as possible, thereby restricting the amount of skin grafting. He recommended introducing barium powder into the acrylic resin to produce a radiopaque mold. Grafting with autogenous hyoid bone was also recommended as a means of enhancing the laryngeal lumen.[9] Around the same period, McNaught introduced the use of tantalum steel as a keel for the repair of anterior laryngeal webs. In the 1960s and 1970s, other inert substances were recommended for the manufacture of indwelling laryngeal stents. Materials such as acrylic (Lucite), polyethylene, silicone rubber, polytetrafluoroethylene (Teflon), and polyvinyl chloride were used by various investigators to manufacture indwelling laryngeal stents.[10]

In the early 1950s, Conley[11] was the first to recommend cricoid resection and thyrotracheal anastomosis for the management of severe subglottic stenosis. Later, in the 1960s, a method of tracheal mobilization including intrathoracic release was developed by thoracic surgeons.[12] This facilitated a tension free end-to-end anastomosis after resection of a stenotic portion. Ogura, Dedo, and Montgomery[13–16] refined the technique of laryngeal release, which became the basic maneuver in mobilization for laryngeal-tracheal or tracheal-tracheal anastomosis. Extensive damage to the laryngotracheal complex caused by the loss of much of the cartilaginous framework and prominent fibrosis required a return to the old laryngostomy, open-trough method, with some modifications.[17] Bryce and his co-workers[18] recommended a multistage surgical procedure, utilizing autogenous materials buried in skin flaps and creating a laryngotracheal trough. This complex repair is necessary in rare situations where the damage is extensive and the distance between larynx and trachea is too great, making a laryngotracheal anastomosis impossible. Variations of the laryngotracheal trough method, involving the use of inert plastic materials imbedded in the skin flaps, have been recently introduced by various authors.[19] Marlex mesh is a favorite material for this purpose. A multistage procedure is still required to prepare the skin flap and incorporate the Marlex mesh to replace the missing anterior wall of the laryngotracheal trough.

CAUSES AND PREVENTION

Some causes of acquired laryngeal stenosis were mentioned briefly earlier in this chapter.

Various factors can be conveniently separated into two categories. The first group consists of all those cases resulting from external injury to the neck and larynx. The second category consists of the cases that arise from internal damage.

EXTERNAL INJURY

External trauma from vehicular injuries, suicide attempts with ropes and sharp objects, blows to the neck during altercations, industrial and battlefield explosions, and sporting events causes laryngeal stenosis less often than does the internal variety. If recognized early, most cases of external injury, whether blunt or sharp, can be repaired successfully without the sequela of laryngeal stenosis. External trauma is virtually unheard of in the prepubertal youngster and rarely occurs until adolescence or adulthood. Cases of external trauma with significant comminution of the laryngeal cartilages (especially the cricoid cartilage) are more likely to result in laryngeal stenosis than are less complicated, minimally displaced laryngeal fractures. A relatively high incidence of subglottic stenosis following external laryngeal fracture can be avoided by reducing those factors that lead to external neck trauma. Efforts to achieve vehicular safety with lower speed limits and mandatory passive safety restraints will significantly reduce automobile injuries. Better supervision of youngsters in the playground and during the use of recreational vehicles will also reduce external laryngeal trauma. Finally, greater alertness of ambulance personnel and emergency room teams should lead to the early diagnosis and successful management of external laryngeal trauma and, thereby, to the prevention of acquired laryngeal stenosis.

INTERNAL INJURY

As mentioned earlier, internal injury to the laryngotracheal complex has risen along with advances in respiratory care. Virtually all pediatric cases of acquired laryngeal stenosis can be traced to prolonged endotracheal intubation. Similarly, laryngeal stenosis as a complication of prolonged intubation and ventilatory assistance has become a more common etiology in the adult age group. Less common today are the late endolaryngeal complications of infectious diseases such as syphilis or tuberculosis. These diseases are usually diagnosed and treated before laryngeal complications can develop. Occasional instances of severe supraglottic injury are seen after accidental or suicidal ingestion of lye or sulfuric acid. Direct exposure to chemical fumes generally causes an acute mucosal injury with edema and copious secretions but rarely progresses to stenosis.

Rare instances of partial laryngeal stenosis, usually at the glottic level, can be seen after injudicious endolaryngeal vocal cord surgery or partial laryngectomy. Another rare but unusually severe iatrogenic cause of stenosis is extensive transglottic damage from radiation-induced chondritis.

Laryngeal stenosis as a by-product of prolonged peroral intubation and ventilatory assistance can be avoided by understanding some of the variables that dispose the larynx to this problem. The duration of intubation is critical, especially in patients treated with nasotracheal or oral endotracheal tubes. After three to five days of continuous intubation, a patient should be reevaluated and considered for a tracheotomy. This may allow adequate ventilatory assistance as well as control of secretions without the hazard of a subglottic stenosis. Selecting the appropriate endotracheal tube size for the patient's size and age is another important factor in reducing the intraluminal damage. Cuffed endotracheal tubes should be avoided whenever possible; if they are needed for effective positive pressure artificial ventilation, then they should be of the low pressure, minimally reactive variety. Other factors that should be controlled to avoid the complications of prolonged intubation are meticulous asepsis of the endotracheal tube and its connections and avoidance of excessive traction or motion of the tube itself. Finally, careful periodic monitoring of the pressure in the endotracheal tube cuff, keeping it below 25 mm of mercury, will help reduce the hazard of cuff over-expansion and the well-known sequelae of pressure necrosis followed by fibrosis and stenosis.

PATHOPHYSIOLOGY OF LARYNGEAL STENOSIS

Following external trauma to the larynx, scarring will occur as part of the normal healing process. Blunt or penetrating injuries to the larynx can produce comminuted fractures and dislocations with contusions and tears of the laryngeal soft tissues. Extensive intralaryngeal soft tissue trauma involving tears in the mucosa and the muscle, if not properly restored, will lead within a week or ten days to an intraluminal granuloma or a web, or to submucosal fibrosis. Extensive fibrosis will fix a malpositioned laryngeal fracture fragment or a dislocated epiglottis or arytenoid cartilage. An infection, leading to chondritis of the laryngeal cartilages, can result in extensive loss of laryngeal cartilage with scar tissue replacement. This is especially true in the debilitated patient suffering from a systemic disease as well as in contaminated injuries. Other factors that may complicate a laryngeal injury and enhance the possibility of laryngeal stenosis are previous irradiation, tumor invasion, or partial surgery for carcinoma.

A model for laryngeal stenosis resulting from internal trauma is the sequela of endotracheal intubation. We know from animal and from human cadaver experiments that even the gentle passage of an endotracheal tube by a skilled operator can result in extensive damage to the respiratory epithelium, including the loss of cilia.[20] Prolonged friction between an intraluminal tube and the surrounding respiratory mucosa will eventually lead to erosion of the mucosa. Damage from an inflated endotracheal tube cuff is of a much greater magnitude than the damage usually associated with the tube itself.[21, 22] After an initial breakdown in the laryngotracheal mucosa, further erosion can expose underlying cartilage and may progress to a perichondritis with cartilage resorption after invasion by pathogenic bacteria. During the initial healing process, the necrotic debris is removed and replaced by granulation tissue. Eventually, a fibroblastic response results in extensive scarring and constriction of the laryngeal lumen. As a tubular structure, the laryngeal lumen is especially susceptible to circumferential stricture and loss of airway patency. Mucosal injury from nasotracheal and orotracheal intubation occurs most often at the cricoid level and may cause circumferential cicatrization. Occasionally, webs and submucosal fibrosis in the posterior commissure can also result from intubation injury.

PROGNOSIS OF LARYNGEAL STENOSIS

Clinical symptoms of acquired laryngeal stenosis may begin immediately after removal of the endotracheal tube or may be delayed for as long as 90 days. Initial symptoms may be mild and include various degrees of hoarseness or aphonia, dyspnea on exertion, or difficulty in clearing mucous secretions. Symptoms may develop after an acute upper respiratory infection. Sometimes the onset of difficulty is dramatic, with severe respiratory stridor leading rapidly to asphyxiation. Disturbances of deglutition may be present if the hypopharyngeal structures and cervical esophagus have been damaged. The diagnosis can readily be established at the bedside with either indirect laryngoscopy or flexible fiberoptic direct laryngoscopy. After the patient has been stabilized by establishing an emergency airway, further evaluation can proceed.

Radiographic evaluation of the larynx, as discussed in Chapter 5 of this volume, can reveal valuable clues to the location and extent of the laryngeal stenosis and any other associated injury. Plain soft tissue lateral x-rays of the neck, lateral neck xeroradiographs, computer assisted tomography (CAT) scans, laryngograms, and retrograde tracheograms are very valuable in studying these problems. Blind pouches in the larynx, fistulas, loss of cartilage, and the length of a stenotic segment can be accurately assessed radiographically.

Endoscopic study can then follow, including direct laryngoscopy, tracheoscopy, and cervical esophagoscopy. If a tracheotomy has been established, retrograde laryngoscopy through the tracheotomy site with a nasopharyngoscope or fiberoptic flexible laryngoscope will reveal valuable information about subglottic stenosis. The location and thickness of the cicatrix can be assessed, as can missing or displaced parts and vocal cord motility.

TREATMENT OF ACQUIRED LARYNGEAL STENOSIS

Laryngeal stenosis is conveniently classified according to the anatomical subdivisions of the larynx in much the same way as laryngeal tumors are classified. The three basic types of laryngeal stenosis are supraglottic, glottic, and subglottic. Cases of extensive laryngeal stenosis can be described as transglottic. Most cases of laryngeal stenosis in children and adults are subglottic. Laryngeal stenosis of the supraglottic type usually follows external trauma and occasionally develops as the sequela of an infection (e.g., tuberculosis or a mycosis). A supraglottic stenosis is, very rarely, encountered in a child following the accidental ingestion of a caustic substance. Occasionally, in adults and children, a posterior commissure stenosis is seen in association with a subglottic stenosis, usually related to endotracheal intubation. Rarely, anterior glottic webs are encountered in adults or children. Less common is a complete glottic atresia secondary to a severe, undiagnosed, external laryngeal fracture. Fortunately, the most severe laryngeal stenosis of the transglottic type occurs rarely. It is seen most commonly in adults after severe, complicated, external injuries with considerable loss of soft tissue and cartilaginous framework.

PEDIATRIC TREATMENT

Conservative Management. Laryngeal stenosis in children, particularly the prepubertal youngster, should be managed conservatively. If the laryngeal stenosis is in the granulomatous stage, judicious endoscopic removal of granulations with microdissection and the carbon dioxide laser and intralesional injection of steroids, such as triamcinolone acetonide (Kenalog), can be effective. Careful laryngoscopic removal with preservation of mucosa, under microscopic control, can be repeated on a weekly basis until adequate healing has corrected the problem. Gentle bougienage with soft dilators can accompany the conservative management. Chronic cases of stenosis do not respond to dilations and steroid injections. Only temporary airway improvement can be obtained with conservative means. Furthermore, traumatizing a dense, mature scar may enhance scar deposition.

Open Procedures in Children. In children with chronic laryngeal stenosis, it is probably best to allow the youngsters to grow so that the larynx dimensions will be more suitable for an open exploration. The best age at which open exploration can be attempted is still debatable. Although experimental work with animals suggests that a carefully done median thyrotomy does not disturb the growth of the infant larynx, no evidence exists that the same applies to humans.[23] The principal concern is that an open procedure for correction of a laryngeal stenosis in a child may interfere with future growth of the child's larynx.

The method of Evans and his co-workers[24] has some merit as applied to children. Children in the first year of life with severe subglottic stenosis were treated with laryngotracheo-

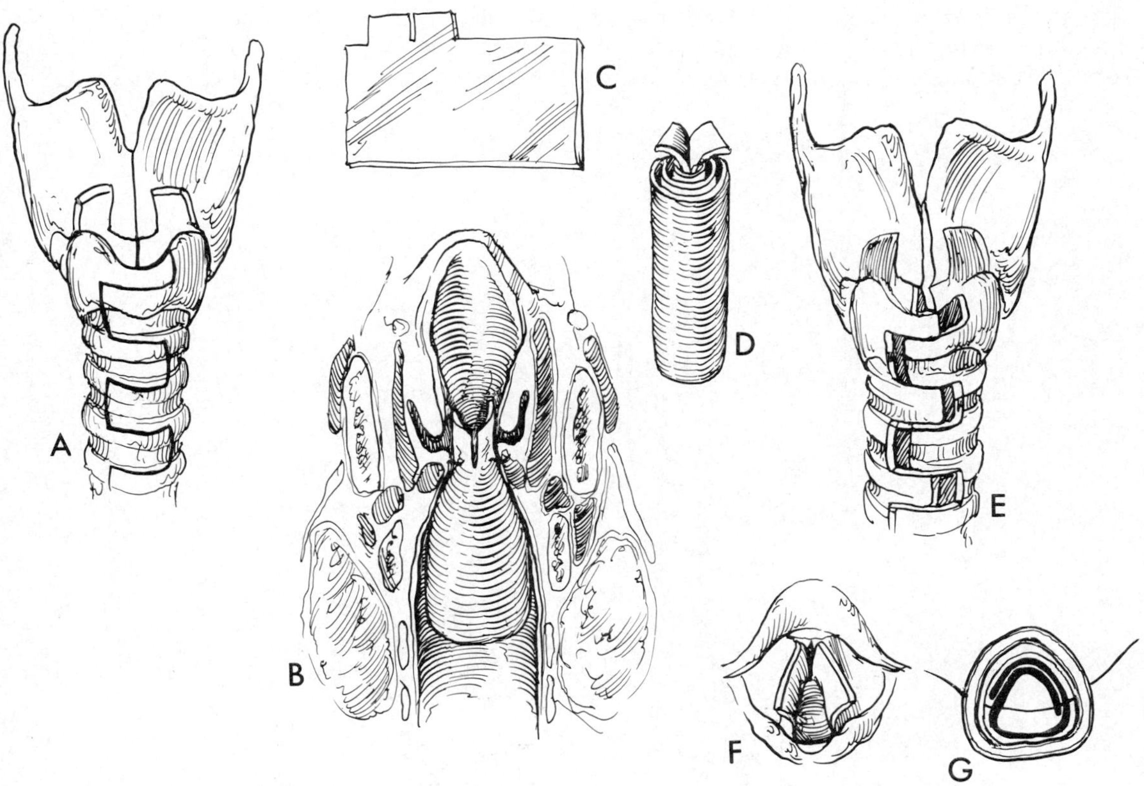

Figure 10–1. Laryngotracheoplasty in infants with subglottic stenosis (see text).

plasty. Each of the children had required a previous tracheotomy for a severe airway problem. In the first stage, under guidance of the operating microscope, the thyroid cartilage is split in the midline and down through the cricothyroid membrane. The cricoid and first four tracheal rings are split in a steplike fashion (Fig. 10–1A). The subglottic stenosis is then resected under direct vision, with the operating microscope in the submucosal plane just internal to the surrounding cartilage (Fig. 10–1B). Following removal of the subglottic scar, a piece of silicone rubber (Silastic) No. 5001 sheeting is fashioned by curling it on itself like a swiss roll and inserting it into the upper trachea with flanges projecting through the glottis (Fig. 10–1, C and D). Care is taken to avoid a supraglottic placement of the roll. A variation suggested by Gates involves the use of a silicone rubber (Silastic) core mold, followed by a Montgomery T-tube.[25] The cartilaginous interdigitations are retracted and sutured in their new positions with number 5-0 stainless steel wire (Fig. 10–1E). The Silastic roll is held anteriorly by a transfixation suture threaded through a small polyethylene tube held externally (Fig. 10–1, F and G). The patients in this series were hospitalized for an average of two months. After approximately six weeks, the Silastic roll was removed as an endoscopic procedure. In this small series of patients, all were decannulated successfully and no vocal cord damage was encountered. The patients were reported to have excellent airways and voices. This procedure may have clinical usefulness in the future, but more experience and follow-up are needed. The hazards of a prolonged tracheotomy in an infant are well known and efforts to reduce these dangers are essential. Another approach in managing subglottic stenosis in children has been the use of autologous tissue to widen the cricoid arch. Some surgeons have employed a free cartilaginous graft of rib, nasal-septal cartilage, or a pedicle flap of thyroid cartilage placed between the cut ends of the cricoid.[26–28] Another method is the use of a free or muscle-pedicled hyoid bone graft (Fig. 10–2).[28–31]

Fearon and Cotton used a method involving the interposition of an anterior wedge of autogenous costal cartilage to correct acquired subglottic stenosis.[27, 28] An elliptical wedge of costal cartilage is harvested from a lower rib. The size of the wedge is designed to correspond to the dimensions of the pediatric patient's anterior cricoid arch and first two tracheal rings. The thyroid and cricoid cartilage of the larynx and first two tracheal rings are divided anteriorly in the midline (Fig. 10–3). The cartilage graft is placed so that the perichondrial lining faces the lumen, and the edges of the graft are beveled to prevent it from settling into the lumen. The largest width of the elliptical graft is wedged at the anterior cricoid arch with the

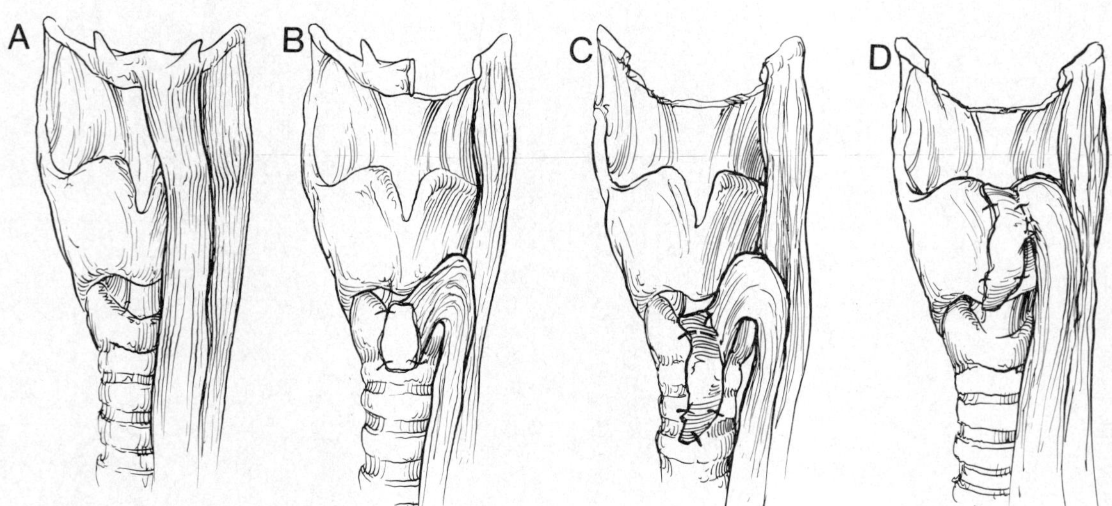

Figure 10–2. Hyoid-muscle pedicle flap.

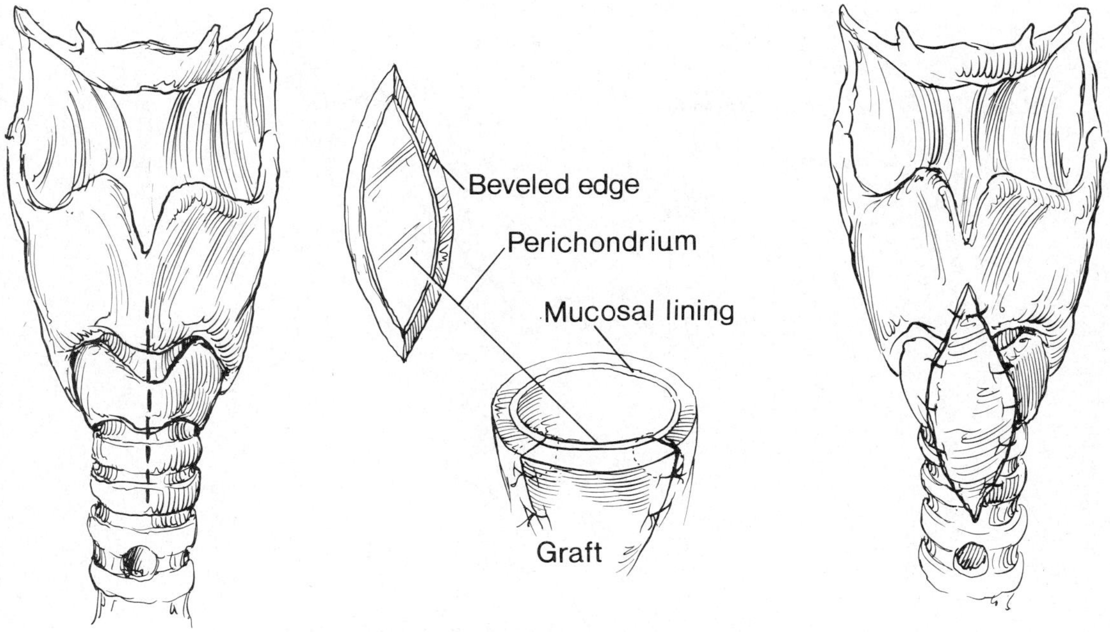

Figure 10–3. Costal cartilage graft—subglottic stenosis.

tapered ends at the thyroid cartilage and tracheal ring levels. Polypropylene (Prolene) 5-0 mattress sutures are placed extramucosally to sew the graft in place. A Montgomery laryngeal stent is placed within the lumen.

Whether open procedures in children will stand the test of time is uncertain, and it is probably best to wait until a child is at least six or seven years old before considering such measures. In the meantime, good tracheotomy care, Silastic tracheotomy tubes, periodic endoscopic inspection, and gentle dilation are the best approaches in infants whenever possible.

ADULT TREATMENT

Conservative management in adult cases is similar to that described for children. Early laryngeal stenosis, especially granulomas, can be managed with endoscopic removal, gentle dilation, and intralesional injection of steroids. Mild cases of stenosis and thin or moderate webs will also respond to dilation and intralesional steroids. Cases of chronic laryngeal stenosis can only be aggravated by improper endoscopic manipulation and dilation. An open procedure is necessary for definitive management of a chronic laryngeal stenosis.

CHRONIC ACQUIRED SUPRAGLOTTIC LARYNGEAL STENOSIS

Cases of high supraglottic hypopharyngeal stenosis can be approached through a transverse incision in the upper neck at the level of the hyoid bone.[32, 33] The transhyoid pharyngotomy approach is then applied (Fig. 10–4). The pharynx is entered either above or below the hyoid bone, and the body of the hyoid can be resected for better exposure. The epiglottis may be retrodisplaced posteriorly and superiorly while remaining firmly adherent to the lateral and posterior pharyngeal walls. The adhesions are incised and the epiglottis is freed from its laryngeal wall attachments. The pharyngeal mucosa is approximated with interrupted absorbable sutures, and the edges of the epiglottis are similarly repaired. Large defects in the pharyngeal wall after scar excision can be repaired with advancement flaps mobilized from the contiguous areas. Stenting with a prefabricated Negus esophageal tube or a fitted sponge is recommended for approximately two weeks. The patient is usually fed through a gastrostomy before and after this procedure until the stent is removed.

More severe cases of supraglottic stenosis

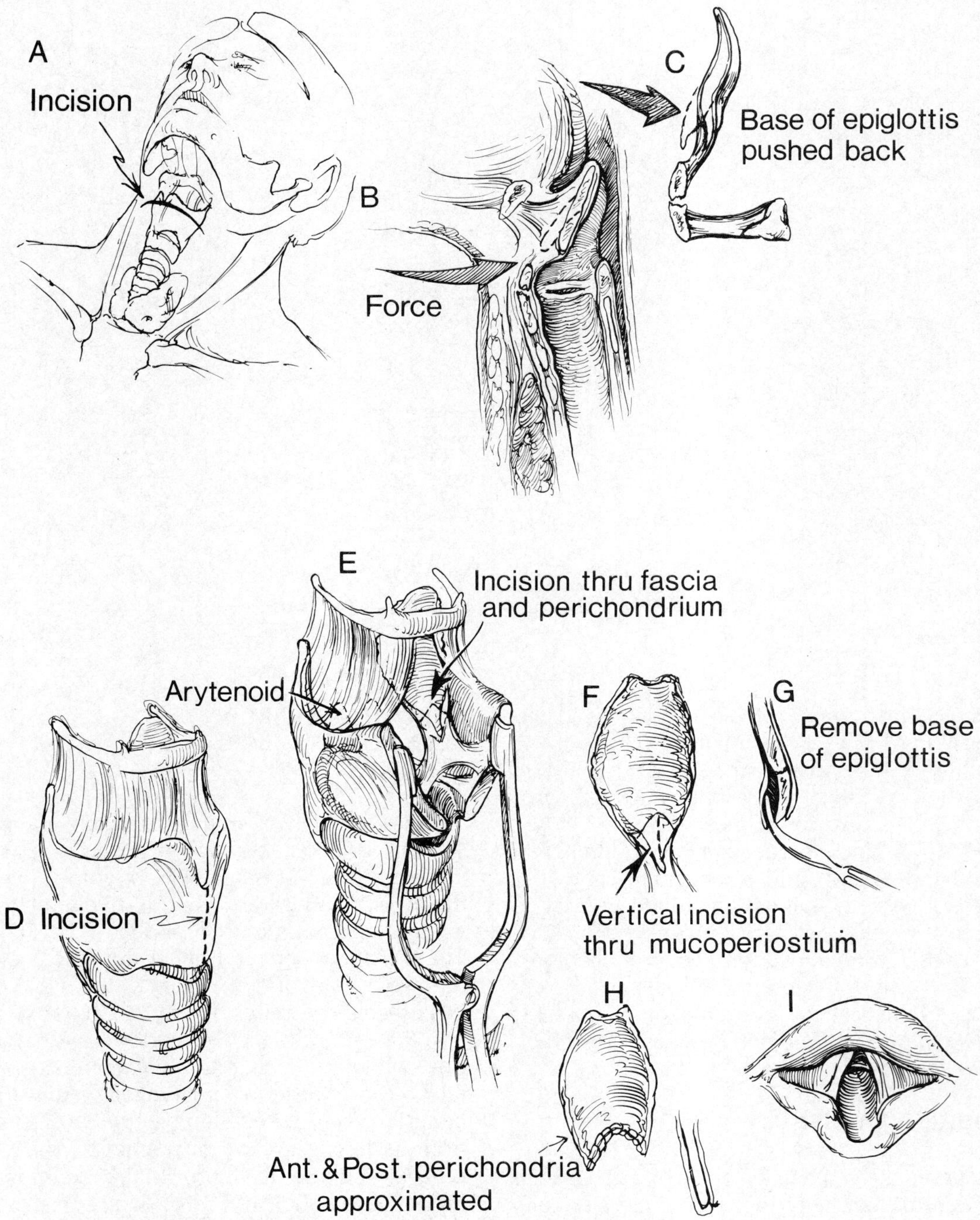

Figure 10–4. Repair of supraglottic stenosis.

require not only a transhyoid pharyngotomy but also a median thyrotomy. Furthermore, the subtotal supraglottic resection approach, as used in conservation surgery for laryngeal cancer, may be necessary in very advanced cases (Fig. 10–5).[34] A collar incision exposes the hyoid bone, thyrohyoid membrane, thyroid cartilage, and cricothyroid membrane before the transhyoid pharyngotomy is performed. The base of the epiglottis, fragments of hyoid bone, and thyroid cartilage may be displaced posteriorly by the injuring force. The minimum procedure needed is resection of the base of the epiglottis after elevating and preserving the perichondrium. Displaced fragments of hyoid bone are removed. The supraglottic structures may be so severely displaced posteriorly as to make it difficult to identify the arytenoid cartilages. The arytenoid is commonly displaced superiorly and posteriorly into the pharynx in these

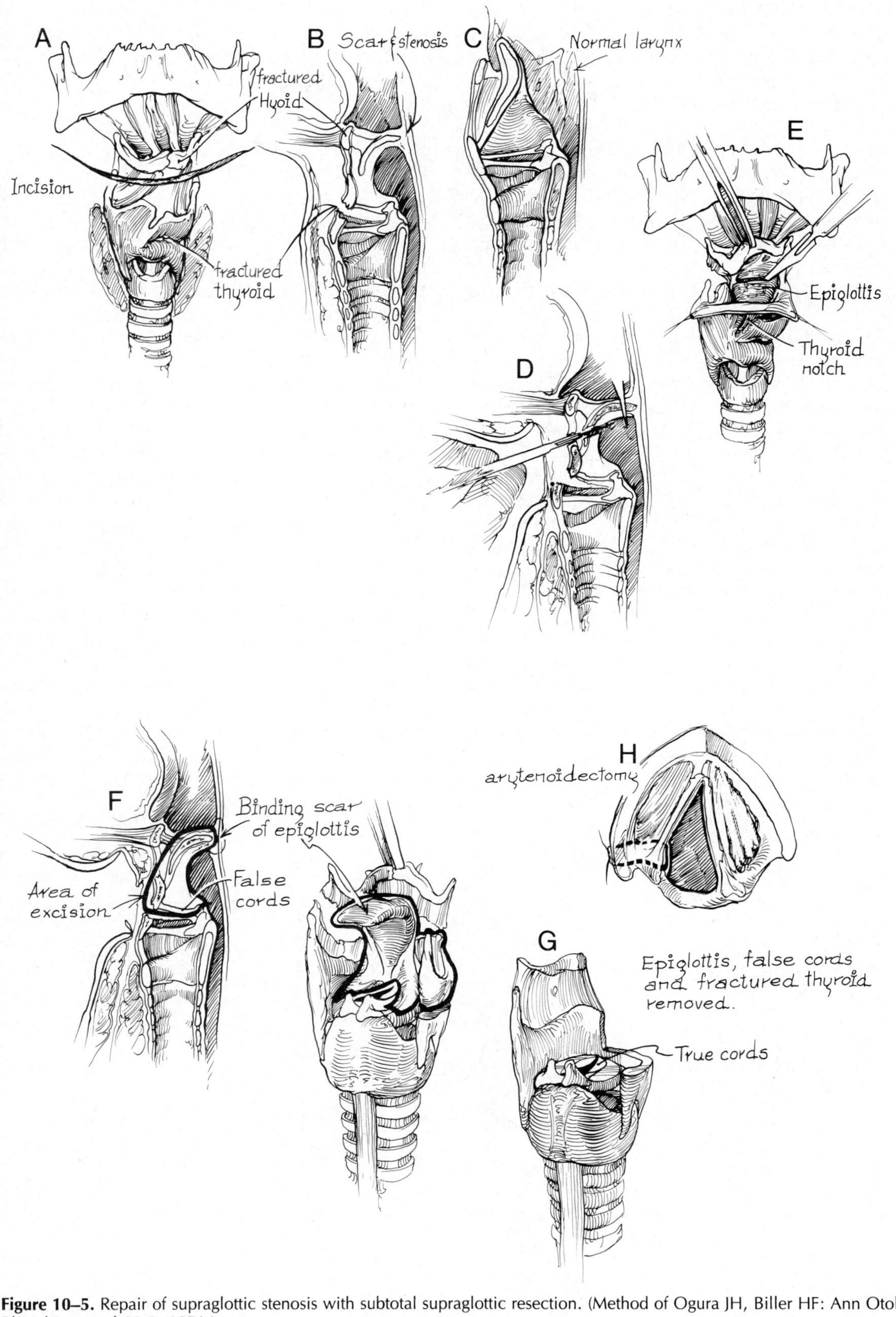

Figure 10–5. Repair of supraglottic stenosis with subtotal supraglottic resection. (Method of Ogura JH, Biller HF: Ann Otol Rhinol Laryngol 80:2, 1971.)

severe cases. A modified supraglottic laryngectomy may be required to establish adequate airway patency. This procedure will involve resection of portions of the superior aspect of the thyroid cartilage as well as the entire epiglottis, aryepiglottic folds, and false cords. The external thyroid cartilage perichondrium is approximated to the base of the tongue for final closure. When significant arytenoid dislocation is present, an arytenoidectomy with vocal cord lateralization may be required to establish glottic patency.

After the open repair is completed, stenting with a prefabricated silicone or polyvinyl chloride prosthesis is necessary in severely fractured larynges with cartilage displacement. Numerous commercial stents are available, made of such substances as acrylic, silicone, rubber, and polyvinyl chloride. The ideal stent should be fashioned to suit the laryngeal dimensions and be both pliable enough to cause minimal mucosal damage and yet rigid enough to support the repair after injury. The Montgomery silicone rubber stent, molded from cadavers, is quite suitable for this purpose, but a simpler alternative is an appropriately sized polyvinyl chloride endotracheal tube, crimped at an edge with a Carmalt clamp and steam autoclaved for 30 seconds. These prostheses are thought to minimize granulation tissue development. The prosthesis is left in place for four to six weeks and then removed endoscopically. Nutrition is maintained through either a nasogastric tube or a gastrostomy. Decannulation is completed one to two weeks after removal of the indwelling stent and may require endoscopic removal of granulations with steroid injections locally, or systemic steroids, or both.

MANAGEMENT OF ACQUIRED GLOTTIC STENOSIS

Anterior commissure webs, either alone or in association with supraglottic fractures, are managed with the median thyroidotomy approach and placement of an anterior keel (Fig. 10–6). The original anterior keel of tantalum steel was developed by McNaught.[10] More recently, Montgomery has introduced an umbrella-like silicone keel that appears to minimize granulation tissue formation (Fig. 10–7).[33] These anterior commissure keels are removed with a minor open procedure under local anesthesia approximately three weeks after placement. Very small anterior commissure webs can also be removed endoscopically with microscope control, especially using the carbon dioxide laser.[35] A polytetrafluoroethylene (Teflon) keel can then be placed endoscopically in small anterior webs.[36] Posterior glottic stenosis is also approached through a median thyrotomy (Fig. 10–8). After the lesion is identified, the scar is excised in the posterior commissure and usually the interarytenoid muscle is divided. The excised area is then covered with mucosal advancement flaps elevated from the hypopharynx, usually from the pyriform sinus re-

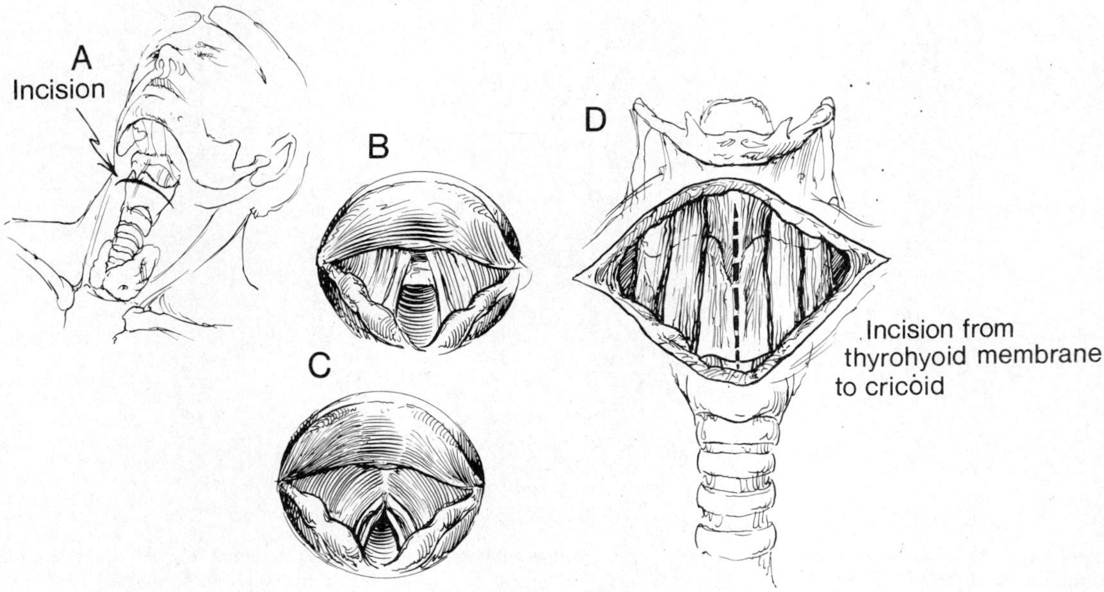

Figure 10–6. Anterior glottic web.

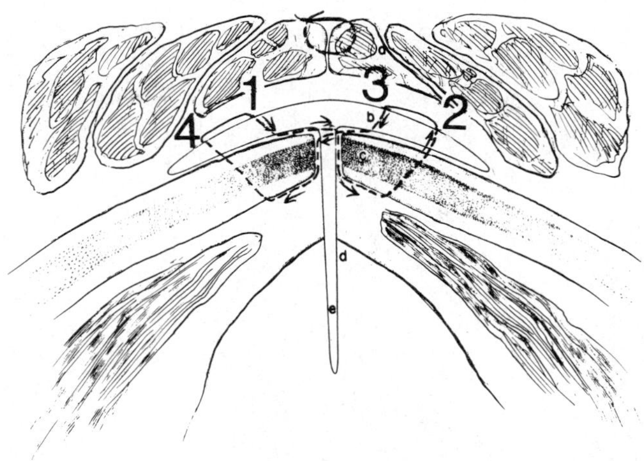

Figure 10–7. Stent for anterior web. Tight closure of the thyroid laminae and fixation of the silicone keel are best accomplished by using a figure-of-eight suture (#4-0 polyethylene). This suture is placed first through the extralaryngeal portion of the keel (1), then through the base of the intralaryngeal extension, and continues through the thyroid laminae and extralaryngeal portion of the keel on the opposite side (2). The second half of the suture (3 and 4) is placed in the reverse direction. The figure-of-eight sutures must be completed before the keel is inserted. Sutures are placed through the thyroid laminae above and below the keel, and the sternohyoid muscles are approximated in the midline over the keel (a, sternohyoid muscles; b, extralaryngeal portion of keel; c, thyroid laminae; d, anterior commissure; e, intralaryngeal portion of keel). (From Montgomery WW: Surgery of the Upper Respiratory System. Vol 2. Philadelphia, Lea & Febiger, 1973, p 570.)

gion. These mucosal flaps are sutured in position to entirely cover the denuded area. In uncomplicated cases, internal stents are unnecessary, but if the vocal cords and the cricoarytenoid joint have sustained significant injuries, an indwelling stent similar to that described in the preceding section can be employed.

A complete glottic stenosis is approached through a low collar incision that will provide access to the entire thyroid cartilage as well as the cricothyroid membrane and cricoid cartilage (Fig. 10–9). After the superior cervical flap is elevated, the laryngeal cartilages are exposed by incising the cervical fascia and retracting the strap muscles laterally. An exact midline thyrotomy is necessary, starting from the level of the cricothyroid membrane in the paralyzed patient. A Kelly clamp is introduced to partially retract the arytenoid cartilages laterally as a precise cut with a scalpel blade or button end knife is made between the two true vocal cords. After the larynx is opened, the stenotic area is excised, with care taken to preserve as much mucous membrane as possible. If the area devoid of mucosa is minimal, posterior advancement flaps elevated from the pharynx, usually at the level of the pyriform sinus, are brought to cover denuded areas in the posterior commissure (Fig. 10–10).[33, 34] If there is an extensive mucosal defect, a very thin split-thickness skin graft or mucosal graft from the nasal septal area or oral cavity can be used. The very thin split-thickness skin graft is obtained from a non-hairbearing area and cut to suit the intralaryngeal defect. The free graft is then wrapped around an appropriate intralaryngeal stent of the variety discussed previously (Fig. 10–9, B and C). The graft is sutured to itself around a stent and the raw area is placed externally to face the denuded area of mucosa. The stent, with its attached free graft, is held in position with two 0 nylon transverse sutures that are brought through skin, soft tissue, thyroid cartilage, and finally, through the stent itself, which is held externally in the neck by the buttons (Fig. 10–9D). The extreme anterior edges of the true vocal cords are advanced to the thyroid cartilage and held in position with some horizontal mattress sutures. The thyrotomy incision is closed by approximating the thyroid cartilage with multiple interrupted 4-0 polyglycolic acid (Dexon) sutures placed through the external perichondrium. The strap muscles are similarly approximated in the midline. The stent is usually left in position for approximately four weeks and removed as an endoscopic procedure. An anterior keel may need to be placed at a later date if anterior web formation develops. If a portion of the anterior aspect of the thyroid cartilage is missing as part of the complete glottic stenosis, autogenous tissue, such as a free hyoid bone graft, can be used to increase the anterior-posterior dimension of the thyroid cartilage.[37] This bone graft can be contoured to the defect and approximated to the edges of the thyroid cartilage with

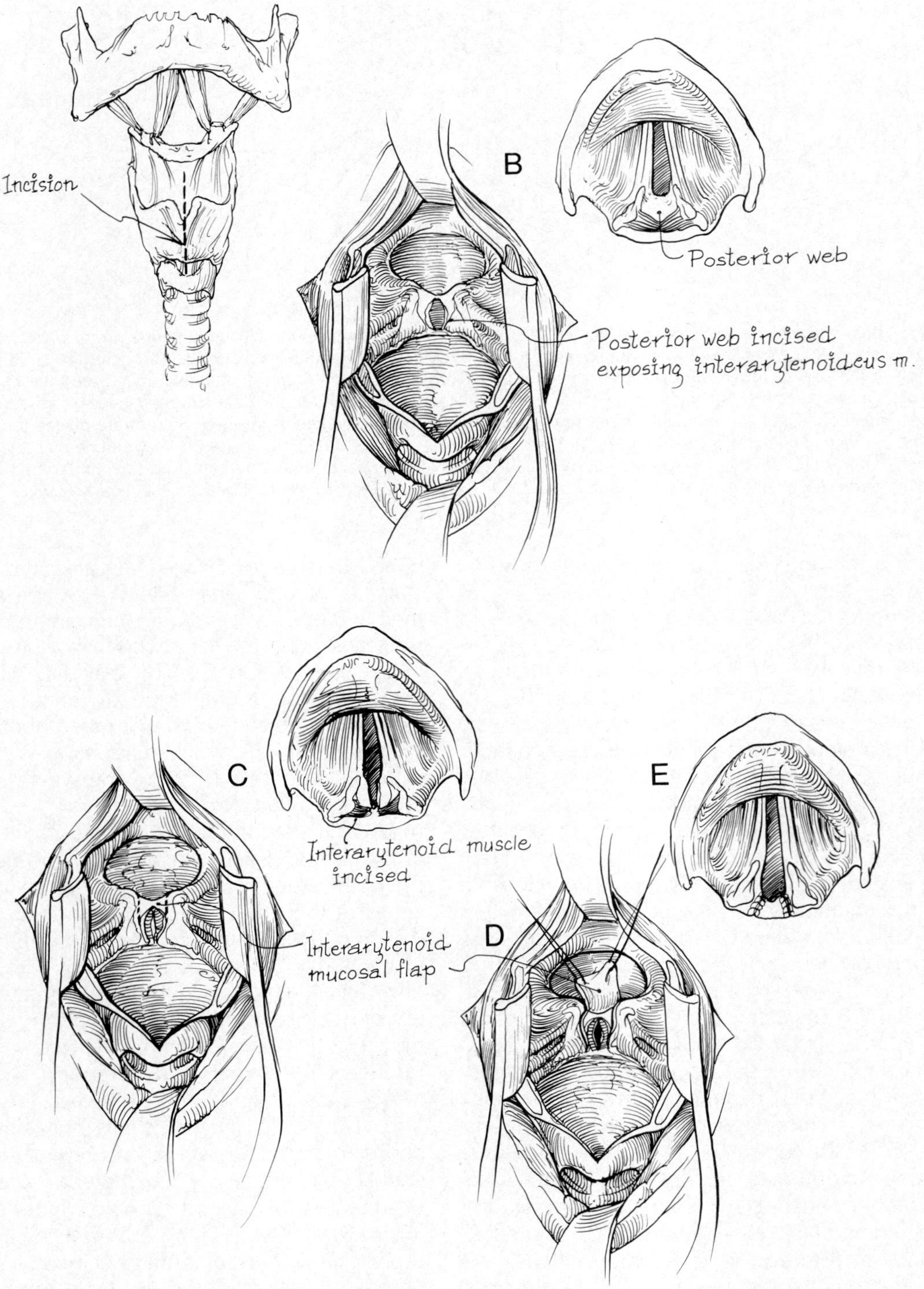

Figure 10–8. Repair of posterior commissure web.

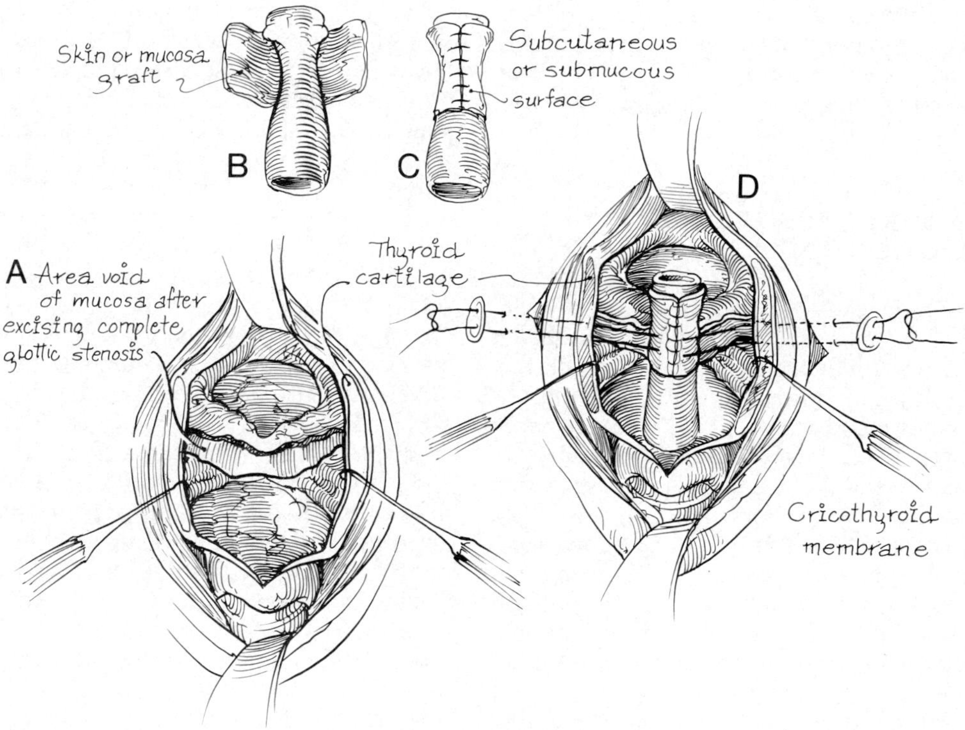

Figure 10–9. Repair of glottic stenosis.

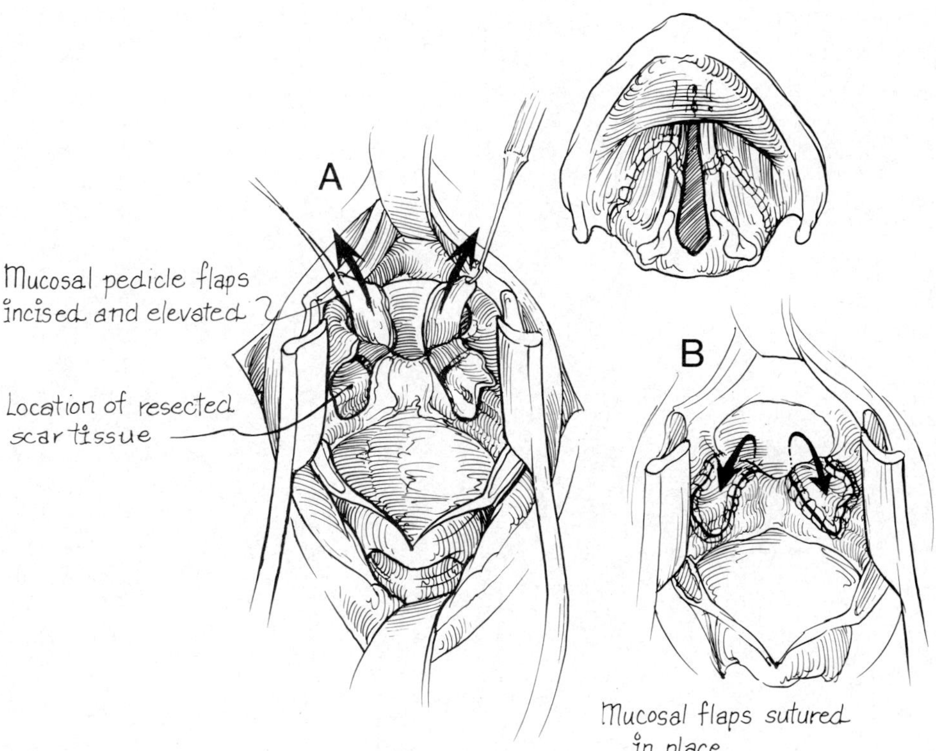

Figure 10–10. Incisions for pedicled mucosal flaps—complete glottic stenosis.

multiple interrupted 3-0 Prolene sutures or No. 5 braided, stainless steel wires. In situations requiring this anterior-posterior lengthening of the thyroid cartilage, some blunting of the anterior commissure is inevitable.

TREATMENT OF ACQUIRED SUBGLOTTIC STENOSIS

Exposure for the open treatment of subglottic stenosis is similar to that employed in glottic stenosis. A low collar incision is made and the superior flap is elevated. The thyroid cartilage, cricothyroid membrane, cricoid cartilage, and the first two tracheal rings are exposed. A tracheotomy should be placed at least at the level of the third or fourth tracheal ring. A vertical incision is made from the first tracheal ring extending through the anterior cricoid arch to the level of the thyroid cartilage. The area of subglottic stenosis is inspected. If the stenotic portion extends to the undersurface of the true vocal cords, a median thyrotomy will be required for exposure. In cases of partial, or minimal, areas of stenosis, the area involved can be resected submucosally, leaving a very narrow mucosal defect (Fig. 10–11). An indwelling stent is then fashioned to maintain the lumen and is held in place for approximately four weeks, after which it is removed as described previously.

In the presence of large mucosal defects, a split-thickness skin graft (0.010 to 0.015 inch thick) like those used in complete glottic stenosis can be placed around the indwelling stent (Fig. 10–9, B–D). If the cricoid cartilage is very small or a portion of the anterior arch is missing, a free graft of hyoid bone or a free nasal septal composite graft of cartilage and mucosa can be placed either to replace a missing part or to splint widely the cricoid cartilage (Fig. 10–2).[26, 37] An autogenous graft of bone or cartilage has an excellent chance of survival and provides a much larger subglottic diameter.

Massive destruction of the subglottic region, especially of the cricoid cartilage, may require a thyrotracheal anastomosis (Fig. 10–12).[11, 14] This generally assumes that the architecture of the cricoid ring is so completely destroyed that any efforts at grafting to replace the missing parts would be impossible. It is also essential to ascertain whether vocal cord motion is lost prior to thyrotracheal anastomosis because the mobilization required for this procedure jeopardizes the recurrent laryngeal nerve. Prior to thyrotracheal anastomosis, the area of subglottic stenosis is resected immediately beneath the thyroid cartilage and posteriorly to the anterior wall of the esophagus. This resection includes most of the cricoid cartilage, especially its anterolateral aspects. If a tracheal ring is involved in the stenosis, it is similarly resected. An effort is made to resect the cricoid area

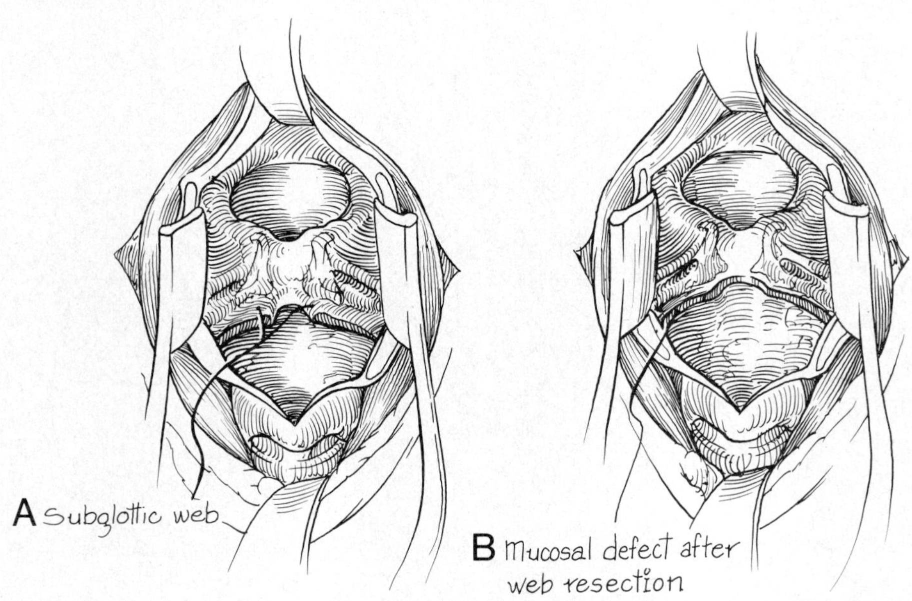

Figure 10–11. Laryngeal stenosis, subglottic web.

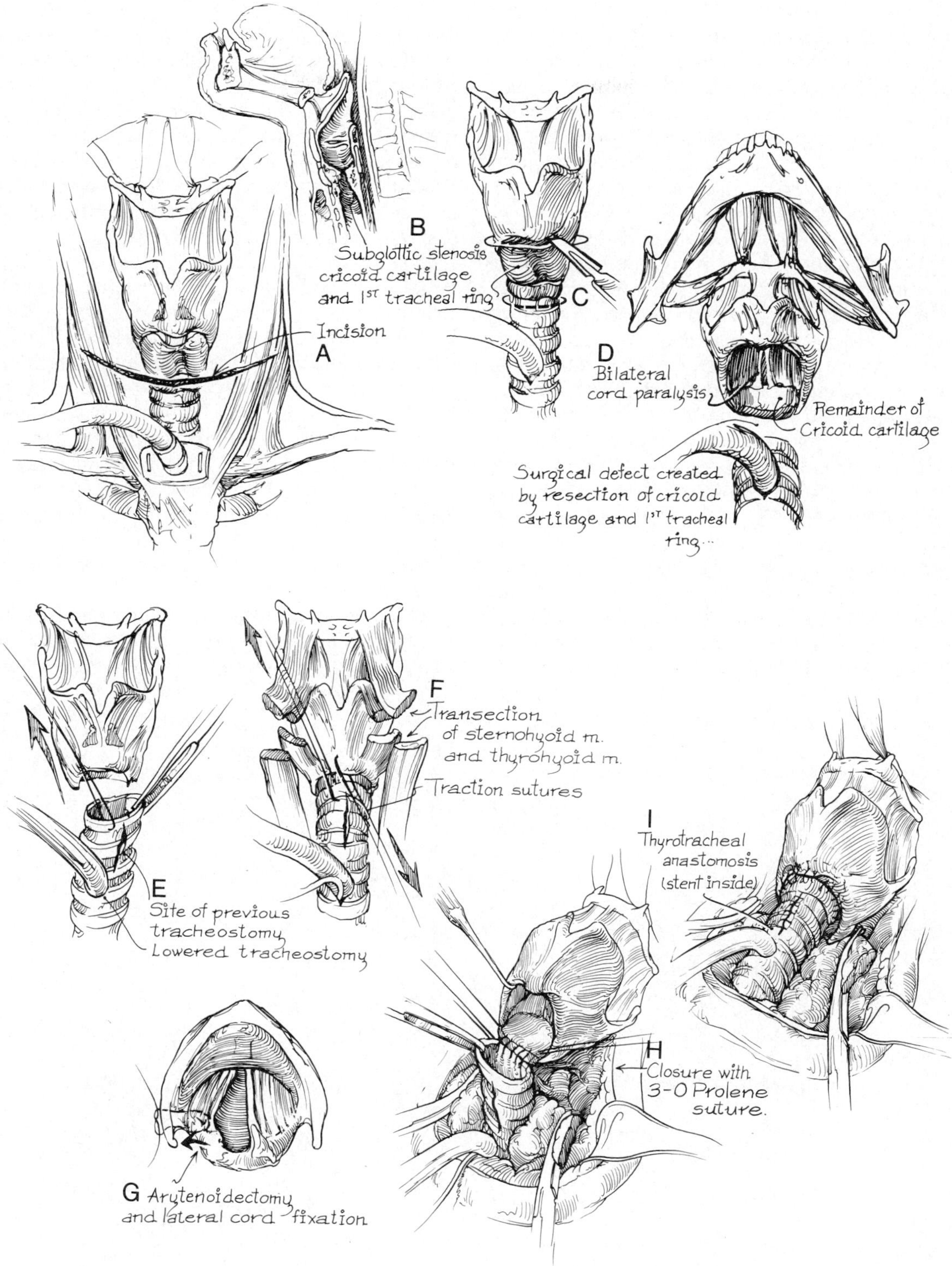

Figure 10–12. Laryngeal release and tracheal mobilization for subglottic resection and thyrotracheal anastomosis.

subperichondrially, which may be very difficult because of extensive scarring and missing cartilage. After the stenotic segment has been widely resected, the larynx is mobilized from above by transecting the sternohyoid and thyrohyoid muscles and portions of the thyrohyoid membrane (Figs. 10–13 and 10–14). Some of the superior constrictor muscle attachments to the superior horn of the thyroid cartilage can also be mobilized. This allows the larynx to drop and, depending on the age of the patient, can provide 4 to 5 cm of relaxation.[38] In the younger patient, greater amounts of relaxation are possible, especially in the long-necked individual. In older patients with stiff structures, less relaxation and mobility will be obtained.

Some additional relaxation and mobility for an anastomosis can be obtained by freeing the trachea from the mediastinum with some anterior and posterior dissection of the trachea. Care must be taken to avoid extensively freeing the trachea laterally because its main blood supply enters from its lateral aspect. After suitable relaxation is obtained, the thyroid cartilage is approximated to the next intact tracheal ring with multiple interrupted 3-0 Prolene or No. 5 braided stainless steel wire sutures. The sutures are all tied with their knots outside the lumen.

An intralaryngeal stent is usually unnecessary unless there is associated malacia to a significant degree or a need for internal grafting of denuded areas. To flex the patient's neck while the anastomosis is being completed is helpful. Also, the thyrotracheal sutures should be placed all around the circumference of the anastomosis prior to tying a single suture. The sutures can then be tied individually while an assistant crosses the next suture line and provides a watertight seal.

In all cases of open repair of subglottic stenosis, it is essential that the tracheotomy be repositioned; if necessary, the tracheotomy should be placed at a lower level, sometimes as low as the fourth or fifth tracheal ring, so that it is distant from the site of repair.

Cases with associated abductor paralysis, in which both vocal cords are immobile and in a midline position, should be managed concomitantly with a vocal cord lateralization. This is especially true in a case requiring a thyrotracheal anastomosis, because it will be very difficult to perform this procedure at a later date in a heavily scarred neck. An arytenoidectomy can be performed and the vocal process lateralized by fixation to the inferior horn of the thyroid cartilage after the interarytenoid muscle has been severed. This cord lateralization procedure, as described by Woodman, appears to be the most satisfactory.[39]

An alternative procedure, recommended by Tucker, is reinnervation of the vocal cord by nerve-muscle pedicle from the ansa cervicalis

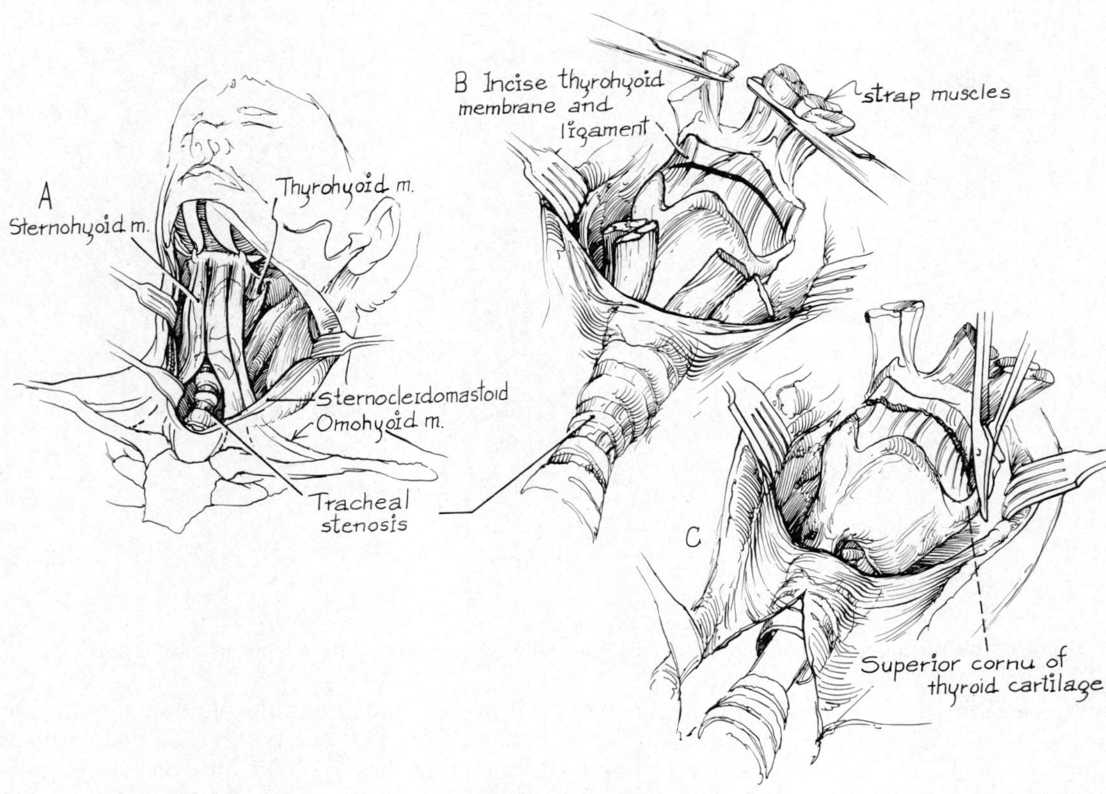

Figure 10–13. Infrahyoid release.

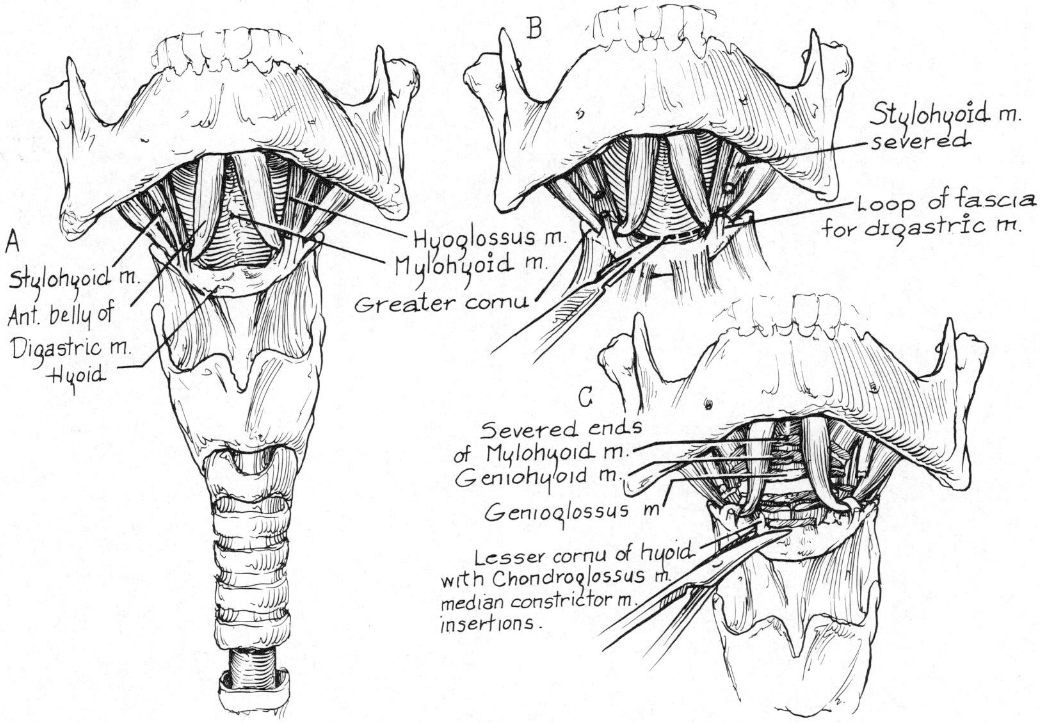

Figure 10–14. Suprahyoid release.

and omohyoid muscle. The nerve-muscle pedicle is then sutured to the posterior cricoarytenoid muscle after this muscle is exposed by retracting the thyroid cartilage and dissection of the inferior constrictor muscle.[40] This procedure, however, is relatively new and more demanding than the Woodman procedure and is not widely used at this time. Heavy scarring in the neck may preclude isolation of the critical nerve-muscle pedicle.

TREATMENT OF ACQUIRED EXTENSIVE TRANSGLOTTIC STENOSIS

In acquired extensive transglottic stenosis, very little supporting structure of the larynx and upper trachea is left. A time-honored procedure developed in the 1930s by LeJeune, "the trough method," may be necessary.[17] Rarely is the destruction of the thyroid and cricoid cartilage so extensive that simple repairs are infeasible. These injuries also commonly involve the upper cervical trachea. The extent of the stenosis is usually 5 cm or greater. A complex, multistage procedure, the laryngotracheal trough, is necessary to reestablish an airway and a functioning larynx. A basic requirement for the success of this procedure is that the posterior and lateral portions of the larynx and trachea remain intact. The laryngotracheal trough technique basically provides a new anterior laryngotracheal wall.[18, 19]

In the first stage of the laryngotracheal trough technique, a T-shaped incision is made in the neck (Fig. 10–15). Through the vertical portion of the T incision, a laryngofissure through the laryngeal and tracheal remnant is completed. All the stenotic areas and granulation tissue are excised. The lateral laryngeal and tracheal remnants are then approximated anteriorly to the skin, which is advanced into the lumen. The trough is kept open with gauze packing impregnated with antibiotic ointment or with an indwelling stent covered by a split-thickness skin graft. The tracheotomy is placed as distal as possible from the trough, usually at the level of the sternal notch.

After one month of healing, a medially based skin flap is created immediately adjacent to the trough. Strips of Marlex mesh are imbedded beneath the skin flap superficial to the strap muscles. The skin flap is then returned to its original bed. One month later the skin flap, with the Marlex reinforcement, is elevated and rotated to cover the laryngotracheal trough and become the new anterior wall. It is essential that the strap muscles be included with the skin

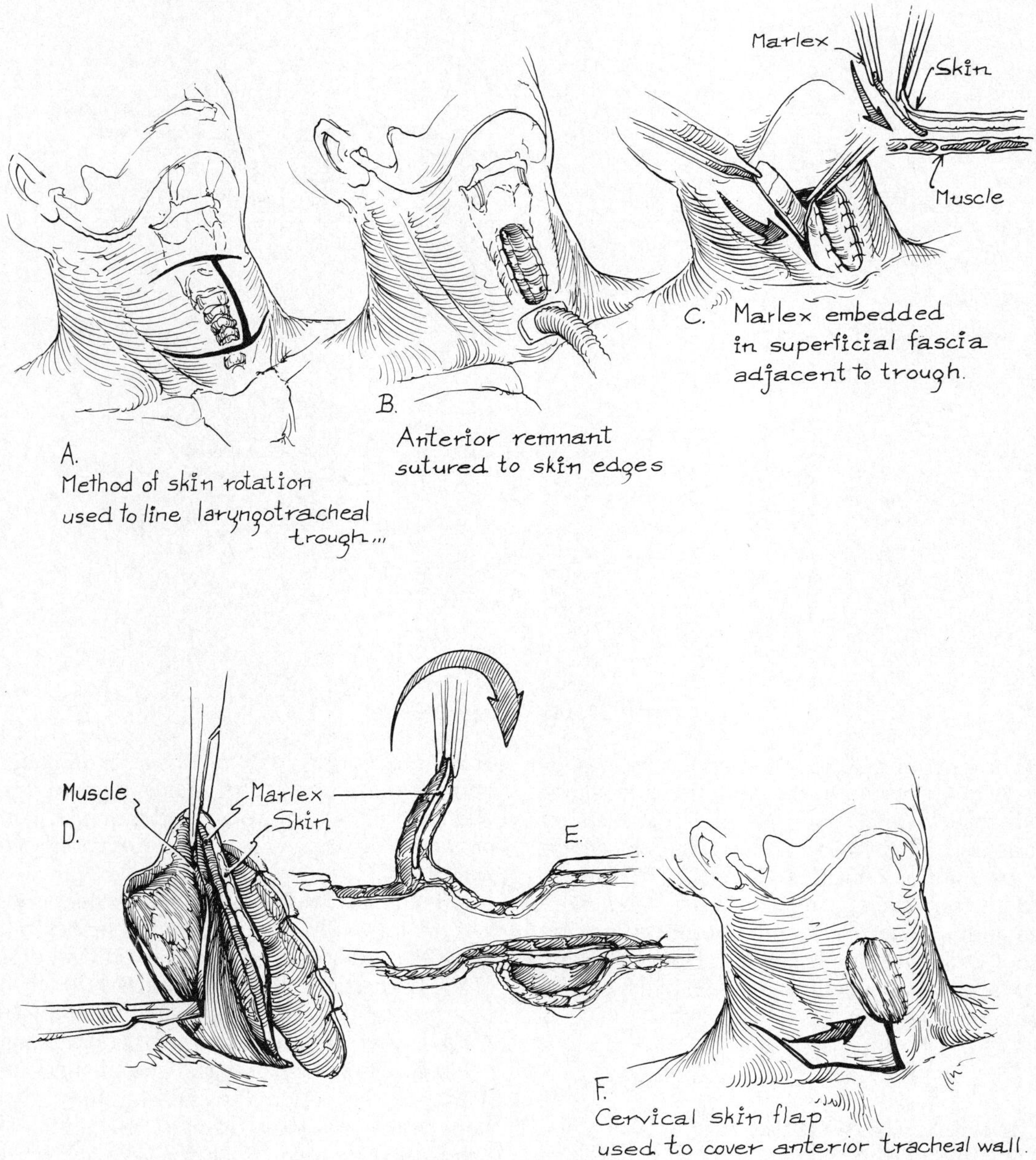

Figure 10–15. Marlex for laryngeal trough.

flap to prevent any exposure of the Marlex mesh, which must be carefully placed in the superficial cervical fascia plane. These strips of Marlex, 0.5 cm in size, are usually adequate for reinforcement. After the composite skin flap is in position, a superiorly based cervical skin flap is rotated to cover the new anterior tracheal wall.

An alternative form of the laryngotracheal trough technique embeds rib bone and cartilage in a laterally based chest flap, which is tubed and placed proximal to the laryngeal opening of the trough. The laterally based chest flap may be necessary in situations where severe scarring of the cervical skin prevents successful implantation of alloplastic material or autogenous tissue. Although these techniques have limited applicability, they should be considered in extreme situations.

COMPLICATIONS OF SURGICAL TREATMENT

The principal complication in the management of acquired laryngeal stenosis is reformation of the stricture and the return to the original condition. Restenosis is especially likely after inadequate surgery for an uncomplicated stenosis or after extensive surgery in the complicated cases. This complication requires reassessment and probable reexploration. After extensive surgery, an infection may develop, leading to loss of vital cartilaginous-supporting structures from chondritis and reabsorption. Another delayed complication is a pharyngoesophageal stricture resulting from surgical exploration. The more immediate complications include laryngopharyngeal fistula, pneumothorax, and damage to the recurrent laryngeal nerves.

During the early postoperative period, especially in patients with intralaryngeal stents, inadvertent decannulation can lead to asphyxia and death. Occasionally, the internal stent can break loose and lodge in a main stem bronchus, producing serious respiratory distress.

References

1. Alonso WA: Surgical management and complications of acute laryngotracheal disruption. Otolaryngol Clin North Am 12:753–760, 1979.
2. Cracovaner AJ, Chodosh PL: Laryngotracheal trauma. *In* Maloney W (ed): Otolaryngology Vol 4. Hagerstown, MD, Harper and Row, 1975.
3. Jackson C: Laryngostomy. Laryngoscope 9:690, 1909.
4. Schmiegelow E.: Stenosis of the larynx: A new method of surgical treatment. Arch Otolaryngol 9:473–493, 1929.
5. Arbuckle MF: Cicatricial stenosis of the larynx. Arch Otolaryngol 8:686, 1928.
6. Figi FA: Chronic stenosis of the larynx with special consideration of skin grafting. Ann Otol Rhinol Laryngol 49:394, 1940.
7. Negus VE: Treatment of chronic stenosis of larynx with special reference to skin grafting. Ann Otol Rhinol Laryngol 47:891, 1938.
8. Woodward FD: The surgical correction of cicatricial stenosis of the larynx. Ann Otol Rhinol Laryngol 59:488, 1950.
9. Looper FA: The use of the hyoid bone as a stent in laryngeal stenosis. Arch Otolaryngol 28:106–111, 1938.
10. McNaught RC: Surgical correction of anterior web of the larynx. Laryngoscope 60:264–272, 1950.
11. Conley JJ: Reconstruction of the subglottic air passage. Ann Otol Rhinol Laryngol 62:477, 1953.
12. Grillo HC: Surgery of the trachea. *In* Current Problems in Surgery. Chicago, Yearbook Medical Publishers Inc., 1970, pp 1–60.
13. Ogura JH, Rogers CL: Surgical correction of traumatic stenosis of the larynx and pharynx. Laryngoscope 74:468–480, 1962.
14. Ogura JH, Powers WE: Functional restitution of traumatic stenosis of the larynx and pharynx. Laryngoscope 74:1081–1110, 1964.
15. Dedo HH, Fishman HC: Laryngeal release and sleeve resection for tracheal stenosis. Ann Otol Rhinol Laryngol 78:285, 1970.
16. Montgomery WW: Suprahyoid release for tracheal stenosis. Arch Otolaryngol 99:255, 1974.
17. LeJeune F, Owens N: Chronic laryngeal stenosis. Ann Otol Rhinol Laryngol 44:354–363, 1935.
18. Bryce DP, Lawson VG: The trough method of laryngotracheal reconstruction. Ann Otol Rhinol Laryngol 76:793–803, 1967.
19. Friedman WH, Biller HF, Som ML: Repair of extended laryngotracheal stenosis. Arch Otolaryngol 101: 152–156, 1975.
20. Hilding AC: Laryngotracheal damage during intratracheal anesthesia. Trans Am Broncho-Esopha Assoc 51:157–173, 1971.
21. Pearson FG et al.: A prospective study of tracheal injury complicating tracheostomy with a cuffed tube. Ann Otol Rhinol Laryngol 77:867–882, 1968.
22. McGovern FH et al.: The hazards of endotracheal intubation. Ann Otol Rhinol Laryngol 80:556–564, 1971.
23. Calcaterra T et al.: Effects of laryngofissure on the developing canine larynx. Ann Otol Rhinol Laryngol 83:810–813, 1974.
24. Evans JNG, Todd GB: Laryngotracheoplasty. J Laryngol 88:589–597, 1974.
25. Gates GA, Fernandez AT: Laryngotracheoplasty for acquired subglottic stenosis in infants and children: Experience with six cases. Laryngoscope 88: 1468–1476, 1978.
26. Toohil RJ et al.: Repair of laryngeal stenosis with nasoseptal graft. Ann Otol Rhinol Laryngol 85:600, 1976.
27. Fearon B, Cotton R: Surgical correction of subglottic stenosis of the larynx in infants and children: Progress report. Ann Otol Rhinol Laryngol 83:428–431, 1974.
28. Cotton R: Management of subglottic stenosis in infancy and childhood: Review of a consecutive series of cases managed by surgical reconstruction. Ann Otol Rhinol Laryngol 87:649–657, 1978.
29. Alonso WA et al.: Clinical experiences in hyoid arch transposition. Laryngoscope 86:617–624, 1976.
30. Wong MF et al.: Vascularized hyoid interposition for subglottic and upper tracheal stenosis. Ann Otol Rhinol Laryngol 87:491–497, 1978.
31. Ward PH et al.: Composite hyoid sternohyoid muscle grafts in humans. Arch Otolaryngol 103:531–534, 1977.
32. Montgomery WW: The surgical management of supraglottic and subglottic stenosis. Ann Otol Rhinol Laryngol 77:534–547, 1968.
33. Montgomery WW: Surgery of the Upper Respiratory System Vol 2. Philadelphia, Lea and Febiger Inc, 1973.
34. Ogura JH, Biller HF: Reconstruction of the larynx following blunt trauma. Ann Otol Rhinol Laryngol 80:492–510, 1971.
35. Strong MS et al.: Endoscopic management of laryngeal stenosis. Otolaryngol Clin North Am 12:797–805, 1979.
36. Dedo HH: Endoscopic Teflon keel for anterior glottic web. Ann Otol Rhinol Laryngol 88:467–473, 1976.
37. Alonso WA: Hyoid arch transposition. Otolaryngol Clin North Am 12:903–908, 1979.
38. Alonso WA et al.: Complications of laryngotracheal disruption. Laryngoscope 84:124–129, 1974.
39. Woodman DG: A modification of the extralaryngeal approach to arytenoidectomy for bilateral abductor paralysis. Arch Otolaryngol 93:63, 1946.
40. Tucker HM: Human laryngeal reinnervation: Long-term experience with the nerve-muscle pedicle technique. Laryngoscope 88:598–604, 1978.

11

Congenital Lesions of the Larynx

William Lawson, M.D., D.D.S.
and Hugh F. Biller, M.D.

Congenital disorders of the larynx account for many of the cases of respiratory distress in the newborn and infant. Other causes include obstruction anywhere in the aerodigestive tract as well as various neurologic, cardiac, and metabolic disorders.[1]

Developmental abnormalities of the larynx disturb its respiratory, phonatory, and protective functions and may cause symptoms that range in severity from minimal to life-threatening. Clinical manifestations may be present at birth or may not appear for weeks, months, or years. Although the clinical findings may suggest involvement of some segment of the larynx, they are generally nonspecific and require direct laryngoscopy for definitive diagnosis and management.

Table 11–1 lists the types and relative incidence of the various congenital disorders of the larynx described in major reported series.[2–4] All but one are anatomic abnormalities of the supraglottic, glottic, and subglottic larynx that reflect altered organ morphogenesis; in the exception, vocal cord paralysis, a neurogenic disorder, affects laryngeal function.

LARYNGOMALACIA

Laryngomalacia, the commonest abnormality of the neonatal larynx, is also known as congenital laryngeal stridor[5] and exaggerated infantile larynx.[6] The etiology of this condition is not known. It has been variously interpreted as a malformation representing retarded laryngeal development, with softness and loss of rigidity of the laryngeal framework, and as a true anomaly, presumably by an increased contribution of the third branchial arch producing a redundant supraglottic larynx.[2]

The clinical presentation is typically an intermittent, high-pitched, inspiratory stridor, crowing in character, which often accompanies increased activity, crying, and feeding. It generally varies with position, being more pronounced while the infant is supine and diminishing when the infant is lying prone. Similarly, flexing the head increases the stridor, while extension of the neck reduces it. The voice and cry are normal. There is no associated cyanosis, feeding difficulties, evidence of aspiration, or failure to thrive. The stridor generally begins a few weeks after birth and may persist until the child is one to one and one-half years of age, when it spontaneously disappears.

Direct laryngoscopy establishes the diagnosis. Characteristically, an elongated floppy epiglottis appears to be curled on itself; the aryepiglottic folds are closely approximated and, on inspiration, are sucked tightly toward each other. The arytenoids may also appear to flutter with respiration. Elevating the epiglottis

Table 11–1. INCIDENCE OF CONGENITAL LARYNGEAL DISORDERS

Congenital Disorder	Number of Cases		
	Holinger, Brown (1967)	*Fearon, Ellis (1971)*	*Tucker et al. (1978)*
Laryngomalacia	650	293	1415
Subglottic stenosis	53	84	278
Webs	32	9	224
Atresia	1	—	43
Cysts	8	3	52
Laryngoceles	12	—	6
Clefts	2	2	56
Vascular tumors	19	14	95
Vocal cord paralysis	84	28	—
Bifid epiglottis	—	—	8
Absent epiglottis	2	—	2
Cricoid fusion	3	—	—
TOTAL	866	433	2179

eliminates the stridor and permits examination of the remainder of the larynx to rule out other abnormalities. Fearon[1] urged that all infants with stridor be examined by bronchoscopy in addition to laryngoscopy to rule out an associated abnormality lower in the respiratory tract.

Most patients require no treatment because the condition resolves spontaneously; however, some infants develop severe dyspnea and cyanosis and may require tracheostomy.[7] Tucker et al.[4] found only 4 instances of tracheostomy among 1415 reported cases.

No constant correlation exists between laryngomalacia and other congenital anomalies. Holinger[7] stressed its association with the pectus excavatum deformity. Fearon and Ellis[3] reported that 5 per cent of their cases with laryngomalacia also had subglottic stenosis. Tucker et al.[4] cited 8 cases of laryngomalacia with brachiocephalic artery compression of the trachea and 3 with premature calcification of the larynx and trachea, suggesting diffuse cartilaginous abnormalities; however, Cohen et al.[8] found laryngomalacia alone in only 12 of their 33 patients. Twenty-one of their patients had subglottic stenosis or vocal cord paralysis.

SUBGLOTTIC STENOSIS

Congenital subglottic stenosis causes severe airway obstruction with relative frequency in the infant (see Table 11–1). Normally the widest portion of the neonatal larynx,[6] in this condition, the subglottis is variably narrowed from just beneath the true vocal cords to the cricoid region. This condition is believed to represent arrested development of the conus elasticus; however, in rare instances, a cartilaginous malformation may be present also.

Clinically, stridor is often present at birth; however, symptoms may not appear for several weeks or months until a respiratory infection supervenes. The stridor is generally both inspiratory and expiratory. Infants with severe stenosis usually have severe respiratory distress and cyanosis at birth; those with minimal narrowing may have stridor only during respiratory infections. Subglottic stenosis should be suspected in infants with recurrent "croup."[9]

Analysis of 153 cases of subglottic stenosis by Fearon et al.[10] revealed 123 to be clearly congenital, 7 clearly acquired, and 23 of uncertain etiology. The ratio of male preponderance was approximately 2.5:1. Congenital anomalies present in many of the children studied involved the respiratory (47), cardiovascular (47), neuroskeletal (22), neurologic (19), and urogenital (5) systems. Stridor was present in 80 cases but was continuous in only 4. Of 158 cases of subglottic stenosis reviewed by Holinger et al.,[9] 115 were congenital and 43 were acquired. These authors found stridor in 43 per cent of the cases, often associated with a barking cough or hoarseness. Approximately 10 per cent of their cases also had a history of pneumonia or atelectasis. Males predominated in a ratio of 2:1. Fifteen patients had associated laryngotracheal abnormalities that included laryngomalacia (5), anterior glottic web (3), tracheomalacia (2), tracheal stenosis (2), tracheoesophageal fistula (2), and vocal cord paralysis (1). Fourteen patients had rubella or congenital anomalies including imperforate anus, cleft palate, cystic fibrosis, meningomyelocele, and craniostenosis.

Direct laryngoscopy reveals the point of maximal narrowing generally at 2 mm to 3 mm below the superior surface of the true cords, with the involved area appearing firm and nonedematous. While generally presenting as a diffuse circumferential soft tissue narrowing, at times it may appear as a bilateral bulge producing a slitlike lumen; in rare cases, the narrowing is unilateral, mimicking a subglottic hemangioma. Holinger et al.[9] observed the following incidence of these types: circumferential (94 cases), bilateral (5 cases), localized in the anterior or posterior wall (6 cases each), and lateral (4 cases).

Most cases of congenital subglottic stenosis require tracheostomy because the compromised airway may rapidly become totally occluded with a respiratory infection. The resulting inflammation and edema are totally internal because of the circular configuration of the cricoid cartilage. By preventing expulsion of secretions from the lungs, the stenotic segment intensifies the respiratory distress. Holinger[7] found that infants with this laryngeal anomaly were the largest group under one year of age requiring tracheostomy. Moreover, tracheal cannulation must often be maintained for several years. Stenosis causes inadequate ventilation when a 3.5-mm pediatric bronchoscope cannot be passed.[1]

Fearon et al.[10] reported 76 of 153 patients with subglottic stenosis required tracheostomy; 53 were urgent and 23 were elective. Fearon and Ellis[3] found that of 84 tracheotomized patients with subglottic stenosis, 25 were decannulated within one year, 34 between one and two years, and 25 after two years; however, all but a single patient were decannulated by six years of age.

Traditionally, management of congenital subglottic stenosis has been based on the expectation of further laryngeal growth, with most patients outgrowing the condition. After tracheostomy, the most common operative treatment has been repeated dilatation of the stenotic segment using Jackson laryngeal dilators or graduated bronchoscopes at intervals of two to six weeks. Fearon et al.[10] treated only 12 patients without tracheostomy; 54 patients required tracheostomy and procedures for ventilation. Narrow stenotic segments respond best to dilatation. Complications of this procedure, including pneumothorax and pneumomediastinum, occur rarely.

External laryngeal surgery is controversial, being employed generally with acquired subglottic stenosis secondary to endotracheal intubation when the pathology is more extensive and the prognosis poorer. Holinger et al.[11] reported that 44 per cent of the patients with the congenital type required tracheostomy, with 2.1 per cent mortality and decannulation failure of 10.8 per cent. They found that 97 per cent of the patients with the acquired type required tracheostomy, with 11 per cent mortality and 27.6 per cent rate of decannulation failure. Open surgery has also been recommended for those congenital cases that have not responded to repeated serial dilatations, those with extensive areas of dense stenosis involving the glottis or upper trachea, or those with cricoid abnormalities in which spontaneous improvement is highly unlikely. An open operative approach in pediatric patients is also based on evidence that surgery on the developing larynx does not interfere with its subsequent growth. This has been shown experimentally with the canine[12] and primate larynx[13, 14] as well as clinically and radiographically in man.[15] Fearon and Cotton[10, 15] divided the cricoid cartilage anteriorly in the midline and inserted a portion of the thyroid lamina or autogenous costal cartilage between the cut ends without endolaryngeal stenting. Grahne's method,[16] employed for very extensive stenosis, involves median section of the lower portion of the thyroid and cricoid cartilages, resection of the scar, median division of the cricoid lamina posteriorly down to the esophagus, and placement of a prosthetic stent for several months through which a tracheostomy tube is inserted. Crysdale and Platt[17] reported success using this method in 3 cases. Cotton[15] claimed that 17 of 18 patients with severe acquired subglottic stenosis could be extubated after surgical reconstruction by these methods.

Evans and Todd[18] reported a method of laryngotracheoplasty entailing laryngofissure with stepped incision of the cricoid cartilage and upper tracheal rings if necessary, submucosal excision of scar tissue, insertion of a rolled silicon rubber (Silastic) sheet, and distraction of the cartilaginous interdigitations with wiring in the new position. Two weeks later, the Silastic was endoscopically removed. They claimed extubation in all five cases of subglottic stenosis so treated; however, they have no long-term follow-up on the effects of this operative procedure on laryngotracheal development.

NEUROGENIC DISORDERS

Congenital vocal cord paralysis may be unilateral or bilateral. Bilateral paralysis is more common and more dangerous because of the increased tendency to airway obstruction. In the unilateral type, the left vocal cord is more often paralyzed because the circuitous path of the left recurrent laryngeal nerve about the aortic arch makes it more susceptible to compression by malformations of the great vessels, cardiomegaly, congenital cysts and tumors of the mediastinum, or anomalies of the tracheobronchial tree. Holinger[7] confirms this in a study of 63 infants under 18 months of age with vocal cord paralysis; he reported that 42 were bilateral, 8 were right sided, and 13 were left sided. In the bilateral group, 17 were complete (13 requiring tracheotomy) and 25 were partial (7 requiring tracheostomy). Two of 21 patients with unilateral vocal palsy also required tracheostomy. Cavanaugh[19] found that

Table 11–2. ANALYSIS OF 149 CASES OF BILATERAL VOCAL CORD PARALYSIS*

Type	Causes
Congenital (82)	*Associated with other anomalies (43)*
	Neurologic (21)
	Cerebral agenesis
	Nuclear hypoplasia
	Congenital hypotonia
	Werdnig-Hoffman disease
	Leukodystrophy
	Charcot-Marie-Tooth disease
	Laryngeal (10)
	Subglottic stenosis
	Laryngomalacia
	Laryngocele
	Cardiac (8)
	Atrial and ventricular septal defects
	Coarctation of aorta
	Transposition of great vessels
	Miscellaneous (4)
	Pneumothorax
	Muscular hypertonia
	Tracheomalacia
	Isolated paralysis (39)
Acquired (59)	*Secondary to congenital anomalies (41)*
	Meningomyelocele, Arnold-Chiari malformation, hydrocephalus (24)
	Hydrocephalus (6)
	Postoperative (11)
	Secondary to acquired conditions (18)
	Infection (7)
	Neoplasm (7)
	Trauma (2)
	Guillain-Barré syndrome (2)
Undetermined (8)	

*Figures in parentheses refer to number of cases. (From data of Holinger LD et al.: Ann Otol Rhinol Laryngol 85:428–436, 1976.

among 37 cases of vocal cord paralysis in infants and children, 10 were bilateral, while 4 were left sided and 23 were right sided. In his series, 11 were asymptomatic at birth, 5 developed symptoms within a few days, and the remainder developed symptoms between several weeks and several years of age. All but 2 cases failed to recover after intervals ranging from several months to seven years. Because the overwhelming number of cases with either type of paralysis is associated with some other congenital or acquired systemic disorder, infants must be carefully studied for the presence of cardiac, respiratory, or other neurologic disease.[6, 20]

Analysis of 389 cases of partial or complete bilateral abductor vocal cord paralysis by Holinger et al.[20] revealed that 149 occurred in infants and children under 12 years of age (see Table 11–2). Of these, 82 cases were congenital, 43 being associated with other developmental anomalies and the remainder having only the isolated laryngeal defect. When the congenital vocal cord paralysis occurred without associated anomalies, it had the better prognosis and many cases tended to spontaneously resolve within weeks or months. In 59 cases, the vocal paralysis was acquired. Of these, in 41 cases, the paralysis was secondary to meningomyelocele, Arnold-Chiari malformation, or hydrocephalus, or occurred after the repair of other congenital lesions; in 18 cases, it followed an infectious, neoplastic, or traumatic disorder. The association between increased intracranial pressure and bilateral vocal cord paralysis is so well established that Holinger et al.[20] advocated that children with increasing stridor be intubated until the increased pressure was corrected. Bluestone et al.[21] analyzed 12 infants with Arnold-Chiari malformation, meningomyelocele, and hydrocephalus with respiratory obstruction, showing that neurosurgical relief of the increased intracranial pressure within 24 hours resulted in early return of vocal cord function. Delayed operative intervention was associated with vocal cord paralysis that persisted as long as one and one-half years. They recommended that infants with vocal cord paralysis be intubated for 48 hours, followed by tracheotomy if respiratory obstruction persisted to prevent acquired subglottic stenosis from prolonged endotracheal intubation. Holinger et al.[20] could not determine the etiology of the bilateral abductor paralysis in 8 patients.

Difficult to recognize clinically, bilateral abductor vocal cord paralysis may create a life-threatening situation.[20] The cry or voice may be normal because the paralyzed and adducted vocal cords passively vibrate equally, as opposed to the hoarseness associated with the unilaterally paralyzed cord; however, a soft or high-pitched inspiratory stridor, which intensifies with exertion, is often present. If the lesion of the vagus nerve involves the superior laryngeal nerve, aspiration also becomes prominent. The superimposition of the edema from an upper respiratory infection may produce acute obstruction or a crouplike state in these patients.

Direct laryngoscopy is imperative for all patients with congenital or acquired persistent stridor. Holinger et al.[20] recommend an endoscopic examination for suspected vocal cord paralysis; this diagnostic procedure should be performed with the Jackson pediatric laryngoscope placed in the vallecula without general anesthesia in the newborn. Passive mobility of the vocal cords and arytenoids should be tested for with a laryngeal spatula to rule out midline vocal cord fixation.

Holinger et al.[20] estimated that 48 per cent of infants and children with bilateral abductor vocal cord paralysis eventually require tracheostomy. The gradual onset of the paralysis in many cases may insidiously produce a marginal airway that is prone to precipitate obstruction. Gacek[22] believes any pediatric patient with significant stridor secondary to vocal paralysis should have a tracheostomy.

A type of heredofamilial bilateral abductor vocal cord paralysis has been described.[22–24] Transmission is sex-linked, involving only males, with onset immediately at birth or delayed until several months or years of age. Failure to perform a tracheostomy when symptoms developed has resulted in death or possible mental retardation secondary to anoxia. Other motor neuron defects may or may not be prominent. The proposed site of the lesion is the midportion of the nucleus ambiguus, where the cell bodies of the motor neurons of the posterior cricoarytenoid muscles lie.[23]

CONGENITAL CYSTS AND LARYNGOCELES

Differential diagnosis of seemingly cystic lesions involving the larynx includes true developmental cysts, simple retention cysts of the lining mucosa, cystadenomas, internal thyroglossal duct cysts, and abnormalities of the ventricle and its appendix. The clinical symptoms are nonspecific and only suggest an obstructing laryngeal lesion. Soft tissue radiographs of the neck may reveal a solid or air-containing mass, suggesting only a cyst or laryngocele. Direct laryngoscopy is diagnostic when aspiration of the mass yields fluid or air.

The laryngocele represents an air-filled dilatation of the ventricular appendix or saccule that communicates with the laryngeal lumen. A laryngocele extends superiorly to produce a swelling that may be limited to the false cord and aryepiglottic fold (internal type), may follow the superior laryngeal neurovascular bundle through the thyrohyoid membrane (external type), or may do both (combined type). Rarely does the external type occur without an internal component. A saccular cyst or laryngeal mucocele is a mucus-filled dilatation of the saccule that does not communicate with the laryngeal lumen. The lateral type extends posterosuperiorly into the false cord and aryepiglottic fold; the anterior type extends medially and posteriorly between the true and false cords.[25]

The variable nomenclature of congenital cysts reflects the uncertain histogenesis of these lesions. The congenital cyst (also called the embryonic, dysembryoplastic, dysontogenetic, or laryngeal dermoid cyst, or cyst of the newborn) is a lesion of the supraglottic larynx. The cyst may vary from a few millimeters to 7 cm in diameter, occasionally having an extralaryngeal extension into the anterior neck. Laryngeal cysts may become symptomatic any time from the neonatal period to advanced age, with most reported cases arising in the sixth decade.[26] Symptoms depend on the size and location of the cyst and on thé patient's age; they include respiratory distress that may be aggravated by head position or feeding, stridor, an altered cry, and the presence of a neck mass in some cases. Pathogenesis of these cysts is unclear; theories of origin include branchial cleft abnormalities, disturbances of the laryngeal saccule, derivation from laryngoceles or obstructed mucous glands, or derivation from displaced thyroid tissue.[26] Histologically, more than half the cysts are lined by respiratory epithelium; the remainder have a stratified squamous, columnar, or cuboidal epithelium, or some combination of these. Scattered or follicular aggregates of lymphocytic tissue have also been observed in about half the cases. The presence of lymphocytic tissue is not diagnostic of this lesion and does not support a branchial origin for these cysts because the larynx develops medial to the visceral pouches.

DeSanto et al.,[26] after analysis of 238 laryngeal cysts, reclassified congenital cysts into saccular cysts (24 per cent) and mucous retention cysts (76 per cent). Mucous retention cysts, later termed ductal cysts (except for one case of thyroid cartilage foraminal cyst), may arise anywhere within the larynx. They tend to be smaller than saccular cysts and rarely present clinical manifestations unless infected. They also tend to be more superficial, lying within the mucosal lining. About one-third of saccular cysts contain granular oxyphilic columnar lining cells and have been subclassified as oncocytic cysts.

Holinger[7] reported on 9 children among 21 patients with laryngoceles; 8 were infants under two months of age and 1 was three years old, symptomatic since birth. He initially divided these laryngoceles into an internal type (which extended from the sinus of Morgagni into the aryepiglottic fold to form an obstructive cystic lesion at the laryngeal inlet) and eventration of the ventricle (in which a cystic mass appeared to protrude from the ventricle into the laryngeal lumen just above the true cords). Holinger and Brown[2] next classified 20 such lesions into 5 internal thyroglossal duct cysts, 3 glottic cysts, 5 ventricular laryngoceles, and 7 arytenoid and aryepiglottic fold laryngoceles. While 12 laryngoceles appeared in children (9 younger than six months of age), 51 laryngoceles were seen in adults. Later, Holinger et al.[25] reported 12 children under three years of age in a series of 42 patients with lesions of the laryngeal ventricle. They were now classified as 10 saccular cysts (6 lateral and 4 anterior) and 2 laryngoceles. All of the patients with cysts presented with respiratory distress, principally inspiratory stridor, with 5 having retractions, 4 an inaudible or muffled cry, 3 cyanosis, and 3 dysphagia. Two patients had other laryngeal abnormalities, which included laryngomalacia and bilateral vocal cord paralysis. All 10 patients received needle aspirations and 5 had unroofing of the cyst. In 6 cases, tracheostomy was performed and maintained for an average of 17 months. Direct laryngoscopy was performed on each infant during the treatment period a mean of 7.5 times. The 2 infants with laryngoceles presented with hoarseness or a weak cry. With direct laryngoscopy, aspiration of the mass failed to yield fluid and no treatment was required.

While aspiration, incision, and drainage are diagnostic and provide temporary relief, the cyst will generally refill. Holinger et al.[25] advocated needle aspiration as the initial treatment of saccular cysts in infants; however, with repeated recurrence, the cyst should be endoscopically unroofed. Temporary tracheostomy may be required in those infants with severe airway obstruction. Fearon[1] also recommended endoscopic resection of the cyst wall.

CLEFT LARYNX

Review of the world literature by Cohen[27] revealed about 30 cases of cleft larynx, to which he added 7 more. Most cases are laryngotracheoesophageal clefts, while only a small number are limited to the posterior larynx. Developmentally, the defect arises from failure of rostral advancement in the formation of the tracheoesophageal septum and fusion of the dorsal laminae of the cricoid cartilage.[28]

The more extensive clefts require surgical correction for survival, whereas those of the cricoid lamina alone can be managed medically. The principal symptom of cleft larynx is aspiration, which is proportional to the extent of the defect, occurs especially with liquids, and results in coughing, choking, cyanosis, and recurrent episodes of pneumonia. There may be some associated voice change. Chest x-ray will reveal evidence of aspiration pneumonitis. A cine-esophagram contrast study should be performed, either by swallowing or catheter injection, to show spillage of the dye into the trachea. Definitive diagnosis, however, requires endoscopic examination. Because of numerous instances in which the diagnosis has been missed, Pillsbury and Fischer[28] devised a measuring probe for use at the time of direct laryngoscopy.

With the posterior cleft larynx, lateral and posterior displacement of the arytenoids is caused by a deficient interarytenoid muscle, with unopposed function of the posterior cricoarytenoid muscles. The laryngotracheoesophageal cleft presents a more extensive posterior midline defect. Bronchoscopy and esophagoscopy must be performed in all cases since most patients with this condition also have associated anomalies of the aerodigestive tract. These include esophageal atresia, tracheoesophageal fistula, and laryngeal, tracheal, and bronchial stenosis. The most common associated congenital defect is tracheoesophageal fistula, with or without atresia.[27] Burroughs and Leape[29] reviewed 33 cases and estimated that 15 had additional congenital defects including facial anomalies and defects of the respiratory, digestive, genitourinary, and cardiovascular systems.

The posterior cleft larynx is treated with a feeding gastrostomy. Tracheostomy is reserved for those individuals who aspirate their oral secretions. The more extensive laryngotracheoesophageal cleft requires prompt surgical repair. A lateral pharyngotomy may be employed,[30] with rotation of the larynx forward and repair of the cleft in the larynx and tracheoesophageal septum. Pillsbury and Fischer[28] stressed the importance of a two-layer staggered closure to resist the shearing force of vigorous crying in the infant. Burroughs and Leape[29] incorporated a portion of the esophagus into the trachea to strengthen the repair. An anterior approach to the defect by laryngofissure, cricoidotomy, and median section of the upper trachea also has been employed successfully.[31] More extensive clefts may also require a thoracotomy. Burroughs and Leape[29] estimated that only 8 of 16 operated patients survived, 2 of whom required secondary reconstruction. All required tracheostomy for one to four years.

ATRESIA OF THE LARYNX

Congenital laryngeal atresia is characterized by complete absence of the laryngeal lumen. Review of the literature by Cohen[32] revealed only 26 reported cases, of which only 4 were not associated with other severe anomalies and only 2 survived the neonatal period. Holinger and Brown[2] reported a single case among 866 laryngeal lesions. Fox and Cocker[33] found 1 case in 50,000 births. They classified 16 cases reported into three groups. In group A (2 cases), laryngeal atresia was associated with numerous unrelated congenital abnormalities; group B (4 cases) had deformities of the trachea and esophagus; and in group C (10 cases), the laryngeal atresia was the only congenital anomaly or was accompanied by only a simple cardiac or intestinal anomaly. After analyzing 9 cases, Smith and Bain[34] classified the defect anatomically into three groups: type I showed combined supraglottic and subglottic atresia; type II was only subglottic; and type III was only glottic.

Clinically, fetal distress is not evident; however, upon the clamping of the umbilical cord, cyanosis and severe respiratory distress with marked retractions appear, without stridor or an audible cry. The vigorous attempts at respiration, accompanied by progressive cyanosis, may be confused with central nervous system, cardiac, or pulmonary disease. The fatal nature of this malformation requires that it be recognized immediately. The infant will survive less than 20 min if tracheostomy is not performed. Endotracheal intubation will be unsuccessful. Direct laryngoscopy is diagnostic of this condition. Findings depend on the type of atresia present. A lumen may be totally absent or a dimple representing the pharyngotracheal duct may be present.

Tracheostomy is mandatory for survival because the nature of the atresia prohibits insertion of an endotracheal tube or perforation with a bronchoscope. Cohen[32] reported a case with endolaryngeal correction accomplished with biting forceps and the insertion of a Silastic tube.

SUBGLOTTIC HEMANGIOMA

Congenital vascular malformations of the larynx may occur as isolated defects, but they arise in association with cutaneous tumors in an estimated 25 per cent to 50 per cent of the patients. In the infant larynx, this defect presents as a sessile, smooth, soft, compressible subglottic mass and is uncommonly bluish or discolored. The presenting features, airway obstruction and stridor, may be exacerbated by vascular engorgement from crying or respiratory infection. Subglottic hemangioma is the prime diagnostic possibility in any infant with respiratory distress and a vascular skin lesion; it must also be considered in the differential diagnosis of recurrent croup. Onset occurs generally within the first days, weeks, or months of life depending on the size of the lesion, with most infants requiring tracheostomy for the marked airway obstruction. Fearon and Ellis[3] reported that 9 of 15, Holinger and Brown[2] 12 of 13, and Benjamin[35] 10 of 11 infants with subglottic hemangioma required tracheostomy.

Ferguson and Flake[36] reviewed 24 published cases and 17 cases of their own. They found a female preponderance of 2:1. About 90 per cent of the cases were diagnosed in the first six months of life. Usually unilateral, the lesion may extend to involve the opposite side. It characteristically involves the subglottic region from just below the true cord down to the cricoid cartilage but, in rare instances, may extend onto the true cord[36] or into the trachea.[37] Holinger and Brown[2] also reported 6 cavernous hemangiomas of the larynx at other sites: 3 on the arytenoid, 1 on the false cord, and 2 on the aryepiglottic fold and lateral pharyngeal wall.

Soft tissue x-rays of the neck may reveal the tumor as a shadow in the subglottic space. A barium swallow may show an increased thickness of the wall between the esophagus and the airway. Direct laryngoscopy will show only a mass covered by a normal mucosa in the subglottis; this mass may shrink with application of topical phenylephrine hydrochloride (Neo-Synephrine) or with subcutaneous injection of epinephrine (Adrenalin).[38] Biopsy and needle aspiration will yield blood; however, this procedure is not generally performed because of the danger of hemorrhage into the airway.

Because hemangiomas tend to involute with age, treatment often consists of tracheostomy and observation, waiting for spontaneous regression to occur; however, some clinicians report rapid and complete regression with radiotherapy in doses as low as 300 to 500 rads[1, 6, 36] and advocate its use to eliminate the hazards and complications of long-term tracheostomy in infants. Radioactive gold grains have been inserted into the lesions to minimize irradiation of the thyroid with the attendant risk of inducing malignant change,[35, 39] but many workers will not risk the long-term effects of radiotherapy in a self-limiting lesion.[37, 40] Calcaterra[40] reported that histologic study of an autopsy specimen of an irradiated pediatric larynx with a subglottic hemangioma showed no significant effect of radiotherapy.

Sclerosing solutions have also been injected into these tumors but carry the risk of scarring and producing subglottic stenosis.[38] Other workers report excellent results using systemic steroids to induce regression of the lesion.[41] Cryosurgery has been employed with limited success.[42] Surgical excision through a laryngofissure has also been performed[43] but is not the generally accepted mode of therapy in the infant larynx.

OTHER TUMORS

Lymphangioma. The cystic hygroma or congenital lymphangioma, when extensive, may displace or encroach on the lumen of the larynx and trachea, producing airway obstruction that may require tracheostomy. Six of the 19 congenital vascular lesions in the series of Holinger and Brown[2] were laryngeal extensions of cystic hygromas. While surgical excision is the treatment of choice for these lesions, this may be technically difficult or virtually impossible with large tumors that extensively infiltrate the soft tissues of the neck.

Papilloma. While laryngeal papillomas generally appear between two and four years of age, rare cases have their onsets in the neonatal period. Most neonatal lesions are associated with maternal genital warts. As the tumor grows, hoarseness, crouplike cough, dyspnea, and wheezing develop. The lesions may achieve sufficient bulk to produce airway obstruction and cyanosis. They may also bleed and become secondarily infected, adding to the respiratory difficulty. While the papillomas often regress at puberty, they may persist into adult life. Although laryngeal papillomas are benign and neither invade the submucosal tissues nor metastasize, they may show extensive multicentric origin and be implanted in the trachea and even the bronchi.

Various therapeutic modalities employed with limited success include surgical excision, implant and beam radiotherapy, fulguration, escharotic agents, hormonal therapy, autogenous vaccines, ultrasound, cryosurgery, and laser therapy.[11, 44] Endoscopic removal must be done with extreme care to prevent mucosal erosions and implantation. Tracheostomy is reserved for cases with extensive papillomas with airway compromise that will require repeated procedures. Tracheostomy carries the danger of implantation of tumor farther into the tracheobronchial tree.

CONGENITAL WEBS

A web may traverse the larynx at any level. Webs are most commonly glottic, followed by subglottic and supraglottic webs. McHugh and Loch[45] reviewed 133 cases of which 75.2 per cent were glottic, 7.5 per cent subglottic, 1.5 per cent supraglottic, 3.7 per cent posterior, and 5.26 per cent completely atretic. In the series of 32 webs reported by Holinger and Brown,[2] 24 were glottic, 4 were subglottic, and 4 were supraglottic. Fearon and Ellis[3] described 9 laryngeal webs of which 3 were glottic and 6 were subglottic. Double webs involving the supraglottic and glottic areas have been reported but are extremely rare.[46]

Webs also vary in length and thickness. The typical glottic web appears as a thin, transparent U-shaped membrane covering the superior surface of the anterior two-thirds of the true vocal cords, ending at the vocal processes laterally, and arching toward the midline. Variants include an extremely thin membrane above the cords and actual fusion of the anterior half of the true cords. Abnormalities of the cricoid cartilage generally accompany subglottic webs. Supraglottic webs involve fusion of the false cords for varying distances backward from the anterior commissure. Clinically, the symptoms vary with the position and extent of the web. Since most are cordal, both the airway and phonation are impaired. In addition to stridor, a weak cry, hoarseness, and even aphonia may be encountered.

Treatment depends on the type of the laryngeal web. Thin webs should be incised endoscopically and dilated serially for two weeks until epithelialization has occurred to prevent re-formation. Thick webs that cannot be readily excised may respond to serial dilatation, generally after tracheostomy; however, they may require lysis and the placement of a keel at the anterior commissure, which may be performed either externally or endoscopically. McNaught[47] describes an external approach that employs insertion of a tantalum keel through a median laryngofissure. In the closed method, a Silastic keel is inserted through a laryngoscope and maintained in position by external loop sutures passed through the thyrohyoid and cricothyroid membranes.[48]

CRI DU CHAT SYNDROME

LeJeune et al.[49] initially reported a condition in which infants had a weak, catlike cry. The glottic chink had a characteristic diamond-shaped appearance during inspiration on laryngoscopy, with deficient adduction posteriorly on phonation. The epiglottis was extremely long and flaccid. Respiratory obstruction with inspiratory stridor may be prominent at birth, presumably due to inward prolapse of the tubular epiglottis. As the child grows older, both the appearance of the larynx and the voice quality tend to become normal.[50]

Other associated congenital anomalies present in this syndrome include microcephaly, hypertelorism, myotonia, low-set ears, epicanthal folds, strabismus, midline oral clefts, severe mental retardation, and birdlike facies. An increased incidence occurs in females. Chromosome studies have revealed a partial deletion of the short arm of the fifth chromosome.[49]

RARE ANOMALIES

Bifid Epiglottis. In this rare condition, the epiglottis is generally cleft to just above the tubercle. The two portions are well supported and, while respiratory obstruction is generally absent, aspiration may be present. Healy et al.[51] accepted only 7 of the 18 reported cases as true examples of this defect. Other laryngeal anomalies that had been reported with this condition include subglottic stenosis and multiple laryngeal cysts. In 44 per cent of the cases, polydactyly was also present.[4]

Absent Epiglottis. Absent epiglottis is the rarest laryngeal anomaly. Only two cases have been reported, both of which had severe subglottic stenosis.[2]

Cricoid Arch Abnormalities. Holinger and Brown[2] reported three cases in which a cartilaginous plate filled the inner aspect of the cricoid cartilage, leaving only a small posterior opening. These patients all required tracheostomy.

Duplication of the Cords. Duplication of the cords is a rare anomaly consisting of the presence of an accessory vocal fold below the normal glottis. Holinger and Brown[2] mention it as a cause of hoarseness.

TRACHEOSTOMY IN INFANCY

In the pediatric population, the otolaryngologist often encounters airway obstruction requiring tracheostomy some time during the clinical course of the disease. The operative technique, complications, and decannulation present special problems in this age group.

Various factors including prematurity, congenital disorders, neurologic diseases, and infectious and inflammatory conditions may produce airway obstruction in early life. Markus et al.[52] reported that 48 of 153 infants younger than one year of age who required tracheostomy had congenital anomalies of the respiratory tract. These anomalies included laryngeal web and stenosis (15), vocal cord paralysis (24), laryngomalacia (4), and miscellaneous anomalies (5). Parkin et al.[53] reported only 3 cases of congenital subglottic stenosis among 603 patients in a newborn intensive care unit. Most of the infants were premature and had respiratory distress syndrome or significant cardiovascular disease. Cohen et al.[8] found that 30 of 124 neonates undergoing endoscopy required tracheostomy. Indications for tracheostomy in their series included vocal cord paralysis (13), laryngeal cyst (1), cystic hygroma (1), subglottic stenosis (4), tracheal stenosis (4), cleft larynx (1), bronchial suppuration (5), and aspiration pneumonia (1).

While a variety of inflammatory diseases can produce laryngeal stenosis,[54] at present, most cases are iatrogenic. Although endotracheal intubation has been recommended as a substitute for tracheostomy for acute airway obstruction, prolonged intubation, especially with ventilatory assistance by a respirator, can produce significant damage to the supraglottic, glottic, and subglottic larynx and trachea. The mechanisms of injury are mucosal ulceration by pressure, secondary infection with the development of chondritis and granulations, and cicatrization. Opinions differ as to how long intubation can be safely maintained before tracheostomy should be performed; different authors report widely disparate findings. Fearon et al.[55] reported laryngeal stenosis in 7 of the 29 survivors in a series of 72 infants undergoing prolonged endotracheal intubation. In another study, Fearon et al.[10] found that 16 of 20 patients with acquired subglottic stenosis had been intubated less than 6 days (mean 4.8 days), all with polyvinyl chloride tubes having an average diameter of 3.8 mm. Allen and Steven[56] had no instance of tracheal stenosis among their last 200 intubated infants and children, while employing a narrow tube and giving careful postoperative care. In infants with neurologic disease and congenital laryngeal disorders who expectedly require prolonged airway cannulation, tracheostomy should be performed immediately. Parkin et al.[53] reported the incidence of subglottic stenosis to be twice as great in intubated newborn patients with respiratory distress.

Technique of Tracheostomy. Wherever possible, tracheostomy in children should be performed over an endotracheal tube or bronchoscope to eliminate the problems and morbidity accompanying the emergency tracheostomy. A vertical incision should be made through the third and fourth tracheal rings, generally with a small horizontal incision at the upper end. Incisions made above the second tracheal ring are often accompanied by prolonged subglottic edema, which increases the duration of cannulation. Fearon and Ellis[3] recommended that the younger the patient, the farther from the cricoid the tracheal incision be made—even as low as the sixth or seventh ring. Silk traction sutures are placed in either side of the tracheal incision to facilitate tube placement at the time of surgery and postoperatively, as well as to serve as a guide to the trachea in the event of accidental decannulation. A Silastic or metal tracheostomy tube is placed, its size depending on the age of the infant (Table 11–3). The tube should be changed daily for the first week. Some authors advocate performing the first tracheostomy change in the operating room. Silastic tubes have the advantage over metal tubes of being more flexible; they have a universal adapter for attachment to a respirator, and have a larger lumen. They have, however, the disadvantage of being a monoluminal tube and present more difficulty in thorough cleaning.

The patient should be moved postoperatively to a surgical intensive care unit. Humidification should be delivered by a collar or tent and frequent and careful suctioning should be performed. A chest x-ray should be performed to detect the presence of pneumothorax or pneumomediastinum and to verify the position of the tracheostomy tube above the carina.

Table 11–3. RECOMMENDED PEDIATRIC TRACHEOTOMY TUBE SIZE AND BRONCHOSCOPE SIZE*

Age	Holinger Tracheotomy Tube Size (mm)	Bronchoscope Size (mm)
Premature—under 4 lb	000 × 26	
Premature—over 4 lb	00 × 26–33	3
0–6 months	0 × 33–40	3.5
6–12 months	1 × 40–46	
12–18 months	1 × 46	4
18 months to 4 or 5 years	1–2 × 46–50	
4 or 5 to 10 years	2–3 × 50–55	5
10 years	3–5 × 50–68	6

*From Fearon B, Ellis D: Ann Otol Rhinol Laryngol 80:670, 1971.

Decannulation. Decannulation should be performed as soon as possible to eliminate the complications of the prolonged presence of an intraluminal tube and so as not to interfere with laryngotracheal growth and development.[57] Decannulation should be attempted only in an operating room after direct endoscopic examination to determine the patency of the airway. Some clinicians advocate administering systemic steroids prior to and following decannulation to minimize laryngotracheal edema.[53] Racemic epinephrine has also been employed by nebulization to reduce edema.[53, 58] Endotracheal intubation has been used posttracheostomy to temporarily stent the airway.[59] Because of the ability of children to breathe relatively well through a narrowed lumen until a respiratory infection occurs, Fearon et al.[10] placed a small obturator in the tracheostoma for three months before total decannulation of patients with subglottic stenosis.

Complications of Tracheostomy. The surgeon should be careful to avoid injuring a bulging pleural apex, especially in the intubated patient with ventilatory assistance. The unusually high innominate artery adds a serious risk. To prevent fistula formation, care must be taken during the actual tracheal fenestration not to injure the membranous posterior tracheal wall. Immediate postoperative complications include subcutaneous and mediastinum emphysema, pneumothorax, and pneumomediastinum. Late postoperative complications include delayed decannulation and permanent airway stenosis. The interval of cannulation is related to the nature of the underlying disease. While patients with inflammatory lesions such as acute laryngotracheobronchitis are generally decannulated in two to three weeks, those with congenital abnormalities and neurologic disorders often wear tubes for one to two years.[52] Some patients, however, will develop tracheomalacia with bulging of the anterior wall of the trachea inward, which may require endoscopic dilatation or the placement of a nasal endotracheal tube to push the softened segment outward.[60] Where extensive granulations develop at the stoma, single or repeated endoscopic removals may be necessary. Occasionally, a persistent tracheocutaneous fistula will develop and require closure. A small but significant number of patients will also acquire subglottic stenosis that will require operative correction as outlined in the chapter on management of acquired laryngeal stenosis.

Additionally, there is a significant mortality in tracheostomized infants. Markus et al.[52] reported a 50 per cent mortality (77 cases in a series of 153 tracheostomized infants). The majority of deaths were related to the underlying systemic pathology; however, in 7 cases, death could be attributed to the tracheostomy, principally through plugging of the tube. Fearon and Cotton[14] had a 25 per cent mortality among 25 children with subglottic stenosis having a tracheostomy in position.

References

1. Fearon B: Respiratory distress in the newborn. Otolaryngol Clin North Am 1:147–169, 1968.
2. Holinger PH, Brown WT: Congenital webs, cysts, laryngoceles and other anomalies of the larynx. Ann Otol Rhinol Laryngol 76:744–752, 1967.
3. Fearon B, Ellis D: The management of long-term airway problems in infants and children. Ann Otol Rhinol Laryngol 80:669–677, 1971.
4. Tucker JA et al.: Clinical correlation of anomalies of the supraglottic larynx with the staged sequence of normal human laryngeal development. Ann Otol Rhinol Laryngol 87:636–644, 1978.
5. Kelemen G: Congenital laryngeal stridor. Arch Otolaryngol 58:245–268, 1953.
6. Ferguson CF: Congenital abnormalities of the infant larynx. Otolaryngol Clin North Am 2:185–200, 1970.
7. Holinger PH: Clinical aspects of congenital anomalies of the larynx, trachea, bronchi, and oesophagus. J Laryngol Otol 75:1–44, 1961.
8. Cohen SR et al.: Endoscopy and tracheostomy in the neonatal period: A 10-year review. Ann Otol Rhinol Laryngol 86:577–583, 1977.
9. Holinger PH et al.: Subglottic stenosis in infants and children. Ann Otol Rhinol Laryngol 85:591–599, 1976.
10. Fearon B et al.: Subglottic stenosis of the larynx in the infant and child: Methods of management. Ann Otol Rhinol Laryngol 87:645–648, 1978.
11. Holinger PH et al.: Laryngeal papilloma: Review of etiology and therapy. Laryngoscope 78:1462–1474, 1968.
12. Calcaterra TC et al.: Effect of laryngofissure on the developing canine larynx. Ann Otol Rhinol Laryngol 83:810–813, 1974.
13. Fearon B, Cotton R: Surgical correction of subglottic stenosis of the larynx: Preliminary report of an experimental surgical technique. Ann Otol Rhinol Laryngol 81:508–513, 1972.
14. Fearon B, Cotton R: Surgical correction of subglottic stenosis of the larynx in infants and children: Progress report. Ann Otol Rhinol Laryngol 83:428–431, 1974.
15. Cotton R: Management of subglottic stenosis in infancy and childhood: Review of a consecutive series of cases managed by surgical reconstruction. Ann Otol Rhinol Laryngol 87:649–657, 1978.
16. Grahne B: Operative treatment of severe chronic laryngeal stenosis in infants up to three years. Acta Otolaryngol 72:134–137, 1971.
17. Crysdale WS, Platt LJ: Division of posterior cricoid plate in young children with subglottic stenosis. Laryngoscope 86:1451–1458, 1976.
18. Evans JN, Todd GB: Laryngotracheoplasty. J Laryngol Otol 88:589–597, 1974.
19. Cavanaugh F: Vocal palsies in children. J Laryngol Otol 69:399–418, 1955.
20. Holinger LD et al.: Etiology of bilateral abductor vocal cord paralysis: A review of 389 cases. Ann Otol Rhinol Laryngol 85:428–436, 1976.
21. Bluestone CD et al.: Airway obstruction due to vocal cord paralysis in infants with hydrocephalus and meningomyelocele. Ann Otol Rhinol Laryngol 31: 778–783, 1972.
22. Gacek RR: Hereditary abductor vocal cord paralysis. Ann Otol Rhinol Laryngol 85:90–93, 1976.
23. Plott D: Congenital laryngeal abductor paralysis due to nucleus ambiguus dysgenesis in three brothers. New Engl J Med 271:593–597, 1964.
24. Watters GV, Fitch N: Familial laryngeal abductor paralysis and psychomotor retardation. Clin Genet 4:429–433, 1973.
25. Holinger LD et al.: Laryngocele and saccular cysts. Ann Otol Rhinol Laryngol 87:675–685, 1978.
26. DeSanto L et al.: Cysts of the larynx: Classification. Laryngoscope 80:145–176, 1970.
27. Cohen SR: Cleft larynx: A report of seven cases. Ann Otol Rhinol Laryngol 84:747–756, 1975.
28. Pillsbury HC, Fischer ND: Laryngotracheoesophageal cleft: Diagnosis, management, and presentation of a new diagnostic device. Arch Otolaryngol 103: 735–737, 1977.
29. Burroughs N, Leape LL: Laryngotracheoesophageal cleft: Report of a case successfully treated and review of the literature. Pediatrics 53:516–522, 1974.
30. Shapiro MJ, Falla A: Congenital posterior cleft larynx. Ann Otol Rhinol Laryngol 75:961–967, 1966.
31. Bell DW et al.: Laryngotracheoesophageal cleft: The anterior approach. Ann Otol Rhinol Laryngol 86:616–622, 1977.
32. Cohen SR: Congenital atresia of the larynx with endolaryngeal surgical correction: A case report. Laryngoscope 81:1607–1615, 1971.
33. Fox H, Cocker J: Laryngeal atresia. Arch Dis Child 39:641–645, 1964.
34. Smith II, Bain AD: Congenital atresia of the larynx. Ann Otol Rhinol Laryngol 74:338–349, 1965.
35. Benjamin B: Treatment of infantile subglottic hemangioma with radioactive gold grain. Ann Otol Rhinol Laryngol 87:18–21, 1978.
36. Ferguson CF, Flake CG: Subglottic hemangioma as a cause of respiratory obstruction in infants. Ann Otol Rhinol Laryngol 70:1095–1112, 1961.
37. Feuerstein SS: Subglottic hemangioma in infants. Laryngoscope 83:467–475, 1973.
38. Pierce MK: Subglottic hemangiomas in infants: A presumption clinical test for diagnosis. Ann Otol Rhinol Laryngol 71:1057–1062, 1962.
39. Holborow CA, Mott TJ: Subglottic hemangioma in infancy. J Laryngol Otol 87:1013–1017, 1973.
40. Calcaterra TC: An evaluation of the treatment of subglottic hemangioma. Laryngoscope 78:1956–1964, 1968.
41. Cohen SR, Wang CI: Steroid treatment of hemangioma of the head and neck in children. Ann Otol Rhinol Laryngol 81:584–590, 1972.
42. Schechter G, Biller HF: The limitations of corticosteroids and cryotherapy for subglottic hemangioma. Trans Am Acad Ophthalmol Otolaryngol 76: 1360–1362, 1972.

43. Mawson S: Subglottic hemangioma of the larynx treated by excision. J Laryngol Otol 757:1076–1081, 1961.
44. Singleton GT, Adkins WY: Cryosurgical treatment of juvenile laryngeal papillomatosis: An eight year experience. Ann Otol Rhinol Laryngol 81:784–790, 1972.
45. McHugh H, Loch J: Congenital webs of the larynx. Laryngoscope 52:43–65, 1942.
46. Holinger LD et al.: Simultaneous glottic and supraglottic laryngeal webs. Arch Otolaryngol 101: 496–497, 1975.
47. McNaught RC: Surgical correction of anterior web of the larynx. Laryngoscope 60:264–272, 1950.
48. Hardingham M, Walsh-Waring GP: The treatment of a congenital laryngeal web. J Laryngol Otol 89:273–279, 1975.
49. LeJeune J, LaFourcade J, Berger R: Trois cas de deletion partielle du bras court d'un chromosome 5. CR Acad Sci (Paris) 257:3098–3102, 1963.
50. Ward PH et al.: The larynx in the cri du chat (cat cry) syndrome. Trans Am Acad Ophthalmol Otolaryngol 72:90–102, 1968.
51. Healy GB et al.: Bifid epiglottis: A rare laryngeal anomaly. Laryngoscope 86:1459–1468, 1976.
52. Markus NJ et al.: Tracheostomy in the first year of life. Trans Am Acad Ophthalmol Otolaryngol 82:466–477, 1976.
53. Parkin JL et al.: Acquired and congenital subglottic stenosis in the infant. Ann Otol Rhinol Laryngol 85:573–581, 1976.
54. Baker DC: Chronic laryngeal stenosis. Ann Otol Rhinol Laryngol 78:751–756, 1969.
55. Fearon B et al.: Airway problems in children following prolonged endotracheal intubation. Ann Otol Rhinol Laryngol 75:975–986, 1966.
56. Allen TH, Steven IM: Prolonged nasotracheal intubation in infants and children. Br J Anaesth 44:835–840, 1972.
57. Freeland AP et al.: Developmental influences of infant tracheostomy. J Laryngol Otol 88:927–936, 1974.
58. Jordan WS et al.: New therapy for postintubation laryngeal edema and tracheitis in children. JAMA 212:585–588, 1970.
59. Greenberg LM et al.: Method for difficult decannulations in children. Arch Otolaryngol 81:72–76, 1965.
60. Crysdale WS: Nasotracheal intubation in management of delayed decannulation. Ann Otol Rhinol Laryngol 83:802–809, 1974.

12

Pediatric Laryngology

John K. Jones, M.D.

ANATOMY

The larynx of the neonate differs from that of the older child and adult in a number of practical ways. It is obviously a smaller structure and affords a relatively even smaller airway. In the infant, the larynx is located higher in the neck. The epiglottis lies opposite the body of the first cervical vertebra and the cricoid is at the level of the fourth cervical vertebra. The larynx gradually descends in the neck during childhood. By age six years, the cricoid lies opposite the fifth cervical vertebra. By the age of 12 to 13 years, the cricoid has finally achieved its adult level opposite the sixth cervical vertebra.[1] The larynx of the fetus is cephalic to the hyoid arch. At birth, the hyoid cartilage is close to the thyroid cartilage; in the adult, the hyoid is considerably superior to the thyroid cartilage. The cricoid cartilage is closely related to the lower border of the thyroid cartilage; thus, the cricoid membrane is very short and does not offer such easy access to the airway as in the adult. The cartilaginous skeleton in the neonate is softer and gives less support to the mucosa and musculature of the larynx. In the infant, the epiglottis is generally more tubular and relatively longer than in the adult. The aryepiglottic folds are, therefore, closer to the midline and the supraglottic area of the larynx takes on a funnel shape. The glottis is tilted downward and anteriorly and is protected from the endoscopist's view by the base of the tongue and the epiglottis. The epithelium and connective tissue are more loosely attached in the infant's larynx, allowing edema to spread more easily. Because of this and the smallness of the lumen, the infant's airway is more easily compromised.

Holinger[2] described the glottis of the newborn as having an anteroposterior dimension of 7 mm with a 4 mm posterior transverse dimension. Tucker,[3] in 1932, published his measurements of the subglottic diameter as being 6 mm in the normal larynx. In 1953, Wilson[4] noted a normal range from 4.5 to 5 mm. In 1972, Fearon and Cotton[5] determined from autopsy specimens that the normal intercartilaginous diameter was 5.5 mm and the normal intermucosal diameter was 4.5 mm.

Any swelling of the subglottic area can expand only into the lumen, to the detriment of the airway. Table 12–1 indicates the size of the laryngeal lumen as it applies to the passage of

Table 12–1. SUITABLE SIZE OF BRONCHOSCOPES TO PASS THROUGH LARYNX*

Age	Size (mm)
Premature—< 5 lb	3
0–6 months	3–5
6 months–3 years	4
3 years–12 years	5
12 years and over	6

*From Fearon B, Ellis D: Ann Otol Rhinol Laryngol 80:669, 1971.

bronchoscopes at different ages. Fearon[6] has endoscopically measured the distance from the glottis to the carina as 5.7 cm at birth and 8.1 cm in the child of 12 to 18 months. The laryngeal airway grows steadily from birth to adult life. Freeland[7] measured the cricoid diameter by radiographic means in a group of children and found a growth rate of 0.5 mm per year. The diameter at 3 months was 6.3 mm, increasing to 12.5 mm at twelve years of age. Following this, rapid growth at puberty achieves the adult dimensions.

CLINICAL ASSESSMENT

Congenital anomalies and acquired diseases of the larynx generally manifest themselves by disturbing laryngeal function. The airway may be obstructed and produce stridor; the voice or cry may change. The protective sphincteric action may be altered and lead to choking spells during feeding. If the airway is obstructed, the physician must decide whether to take immediate action to relieve the obstruction or to take a more deliberate approach. The physician should inquire into the circumstances surrounding the onset of symptoms. Congenital lesions such as laryngomalacia, subglottic stenosis, and paralysis of the vocal cords will become evident at birth or in the first few months of life. Infective laryngitis may appear gradually after the onset of a cold, as in croup, or more rapidly and severely, as in epiglottitis. A foreign body should be suspected when the onset of respiratory obstruction is sudden.

The child who has severe respiratory obstruction should be moved as little as possible. Any clothing covering the chest and neck should be removed. The nature of any stridor should be recorded. Inspiratory stridor is due to laryngeal obstruction, expiratory stridor emanates from the lower respiratory tract, and two-way stridor may be seen in tracheal or subglottic lesions. If the stridor has a wet, rough sound, it is more likely to be caused by a supraglottic obstruction, whereas dry and raspy stridor is more likely to come from a lesion at the glottic or subglottic region. The child's pulse, respiratory rate, and color should be noted and recorded. The distress of a child can be assessed by viewing the amount of supraclavicular, intercostal, and substernal indrawing as well as the degree of tracheal tug. If the respiration changes from a rapid marked inspiratory effort to a slow rate of breathing associated with cyanosis or pallor and increased tachypnea, the child is in imminent danger of asphyxiating. Immediate measures must be taken under these circumstances to relieve or bypass the obstruction.

The voice or cry of the child should be assessed, since this may indicate the underlying pathology. Does the child have a brassy cough as in croup, where the cords are held apart by the swelling in the subglottic region? Is the voice husky and breathy, as in papilloma of the glottic region? Is the cry weak, as in bilateral vocal cord paresis in the neonate?

The child with respiratory obstruction has considerable difficulty acquiring the successful coordination of pharyngeal and laryngeal musculature necessary for competent swallowing. Children who have a central cause for their vocal cord paralysis usually have an associated paralysis of the pharyngeal musculature. A laryngeal cleft is a much rarer cause of aspiration and a differential diagnosis must be made between that and tracheoesophageal fistula.

At this stage, the physician should suspect whether or not the larynx is involved in the child's respiratory distress. He also should try to clarify whether this is a congenital or an acquired lesion and whether there is a mechanical obstruction or the child has a neurologic etiology for the airway distress.

If the child's condition necessitates hospital admission, certain baseline observations are recorded: respiratory rate, presence or absence of indrawing of accessory respiratory muscles, presence or absence of cyanosis, pulse rate, temperature, and hydration of the patient. Specific investigations and treatments can then be instituted as the clinical situation dictates.

Specific examination of the larynx can be achieved by indirect or direct laryngoscopy. A cooperative four-year-old can be examined with a mirror. This involves a certain amount of reassurance by the physician and requires the presence of a nurse to steady the child's head. A No. 2 mirror is more easily accepted than the normal laryngeal mirror used on adults. The same technique is used as in adults. The tongue is protruded, and it is grasped by the examiner in a piece of gauze held by the thumb and middle finger. The child is told to push out his tongue and breathe through the mouth. The mirror is then introduced with confidence and the larynx visualized. Anesthetic sprays are not liked by children. The flexible fiberoptic laryngoscope has become very valuable for examination of the larynx in both infants and older children. The flexible laryngoscope should be used with caution in children who have compromised airways. Laryngospasm is a hazard in such cases. The infant is immobilized, and the instrument can be introduced without local anesthetic. I prefer to use a pledget of cotton soaked in cocaine and then wrung out. The cocaine pledget is placed in the nasal cavity with the child in the reclining position. Ten minutes later it is removed, and the flexible laryngoscope is passed through the nose and nasopharynx into the oropharynx and hypopharynx. At this stage, a view of the larynx is obtained. The supraglottis and glottis are seen very well, but the subglottic larynx is not as well visualized. The great advantage of the flexible laryngoscope is that it shows the larynx without any distortion of anatomy caused by the instrument, allowing accurate assessment of the movement of the larynx.

Plain x-rays of the neck are generally useful in assessment of the pediatric airway; however, their value in supraglottitis should be measured against the dangers of the child obstructing in an area where resuscitative measures are not at hand. This will be considered further in the discussion of epiglottitis. If an x-ray is indicated, it is essential that the child be in the correct position with head and neck extended. This straightens the larynx and trachea. If this is not done, the trachea may appear to be pushed away from midline by the aorta and the retropharyngeal tissue may give the erroneous

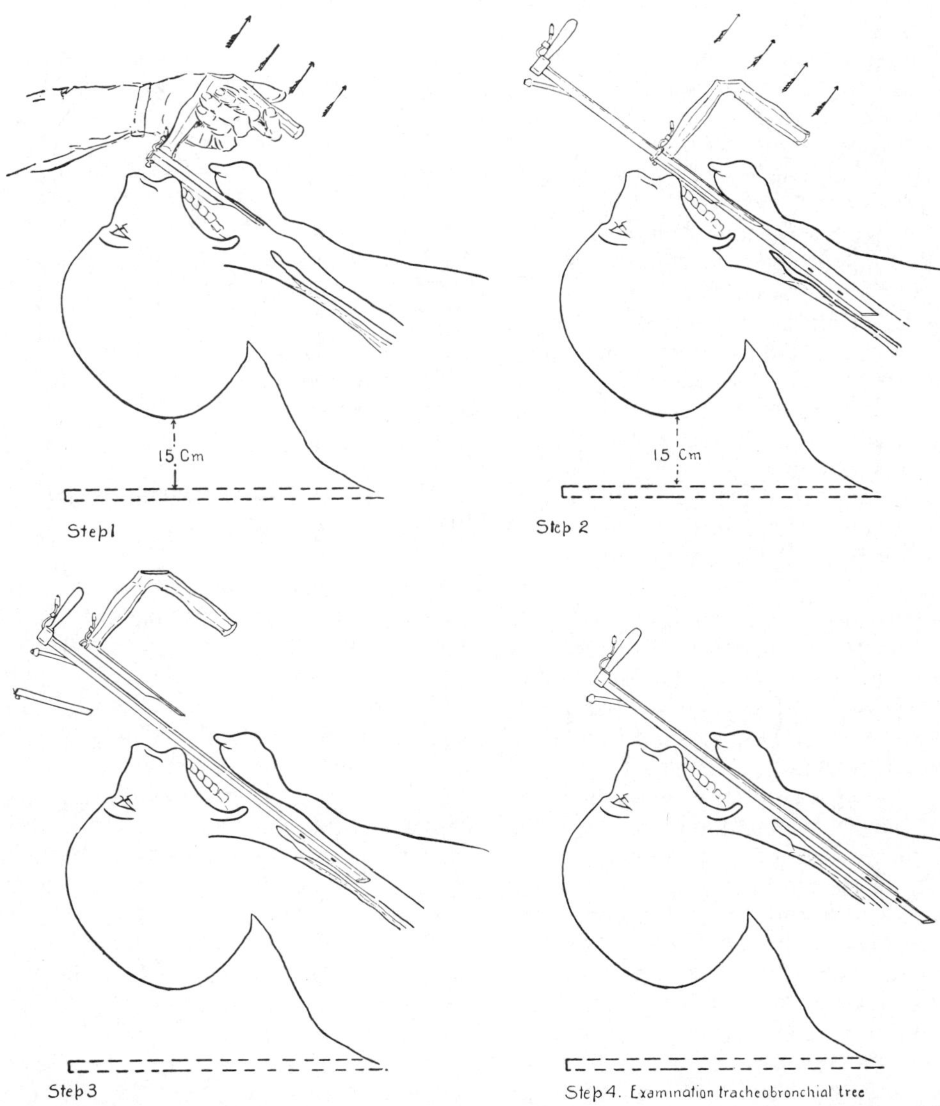

Figure 12–1. Technique of introduction of bronchoscope through the laryngoscope; *arrows,* direction of lifting the head. (From Jackson C, Jackson CL: Bronchoesophagology. Philadelphia, WB Saunders Company, 1950, p 1237.)

impression of being swollen as in a retropharyngeal abscess.

Fluoroscopy is useful in observing the movement of the larynx. Some pediatric radiologists state that they can recognize vocal cord paralysis with this technique. Contrast studies are useful in demonstrating a laryngeal cleft or tracheoesophageal fistula. They also show evidence of an anomalous course of the innominate artery or a vascular ring. These latter conditions can then be verified by arteriography. Some departments use xerograms, which give a high resolution of soft tissue but have the disadvantage of exposing the child to higher levels of irradiation.

Examination of the larynx by a rigid endoscope is best achieved using general anesthesia. The Holinger and Jackson laryngoscopes are ideally suited for the neonate, infant, and small child. The anterior commissure laryngoscope provides a way to accurately assess the subglottic region. The Hopkins telescope can be passed through the laryngoscope to view the subglottic area and trachea. This instrument provides magnification and excellent illumination. The tracheoesophageal septum is seen well with this instrument and should not be confused with a hemangioma. The Jackson slide laryngoscope provides a general view of the hypopharynx and larynx. It also facilitates the passage of a bronchoscope (Fig. 12–1). The Jako and Dedo laryngoscopes provide a binocular view of the larynx. The advantage of binocular vision is, of course, lost if the examiner does not keep his eye more than 18 inches from the instrument. Microsurgical techniques and laser surgery are best done with these laryngoscopes.

The standard anesthetic technique used at our institution consists of a period of preoxygenation and face mask induction. Muscle relaxants are not used unless an airway has been secured, as with an already existing tracheostomy. Although techniques of introducing the instrument vary, the technique described by Jackson (Fig. 12–2) is recommended. The procedure should be carried out carefully, and tissue should be treated gently. Excessive suction is avoided. Instruments of the appropriate size must be used. Iatrogenic edema of the subglottic area will lead to a compromised airway and should be prevented by taking the above precautions and avoiding unnecessary prolonged instrumentation. Following the procedure, the surgeon should be satisfied with the adequacy of the airway. Humidification, racemic epinephrine nebulizers, and dexamethasone (Decadron) are all useful in postoperative management.

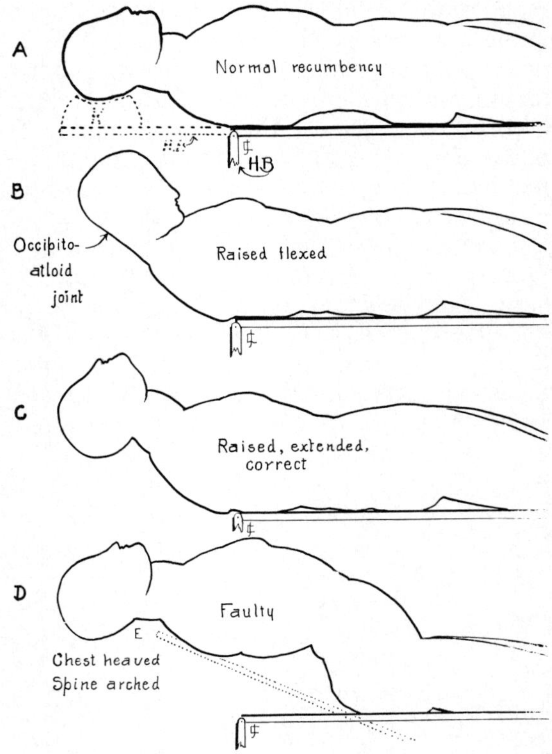

Figure 12–2. Positions for laryngoscopy or bronchoscopy. C, best position. (From Jackson C, Jackson CL: Bronchoesophagology. Philadelphia, WB Saunders Company, 1950, p 1236.)

CONGENITAL DISORDERS OF THE PEDIATRIC LARYNX

Laryngomalacia. Laryngomalacia is the most common congenital cause of stridor in infants.[8] Anatomically, this is an infantile larynx, representing delayed development of the larynx with no softening process of the laryngeal cartilages. The larynx has a floppy cartilaginous support and loosely attached soft tissues, which are thought to collapse inward with inspiration and create a stridulous sound. The stridor is inspiratory and usually is present at birth or soon after. It is typically worse when the head is flexed and improves when the head is extended and the mandible held forward. It may be brought on by agitation with rapid breathing and by decrease in muscle tone during sleep. The obstruction created is seldom severe. Each patient should have a diagnostic direct laryngoscopy. The epiglottis may have an omega or spatula shape when seen at direct laryngoscopy. It is important to remember that there may be other concomitant abnormalities of the airway. Thus, a tracheoscopy and bronchoscopy are indicated. Supportive treatment is provided to the patient and parents. The child normally will be expected to outgrow this condition and a tracheostomy is rarely necessary.

Congenital Subglottic Stenosis. Congenital subglottic stenosis, the most common cause of severe respiratory obstruction, ranks as the third most common congenital laryngeal anomaly following laryngomalacia and vocal cord paralysis.[8] It results from incomplete canalization of the airway at the level of the sixth branchial arch. The stenosis can vary in severity and is usually seen as a circumferential swelling, which is maximal 2 to 3 mm below the superior border of the vocal cords. Occasionally it is seen as an anterior and posterior bulge or anteroposterior slit. The child with subglottic stenosis usually presents immediately at birth with stridor and airway obstruction, which are more evident when the child is stressed. Some children, however, do not have symptoms until a few months later. This late presentation may develop gradually over a period of months. One explanation suggests that the child's physique and activity increase disproportionately to the stenosed larynx, which cannot cope with the demand for increased passage of air.[9] Respiratory infections will exacerbate the symptoms and also reveal a previously unsuspected stenosis. The child who has an abnormally prolonged bout of croup or recurrent episodes of croup should be investigated for subglottic stenosis. In the latter situation, the sum of the edema accompanying the infection and the asymptomatic anatomic narrowing causes sufficient obstruction to compromise the airway. The dry, raspy stridor produced by subglottic stenosis has both inspiratory and expiratory components. In Paul Holinger's series of 115 patients with congenital subglottic stenosis, stridor was the initial symptom in 43 per cent and was accompanied by dyspnea, a barking cough, or hoarseness.[8] Prolonged or recurrent croup was the first indication of stenosis in 35 per cent of the patients in this series. Other symptoms were recurrent pneumonia, atelectasis, postextubation stridor, noisy breathing, and a hoarse cry.

Plain x-rays of the neck help to demonstrate the presence and length of the stenosis. More information can sometimes be gleaned from fluoroscopy. The definitive method of making the diagnosis is by direct laryngoscopy, at which time the subglottic area can be assessed very well with a Hopkins telescope; the length of the stenosis should be estimated and a differentiation of whether this is a cartilaginous stenosis or a soft tissue stenosis should be made. The likelihood of success in treating soft tissue stenosis using dilatation or endoscopic methods is much higher than that treating cartilaginous stenosis. Indications of a subglottic stenosis leading to airway embarrassment are a subglottic opening less than two-thirds of the diameter of the glottis[9] or an opening that will not easily allow the passage of a 3 mm Holinger bronchoscope (external dimensions 4 mm by 4.5 mm).[8] Caution should be exercised during instrumentation, since any trauma to the subglottic stenosis may be followed by swelling and obstruction that may precipitate a tracheostomy.

Treatment depends on the severity of the stenosis and reflects the fact that most children eventually outgrow the stenosis. Upper airway infection should be treated vigorously and a low humidity in the child's bedroom should be avoided. Forty-four per cent of the patients in Holinger's series required tracheostomy, maintained for an average of 18 months. Periodic laryngoscopy and initial dilatation are advocated during this period. Some surgeons also administer local injections of steroids following the dilatation. The shorter the stenosis is in length, the greater is the likelihood of success with this method. More recently, endoscopic laser excision of the subglottic stenosis has been advocated with reasonably good results. The advantage of this method is that tracheostomy is avoided.[10] It should be stressed that the expectation for this condition is usually quite different from that of an acquired subglottic stenosis.

Neurogenic Disorders. Paralysis of the vocal cords in the newborn may be bilateral or unilateral and complete or partial. Familial bilateral abductor paralysis has been described,[11, 12] but patients with this problem comprise a small minority of the total cases. Some patients have transient paralysis, which usually subsides within four to six weeks of birth.[1] This condition is thought to occur at birth as a result of trauma to the recurrent laryngeal nerve where it crosses the cricothyroid joint. Bilateral vocal cord paralysis is more common than unilateral. L. Holinger reviewed 389 cases of bilateral abductor vocal cord paralysis.[13] Eighty-two of these were congenital. Twenty-one of these were associated with a central neurologic disorder, eight with cardiac anomalies, ten with other laryngeal pathology, and four with miscellaneous other anomalies. Thirty-nine had no other associated anomalies and, in most of this group, the problem resolved spontaneously over a period of weeks or months. Patients with cerebral agenesis and cranial nerve palsies formed the majority of the group with central neurologic pathology. Ventral septal defect, coarctation of the aorta, and transposition of the ventricle were the most common thoracic causes. Subglottic stenosis was the most common concomitant laryngeal pathology.

Symptoms of cord paralysis vary from inspiratory stridor that is only present on exertion to persistent inspiratory stridor and marked respiratory obstruction. The cry sounds normal in the bilateral cord paralysis but may be diminished in volume. In the unilateral paralysis, the cry is commonly weak.

Because of the correlation with other pathology, children with vocal cord paralysis should be investigated for intrathoracic and intracranial pathology. Definitive diagnosis is made by viewing the cords when the patient is awake. This can best be done with a flexible laryngoscope. If the flexible laryngoscope is not tolerated, cord mobility can be assessed by direct laryngoscopy during examination of the remainder of the respiratory tract. Cord movement is assessed with a Jackson laryngoscope placed in the vallecula. Care should be taken not to reduce the mobility of the larynx by inadvertently placing the tip of the laryngoscope on either the false or true vocal cords. The passive movement of the cords can also be assessed. At the same procedure, the subglottic area of the larynx should be inspected for concomitant subglottic stenosis. In some patients, the arytenoids are observed to move, yet the membranous cords do not abduct. In the author's experience and from observations by others,[13] these patients tend to show resolution of their symptoms and develop full cord movement.

Patients with bilateral paralysis and respiratory obstruction will require a trachéostomy. Surgical attempts to give the patient a normal airway, whether by lateralization of the vocal cord, arytenoidectomy,[14] or a Tucker procedure, are delayed until just before the child reaches school age.

Laryngeal Web. In a series of 866 laryngeal abnormalities, Paul Holinger described 32 cases of laryngeal webs.[15] The majority (approximately 75 per cent) occurred at the level of the true vocal cords. About one-half of the remainder were supraglottic, the other half subglottic. The web formation results from failure of the lateral masses to dissolve, which usually occurs at about the tenth week of fetal life. The webs of the supraglottic level are usually seen as a fusion of the false cords. The subglottic webs are more frequently associated with cartilaginous deformities of the cricoid. Most glottic webs are membranous, extending posteriorly to the anterior extent of the vocal processes of the arytenoids. The extent of the involvement of the glottis may vary from a small anterior commissure web to the more common membranous web, which extends posteriorly as described above. In two cases in Holinger's series and one case treated by the author, the membranous vocal cords were fused. Symptoms usually appear at birth and vary according to the amount of occlusion of the airway and the mobility of the vocal cords. Stridor results from partial occlusion and the cry is weak. In some cases, the infant may be aphonic. Thin webs can be treated through the laryngoscope using sharp dissection, laser surgery, or laryngeal dilation. Tracheostomy is sometimes necessary. In cases where the web reforms or in the thicker web, a midline thyrotomy with insertion of a keel is indicated.

Atresia. Atresia implies complete obstruction of the larynx. It results from failure of canalization of the fetal larynx, a step that occurs at about the tenth week of embryologic development. The condition is incompatible with life. Ferguson refers to a case described by Jackson in which the completely obstructing membrane was perforated by a 3 mm bronchoscope.[1] Obviously, rapid identification of the cause of this obstructive respiratory failure is necessary and either perforation of the atresia or a tracheostomy must be performed immediately.

Cysts and Laryngoceles. Cysts and laryngoceles are rare causes of laryngeal symptoms in the infant. Laryngoceles are air-containing and communicate with the lumen, usually through the ventricle. In Holinger's series of twelve laryngoceles,[15] the sac was ventricular in five and extended posteriorly to the aryepiglottic fold. The symptoms of obstruction and interference with the voice vary with the size of the sac. A laryngocele can be diagnosed by x-ray. In the one case of a small laryngocele in the author's experience, the findings at laryngoscopy were normal, but a laryngocele can enlarge considerably to produce an obvious swelling in the larynx.

Cysts contain fluid and are more obvious, appearing as swellings of the larynx that may obliterate the normal anatomy. They often show prominent blood vessels crossing over their surface. The cysts are treated either by repeated aspiration or by marsupialization. Tracheostomy may be required to safeguard the airway. Another cyst that sometimes impacts on the larynx is a thyroglossal duct cyst; this cyst can present internally in the vallecula and push the epiglottis downward and posteriorly, causing occlusion of the larynx. The ensuing symptoms of obstruction are much more evident when the child is supine.

Laryngotracheoesophageal Cleft. Laryngotracheoesophageal cleft is a very rare condition that results from failure of the posterior plate of the cricoid to fuse. The posterior split in the larynx may extend inferiorly to a variable level of the trachea. The infant aspirates its own secretions as well as its food, giving rise to cyanotic attacks and aspiration pneumonia. Because the larynx is split posteriorly, the cry is weak. The defect in the laryngeal area can be repaired through a lateral pharyngotomy approach if it does not extend far inferiorly.

Cri du Chat Syndrome. LeJeune[16] in 1963 described a multiple congenital syndrome associated with the deletion of the short arm of chromosome 5 in the B group. The child typically has a cry that sounds like the meowing of a cat, microcephaly, micrognathia, antimongoloid epicanthic folds, hypertelorism, strabismus, and low-set ears. Midline oral clefts and a beaklike profile are features of the syndrome. Physical and mental development is retarded. Ward[17] described the laryngeal appearance as a diamond-shaped glottis. Adduction occurs in the anterior glottis but not in the posterior. The child loses the catlike cry as he becomes older.

Hemangioma. These vascular tumors of the larynx in infants are usually of the capillary type and are most commonly situated in the subglottic region. They predominate in females in a ratio of about 5:1. The natural history of the tumor involves enlargement during the first three months of life, by which time 90 per cent of the infants will have symptoms.[18] Approximately 50 per cent of laryngeal hemangiomas will be associated with hemangiomas of the skin and other organs.[19] Size continues to increase during the first six months of life, after which the cutaneous hemangiomas show spontaneous regression.[20] This regression is also sometimes seen in laryngeal tumors. The infant will present with biphasic stridor and dyspnea. A prolonged episode of apparent croup may be the presenting feature. The symptoms tend to fluctuate in character. The distress varies with excitement and aggravation. This last feature, which should cause the observer to strongly suspect the presence of a hemangioma, is thought to be caused by variation in size of the hemangioma following changes in venous pressure.[21]

The tumors can be demonstrated by soft tissue x-rays, fluoroscopy, and contrast studies. Definitive diagnosis is made by direct laryngoscopy. The tumor is seen in the posterior subglottic area and may extend to involve the lateral walls. It is easily compressed. The covering of mucosa and submucosa often obscures the tumor's vascularity.

Various modalities of treatment have been offered.[21] Healey[22] has described laser excision as a successful and safe means of treatment. Ferguson and Flake[23] advocated radiotherapy at a dosage of 200 to 500 rads. Benjamin has recorded success with radioactive gold grain implants[24]; however, this carries a risk of thyroid cancer following radiotherapy.[25] Another modality that has been used is steroids in a dose of 60 mg of prednisone per square meter of body surface area.[26] All of these therapies have been advocated in addition to protection of the airway by tracheostomy because death poses a real threat if the tumor increases in size. Because spontaneous regression is usually seen in these tumors, treatment other than tracheostomy to maintain a safe airway is not always necessary.

ACQUIRED DISORDERS OF THE LARYNX

Inflammatory Disease of the Larynx. Croup and epiglottitis are life-threatening inflammatory processes that involve the larynx. The term *croup* includes laryngotracheobronchitis, laryngotracheitis, and spasmodic croup. The inflammation involves the subglottic area. Epiglottitis, on the other hand, involves the supraglottic structures only and should more correctly be called supraglottitis. Laryngotracheobronchitis is the most common cause of acute laryngeal obstruction. Over a six-year period, 5,000 children were admitted to Sick Children's Hospital in Toronto with inflammatory disease of the larynx. Only 100 of the cases had confirmed supraglottitis.[27]

Croup. Laryngotracheobronchitis and laryngotracheitis occur predominantly in the age group between six months and three years old. Croup may occur throughout the year and is more common at times of increased viral respiratory infections. The most common etiologic agent is the type 1 parainfluenza virus. Respiratory syncytial virus, type 2 and 3 parainfluenza viruses, and influenza viruses are also important causes. Adenoviruses, rhinoviruses, and measles may infrequently cause croup. A bacterial tracheitis has been described,[28] involving the same anatomic areas as do the viral agents. The implicated bacteria are *Staphylococcus aureus,* group A streptococci, and *Haemophilus influenzae.* The clinical picture in bacterial croup is more severe than in the viral form, and the patient exhibits the same systemic manifestations as are seen in supraglottitis. Laryngotracheitis and laryngotracheobronchitis show an inflammatory process in the subglottic and tracheal areas. As the swelling increases, the airway decreases. This is particularly evident in the subglottic region. The airway becomes more compromised as a fibrinous exudate accumulates. This exudate is difficult for the child to clear. The symptoms of airway obstruction are gradual in onset and are usually preceded by symptoms of a cold. Hoarseness and a barking cough develop. As the subglottic edema develops, inspiratory and expiratory stridor can be heard. Intercostal, supraclavicular, and substernal indrawing occurs. The development of hypoxemia will produce restlessness, anxiety, tachypnea, and tachycardia well before cyanosis appears. A particularly dangerous situation may occur when exhaustion decreases the respiratory effort and, thus, the intensity of the stridor. The pulse rate continues to rise, but less air is being moved, as shown by quieter breath sounds. This quietness of the stridor may be misinterpreted as clinical improvement, but it is in fact the prelude to death and necessitates assisted respiration via an artificial airway. Examination of the larynx at this time shows a red, angry swelling in the subglottic area. Radiographs of the neck show a wine-bottle appearance of the trachea and subglottic area (Fig. 12–3). Croup may recur in up to 5 per cent of cases,[29] requiring a search for an underlying anatomic anomaly.

Spasmodic croup typically occurs at night and without a preceding infection. The child awakens with stridor, cough, and dyspnea. The symptoms usually settle rapidly. Exposure to humidified air, as in the shower or in the cold night air during the rush to the hospital, have resulted in resolution. The etiology is unknown and may be noninflammatory edema of the subglottic area.[30]

Supraglottitis. Supraglottitis occurs in a slightly older age group than does croup and is occasionally seen in adults. *Haemophilus influenzae* type b, the most common causative agent, can occur throughout the year and is particularly prevalent at times of increased hospital admission for respiratory infections.[29] Pres-

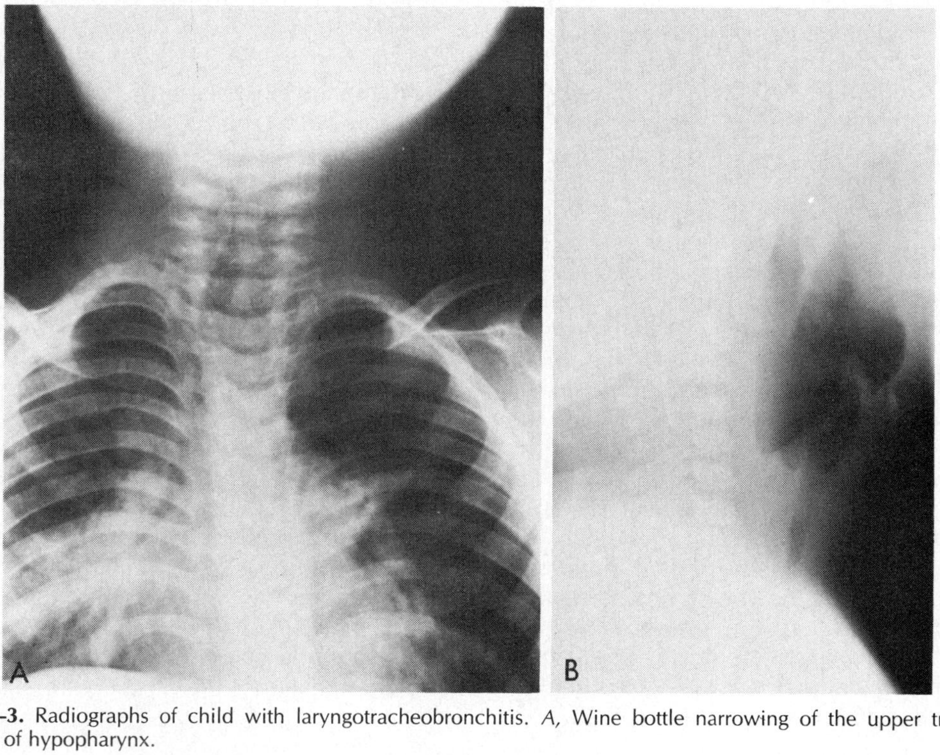

Figure 12–3. Radiographs of child with laryngotracheobronchitis. *A,* Wine bottle narrowing of the upper trachea. *B,* Distention of hypopharynx.

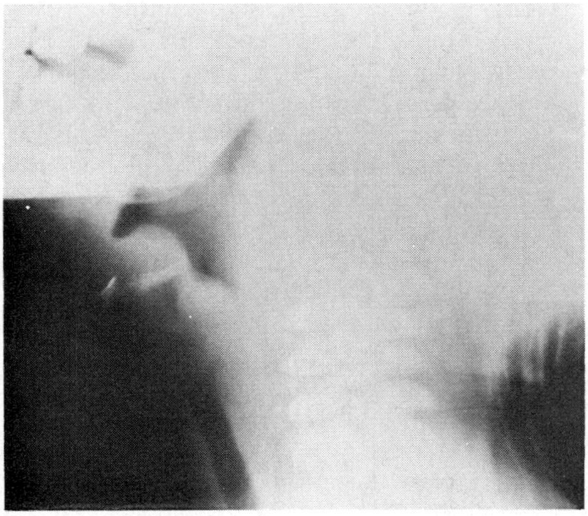

Figure 12–4. Epiglottitis showing swelling of the supraglottic structures.

entation is acute. In the early stage of the disease, inflammatory edema arises on the lingual surface of the epiglottis, later progressing to the ventricular bands, the aryepiglottic folds, and the mucosa over the arytenoids. The airway obstruction is proportionate to the amount of supraglottic swelling. Initially, the child will complain of a sore throat. Examination at this time is often unremarkable and, when seen at this stage, the child will often be treated for uncomplicated pharyngitis. The disease progresses rapidly over the next twelve hours, but severe obstruction may develop within only two to four hours. The child does not tolerate lying down and prefers to sit up, thrusting the chin upward and forward. He appears pale, toxic, and lethargic. The voice is muffled, a low-pitched stridor may be present, swallowing is difficult, and drooling will occur in the later stages. The barking cough of croup is absent. A fever is present together with tachycardia. Cervical adenopathy is marked. Examination of the throat reveals red swelling of the epiglottis and other supraglottic structures. Lateral radiographs reflect the pathology (Fig. 12–4). Sudden complete airway obstruction may occur, precipitated by movement, as by depressing the tongue with a tongue blade or by taking blood. The presence of means to achieve an emergency airway should be confirmed before performing any of the above maneuvers. Although the diagnosis of supraglottitis and croup may be clear, the two diseases are difficult to differentiate in some patients.

Conservative Management of Croup and Supraglottitis. Successful management of children with croup or with supraglottitis involves a planned team approach. Barker[29] discusses the rationale for various forms of treatment.

Most children with croup can be managed on an outpatient basis. If home care is to be instituted, the parents should be conscientious and reliable and they should live within a reasonable distance of the hospital. They are instructed to humidify the air using mist or steam. Approximately five to ten per cent of children with croup are admitted to the hospital because of significant airway obstruction.[31] Indications for hospitalization are either a significant problem in moving air or anxiety and restlessness that suggest hypoxemia.

As in the home, so in the hospital, where the child is usually more ill, disturbance must be kept to a minimum. The infant is nursed in a crib under nebulized oxygen mist. Hydration is usually achieved by oral feeding, but, if this is not possible, an intravenous line should be established. The child must be examined regularly and carefully. The drawing of blood for arterial blood gas levels is disturbing to the child and should be done only when absolutely necessary. An excellent correlation exists between rising pulse rate and respiratory rate with a falling arterial oxygen tension;[32] however, hypercapnia, which develops late, is difficult to determine clinically.

If the child does not respond well to humidification, the question of using corticosteroids and racemic epinephrine arises. The use of corticosteroids in treating laryngotracheobronchitis generates considerable controversy. Many clinical trials have been conducted that involve scoring the severity of the croup and using different dosage regimens. Despite these, the controversy still rages. At present, we have no evidence that a short course of steroids is harmful.[29] Leipzig[33] performed a double blind prospective study on 16 patients who received two doses of dexamethasone (0.3 mg per km intramuscularly) and 14 who received saline placebo. He demonstrated a more rapid improvement in the dexamethasone group, shown by the "croup score," number of administrations of racemic epinephrine, and length of hospital stay, and concluded that this drug could be used beneficially to treat croup. Cherry,[30] in his editorial, argued against this conclusion. Adair[34] showed a reduction of the tracheostomy rate to zero over a ten-year experience during which racemic epinephrine was applied with positive pressure breathing using a face mask. Racemic epinephrine is known to have a vasoconstrictive effect; however, we do not fully understand why the racemic form should be more effective than the l-isomer alone. This drug can be applied by intermittent positive pressure breathing or via a nebulizer. The action of assisted respiration may in itself aid the infant by opening up collapsed segments of the airway. Racemic epinephrine should not be used in children with tetralogy of Fallot because it may cause a sudden decrease in cardiac output by increasing the degree of outflow obstruction.[35]

When considering conservative management, remember that supraglottitis may cause a sudden respiratory arrest. Significant mortality accompanies this disease. Cantrell[36] reviewed 749 cases of epiglottitis, treated as follows: tracheostomy—348 (3 deaths, 0.8 per cent); endotracheal intubation—216 (2 deaths, 0.92 per cent); and medical management with no artificial airway—214 (13 deaths, 6.1 per cent). Cantrell concluded that an artificial airway should be used in all children with supraglottitis. Adults with supraglottitis can be treated without an artificial airway; however, in the author's personal experience, one adult male had a sudden respiratory arrest in the emergency room when his pharynx was being examined and an emergency tracheostomy was required. The team approach of otolaryngologist, anesthesiologist, and pediatrician is very important. If the diagnosis of supraglottitis is suspected, the child should be taken to the operating room as soon as possible. There the diagnosis can be made and an airway established. Only after this should blood studies and intravenous therapy be instituted. Lateral radiographs of the neck have been used to aid in the diagnosis. To send a child with supraglottitis out of an area where an airway can be rapidly secured is a dangerous practice.

The Artificial Airway in Croup and Supraglottitis. Prior to the 1960s, the preferred treatment for airway obstruction was tracheostomy. Allen and Steven[37] substantiated their earlier claims citing the efficacy and safety of nasotracheal intubation. Subsequently, the principle of using a smaller tube than would normally be used, together with gentle intubation, careful monitoring of movement of the tube, and hydration of the patient, has made this method acceptable in most institutions.

Indications for an artifical airway have been mentioned. Humidification and tracheal and bronchial toilet are important in the continued management. Because of the danger of subglottic stenosis in laryngotracheobronchitis, the tube should not be left in for a prolonged period. Tracheostomy should be performed if no resolution occurs after two days.

As has been discussed, supraglottitis in children is an absolute indication for an artificial airway, to be achieved preferably in the operating room. Facilities for intubation, bronchoscopy, and tracheostomy should be immediately available. In the hands of a skilled pediatric anesthesiologist, general anesthesia is usually safe and more humane than attempting to intubate an awake, struggling, and hypoxic patient. Anesthesia is induced using assisted ventilation via a face mask with halothane and oxygen.[29] The patient is allowed to remain sitting. If the patient is obstructed, the airway can usually be maintained by this method. Muscle relaxants and respiratory depressants should not be used. A laryngoscopy is then performed to confirm the diagnosis and an endotracheal tube is introduced. After the oral endotracheal tube has been passed, the anesthesia is deepened and the oral tube is replaced by a nasal tube, which is taped securely in place. If the tissues are so edematous and stiff as to prevent passage of an endotracheal tube, a rigid ventilating bronchoscope is introduced and a tracheostomy is performed. Now that the airway has been established, intravenous therapy is instituted and throat culture and blood cultures are taken. Because of the growing incidence of ampicillin-resistant *Haemophilus influenzae,* both ampicillin (200 to 400 mg per kg per day) and chloramphenicol (100 mg per kg per day) are used intravenously until antibiotic sensitivity test results are available; then, a full course of the appropriate antibiotic should be given.

The decision as to whether to treat with intubation or tracheostomy depends on the facilities and skills available in the individual institution. Constant nursing supervision to prevent blockage or extubation of the tracheal tube is required. A physician capable of reintubating the child must be available 24 hours a day. Accidental decannulation of a tracheostomy tube can be just as disastrous as decannulation of an endotracheal tube. In the case of laryngotracheobronchitis treated with an endotracheal tube, the tube will have compressed the subglottic edema, providing the child with a few minutes after accidental extubation before the airway becomes inadequate again. This is not so in decannulation of a tracheostomy, where the edema may still be considerable; however, the care of a tracheostomy is somewhat less demanding than that of an endotracheal tube and it appears advisable to opt for a tracheostomy if facilities and staff are not available.

Planned extubation can be performed when the swelling has subsided. This takes less time in epiglottitis (24 to 36 hours) than in croup (2 to 4 days). Resolution of fever, clear tracheal secretions, air leak around the endotracheal tube, absence of atelectasis, and observation via a laryngoscope are all determinates to the decision of when to extubate. After extubation, the child should be observed closely in case reintubation is required. He is nursed in a mist tent until the physician is satisfied with the condition of the airway.

Trauma. Internal trauma of the larynx is more common than external trauma in the pediatric age group. Since the practice of prolonged intubation has become more widespread, glottic and subglottic stenosis has increased. In Holinger's series[8] of 43 cases of acquired subglottic stenosis, endotracheal intubation accounted for 37 cases (86 per cent). The subglottic area is completely enclosed by the cricoid ring. Any swelling must encroach on the lumen of the airway. The tube causes irritation of the respiratory epithelium, resulting in inflammatory edema, ulceration, and infection followed by formation of granulation tissue. The inflammatory process may progress to involve the perichondrium of the cricoid and then the cricoid cartilage itself. The airway is thus compromised and the child has difficulty in moving air when the tube is removed. Scarring may then occur at the glottic and subglottic level with severe decrease in the cross-sectional area of the airway. Scarring in the glottic region is usually in the interarytenoid region where the tube has lain. In the subglottic area, scarring is usually circumferential with the predominant amount in the anterior part of the larynx. The effects of a 1 mm swelling in the neonate are severe. The airway will be reduced to 32 per cent of its former cross-sectional area.[8]

The factors in production of stenosis are related to the tube and to the host. Polyvinyl chloride tubes are the most acceptable at present; however, residue of ethylene oxide (used to sterilize them) has been shown to injure the mucosa.[38] The tube's size, introduction, number of times changed, and movement in the larynx are all factors. Cuffed tubes are not used in the young child; thus, the vocal cords must grip the tube to provide an airtight seal when a ventilator is used. This in itself is conducive to mucosal irritation, infection, and acquired stenosis. In the older age group, a cuffed tube may be used. The cuff should be placed in the trachea; placement in the glottic or subglottic region predisposes to stenosis.

The status and age of the host are considerations in deciding the length of time that the tube may be left in the airway. Prolonged intubation in neonates is commonly measured over a period of weeks, whereas in adults it is commonly measured in days. The laryngeal cartilages of neonates are more flexible than those in the older child. Hawkins[39] has shown that there is less territorial matrix in the neonate. This matrix gives the cartilage its rigidity; it increases as the child grows older. Local and systemic infection as well as local blood perfusion are factors to consider. Intubation in the treatment of inflammatory croup still gives rise to concern. In Cotton's series of 27 cases of acquired subglottic stenosis, published in 1978, 6 children had been intubated for treatment of croup.[40]

Acquired subglottic stenosis in children is a more severe problem than is congenital subglottic stenosis. In Holinger's series,[8] 97 per cent of the group with acquired stenosis required tracheostomy. A mortality rate of 11 per cent was ascribable to the tracheostomy in those patients.[8] Of the congenital group, 44 per cent required tracheostomy, and the mortality rate from the tracheostomy was 2.1 per cent. Fearon and Cotton found a mortality rate of 24 per cent in these patients treated with tracheostomy for acquired subglottic stenosis.[41]

Treatment of acquired subglottic stenosis starts with its prevention. Each patient should be treated individually. The factors discussed here should influence management of the airway. Unfortunately, subglottic stenosis still occurs, even with conscientious application of principles aimed at its avoidance. Initial assessment of a patient suspected of subglottic stenosis is achieved by x-ray and by direct inspection of the larynx, trachea, and mainstem bronchi to prevent the embarrassment of missing a secondary pathology lower in the airway. The CT scan is now providing useful information in this area. Extent of the stenosis and the degree of cartilaginous and soft tissue involvement must be assessed. As with congenital stenosis, these factors assist in the logical choice of treatment. If the degree of stenosis is sufficient to cause significant airway obstruction, a tracheostomy is performed at this stage. Various management regimens have been advanced for treatment of acquired subglottic stenosis. Traditionally, open surgical techniques have been avoided because of the unknown effect on the growth of the cartilage. Calcaterra demonstrated in dogs that a midline incision of the larynx, as in a laryngofissure, did not affect the growth, eventual weight, or size of the laryngeal lumen.[42]

Cotton and Seid[43] introduced the technique of the anterior cricoid split in an attempt to abort scarring in the subglottic region. This was initially applied to the neonate or infant who had edematous swelling of the subglottic region following intubation. The operation is quite simple and involves a vertical cut through the cricoid and upper two rings of the trachea. The incision is taken down to the indwelling endotracheal tube. This theoretically drains the edematous submucosal area and releases the cricoid, which in itself increases the lumen. Successful decannulation occurs two to three weeks later. The advantage of this procedure lies in the prevention of scarring and the avoidance of a tracheostomy.

Direct laryngoscopy and repeated dilatations have been used, with or without the injection of steriods. If the vertical extent of the stenosis is short, the dilatations are usually effective. If, however, the stenosis is more extensive, success with dilatations is less likely. Nonetheless, many patients have been treated successfully by this method.[8, 41] The laser has also been useful in treating the short, soft stenosis.[10]

An open surgical approach is indicated in children for whom repeated dilatations have shown no improvement in the airway. Children who have a long or particularly dense stenosis fall into this category. If the cricoid cartilage is abnormally thickened, dilatation is doomed to failure. The operation devised by Fearon and Cotton has been demonstrated successfully in numerous patients.[40, 44] This operation is particularly suited to situations where stenosis does not involve the vocal cords, the stenosis is long, or the cartilage of the anterior wall of the trachea and cricoid is deficient. A midline vertical incision is made from the cricoid to the lower extremity of the stenosis (Fig. 12–5). The scar is not removed. A beveled boatlike piece of rib cartilage is inserted into the defect, which is thus opened outward. The laryngotracheoplasty of Evans and Todd[45] also strives to expand the airway without removing the scar (Fig. 12–6). This operation can be used in both glottic and subglottic stenosis. The rings of the trachea and cricoid are cut horizontally and held apart by rolled Silastic sheeting. In situations where the posterior glottic and subglottic larynx are predominantly affected, Rethi's operation is used.[46] In this situation, the scar is excised and the cricoid is divided vertically in the midline , both anteriorly and posteriorly. A stent is then left in position.

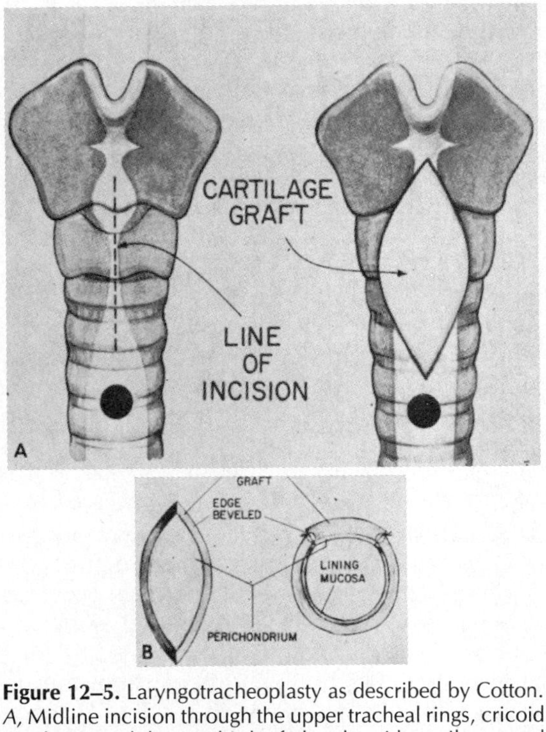

Figure 12–5. Laryngotracheoplasty as described by Cotton. *A*, Midline incision through the upper tracheal rings, cricoid cartilage, and lower third of the thyroid cartilage, and through the corresponding length of stenosis to enter lumen of airway. *B*, Details of fashioning graft, demonstrating extramucosal placement of 5-0 Prolene sutures. (From Cotton R: Ann Otol Rhinol Laryngol 87:652, 1978.)

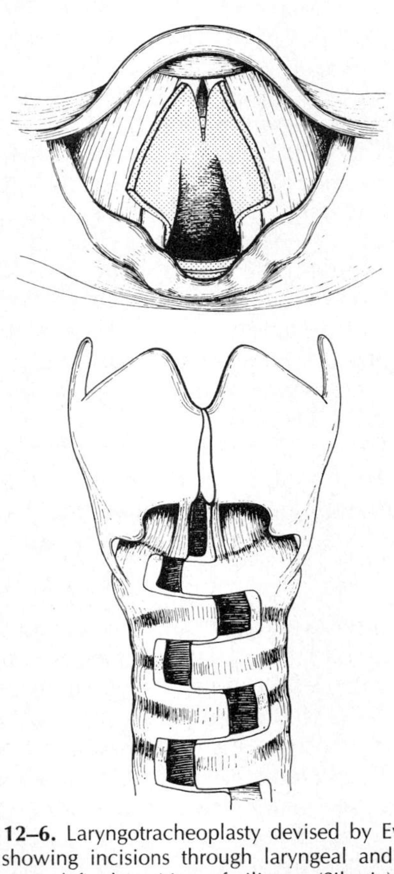

Figure 12–6. Laryngotracheoplasty devised by Evans and Todd, showing incisions through laryngeal and tracheal cartilages and final position of silicone (Silastic) sheeting before suturing. (From Evans JGN, Todd GB: J Laryngol Otol 88:593, 1974.)

Goode has also achieved success with long-term stenting for an average time of 7.7 months.[47] The child has a tracheostomy to maintain the airway. The stenosis is dilated and the stent is introduced with the aid of a bronchoscope. The stent is held in position attached to the tracheostomy tube.

Thermal and chemical burns of the larynx are seen occasionally. Thermal blasts tend to affect mainly the supraglottic and glottic part of the larynx, as the glottis reflexly closes to protect the lower airway. Chemicals will, however, affect both the upper and lower airway. The patient should be treated expectantly, being observed closely for evidence of obstruction. The larynx can be examined directly. Humidified oxygen is used. If obstruction occurs, an endotracheal tube is the treatment of choice unless the larynx has sustained severe mucosal damage, in which case a tracheostomy should be performed.

External trauma is seen less frequently in the young child. Infants and toddlers are seldom exposed to the vehicular injuries seen in adolescents and adults. Anatomically, the pediatric larynx is less susceptible to injury because it is higher in the neck and more mobile; the cartilages are more flexible and less likely to fracture, although the intercartilaginous membrane may well rupture. The diagnosis and management of external laryngeal trauma is dealt with in Chapter 9 of this volume.

Foreign Bodies. Laryngeal foreign bodies comprise a small proportion of the endoscopic experience. Two series quote laryngeal foreign bodies to be 2 per cent and 4 per cent of the total foreign bodies in the larynx and tracheobronchial tree.[48, 49] They are, however, much more likely to obstruct the airway and lead to asphyxiation and death. Immediate first aid such as pounding on the back, finger probing the throat, turning the patient upside down, and the Heimlich maneuver should be used only when the airway is completely obstructed and the patient is in imminent danger of dying. If the airway is only partially obstructed, these procedures may convert a partial obstruction to a total one. Laryngeal foreign bodies should be removed as soon as possible, because edema or repositioning of the foreign body may result in complete obstruction. The patient with a suspected foreign body should be assessed immediately by a team consisting of the endoscopist, anesthesiologist, and pediatrician. Removal of a foreign body should be done in the operating room where life support facilities and provision for tracheostomy are available. A decision should be reached regarding safety of inducing the child with a general anesthetic. If the airway is severely compromised, anesthesia may precipitate obstruction. In this situation, the child is mummified and the foreign body removed in the awake child. In the less severe cases, the child can be anesthetized. A slow halothane induction is used. The foreign body is then removed through the laryngoscope with appropriate forceps. Care must be taken not to impact the foreign body in the larynx, producing a complete obstruction. Postoperative humidification is used. Decadron and racemic epinephrine will reduce laryngeal edema.

Tumors. The great majority of tumors of the pediatric larynx are benign.

Papilloma. Recurrent respiratory papilloma are the most common tumors of the larynx in the pediatric age group. They have been diagnosed from infancy onwards and are usually multiple in children. They appear as warty growths. They may have a fleshy grapelike look or a more firm cornified appearance (Fig. 12–7). They have a predilection for the larynx but are also found in the nasal and oral cavities, pharynx, trachea, and bronchi. They may involve only a small portion of the membranous vocal cord or may exist as a bulky tumor, which appears to involve all of the glottic and supraglottic larynx. The greater the mass of the papilloma, the more likely the airway is to become obstructed. The relationship of the patient and the papilloma varies from individual to individual. The tumor often appears more aggressive in patients less than five years old, where the likelihood of respiratory embarrassment is increased. This, of course, may also be

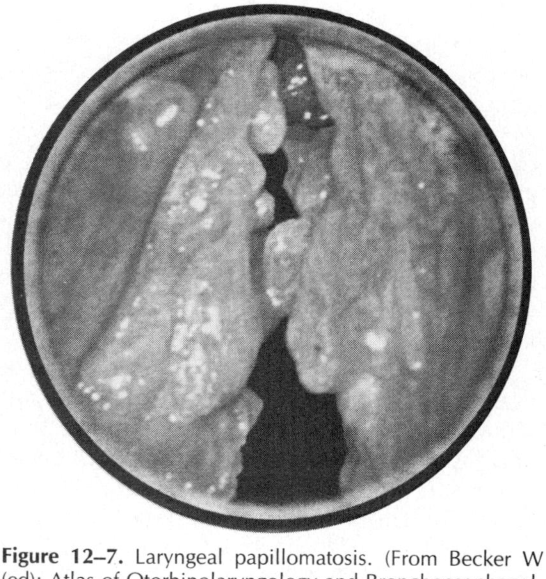

Figure 12–7. Laryngeal papillomatosis. (From Becker W (ed): Atlas of Otorhinolaryngology and Bronchoesophagology. Philadelphia, WB Saunders Company, 1969, p 247.)

a reflection of the size of the larynx in this age group. The reponse to therapy also varies. Some patients may need only two or three laser excisions after which the tumor is well controlled or ceases to manifest itself. Another patient may require laser excision every two to three weeks to maintain an airway. It is often stated that papillomas regress at puberty; however, a number of our patients improved around the age of seven to eight years, at which time they required less frequent treatment. Unfortunately, papilloma does continue into adult life in some patients. These characteristics make for an uncertain and trying time for patient and parents. The impact on the activity, psychologic makeup, and education of the child is considerable. The parents also suffer with their child. The financial commitment by parents, state agencies, and institutions is considerable. Etiology of the papilloma is thought to be viral. Ulman[50] in 1923 reported that a cutaneous wart appeared at the site of injection of laryngeal and condyloma extracts in his skin and that of his co-worker. Evidence suggests that cutaneous warts, respiratory papillomas, and condylomata are caused by DNA viruses of the papovavirus group, i.e., human papillomavirus; however, it is thought that if laryngeal papilloma has a viral etiology, the agent is a different species from that causing cutaneous warts. Quick,[51] in his series of patients, finds a 60 per cent positive history of vaginal condylomata in the mothers of children with respiratory papillomas. He goes on to suggest that the causative agent is a papovavirus, which exists in the DNA form in the cell and not in its more easily recognized crystalloid form.

The clinical presentation is frequently an abnormality of the voice. A hoarse cry or a breathy voice are the earliest symptoms. As the tumor increases in size, the voice becomes weaker and the airway becomes compromised. Diagnosis is achieved by either indirect laryngoscopy or flexible laryngoscopy. The upper aerodigestive tract should be examined for evidence of involvement of other sites. A direct laryngoscopy and biopsy should be performed to obtain histological confirmation of the diagnosis.

Many different modalities of treatment have been tried, including surgical removal of the tumor, ultrasound and cryotherapy destruction, and laser photocoagulation. Local application of caustics and chemotherapeutic agents such as podophyllum have been used; autogenous vaccines have also been used. None of these therapies has resulted in permanent cures. The preferred treatment at present is the laser (for use, see Chapter 6 of this volume). Use of human leukocyte interferon[52] has shown some promise. Interferon causes degeneration of the papilloma; however, recurrence occurs after the interferon treatment ceases. The optimum dose and time schedules are yet to be determined. Tracheostomy is sometimes necessary to maintain the airway; however, as a treatment, it is controversial. Some allege that it causes seeding in the stoma and tracheobronchila tree. Others feel that involvement by papilloma of the lower airway reflects the severity of the disease and obstruction, which necessitates tracheostomy. Malignant change in the papilloma has occurred after the use of radiotherapy[53] and thus is not advised. Spontaneous malignant change has also been seen on one occasion in the author's experience.

Malignant Tumors. Malignant tumors of the larynx in children are very rare and are usually mesodermal in origin. Fibrosarcoma and rhabdomyosarcoma are examples. Epidermoid carcinoma is extremely rare.

Vocal Cord Nodules. Vocal cord nodules are not uncommon in children. They are seen in children who shout or scream. Examples are children with behavior problems and those who have an urge to shout loudest, above the level of noise about them. In all, the condition reflects an undisciplined use of the voice. The nodules are seen at the junction of the anterior and mid one-third of the vocal cords lying directly opposite each other (Fig. 12–8). They may have a soft, immature appearance associated with swelling of the vocal cords or a more mature, firm appearance. The histopathology varies from polypoid to fibrous. The child has a dry, hoarse voice, with reduced pitch. Diagnosis is made by laryngoscopy. Treatment involves the services of a speech pathologist, who endeavors to alter the vocal habits of the

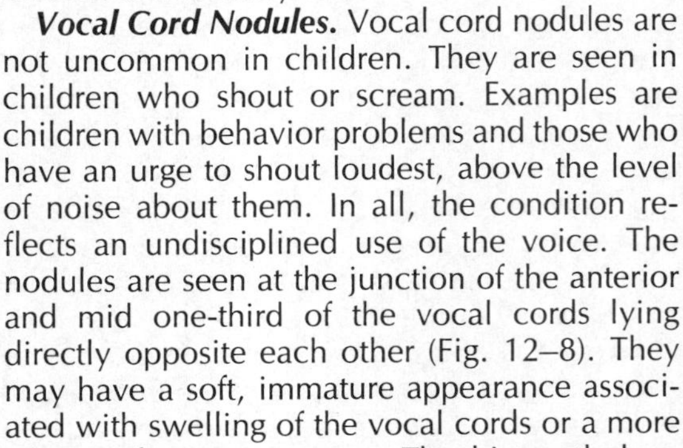

Figure 12–8. Vocal cord nodules. (From Becker W (ed): Atlas of Otorhinolaryngology and Bronchoesophagology. Philadelphia, WB Saunders Company, 1969, p 230.)

child. If this is successful, the nodule will often reduce in size and disappear. Excision of vocal nodules, in children, is rarely indicated. If excision is necessary, it should be done using the microscope to avoid damage to the vocalis muscle. Excision without alteration of vocal misuse will result in reappearance of the nodules.

INTUBATION AND TRACHEOSTOMY

The indications for an artificial airway by intubation or by tracheostomy are often the same. The choice between the two procedures will be made on such factors as specific pathology, expected duration of the problem, and availability of staff capable of maintaining a safe airway. The advantages and disadvantages of the two techniques are summarized in Table 12–2.

The indications for tracheostomy can be classified into three categories, which frequently overlap. These are first, to bypass an upper airway obstruction, second, to provide assisted ventilation, and third, to achieve pulmonary toilet (Table 12–3). Additional effects of tracheostomy include decreased resistance to airflow and reduction of physiologic dead space. Less desirable effects include aphonia, decreased effectiveness of cough, dysphagia, and aspiration.

The best time to provide an artificial airway depends on the severity of the present obstruction and the anticipated progression of the disease. Obviously, the clinician should anticipate this need and keep the number of "crash" intubations and emergency tracheostomies to a minimum. Douglas et al.[54] have produced a table of guidelines based on the mnemonic *TRACHS* (Table 12–4).

Table 12–2. INTUBATION AND TRACHEOSTOMY

Advantages	
Intubation	No operation Usually easier Short-term conditions Better seal for ventilating
Tracheostomy	Long-term conditions Removal of thick secretions
Disadvantages	
Intubation	Displacement of tube Difficult to clear thick secretions Glottic and subglottic trauma Pneumothorax
Tracheostomy	Operative procedure See complications, Table 12–7

Portex endotracheal tubes, which are commonly used, become soft and pliable at body temperature. Cuffed tubes are not used in the small child. For this reason, the clinician should achieve a snug fit at the glottis to decrease air leakage when a ventilator is used. The Silastic tracheostomy tubes have become popular, but many surgeons still use the metal Holinger tubes. The Shiley tracheostomy tube has the advantage of connecting to the ventilator tubing more easily than does the Aberdeen. Choice of the tube size depends on the size of the child.

Table 12–3. INDICATIONS FOR TRACHEOSTOMY

A. *Upper airway obstruction*	
Congenital	Pierre Robin syndrome Subglottic stenosis Laryngeal web, cyst Vocal cord paralysis Laryngomalacia
External trauma	Maxillofacial injuries Cervical soft tissue contusion Laryngeal fractures
Internal trauma	Foreign bodies Burns Instrumentation Prolonged intubation
Infections	Epiglottitis Laryngotracheobronchitis Cellulitis Retropharyngeal abscess Diphtheria
Tumor	Papilloma Hemangioma Lymphangioma
Neurologic	Bilateral vocal cord paralysis
B. *Pulmonary toilet and protection of airway*	
Stagnation of bronchial secretions	
Coma	Encephalitis Head injury Drug intoxication
Cervical cord lesion	Degenerative
Trauma	Burns Crush chest Shock lung
Aspiration	Maxillofacial injury Laryngeal cleft, tracheoesophageal fistula Neurologic—as above
C. *Assisted ventilation*	
Neurologic	Coma Polyneuritis Poliomyelitis
Pulmonary disease	Respiratory distress syndrome
Trauma	Flail chest Pneumothorax, pneumomediastinum

Table 12–4. DEGREE OF EMERGENCY (*TRACHS*)*

	Mild (days)	Moderate (hours)	Severe (minutes)	Extreme (immediate)
Tussive (cough)	Occasional	Hoarse	Bark	Bark or depressed
Retractions	Absent	Suprasternal	Supra- and infrasternal	All accessory muscles
Anxiety	Calm	When disturbed	Restless	Agitated or stuporous
Cyanosis	None	None	In room air	In 40% O_2
Heart rate	Less than 120	Less than 140	Over 140	Over 140
Stridor	Occasional	Inspiratory	Inspiratory and expiratory	Marked or diminished

*From Douglas GS et al.: Ear Nose Throat J 57:159, 1978.

The important measurements are the external and internal diameters. Tables 12–5 and 12–6 indicate the tube size that is age appropriate. For airway problems that necessitate an artificial airway, an experienced anesthesiologist and nursing staff are necessary. The airway should be introduced in the operating room. Thus, if the original plan to introduce an endotracheal tube fails, a tracheostomy can be done. In most situations, the child can be carefully and gently anesthetized; however, certain situations such as a foreign body or highly vascular tumor in the upper airway may necessitate a tracheostomy without general anesthesia. The anesthesia for airway obstruction because of inflammatory disease of the larynx and foreign bodies has been described previously. A methodical approach involving preoxygenation, slow induction, maintenance of oxygenation using mask ventilation, placement of an intravenous line, and the introduction of a tube or ventilating bronchoscope is the key to success. Many surgeons prefer to have a ventilating bronchoscope in the trachea when they do a tracheostomy. The rigidity of the tube and the light shining from the bronchoscope through the tissues are aids to finding the very soft and mobile infant trachea. I find,

Table 12–5. APPROXIMATE GAUGE EQUIVALENTS FREQUENTLY USED IN ENDOTRACHEAL AND TRACHEOTOMY TUBES*
(Based on nearest inner diameter measurement)

Endotracheal[1]			Shiley[2]			Aberdeen[3]				Holinger[4]			
ID (mm)	OD (mm)	FR[5]	ID (mm)	OD (mm)	FR	Size	ID (mm)	OD (mm)	FR	Size	ID (mm)	OD (mm)	FR
2.0	2.9	8											
2.5	3.5	10								00	2.5	4.0	13
3.0	4.2	12	3.1	4.5	14	00				0	3.5	5.0	15
3.5	4.9	15	3.4	5.0	15	0	3.5	5.0	15	1	3.5	5.5	17
4.0	5.5	16	3.7	5.5	17	1	4.0	6.7	20	2	4.0	6.0	18
4.5	6.1	18	4.1	6.0	18	2	4.5	6.7	20	3	4.5	7.0	21
5.0	6.8	20	4.8	7.0	21	3	5.0	7.3	22	4	5.0	8.0	25
5.5	7.4	22	5.0	8.5	26	4				5	5.5	9.0	27
6.0	8.0	24					6.0	8.7	26	6	6.0	10.0	30
6.5	8.7	26											
7.0	9.5	29	7.0	10.0	30	6	7.0	10.7	32				
7.5	10.0	30											
8.0	10.7	32											

*From Stool SE, Eavey R. *In* Bluestone CD, Stool SE (eds): Pediatric Otolaryngology. Philadelphia, WB Saunders Company, 1983, p 1325.

[1]The endotracheal tubes are marked with the internal diameter, usually with the outer diameter, and the length.

[2]The Shiley tube is manufactured by Shiley Laboratories, Irvine, CA. The tube is stamped with the size and inner and outer diameters. The larger sizes are supplied with a low-pressure cuff.

[3]This tube is the Aberdeen design, known also as the Great Ormand Street Tube. It is manufactured by J. G. Franklin & Sons, Ltd., High Wycombe, England. The tube is stamped with the inner diameter.

[4]The Holinger design is manufactured by several companies; therefore, the sizes may vary, and the internal diameter may show considerable variation. These measurements were made on tubes produced by Pilling Company, Fort Washington, PA.

[5]The French number is arrived at by multiplying the outside diameter in millimeters by 3.

Table 12–6. APPROXIMATE SIZE OF ENDOTRACHEAL AND TRACHEOTOMY TUBES FOR INFANTS AND CHILDREN*
(Based on outer diameter or circumference [French No.])†

Age	Endotracheal‡	Shiley	Aberdeen	Holinger
Premature	11–13	00		00
Newborn	14	0	3.5	0
Newborn–3 months	15–16	0	3.5	1
3–10 months	17	1	4.0	2
10–12 months	18	2	4.5	3
13–24 months	20	3	5.0	3
2–3 years	22	4	5.0	4
4–5 years	24	4	5.0	4
6–7 years	26	4	5.0	4
8–9 years	28	4	6.0	5
10–11 years	30	6	6.0	6
12 and over	32	6	7.0	6

*From Stool SE, Eavey R. *In* Bluestone CD, Stool SE (eds): Pediatric Otolaryngology. Philadelphia, WB Saunders Company, 1983, p 1325.
†Usually a larger size tracheotomy than endotracheal tube may be used because the trachea is larger than the subglottic region. The outer diameter or circumference will determine the size of tube that may be used.
‡French Number.

however, a Portex endotracheal tube sufficiently helpful for that purpose.

The technique of tracheostomy in children has certain basic principles (Fig. 12–9). The child is positioned with a small roll under the shoulders. The anesthesiologist holds the chin up with the neck hyperextended. The head, neck, and chest should be lying on a straight vertical axis. The laryngeal and tracheal cartilages are palpated. To differentiate these soft cartilages in children is often difficult. The incision is placed about one finger's breadth

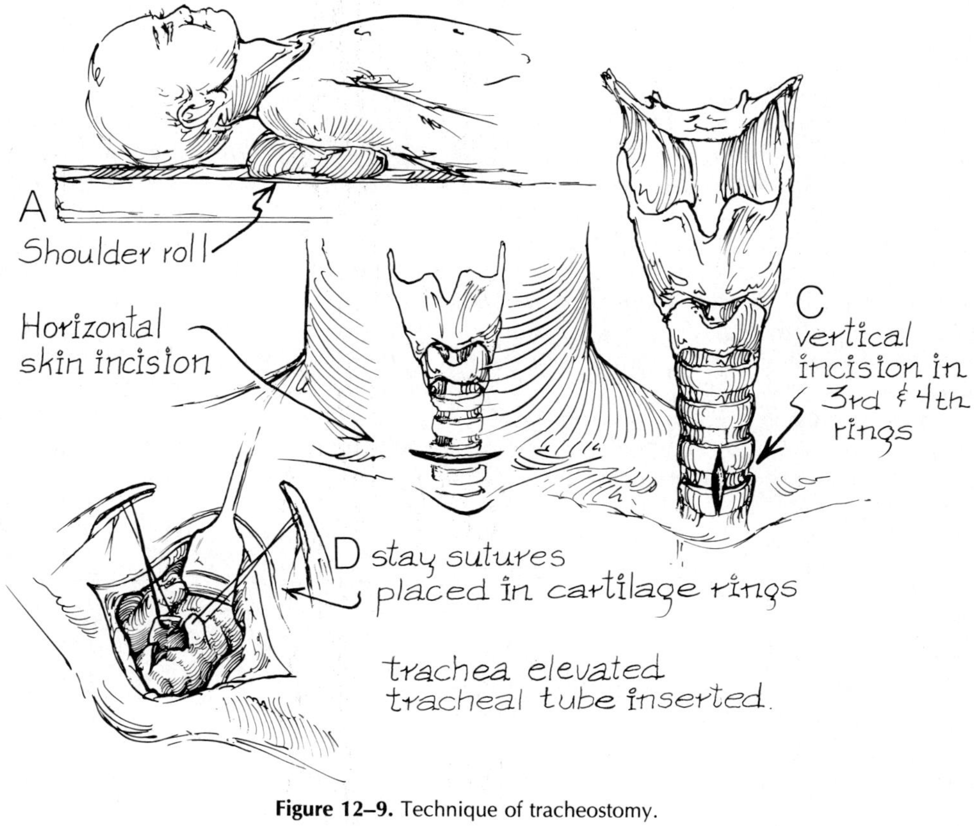

Figure 12–9. Technique of tracheostomy.

above the suprasternal notch, where the trachea usually turns posteriorly in its descent.

A vertical or horizontal incision is permissible. The dissection is taken through the superficial fascia down to the deep investing fascia. From this point, the dissection is kept strictly in the midline by repeatedly palpating the trachea with a finger. The fascia and strap muscles are brought up to the skin level with small hemostats or 3–0 silk stay sutures, providing good retraction and preventing a funnel approach to the trachea. The isthmus of the thyroid gland should be divided if it obstructs the approach to the trachea. The pretracheal fascia should be elevated minimally. Silk stay sutures are placed in the tracheal wall 3 mm from the midline. These sutures are then used to elevate the trachea towards the skin. A vertical incision is made through the third and fourth tracheal ring (some surgeons prefer an inferiorly based U-shaped flap). The endotracheal tube is withdrawn until the tip is visible in the opened trachea and the tracheostomy tube is inserted. Both sides of the chest are auscultated to ensure the tube does not enter the right mainstem bronchus. The endotracheal tube is then removed. The tracheostomy tube is secured with tapes around the patient's neck. The tracheal stay sutures are labeled and taped to the chest. If the tracheostomy tube comes out, the sutures can be used to pull the trachea forward and also open the stoma. This facilitates replacement of the tube. A chest x-ray should be done either in the operating room or immediately upon the child's arrival in the recovery room. The situation of the tube is checked and the presence or absence of a pneumomediastinum or a pneumothorax is ascertained. A tracheostomy tube of the same size and a curved hemostat or tracheal dilator should be kept taped to the crib so that they are immediately at hand if the indwelling tracheostomy becomes displaced.

Emergency tracheostomy is a far more hazardous procedure. Cricothyroidotomy, a vertical incision in the cricoid, and needle intubation using a large IV cannula have been advocated as temporary measures. A "slash" tracheostomy in a child is extremely hazardous since the innominate artery may cross the trachea in the neck. Also, the pleural domes may encroach into the operative field as the child strains for breath; however, when such an extreme situation exists, the physician does the best he can with the available tools.

The complications of tracheostomy are shown in Table 12–7. The early complications seen most frequently are pneumothorax, hemorrhage, and displacement of the tube. Pneumothorax and pneumomediastinum appear to be closely related to an urgent tracheostomy performed without the benefit of an indwelling endotracheal tube. Rabuzzi carefully studied patients for the presence of pneumothorax and pneumomediastinum after tracheostomy.[55] These complications were found in 36 per cent of patients who had an endotracheal tube and 80 per cent who did not. In patients with acute respiratory distress, the complication rate was 39 per cent with an endotracheal tube in place at the time of surgery and 100 per cent without. In all situations, dissection under the pretracheal fascia should be avoided, since this can provide access for air pulled into the mediastinum.

Decannulation should be performed as early as is feasible. The longer a tracheostomy remains patent the more difficult its removal will become. Decannulation should be performed in a gradual manner rather than suddenly. The airway must be assessed radiologically and endoscopically for new or old pathology. The original tracheostomy tube is replaced sequentially by smaller tubes. The tube is then plugged before removal, allowing the child to get used to the increased airway resistance experienced with laryngeal breathing. Some children will not tolerate decannulation. In these cases, a careful investigation for the cause must be made. Minor airway obstruction may be compounded in the infant by indrawing of the soft tracheal rings as the child makes more forceful inspiratory effort. Decannulation was delayed in 44 of 123 pediatric tracheostomies reviewed by Sasaki.[56] Tracheal granulomas are often found in this group and can be removed endoscopically. Posterior displacement of the tracheal ring above the stoma will also provide obstruction. Chrysdale has described his experience in successfully treating this latter problem with an indwelling endotracheal tube.[57] Tracheal and subglottic stenosis will also delay

Table 12–7. COMPLICATIONS OF TRACHEOSTOMY

Hemorrhage
Subcutaneous emphysema, pneumothorax, pneumomediastinum
Tube malposition, displacement, blockage
Infection: wound, perichondritis, tracheitis, pneumonia
Dysphagia, aspiration
Fistula: tracheocutaneous, tracheoesophageal
Delayed decannulation: granuloma, malacia, stenosis
Scar

decannulation. The treatment for these conditions has been reviewed earlier in this chapter.

The long-term effect on the child's physical development is difficult to evaluate; however, Freeland[7] reviewed 23 infants who had been tracheostomized. Those infants who had tracheostomies for less than one week appeared to be normal, whereas the 9 children who had a prolonged tracheostomy showed a tendency to retarded general physical, laryngeal, and tracheal growth. Although verbal communication is always a concern, these children do not seem to have a serious problem in this regard.

References

1. Ferguson CF: Congenital abnormalities of the infant larynx. Otolaryngol Clin North Am 3(2):185, 1970.
2. Holinger PH, Johnson KC: Factors reponsible for laryngeal obstruction in infants. JAMA 143:1229, 1950.
3. Tucker G: The infant larynx: Direct laryngoscopic observations. JAMA 99:1899, 1932.
4. Wilson TG: Some observations on the infantile larynx. Acta Otolaryngol (Stockh) 43:95, 1953.
5. Fearon B, Cotton R: Subglottic stenosis in infants and children: The clinical problem and experimental surgical correction. Can J Otolaryngol 1:281, 1972.
6. Fearon B, Whalen J: Tracheal dimensions in the living infant. Ann Otol Rhinol Laryngol 76:964, 1967.
7. Freeland AP et al.: Developmental influences of infant tracheostomy. J Laryngol Otol 88:927, 1974.
8. Holinger PH et al.: Subglottic stenosis in infants and children. Ann Otol Rhinol Laryngol 85:591, 1976.
9. Fearon B: Respiratory distress in the newborn. Otolaryngol Clin North Am 1(1):147, 1968.
10. Holinger LD: Treatment of severe subglottic stenosis without tracheotomy. Ann Otol Rhinol Laryngol 91:407, 1982.
11. Plott D: Congenitial laryngeal abductor paralysis due to nucleus ambiguous dysgenesis in three brothers. New Engl J Med 27:593, 1964.
12. Gacek RR: Hereditary abductor vocal cord paralysis. Ann Otol Rhinol Laryngol 85:90, 1976.
13. Holinger LD et al.: Etiology of bilateral abductor vocal cord paralysis. Ann Otol Rhinol Laryngol 85:428, 1976.
14. Cohen SR: Arytenoidectomy in children. Laryngoscope 84:1293, 1974.
15. Holinger PH, Brown WT: Congenital webs, cysts, laryngoceles, and other anomalies of the larynx. Ann Otol Rhinol Laryngol 76:744, 1967.
16. LeJeune J: "Cri du Chat" Syndrome. Chromosome deletion causes retardation. JAMA 197:40, 1966.
17. Ward PH et al.: The larynx in the "Cri du Chat" (cat cry) syndrome. Laryngoscope 78:1716, 1968.
18. Tefft N: Radiotherapuetic management of subglottic hemangioma in children. Radiol 86:207, 1966.
19. Littler ER: Asphyxia due to hemangioma in the trachea. J Thoracic Cardiovasc Surg 45:552, 1963.
20. Lister WA: The natural history of strawberry naevi. Lancet 13:1429, 1938.
21. Calcaterra TC: An evaluation of the treatment of subglottic hemangioma. Laryngoscope 78:1956, 1968.
22. Healey GB et al.: Treatment of subglottic hemangioma with the carbon dioxide laser. Laryngoscope 90:809, 1980.
23. Ferguson CF, Flake CG: Subglottic hemangioma as a cause of respiratory obstruction in infants. Ann Otol Rhinol Laryngol 70:1095, 1961.
24. Benjamin B: Treatment of infantile subglottic hemangioma with radioactive gold grain. Ann Otol Rhinol Laryngol 87:18, 1978.
25. Fisher JM: Cancer in the irradiated thyroid. New Engl J Med 292:975, 1975.
26. Cohen SR, Wang CI: Steroid treatment of hemangioma of the head and neck in children. Ann Otol Rhinol Laryngol 81:584, 1972.
27. Fearon B, Cinnamond M: Tracheotomy in acute supraglottitis (epiglottitis): The treatment of choice. Laryngoscope 87:879, 1977.
28. Jones R et al.: Bacterial tracheitis. JAMA 242:721, 1979.
29. Barker G: Current management of croup and epiglottitis. Pediat Clin North Am 26:565, 1979.
30. Cherry JD: The treatment of croup: Continued controversy due to failure of recognition of historic, ecological, etiological and clinical perspectives (editorial). J Pediat 94:352, 1979.
31. Williams HE, Phelan PD: Respiratory Illness in Children. Oxford, Blackwell Scientific Publications, Inc. 1975, p 26.
32. Newth CJL et al.: The respiratory status of children with croup. J Pediat 81:1068, 1972.
33. Leipzig B et al.: A prospective randomized study to determine the efficacy of steroids in treatment of croup. J Pediat 94:194, 1979.
34. Adair JC et al.: Ten year experience with intermittent positive pressure breathing in the treatment of acute laryngotracheobronchitis. Anaesth Anagl 50:649, 1971.
35. Lockhart CH, Battaglia JD: Croup and epiglottitis. Pediat Ann 6:262, 1977.
36. Cantrell RW et al: Acute epiglottitis: Intubation versus tracheostomy. Laryngoscope 88:994, 1978.
37. Allen TH, Steven IM: Prolonged endotracheal intubation in infants and children. Brit J Anaesth 44:835, 1972.
38. Stetson JB, Guess WL: Causes of damage to tissues by polymers and elastomers used in the fabrication of tracheal devices. Anesthesiol 33:635, 1970.
39. Hawkins DB: Hyaline membrane disease of the neonate. Laryngoscope 88:201, 1978.
40. Cotton R: Management of subglottic stenosis in infancy and childhood. Ann Otol Rhinol Laryngol 87:649, 1978.
41. Fearon B, Cotton R: Subglottic stenosis in infants and children: The clinical problem and experimental surgical correction. Can J Otolaryngol 1:281, 1972.
42. Calcaterra TC et al.: Effect of laryngofissure on the developing canine larynx. Ann Otol Rhinol Laryngol 83:810, 1974.
43. Cotton RT, Seid AB: Management of the extubation problem in the premature child. Ann Otol Rhinol Laryngol 89:508, 1980.
44. Fearon B et al.: Subglottic stenosis of the larynx in the infant and child. Ann Otol Rhinol Laryngol 87:645, 1978.
45. Evans JNG, Todd GB: Laryngo-tracheoplasty. J Laryngol Otol 88:589, 1974.
46. Rethi A: An operation for cicatricial stenosis of the larynx. J Laryngol Otol 70:283, 1956.

47. Goode RL, Shinn JB: Long-term stenting in the treatment of subglottic stenosis. Ann Otol Rhinol Laryngol 86:795, 1977.
48. Bothmann DF, Breckman CR: Foreign bodies in the larynx and tracheobronchial tree in children. Ann Otol Rhinol Laryngol 89:434, 1980.
49. Cohen SR et al.: Foreign bodies in the airway. Ann Otol Rhinol Laryngol 89:437, 1980.
50. Ulman EV: On the etiology of the laryngeal papillomata. Acta Otolaryngol (Stockh) 5:317, 1923.
51. Quick CA et al.: Relationship between condylomata and laryngeal papillomata. Ann Otol Rhinol Laryngol 89:467, 1980.
52. Hagland S et al.: Interferon therapy in juvenile laryngeal papillomatosis. Arch Otolaryngol 107:327, 1981.
53. Walsh TE, Beamer PR: Epidermoid carcinoma of the larynx occurring in two children with papilloma of the larynx. Laryngoscope 60:1110, 1950.
54. Douglas GS et al.: Tracheotomy in pediatric airway management. Ear Nose Throat J 57:159, 1978.
55. Rabuzzi DD, Reed GF: Intrathoracic complications following tracheostomy in children. Laryngoscope 81:939, 1971.
56. Sasaki CT et al.: Tracheostomy decannulation. Am J Dis Child 132:266, 1978.
57. Chrysdale WS: Nasotracheal intubation in management of delayed decannulation. Ann Otol Rhinol Laryngol 83:802, 1974.

13

Nonsurgical Conditions of the Larynx*

Roger McNeill, M.D.

For the purposes of this chapter, the term *nonsurgical conditions of the larynx* has been used to encompass a heterogeneous group of disorders, the primary management of which, at least in the initial stages of disease, is by medical rather than operative means. Despite the emphasis on medical therapy, modern developments in endolaryngeal microsurgery have expanded the scope of treatment for many of these conditions, the management of chronic laryngitis and vocal nodules being obvious examples. Medical therapy also does not preclude surgical intervention, which may be indicated for the acquisition of tissue for diagnostic purposes, for airway diversion in cases of upper respiratory obstruction, or for the establishment of airway patency if it is compromised by late effects of the disease process.

It will be evident that the larynx may become secondarily involved in a variety of systemic disorders, inflammatory and noninflammatory. Detailed descriptions of the clinical and histopathologic features of these conditions are necessarily beyond the scope of this chapter, and the reader is therefore directed to more specific discussions of these topics. The various functional and neurologic disorders of the larynx have also been excluded, as they will be discussed elsewhere.

INFLAMMATORY DISEASES

Acute Nonspecific Laryngitis

Acute nonspecific laryngitis is perhaps the most common laryngeal disorder encountered and, because most patients afflicted with this condition do not seek medical attention, its true incidence is not easily documented. Symptoms are usually of abrupt onset and consist mainly of hoarseness, sometimes progressing to almost complete aphonia. Attempts at speaking above a whisper are often associated with discomfort or mild pain in the throat. At times, a dry, irritating, nonproductive cough may be the predominant complaint; shortness of breath and stridor are not usually associated with this disorder in adults. Acute nonspecific laryngitis most frequently occurs as a sequel to upper respiratory tract infection, and a variety of organisms (including viruses, alpha streptococcus, beta streptococcus, *Staphylococcus aureus, Staphylococcus albus,* pneumococci, and *Haemophilus influenzae)* have been iso-

*The author gratefully acknowledges the assistance and consultation provided by James A. Reinarz, M.D., Professor of Internal Medicine and Director of the Division of Infectious Diseases, University of Texas Medical Branch, Galveston, Texas, in the preparation of this chapter.

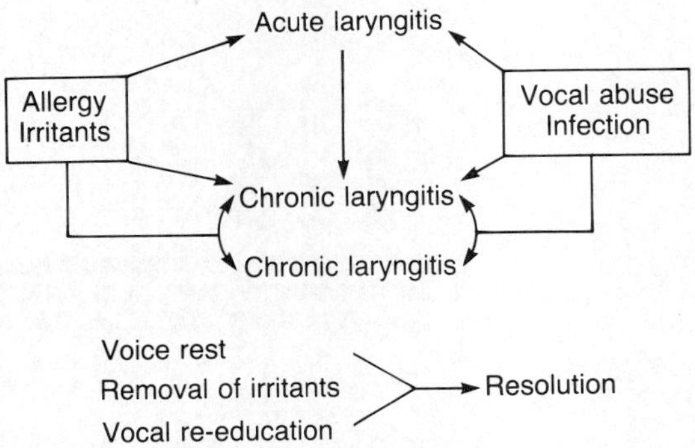

Figure 13–1. Chronic nonspecific laryngitis—interaction of factors responsible for perpetuation of the disease.

lated.[1–3] Undoubtedly, however, a significant proportion of cases are noninfectious in origin and are probably related to other inciting factors such as vocal abuse, allergy, and chemical irritants. Acute inflammation may also occur secondarily to trauma (as from endotracheal intubation) and to thermal or chemical injury resulting from the ingestion or inhalation of noxious substances.

Since most patients with acute laryngitis do not seek medical advice (and of those who do, a significant number do not, in fact, undergo indirect visualization of the larynx), the diagnosis is often a presumptive one based on the acute history, the symptoms, and the self-limiting nature of the disease.

Examination of the larynx in acute nonspecific laryngitis reveals changes confined mainly to the true vocal cords. The changes consist of hyperemia, erythema, and edema of the overlying mucosa. Characteristically, the degree of hoarseness contrasts sharply with the very minimal changes often seen in the appearance of the vocal cords, a feature that surprises the inexperienced observer. Airway compromise and loss of vocal cord mobility are not usually features of this disorder.

The single most effective therapeutic modality in the management of acute laryngitis is voice rest, and the duration of symptomatology appears to be directly related to persistence in the use of the inflamed larynx. Antibiotics are frequently used concomitantly, although it is questionable whether they hasten resolution of the disease. In situations where chemical inhalants are felt to play some etiologic role, attention must be directed at environmental control or modification of such personal habits as smoking. Symptomatic measures such as mild analgesics, gargles, cough suppressants, and humidification are also often beneficial.

Airway obstruction in acute laryngitis rarely develops in adults but may occur in association with thermal or chemical injuries. In severe cases, steroid therapy may be beneficial in averting late complications of laryngeal stenosis because of scarring.

Chronic Nonspecific Laryngitis

The term *chronic nonspecific laryngitis* refers to a long-standing diffuse inflammation involving predominantly the true vocal cords. This disorder may occur as a sequel to an episode of acute laryngitis, or may, as is often the case, develop insidiously in the absence of any dramatic inciting event. Numerous factors have been incriminated in the etiology of this condition and, in most instances, it appears that a combination of insults is responsible, producing a vicious cycle of events from which the lar-

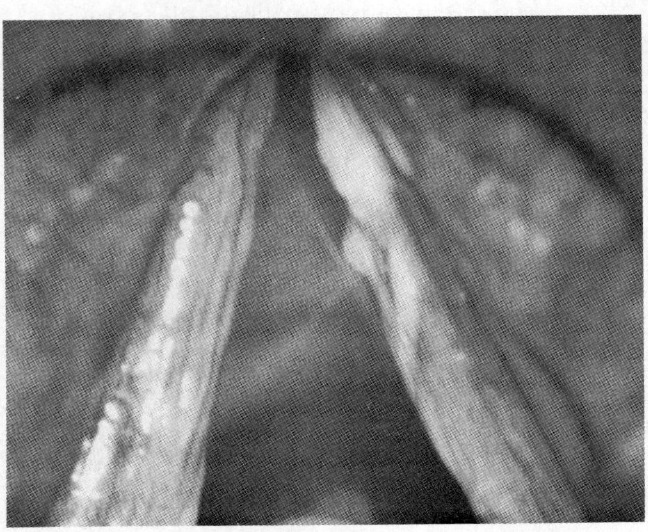

Figure 13–2. Beginning hyperplastic laryngitis, showing patchy keratinization of the epithelium. (From Kleinsasser O: Microlaryngoscopy and Endolaryngeal Microsurgery. Philadelphia, WB Saunders Company, 1968, p 33.)

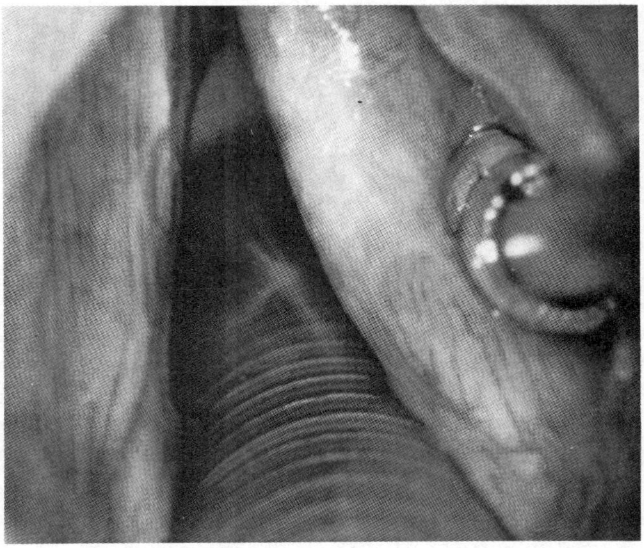

Figure 13–3. Epidermization of the epithelium on the subglottic surface of the vocal cord in chronic hyperplastic laryngitis. (From Kleinsasser O: Microlaryngoscopy and Endolaryngeal Microsurgery. Philadelphia, WB Saunders Company, 1968, p 33.)

yngeal mucosa may fail to recover (Fig. 13–1). The most striking histologic feature of chronic laryngitis is a progressive metaplasia of the endolaryngeal mucosa with subsequent hyperplasia of the lining, often referred to as "epidermization of the laryngeal epithelium" following Kleinsasser[4] (Figs. 13–2 and 13–3). This process progressively involves the epithelium of the true cords, false cords, subglottis, and epiglottis and is accompanied by atrophy of the mucous glands, hyperemia and edema of the mucosa and submucosa, and chronic inflammatory exudation (Fig. 13–4). Epidermization tends to be most pronounced on the true vocal cords, often being accompanied by areas of keratinization (keratoses). Occasionally, this process may develop to such an extent that it produces a heaped-up, thickened pad in the interarytenoid area. The pad is referred to as pachyderma laryngis.

Variants of chronic laryngitis that have been described include:

1. Chronic diffuse hyperplastic laryngitis.
2. Chronic localized hyperplastic laryngitis.
3. Pachyderma laryngis.
4. Laryngitis sicca.
5. Contact ulcer.

These conditions probably represent essentially various forms of the same disease process with respect to the predominant macroscopic and microscopic features.[1, 4, 5]

Epidemiology of Chronic Laryngitis. Numerous factors have been incriminated in the etiology of chronic laryngitis. The role of vocal

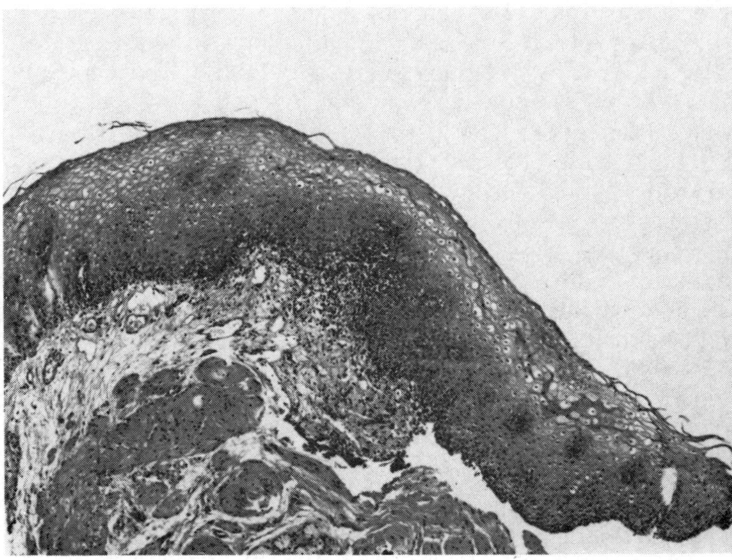

Figure 13–4. Chronic laryngitis. Vocal cord biopsy showing accumulation of chronic inflammatory cells (hematoxylin and eosin stain [H&E], × 100).

abuse certainly appears to be undisputed in some patients, especially those in whom there is an occupational or recreational predisposition. Exposure to various irritant inhalants such as cigarette smoke, dust, and chemical fumes may initiate, exacerbate, or prolong the disorder.[6, 7, 8] Upper respiratory allergy is also felt to be responsible, in some patients, and chronic infection of the upper and lower respiratory tracts has been an associated finding in a significant number of patients with chronic laryngitis.[9, 10] Stell, studying a group of 58 patients with chronic laryngitis, found that 53 per cent had a history of chronic upper or lower respiratory tract sepsis, although the smoking habits of the patients were no different from those of a control group matched for age and sex.[11]

Of interest, also, is the possible relationship of chronic laryngitis to gastroesophageal and esophagopharyngeal reflux. Using the technique of acid barium swallow, as described by Donner,[12] Delahunty was able to demonstrate reflux of gastric contents in all of nine patients with posterior laryngitis.[13] All patients in his series responded to antacids and head elevation during sleep.

Other factors attributed to the etiology of chronic laryngitis are alcohol, chronic mouth breathing, and various systemic and metabolic conditions. Stell and McLoughlin, however, found no association with anemia, diabetes, or renal disease in their series.[11]

Chronic laryngitis is most often reported as being more common in males than females, with a peak incidence in the fourth to sixth decades.

The relationship between chronic laryngitis and carcinoma of the larynx evokes considerable interest and speculation. Gabriel and Jones followed 101 cases of chronic laryngitis occurring over a five-year period and found that 9.9 per cent subsequently developed laryngeal carcinoma.[6] Similarly, they reported that of 51 cases of carcinoma of the larynx occurring during a five-year period, 19.7 per cent gave a previous history of chronic laryngitis. Kleinsasser is also in agreement with the widely expressed feeling that chronic hypertrophic laryngitis is "an important precursor of laryngeal carcinoma."[4] McGavran et al., however, from a study involving close follow-up of 87 patients with isolated laryngeal keratoses, concluded that this is not a distinct precancerous condition.[14]

Clinical Features of Chronic Laryngitis. The predominant symptom in chronic laryngitis is persistent hoarseness. This is not infrequently associated with dry cough and the feeling of a lump in the throat. The appearance of the larynx varies from mild vocal cord edema and hyperemia in the early stages to marked swelling, bogginess, and erythema of the true cords, false cords, and adjacent areas. The airway is not, as a rule, compromised, and mobility of the cords is unimpaired. In long-standing cases, the laryngeal epithelium in certain areas takes on a dull grayish, irregular appearance representing foci of metaplasia and hyperplasia. Hyperkeratotic areas may be evident, particularly on the true vocal cords, presenting an appearance indistinguishable macroscopically from in situ or early invasive carcinoma.

Treatment of Chronic Laryngitis. Treatment is initially conservative and consists of an aggressive program of voice rest together with control of any underlying etiologic factors that may exist. Failure to recognize and eliminate or reduce exposure to offending irritants or allergens will undoubtedly result in failure to produce resolution of the disease. Attempts at modifying speech production through the use of vocal intensity controllers have met with some success.[15] Adjunctive measures such as the use of inhalations and expectorants may also provide symptomatic relief. It is doubtful, however, whether antibiotics provide any benefit in most cases.

Unfortunately, chronic laryngitis of long duration tends to be refractory to therapy. It is unclear whether this is because of a failure to remove specific etiologic factors or whether the persistence of the disorder results from irreversible changes that have occurred in the laryngeal mucosa. Kleinsasser feels that systematic removal of diseased epithelium contributes toward breaking the cycle that perpetuates the disease by allowing regeneration of more normal epithelium. Undoubtedly surgical intervention in the established refractory chronic hyperplastic laryngitis is often indicated to provide microscopic assurance of the absence of malignant disease.

Contact Ulcer (Contact Pachyderma)

Contact pachyderma, first described by Jackson, is a characteristic ulcerated or heaped-up area overlying the vocal process of the arytenoid and, more often than not, occurs bilaterally on opposing surfaces of the vocal processes[16] (Fig. 13–5). Occasionally, the mucosa overlying the medial surface of the body

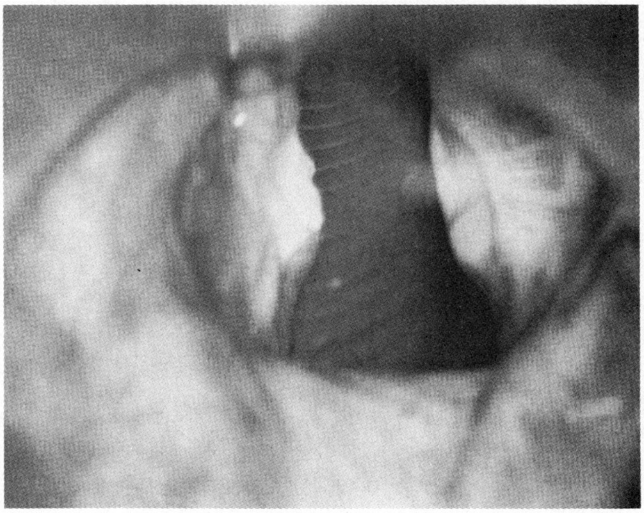

Figure 13–5. Older contact pachyderma with keratinization of the floor of the typical crater. (From Kleinsasser O: Microlaryngoscopy and Endolaryngeal Microsurgery. Philadelphia, WB Saunders Company, 1968, p 43.)

of the arytenoid may be involved. It is generally agreed that the lesions result from trauma, secondary to vocal abuse or misuse, and originally appear as areas of mucosal erythema and edema overlying the vocal processes.[4, 17–19] This is later followed by superficial ulceration and granulation tissue formation. On occasion, the lesion may present as an area of thickened mucosal elevation (contact pachyderma) with central crater formation.[4] Granulation tissue formation may occasionally be so pronounced as to present a microscopic and macroscopic appearance indistinguishable from postintubation granuloma. The underlying submucosa is usually thickened and edematous, with a chronic inflammatory exudate. Rarely, the ulceration may reveal an area of exposed cartilage in the region of the vocal process.

Males appear to be afflicted far more commonly than females, and a history of vocal abuse or misuse is usually not difficult to elicit. Preacher feels that emotional tension may also play some underlying role.[19] Holinger et al. found allergy to be an associated factor in several patients and, in a significant number (28 per cent), symptoms began after an upper respiratory infection.[17] In their series, almost half of the patients were nonsmokers or smoked very little.

The main symptoms associated with contact ulcers and contact granulomas are hoarseness, caused by poor approximation of the vocal cords, and pain that occasionally radiates to the ear. The appearances of the lesions are fairly characteristic on indirect examination of the larynx, and only rarely is clinical differentiation from malignant disease a problem.

The most effective treatment for contact ulcers is generally agreed to be voice therapy. Prior to institution of this modality of treatment, very few patients showed any long-lasting response. Peacher and Holinger found that the lesions failed to heal unless the patient was able to modify his mode of speech production.[18] In their experience, all patients who received voice therapy showed some improvement.

Occasionally the presence of large granulomas may necessitate surgical removal, and Kleinsasser has at times found excision of swollen mucosa (circumcision) around the ulcer or crater to hasten resolution.[4]

Granulomatous Infections

Laryngeal Tuberculosis. Since the advent of chemotherapeutic agents, the incidence of laryngeal tuberculosis has undergone a marked and sustained decline. Table 13–1 shows this decline in incidence, as reported in five studies between 1928 and 1974.[20–24]

Table 13–1. INCIDENCE OF LARYNGEAL TUBERCULOSIS

Author	Laryngeal Involvement (per cent)
Looper and Schneider[20] (1928)	15.5
Weidman and Campbell[21] (1939)	26.0
Myerson[22] (1944)	10.7
Looper and Lyons[23] (1948)	7.7
Rohwedder[24] (1974)	1.3

Epidemiology of Laryngeal Tuberculosis. With few exceptions, occurrence of laryngeal tuberculosis is secondary to advanced pulmonary tuberculosis and results from the exposure of the laryngeal epithelium to contaminated sputum. Accurate statistics as to the frequency of laryngeal involvement in pulmonary tuberculosis, however, are difficult to ascertain as undoubtedly subclinical infections do occur. Auerbach, from a study of 811 tuberculosis autopsy cases, found laryngeal involvement in 37.5 per cent.[25] The frequency of laryngeal involvement in pulmonary tuberculosis has, in earlier studies, been reported to be anywhere from 1.2 per cent to 97 per cent. Present-day methods of antituberculous treatment have certainly reduced the occurrence of this disease to a mere fraction of its previous incidence.

As stated earlier, laryngeal tuberculosis invariably occurs in the presence of active pulmonary tuberculosis, usually advanced. Lell found extensive bilateral pulmonary involvement in 75 per cent of patients,[26] and Rohwedder noted apical cavity disease with endobronchial spread in 75 per cent.[24] Rarely, miliary invasion by the blood stream may occur, producing granular, widespread involvement of the laryngeal mucosa with rapid and extensive ulceration.

Laryngeal tuberculosis reportedly occurs more commonly in males than females, with peak susceptibility in the third and fourth decades. There does not appear to be any specific racial or occupational predisposition. Children and the elderly are much less frequently affected. Malnutrition, debilitation, and silicosis have been incriminated, however, as predisposing factors.

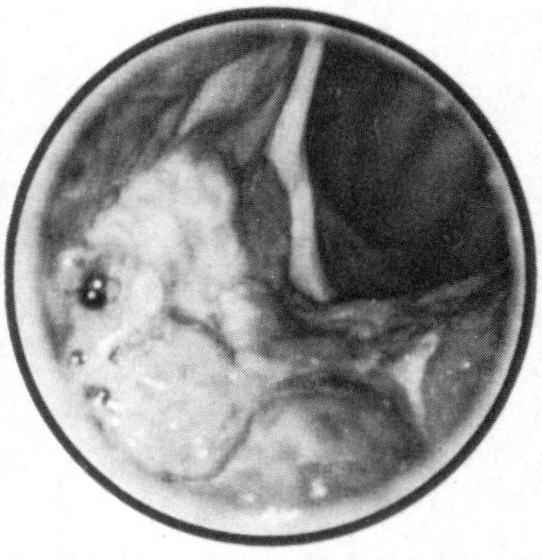

Figure 13–7. Tuberculosis of the larynx. (From Becker W (ed): Atlas of Otorhinolaryngology and Bronchoesophagology. Philadelphia, WB Saunders Company, 1969, p 234.)

Pathology of Laryngeal Tuberculosis. The initial phase of laryngeal involvement is an exudative reaction characterized by diffuse mucosal edema, hyperemia, and cellular infiltration. This is felt to represent an allergic reaction to the tubercle bacillus. The cellular infiltration is predominantly lymphocytic and is soon followed by tubercle formation (Fig. 13–6), giving a granular appearance to the mucosa. Confluence of the tubercles leads to necrosis and ulceration of the overlying epithelium.[21, 22, 24, 27]

The early lesions of tuberculous laryngitis most frequently involve the true vocal cords and posterior commissure (Fig. 13–7). In untreated patients or in the absence of adequate host resistance, the disease later spreads to

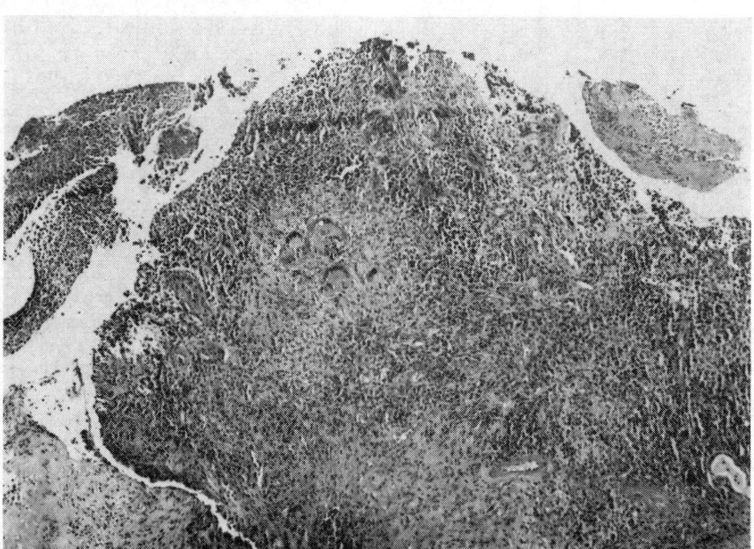

Figure 13–6. Tuberculosis of the larynx; biopsy from true vocal cord. A chronic granulomatous reaction with multinucleate giant cells is present. Special stains and cultures for acid-fast bacilli were positive. (H&E, × 100).

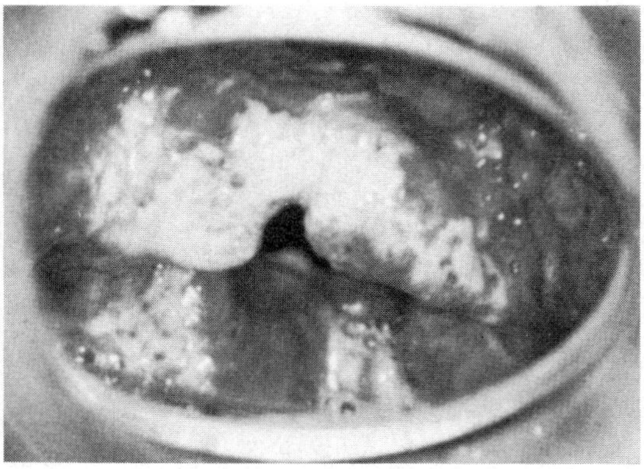

Figure 13–8. Ulcerative laryngeal tuberculosis. (From Becker W (ed): Atlas of Otorhinolaryngology and Bronchoesophagology. Philadelphia, WB Saunders Company, 1969, p 235.)

involve other areas such as the epiglottis, false cords, and aryepiglottic folds (Fig. 13–8). Involvement of the postcricoid and subglottic areas, however, is much less common. The initial mucosal ulceration may be followed by granuloma or tuberculoma formation.

According to Myerson, cartilage necrosis rarely occurs, but perichondritis is frequently seen in advanced tuberculous laryngitis.[22] In lesions with the capacity to heal, this leads to distortion of the epiglottis and fixation of the cricoarytenoid joints. Surprisingly, however, significant upper airway obstruction in tuberculous laryngitis is rarely seen.[21, 22]

Concomitant presentation of mucosal lesions in other areas is also occasionally seen. Myerson reported a 5 per cent incidence of simultaneous tuberculous lesions involving the oral cavity and pharynx and a 2.5 per cent incidence of middle ear and mastoid disease.[22] Interestingly enough, Auerbach found an 88.1 per cent incidence of intestinal tuberculous involvement in 811 tuberculosis autopsy cases.[25]

Symptoms and Diagnosis of Laryngeal Tuberculosis. The commonest symptoms associated with laryngeal tuberculosis are hoarseness and odynophagia. Cough, weight loss, fever, night sweats, and other systemic symptoms are also frequently present and are usually secondary to active pulmonary disease. Hemoptysis, referred otalgia, and (rarely) stridor may be present. The lesions in the larynx are in no way specific, either in appearance or location, and the early diagnosis of laryngeal tuberculosis rests primarily on a high index of suspicion. The presence of a normal chest x-ray makes the diagnosis unlikely.

The differential diagnosis includes carcinoma and other chronic granulomas such as fungal infections, lethal midline granuloma, and Wegener's granuloma. Although the majority of patients with active laryngeal tuberculosis will have positive tuberculin skin tests and sputum smears and cultures that are positive for *Mycobacterium tuberculosis,* specific confirmation of laryngeal involvement depends on the ability to demonstrate acid-fast organisms or typical caseating granulomas in biopsy material.

Treatment of Laryngeal Tuberculosis. Treatment consists essentially of antituberculous drugs. Rohwedder reports that in the presence of upper airway involvement, a longer time is needed for sputum conversion[24]; however, clinical and chest roentgenographic improvement can generally be expected within two to four weeks. Rarely, in the event of airway obstruction, surgical intervention may be indicated for airway diversion or correction of late deformities.

Scleroma. Rhinoscleroma is a chronic granulomatous infection caused by the bacterium *Klebsiella rhinoscleromatis.* Although rarely seen in North America and the United Kingdom, the disease is endemic in certain parts of Europe, the Middle East, Far East, Central America, and South America. Nasal obstruction and deformity due to large granulomatous masses are the usual presenting features in the vast majority of patients with this disease. Laryngeal involvement is allegedly rare, although Acuna reported a 15 per cent incidence in a series of patients from Mexico City.[28] Granulomatous nodules may be present in the larynx, leading to hoarseness and, occasionally, airway obstruction. Induration and distortion with rigid

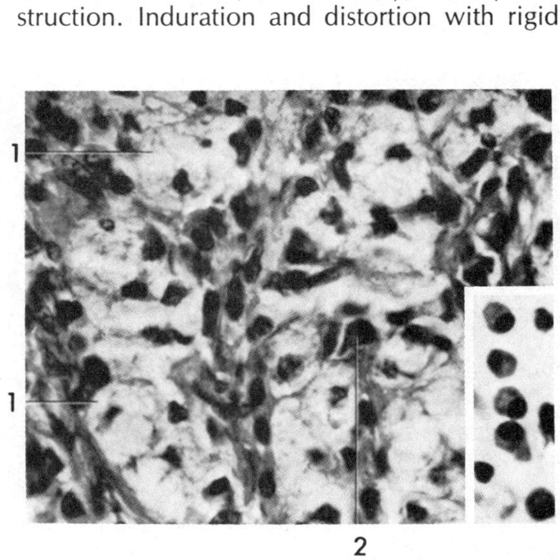

Figure 13–9. Rhinoscleroma involving the larynx. The high-power photomicrograph shows Mikulicz's cells with clear cytoplasm *(1)* and plasma cells *(2).* (From Becker W (ed): Atlas of Otorhinolaryngology and Bronchoesophagology. Philadelphia, WB Saunders Company 1969, p 237.)

stenosis may occur. Associated stenotic lesions in the trachea are also commonly seen. Histologically, the granulomatous lesions contain characteristic large Mikulicz's cells (as seen in Fig. 13–9), Russell's bodies, and gram-negative bacilli.[1, 28, 29] Recommended medical treatment for the laryngotracheal lesions consists of prolonged courses of streptomycin sulfate in conjunction with any of the tetracycline drugs.

Syphilis.[1, 2] Luetic infection of the larynx is now rarely seen. In the secondary stage of the disease, the laryngeal manifestations include diffuse hyperemia and mucous patches similar to those seen on the buccal mucosa. The lesions usually clear within a couple of weeks with or without treatment. Tertiary syphilitic involvement is evident as shaggy, undermined ulcers or gumma formation. Perichondritis, chondritis, and chondronecrosis are late sequelae with subsequent fibrosis, stenosis, and distortion of the larynx.[30] The lesions in congenital syphilis appear in early childhood and are similar to those seen in the tertiary acquired disease. Symptoms include hoarseness, referred otalgia, and occasionally hemoptysis. In the preantibiotic era, surgical intervention was frequently necessary for the relief of upper airway obstruction. The advent of penicillin, however, has relegated syphilis of the larynx almost to obscurity.

Leprosy. Leprosy involving the larynx is also rarely seen. Jackson and Jackson estimated that laryngeal involvement occurs in approximately 10 per cent of patients with tuberculoid leprosy and even less commonly in the lepromatous variety.[2] The lesions are clinically indistinguishable from those of tuberculosis and syphilis. Scarring and distortion of the larynx may occur in the late stages of the disease.

Miscellaneous Granulomatous Infections. Laryngeal involvement has also been reported in granuloma inguinale, yaws, lymphogranuloma venereum,[31] and mucocutaneous leishmaniasis.[32] The latter condition may be mistaken for histoplasma infection as the organisms look much alike with routine staining techniques. These conditions are extremely rare and would obviously present great difficulty in diagnosis.

Mycotic Infections. Fungal infections of the larynx are uncommon and thus are apt to be misdiagnosed for long periods. In recent years, greater awareness of these disorders has resulted in more frequent recognition and, hence, should certainly lead to their inclusion in the differential diagnosis of any chronic nontuberculous granuloma of the larynx. Demonstration of the fungal elements is often difficult and repeated biopsies may be necessary before specific confirmation can be achieved.

Histoplasmosis. *Histoplasma capsulatum* is a deep mycosis of worldwide distribution, occurring endemically in such areas as the Ohio valley and the Mississippi and Missouri valleys in the United States. The fungus exists in mycelial and yeastlike forms, the latter being pathogenic. It is estimated that approximately 31 million Americans have at some time been infected by this organism, as evidenced by pulmonary calcification and cutaneous hypersensitivity.[33] In contradistinction to this benign form, the disease may occur, much less commonly, as a disseminated extrapulmonary form involving most frequently the liver, spleen, bone marrow, and adrenals. Mucosal lesions involving the oral cavity, pharynx, and larynx are being reported with increased frequency and are generally felt to represent manifestations of the disseminated form of the disease rather than primary infections.[33–40]

In most cases, the laryngeal lesions of *H. capsulatum* are grossly indistinguishable from tuberculosis and consist of edema, erythema, nodular thickening, and ulceration.[34, 41] Fixation of the vocal cord has also been described.[35] In contrast to tuberculosis, however, early lesions often have a predilection for the anterior portion of the larynx, especially the epiglottis, and associated oral and oropharyngeal involvement is commonly seen. The microscopic apperance of the lesions is variable and appears to be somewhat dependent on host immunity, with definite granulomas being seen in the localized and the chronic disseminated forms of the disease. In these situations, organisms may be difficult to demonstrate, whereas in the acute disseminated form or in the presence of anergy (for example, lymphoma, immunosuppression), there may be primarily a histiocytic response with preponderance of organisms (Fig. 13–10, A and B).

Histoplasmosis should be considered in the differential diagnosis of any chronic laryngeal inflammation, particularly if ulcerogranular lesions of the oral cavity and oropharynx coexist. Specific confirmation rests with demonstration of the organisms on tissue staining (methenamine-silver) or culture (Sabouraud's medium). Occasionally, organisms may also be identifiable in sputum samples. In the chronic form of the disease, organisms may be difficult to demonstrate, but circumstantial evidence can be provided by positive skin tests, complement fixation tests, or chest x-ray abnormalities. Sub-

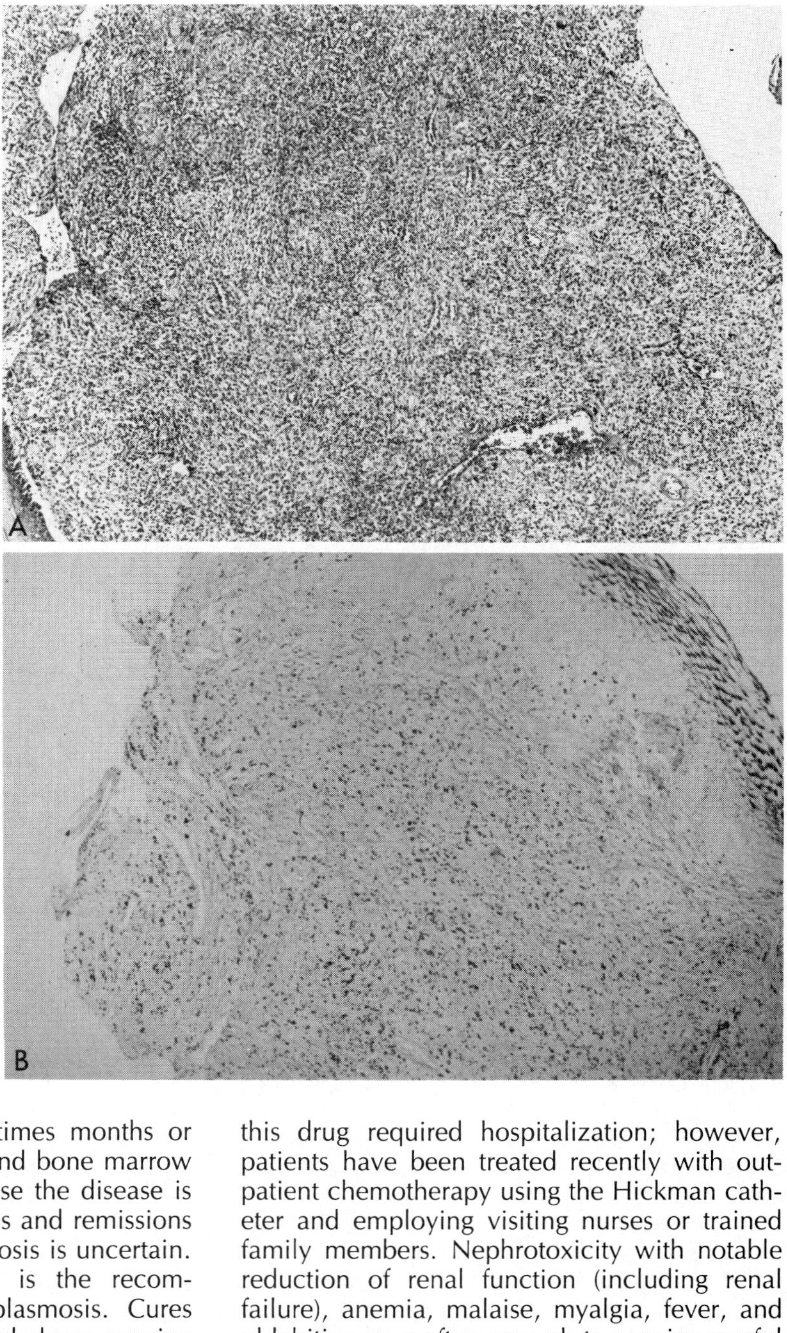

Figure 13–10. Histoplasmosis of the larynx. *A,* Vocal cord biopsy showing chronic granulomatous inflammation with occasional giant cells (H&E, × 100). *B,* Methenamine-silver stain positive for fungal organisms (× 100).

sequent dissemination, sometimes months or years later, to liver, spleen, and bone marrow is reported commonly. Because the disease is characterized by exacerbations and remissions regardless of treatment, prognosis is uncertain. Amphotericin B (Fungizone) is the recommended treatment for histoplasmosis. Cures have been recorded with total doses ranging from 950 to 5000 mg.[40]

Amphotericin B is currently the best available drug for treating histoplasmosis and all the other laryngeal fungal infections. This drug is the standard with which all new drugs are compared, but its use has serious disadvantages. Although usually quite active, amphotericin B is cumbersome to administer, expensive, and highly toxic. Administration usually consists of 30 mg to 50 mg doses given to the patient for 4 to 6 hours daily. In the past, treatment with this drug required hospitalization; however, patients have been treated recently with outpatient chemotherapy using the Hickman catheter and employing visiting nurses or trained family members. Nephrotoxicity with notable reduction of renal function (including renal failure), anemia, malaise, myalgia, fever, and phlebitis occur often enough to require careful monitoring for the development of these complications.

In 1981, ketoconazole (Nizoral) was introduced in the United States. Ketoconazole is the first of a series of imidazoles with broad antifungal activity. Although fungistatic, it is still quite active against disseminated histoplasmosis, mucosal and visceral candidiasis, and mucocutaneous candidiasis. The results are less positive, although encouraging, against coccidioidomycosis, blastomycosis, and cryptococcosis. Ketoconazole is absorbable orally and has minimal toxicity when administered in lower dosage ranges (400 mg) daily. The drug should be administered with a meal (preferably breakfast). Because an acid pH is required for absorption, antacids or H_2 antagonists (e.g., cimetidine) should not be given in conjunction with ketoconazole. Measurements of serum concentrations will determine absorption of the compound and guide the physician in adjusting the total daily dosage.

The principal adverse effects of ketaconazole—anorexia, metallic taste, mild gastrointestinal distress, nausea, and abdominal cramps—affect a small percentage of patients. These problems are usually mild and easily tolerated, especially when compared with the universal toxicity of amphotericin B. Hepatotoxicity, usually only elevations of hepatic enyzmes, has been reported in approximately 1 per cent of patients receiving prolonged treatment or higher dosages. These patients should be monitored for hepatotoxicity. Discretion is suggested when ketoconazole is given to individuals with liver disease or to those receiving other potentially hepatotoxic drugs. At higher doses (usually 800 mg or higher), ketoconazole may diminish testosterone synthesis and may blunt adrenal steroid synthesis, resulting in feminization (impotence, gynecomastia) or potential adrenal insufficiency. Despite these minor disadvantages, ketoconazole is a useful compound that allows prolonged oral outpatient treatment with reduced risk of toxicity. Optimal dosage and duration have not been determined.

Candidiasis. Laryngeal candidiasis, though uncommon, occasionally occurs in association with thrush infection of the oral cavity and pharynx. The fungus, *Candida albicans,* although essentially a saprophyte, may assume a pathogenic role—usually in the presence of debilitating disease, immunoincompetence, or diabetes, or after prolonged usage of antibiotics, corticosteroids, or immunosuppressives. Laryngotracheobronchial infection has also been related to the prolonged use of corticosteroid aerosols. The changes occurring in the larynx include edema and erythema of the mucosa with the appearance of a grayish-white exudate and adherent pseudomembrane. The epithelium is friable and bleeds easily. Biopsy reveals superficial ulceration of the mucosa with chronic inflammatory cells and reactive hyperplasia or hyperkeratosis.[42] The organism is usually easily demonstrated on biopsy, scrapings, or culture. Treatment is with nystatin (Mycostatin, Nilstat), or amphotericin B in resistant cases.

Flucytosine (5-fluorocytosine, Ancobon) is an orally administered, fungistatic antimetabolite that is quite active against *Cryptococcus neoformans* and some *Candida* species. Its activity against *Candida* organisms is unpredictable. Administered in daily doses of 150 mg per kg, flucytosine achieves excellent penetration of tissue and cerebrospinal fluid. Unfortunately, when flucytosine is used as the sole therapeutic agent, cryptococci and other fungi develop resistance rapidly, thus precluding this drug's exclusive use for these serious infections. Fortunately, flucytosine is synergistic with amphotericin B; this combination permits both lower dosage and shorter duration of therapy, thereby delaying emergence of resistance.

Aerosolized nystatin has been valuable for patients with upper airway candidiasis who do not respond to or absorb ketoconazole. This novel and largely unreported form of therapy is achieved by placing 100,000 to 200,000 units of nystatin powder and 4 ml water in a nebulizer (e.g., Bird, De Vilbis) and administering by aerosol inhalation every four to six hours. The patient's response dictates duration of therapy.

Paracoccidioidomycosis. The causative organism of paracoccidioidomycosis (South American blastomycosis) is *Paracoccidioides brasiliensis,* a deep mycosis endemic to South and Central America. The disease usually manifests itself with complaints referable to the lower respiratory tract, the skin, or the mucous membranes of the mouth, pharynx, and larynx. In fact, laryngeal involvement has been reported to be as high as 41 per cent and Stachowsky noted 21 cases of laryngeal infestation in 45 patients with involvement of the ear, nose, and throat regions.[43] It is uncertain whether laryngeal implantation occurs primarily or if it is secondary to pulmonary disease. At any rate, most patients manifest evidence of pulmonary infestation.

The laryngeal lesions appear as ulcerations or vegetations with induration of the underlying tissues. Associated tracheal involvement is often present, with occasional stricture formation.[44] Diagnostic confirmation is obtained by identification of the organisms in biopsy specimens, scrapings, or sputum smears. Serologic and skin tests may provide additional substantiation. Treatment consists of prolonged courses of sulfonamides and amphotericin B.[45]

Coccidioidomycosis. *Coccidioides immitis* is an imperfect fungus occurring endemically in the southwestern United States, particularly the San Joaquin valley in southern California. Primary infections occur commonly and are manifested by mild respiratory illnesses and cutaneous hypersensitivity. The disseminated form of the disease, however, is rare. Until 1977, there appeared in the literature only seven cases of laryngeal involvement. The lesions described have been mainly either heaped-up fungating granulomas or areas of granularity and ulceration that are clinically indistinguishable from tuberculosis or any other chronic granuloma.[46–48]

Ward et al. also described a case of subglottic stenosis due to coccidioidomycosis of the larynx in an infant four and one-half months old. Diagnostic confirmation depends on demonstration of the fungus on biopsy specimens, and clearing of the lesions has been reported after prolonged treatment with amphotericin B.

Miscellaneous Mycotic Infections. Laryngeal involvement by *Blastomyces dermatitidis* (North American blastomycosis)[49, 50] and *Actinomyces israelii* has also been reported and is worthy of mention. Microabscess formation has been frequently described in blastomycosis, in addition to fibrosis, stenosis, fistula formation, and the usual chronic granulomatous inflammation. Cervicofacial actinomycosis with laryngeal involvement occurs but is very rare. Brawny induration of the surrounding tissues and the existence of multiple draining sinuses may raise suspicion as to its presence. Finally, isolated reports of laryngeal infection with *Cryptococcus neoformans* (*Torula histolytica*), *Rhinosporidium seeberi,* and *Aspergillus niger* have also appeared in medical literature.

LARYNGEAL EDEMA

Laryngeal edema may be acute or chronic and, depending on its severity, presents as hoarseness with or without upper airway obstruction. Airway compromise requiring intubation or tracheostomy is more likely to ensue in infants and children than in adults, because of the smaller dimensions of the larynx. In neonates, in fact, it has been estimated that 1 mm of swelling of the mucosa at the glottic inlet produces approximately 65 per cent narrowing of the upper airway. Furthermore, it is in the subglottic area, because of the limitations imposed by the cricoid ring and conus elasticus, that the effects of mucosal edema become most apparent. The causes of laryngeal edema include both local and systemic problems,[53] some of which are listed in Table 13–2.

In the noninfectious forms, the laryngeal mucosa appears pale and boggy, with swelling most apparent in the loose tissues overlying the epiglottis, aryepiglottic folds, and arytenoids. The vocal cords appear boggy and edematous because of extravasation of fluid into Reinke's space. In the presence of infection, the mucosa, however, assumes a reddened hyperemic appearance.[9] Compromise of the endolaryngeal airway may be apparent, depending on the degree of swelling.

Table 13–2. CAUSES OF LARYNGEAL EDEMA

Trauma
External trauma
Intubation
Noxious inhalation
Infection
Allergy
Neoplastic disease
Metabolic dysfunction
Radiotherapy
Hemodynamic dysfunction
Venous obstruction
Lymphatic obstruction
Increased capillary permeability (e.g., anaphylaxis, angioedema, collagen disease)

The treatment of laryngeal edema varies with the underlying cause. Epinephrine (Adrenalin chloride solution, epinephrine HCl ampul, Sus-Phrine), antihistamines, and corticosteroids are usually effective in the allergic laryngeal edema and some forms of angioneurotic edema. Racemic epinephrine (Vaponefrin solution), administered by nebulization, has also been used effectively in acute laryngotracheobronchitis in children. Dexamethasone, a powerful glucocorticoid, when given intravenously in large doses (0.5 mg to 1 mg per kg) appears also to be of benefit in the treatment of acute edema secondary to intubation, trauma, and laryngotracheobronchitis. Adjunctive measures such as hydration, inhalations, and antibiotics are recommended, if indicated.

Angioneurotic edema may involve the larynx, producing sudden and severe upper airway obstruction[54] (Fig. 13–11). This interesting disease has recently been elucidated and manifests itself in these four distinct categories:

1. Hereditary angioneurotic edema.
2. Hereditary allergic angioneurotic edema.
3. Nonhereditary allergic angioneurotic edema.
4. Nonhereditary angioneurotic edema of unknown cause.

Hereditary angioneurotic edema is transmitted as an autosomal dominant and is due to a deficiency in the inhibition of the activated first component of complement (C1 esterase) or a deficiency of C2 or C4 substrates of C1 esterase. The disease is manifested as episodic angio-

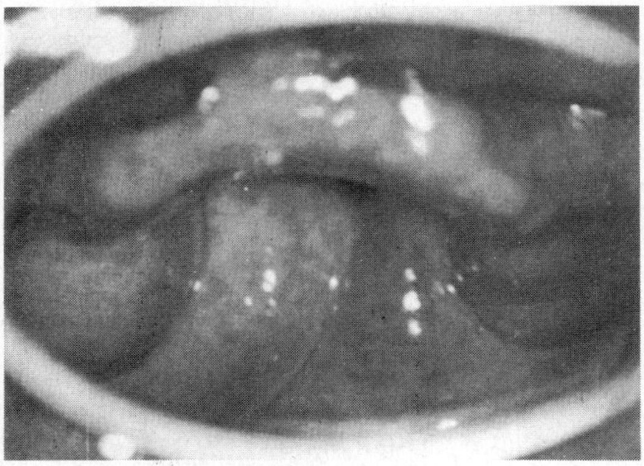

Figure 13–11. Angioneurotic edema of the larynx. Edema of the epiglottis, the aryepiglottic folds, and particularly the arytenoids prevents visualization of the cords. (From Becker W (ed): Atlas of Otorhinolaryngology and Bronchoesophagology. Philadelphia, WB Saunders Company, 1969, p 223.)

edema involving the skin, gastrointestinal tract, and the upper respiratory tract. Exacerbations may be precipitated by trauma and stress such as surgery. Antihistamines, epinephrine, and corticosteroids are often ineffective, but the exacerbations have responded to treatment with aminocaproic acid (Amicar) and tranexamic acid, which can be administered during an acute episode or prophylactically.[55] The mortality from acute airway obstruction in patients with this form of the disease is high. The other variants of angioedema are characterized by the ability to demonstrate an inciting antigen in the allergic types of edema and by the response to epinephrine or antihistamine therapy.

Treatment of other forms of laryngeal edema is largely related to control of the underlying causes, if possible. The necessity for tracheostomy or endotracheal intubation will be dictated by the degree of airway compromise; thus, careful monitoring of the situation is indicated.

CRICOARYTENOID ARTHRITIS

The cricoarytenoid joint is a diarthrodial articulation subject to involvement by local and systemic diseases. Some of the former have already been alluded to in the section devoted to chronic infections of the larynx. Cricoarytenoid arthritis has been described in patients with rheumatoid arthritis,[56–58] ankylosing spondylitis,[59] Tietze's syndrome,[60] mumps,[61] and collagen vascular diseases.[61] Acute symptoms usually include hoarseness, referred otalgia, odynophagia, and a feeling of fullness in the throat. Redness and swelling over the arytenoid cartilage may be evident on indirect laryngoscopy, with decreased mobility of the vocal cord. Frequently, pain may be elicited by palpation over the posterior aspect of the thyroid ala. In a clinicopathologic study of the joint in patients with rheumatoid arthritis, Bienstock found evidence of synovial inflammation, pannus formation, and destruction of articular cartilage. In his series, seven of eight postmortem examinations showed evidence of cricoarytenoid joint involvement.[56] Similarly, Grossman et al. found rheumatoid disease of the joint in five of eleven patients with rheumatoid arthritis on whom autopsies had been performed.[62]

Acute involvement of the cricoarytenoid joint in rheumatoid arthritis or ankylosing spondylitis responds symptomatically to anti-inflammatory agents such as aspirin, phenylbutazone (Azolid, Azolid-A, Butazolidin, Butazolidin alka), or corticosteroids. Intra-articular corticosteroid injections have also been used.[63] Continuation of the disease process may, however, lead to eventual ankylosis of the joint with vocal cord fixation.

PERICHONDRITIS AND CHONDRITIS

Perichondritis and chondritis of the laryngeal cartilages may occur secondarily to a wide variety of causes, some of which are listed in Table 13–3.

In the past, these problems were fairly frequently seen and were most often associated with typhoid fever, diphtheria, and tuberculosis. In 1938, however, Jackson observed a marked reduction in the occurrence of perichondritis of the larynx and attributed this phenomenon largely to improvements in preventive medicine and control of communicable diseases.[64] Florid perichondritis with abscess formation, chondritis, and chondronecrosis, as

Table 13–3. CAUSES OF PERICHONDRITIS AND CHONDRITIS OF THE LARYNX

Trauma
External
Penetrating injury
Surgery
High tracheostomy
Internal
Intubation
Nasogastric tube
Infection
Acute (e.g., typhoid, streptococcus, diphtheria)
Chronic (e.g., tuberculosis, syphilis)
Malignancy
Radiation therapy
Relapsing polychondritis

described earlier in this century, are thus rarely seen today; however, the circumscribed or localized forms are still encountered occasionally, usually in association with radiotherapy to the larynx, external laryngeal surgery, penetrating trauma, or malignancy.[65, 66]

Laryngeal perichondritis may be diffuse or localized. The former is characterized by hoarseness, neck pain, dysphagia, and odynophagia. The endolarynx is erythematous and swollen, which often leads to airway obstruction. Cord fixation is also frequently seen. External swelling and tenderness over the larynx is usually evident. Abscess formation may also occur in untreated cases. In the localized form of perichondritis, the clinical features are less florid and may be manifested only as localized areas of thickening and tenderness over the laryngeal skeleton. Cartilage necrosis may occur; it was frequently seen in the preantibiotic era. The sequelae of this complication are distortion of the laryngeal architecture, stenosis, cord fixation, and draining sinuses. Occurrence of mediastinitis may be secondary to descending infection.

If recognized early, laryngeal perichondritis may respond to specific antibiotic therapy. Surgical intervention, however, may be necessary for airway diversion, drainage of abscess or necrotic cartilage, or for the correction of residual deformities such as stenosis or cord fixation. Following heavy tumoricidal doses of radiotherapy to the larynx, however, the occurrence of these complications is frequently met with unsuccessful attempts at conservative management. The necessity for total laryngectomy is the usual outcome.[66]

MISCELLANEOUS SYSTEMIC DISEASES WITH LARYNGEAL INVOLVEMENT

Hypothyroidism. Laryngeal involvement in hypothyroidism appears early in the course of the disease and is characterized by the accumulation of acid mucopolysaccharides in the submucosa of the true and false vocal cords, similar to that seen in other parts of the body.[67, 68] Early laryngeal symptoms include reduction in vocal strength, as evidenced by difficulty in maintaining pitch, and a reduction in phonation time. Occasionally, a dry cough may be present. This is followed by frank hoarseness, and the voice assumes a low-pitched, coarse, brassy quality that is almost characteristic of the disease. Gross changes in the vocal cords later become evident, and edema or polypoid thickening may appear. Not uncommonly, however, the degree of voice change appears disproportionate to the macroscopic changes evident on laryngoscopy. The treatment is essentially that of the underlying hypothyroid state.

Miscellaneous Endocrine Disorders. Disturbances in the growth and maturation of the larynx may result from prepubertal hormonal imbalances involving the pituitary, thyroid, adrenals, testes, or ovaries.[69, 70] Despite obvious abnormalities in the voice, more often than not laryngoscopic examination is unremarkable. A comparative decrease in the laryngeal dimensions may be evident, however. As occasionally occurs in the pituitary giant or acromegalic patient, marked overgrowth of the laryngeal cartilages and soft tissues may occur.[71]

Changes in vocal quality also have been described in hyperthyroidism, parathyroid deficiency, hyperparathyroidism, hypoadrenalism, Cushing's disease, and pituitary, ovarian, or testicular hypogenitalism. Little data on the pathologic changes occurring in these patients are available, however, and abnormalities in laryngeal function have been mainly attributed to neuromuscular disturbances, impaired development, or infiltrative and edematous changes in the laryngeal soft tissues.[70]

Variations in vocal quality during the premenstrual period, pregnancy, and menopause and following the administration of oral contraceptives have also been observed in female patients.[72, 73]

Sarcoidosis. Lesions of the upper airway in sarcoidosis are relatively uncommon and are most frequently seen involving the nasal mucosa.[74] Associated skin lesions in these patients are usually present. Laryngeal involvement is estimated to occur in approximately 1 per cent of all cases of sarcoidosis[75] and appears as diffuse thickening or edema of the epiglottis (Fig. 13–12), granulomatous masses, or infiltrative and nodular lesions on the epiglottis, false cords, and aryepiglottic folds.[74, 76, 77] Mucosal ulcerations, subglottic granulomas, and laryngeal stenosis due to late contraction and scarring have also been described. Although airway obstruction has been reported, the lesions are usually asymptomatic or productive of hoarseness by true vocal cord involvement.[74, 78, 79] Recurrent laryngeal nerve palsy is also occasionally seen. Invariably, the laryngeal lesions appear in patients with established, long-standing disease rather than as a presenting manifestation of sarcoidosis.

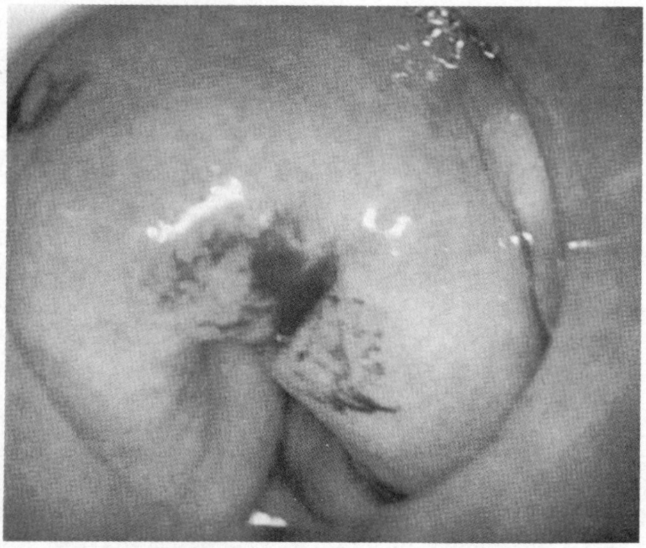

Figure 13–12. Boeck's sarcoid of the epiglottis. Diffuse swelling and tubelike involution of the epiglottis. (From Kleinsasser O: Microlaryngoscopy and Endolaryngeal Microsurgery. Philadelphia, WB Saunders Company, 1968, p 79.)

The diagnosis of sarcoidosis is confirmed by the histologic appearance of the endolaryngeal lesions and by the exclusion of other chronic noncaseating granulomas, as their gross appearance is nonspecific. Administration of large doses of corticosteroids appears to be beneficial and has been effective in averting tracheostomy in some instances. Endoscopic removal of granulomas, however, may be necessary for the treatment of hoarseness or upper airway obstruction.

Amyloidosis. Amyloid deposits may occur in the larynx in diffuse or localized forms. The diffuse variety is quite rare and is associated with primary or secondary generalized amyloidosis.[80] Usually, there are no specific symptoms referable to the larynx in these situations. Localized amyloid deposits occur most commonly in the upper respiratory tract and, although also rare, are being reported with increasing frequency.[81] Lesions in the larynx appear as distinct nodular masses or subepithelial deposits (Fig. 13–13) and may produce hoarseness or airway obstruction necessitating endoscopic removal. It should be mentioned that, occasionally, massive hyalinization in laryngeal polyps may be mistaken for localized amyloid deposits, because the appearance on staining with hematoxylin and eosin is similar. The presence of amyloid, however, may be differentiated by special staining techniques. If generalized amyloidosis is suspected, rectal or renal biopsy is indicated.

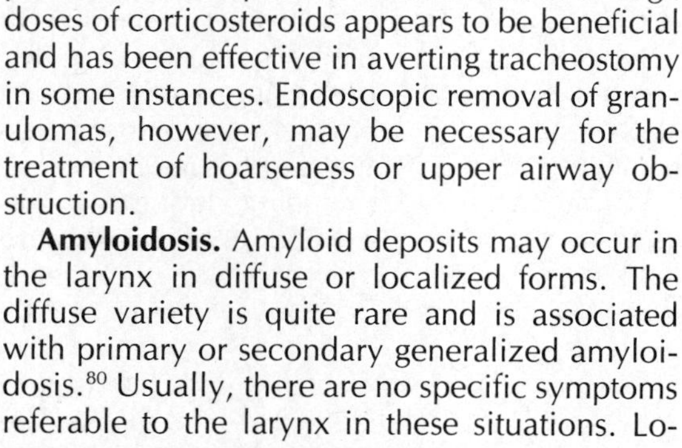

Figure 13–13. Amyloid disease of the larynx. A deposit of the hyaline stage of amyloid is shown consisting of compact amorphous eosinophilic material beneath the ciliated surface epithelium. Numerous inflammatory cells, chiefly lymphocytes, surround the amyloid (From Becker W (ed): Atlas of Otorhinolaryngology and Bronchoesophagology. Philadelphia, WB Saunders Company, 1969, p 239.)

Systemic Lupus Erythematosus. The frequency of laryngeal involvement in systemic lupus erythematosus is unknown but may be as high as 33 per cent.[82] A wide spectrum of lesions has been reported in the medical literature and includes acute epiglottitis, acute laryngitis, laryngitis sicca, chronic hyperplastic laryngitis, ulceration, edema, perichondritis, hemorrhagic bullae, cricoarytenoid arthritis, and vocal cord palsy. Sinclair et al. also reported a case of an isolated vocal cord granulomatous nodule secondary to systemic lupus erythematosus.[83] Occasionally, respiratory tract obstruction may occur. Treatment is essentially that of the underlying disease.

Pemphigus and Pemphigoid. Pemphigus is a disorder of unknown etiology affecting skin and mucous membranes of the upper aerodigestive tract, vagina, and conjunctiva. Not uncommonly, mucosal involvement may precede the onset of skin lesions, although generalized skin eruptions usually become evident within about six months. The unmistakable histologic feature of the disease is the appearance of intraepithelial vesicles and bullae in skin and mucous membranes with separation of the more superficial layers from the basal cell layer.[84] Acantholytic cells may be demonstrated in cytologic smears of the vesicle fluid. The presence of tissue-fixed or circulating antibodies can be demonstrated by immunofluorescent techniques.

Laryngeal lesions, when present, occur usually in association with oral and pharyngeal involvement. Symptoms include dysphagia, odynophagia, referred otalgia, cough, and occasionally hemoptysis.[85–87] Bullous eruptions are usually short lived and often not seen. Rupture of the vesicles and denudation of the lining reveal shallow superficial ulcerations covered by a shaggy membrane or slough (Fig. 13–14). Scarring of the larynx with distortion and stenosis may occur in the healing phase of the disease. The diagnosis is confirmed by biopsy, cytology, or serologic and histologic immunofluorescent studies.

Benign mucous membrane pemphigoid and bullous pemphigoid are thought to be variants of the same disease, as their clinical and histologic manifestations are somewhat similar. Both differ from pemphigus, however, in that the vesicles and bullae are subepithelial rather than intraepithelial. Bullous pemphigoid predominantly affects skin, and mucous membrane involvement occurs only in approximately 15 per cent of cases.[88] Benign mucous membrane pemphigoid, on the other hand, rarely involves skin, but conjunctival involvement is common. Dysphagia and odynophagia may occur because of oral and pharyngeal involvement. Severe scarring resulting in pharyngeal and laryngeal stenosis may later occur.

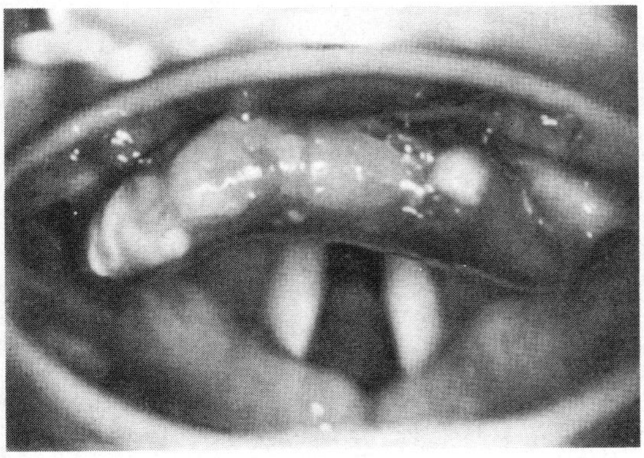

Figure 13–14. Pemphigus of the epiglottis. Ulcerative lesions involving the tip of the epiglottis are present. (From Becker W (ed): Atlas of Otorhinolaryngology and Bronchoesophagology. Philadelphia, WB Saunders Company 1969, p 233.)

The treatment of pemphigus has been revolutionized since the introduction of corticosteroids. Lever (1953) recommended prednisone (180 to 240 mg per day) in moderate to severe cases.[84] More recently, adjuvant immunosuppressive therapy with methotrexate or cyclophosphamide (Cytoxan) has been used effectively in an attempt to reduce the dosage of steroids and thereby avoid the side effects of such high doses.[89] Bullous pemphigoid and benign mucous membrane pemphigoid are both much more benign conditions than pemphigus, and response can usually be achieved with lower steroid doses.

Pemphigus and pemphigoid must be differentiated from other vesicular eruptions that affect the oral cavity and that may, on occasion, involve the larynx. To be considered in the differential diagnosis are herpes simplex, herpes zoster, erythema multiforme, bullous lichen planus, varicella, and epidermolysis bullosa.

Nonhealing Granulomas. McBride's original report in 1897 of a case of relentless, ulcerative midline destruction of the face initiated interest in a group of disorders characterized by granulomatous ulceration of the upper respiratory tract. They continue to be surrounded by controversy to the present time. Detailed descriptions of the so-called lethal midline granuloma (LMG) of the face were further provided by Stewart in 1933. In 1936, Wegener reported on the occurrence of systemic manifestations associated with similar upper respiratory tract lesions. Subsequently, it was felt that LMG represented a local manifestation of Wegener's granuloma.[90] More recently, however, histopathologic distinctions between LMG and Wegener's granulomatosis have been drawn, despite the similarities in clinical presentation. It is now also recognized that LMG may involve other sites such as the lower respiratory tract, lungs, kidney, gastrointestinal tract, and skin.

Wegener's granulomatosis, as classically described, constitutes a triad of necrotizing epithelioid granulomas of the upper and lower respiratory tracts, focal necrotizing glomerulonephritis, and systemic angiitis.[91, 92] Histologically, the mucosal lesions reveal extensive necrosis and ulceration with necrotizing vasculitis and thrombosis affecting small vessels, both arteries and veins. Multinucleate giant cells are usually easily identified (Fig. 13–15). McDonald et al. feel that Wegener's granuloma can be distinguished from LMG by the absence of epithelioid granulomas in the latter and de-

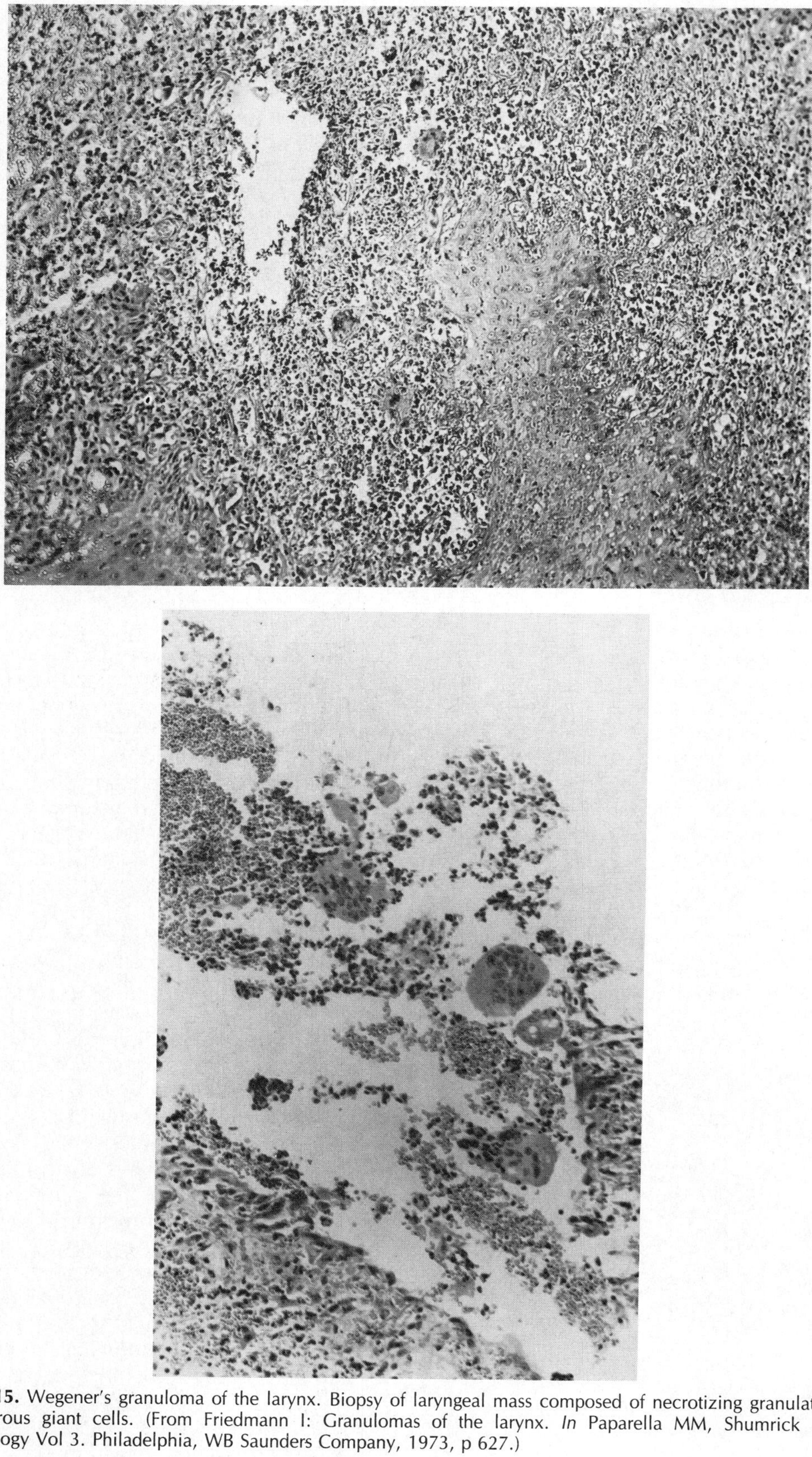

Figure 13–15. Wegener's granuloma of the larynx. Biopsy of laryngeal mass composed of necrotizing granulation tissue with numerous giant cells. (From Friedmann I: Granulomas of the larynx. *In* Paparella MM, Shumrick DA (eds): Otolaryngology Vol 3. Philadelphia, WB Saunders Company, 1973, p 627.)

scribed LMG as a "necrotizing atypical lymphoproliferative lesion" presenting characteristic angiocentric and angioinfiltrative growth patterns.[93] Occlusion or secondary thrombosis of small vessels occurs, leading to extensive necrosis (even more marked than in Wegener's granuloma), and affecting mucosa, submucosa, bone, cartilage, and skin. Renal lesions in LMG also differ from those seen in Wegener's granulomatosis by the absence of necrotizing glomerulitis.

Clinically, there is little to differentiate Wegener's granulomatosis from LMG. In both diseases, early symptoms are usually caused by nasal and paranasal sinus involvement, as evidenced by nasal obstruction, rhinorrhea, and painless progressive destruction of cartilage and facial bones. Laryngeal lesions appear as granulations and ulcerations with an apparent predilection for the subglottic area, although any site may be affected.[94] Subglottic stenosis has also been reported.

Laryngeal involvement invariably occurs in association with concomitant nasal and sinus disease. Pulmonary involvement is usually manifested by cough, hemoptysis, and chest pain with single or multiple nodules appearing in the lower lung fields, mimicking metastatic carcinoma. In both LMG and Wegener's granulomatosis, systemic complaints of fever, malaise, and weight loss are usually prominent, often apparently out of proportion to the severity of the presenting local disease.

The pathogenesis of nonhealing granulomas remains controversial. Aspects worth considering, however, are the possible relationships of Wegener's granulomatosis to periarteritis nodosa, giant cell arteritis, and other vascular hypersensitivity reactions.[29, 30, 95] LMG is considered by McDonald et al. to be an immunoproliferative process closely linked to malignant lymphoma. McDonald and his co-workers stress the importance of the histologic differentiation from Wegener's granulomatosis as the response of both diseases to various modalities of treatment appears to be different.[93] The question of whether LMG and Wegener's granulomatosis are distinct clinical entities, however, remains unanswered. Eichel and Mabery, in a review of 55 patients with an initial diagnosis of LMG, found that 48 patients were later reclassified under a different disease entity, either late in the course of their illness or at postmortem.[96] Similarly, Burston found that five of eleven cases initially diagnosed as LMG were subsequently reclassified.[97]

Although, in the past, a generally fatalistic outlook has usually been adopted for patients with LMG and Wegener's granulomatosis, it would now appear that some measure of success can be achieved with early diagnosis and treatment. The otolaryngologist should be alerted to any nonspecific upper respiratory tract granuloma, particularly if accompanied by marked constitutional symptoms. Repeated biopsies may be necessary, with the use of special stains and cultures to rule out other granulomatous lesions affecting the upper aerodigestive tract (Table 13–4). Hematologic studies such as complete blood count and smear, serum protein electrophoresis, immunoglobulin levels, rheumatoid factor, lupus erythematosus precipitation, and antinuclear antibodies as well as urinalysis and renal function studies should be carried out to exclude other disorders and to assess possible multifocal involvement. Chest and sinus x-rays are also essential. Corticosteroids and immunosuppressive agents have markedly improved the prognosis in patients with Wegener's granulomatosis and may be beneficial in mulitfocal LMG. Localized LMG, involving the upper respiratory tract, appears to respond best to radiation therapy, however.

Table 13–4. DIFFERENTIAL DIAGNOSIS OF GRANULOMATOUS LESIONS OF THE LARYNX

1. Infection
   - Mycobacterial disease (tuberculosis, leprosy)
   - Treponemal disease (syphilis, yaws)
   - Rhinoscleroma
   - Mycotic infection
   - Parasitic infection (leishmaniasis)
2. Sarcoidosis
3. Nonhealing granulomas
   - Lethal midline granuloma
   - Wegener's granuloma
   - Indeterminate type of granuloma
4. Miscellaneous lesions
   - Crohn's disease
   - Chronic granulomatous disease of childhood

Relapsing Polychondritis. Although fairly rare, relapsing polychondritis is of interest to the otolaryngologist because of the frequency of upper respiratory tract and audiovestibular involvement. First described by Jaksch-Wartenhorst in 1923, this disorder has an etiology as yet undetermined. Relapsing polychondritis most commonly presents with episodic arthritis and nonsuppurative inflammation of the auricular cartilages. The frequencies of various organ and structural involvement have been reported as follows: auricular chondritis 89 per cent, arthritis 81 per cent, nasal chondritis 72 per cent, ocular inflammation 65 per cent, respiratory tract chondritis 56 per cent, and audiovestibular damage 46 per cent. Vasculitis and cardiac involvement (including aortic insufficiency, mitral incompetence, and pericarditis) are also seen in 25 per cent of cases.[99] This disorder is characterized by episodic and progressive destruction of cartilaginous structures. Histologically, the basophilic cartilage matrix is replaced by eosinophilic material infiltrated by acute and chronic inflammatory cells. Chondritis is accompanied by perichondrial inflammation, chondronecrosis, and fibrosis.

Laryngotracheal involvement in relapsing polychondritis occurs in slightly more than half of all patients with this disorder and is felt to be the major cause of death. Clinical features include hoarseness and dysphagia with edema, erythema, and tenderness over the laryngeal cartilages. Airway obstruction requiring tracheostomy may occur, caused by laryngeal edema or stenosis. Long-term corticosteroids have mainly been used in the treatment of relapsing polychondritis, the dosage varying with the severity of the disease. Although corticosteroids are generally considered to be beneficial in alleviating acute symptoms, they do not appear to alter the process of progressive cartilage destruction nor to have much effect on the systemic vascular lesions. Anti-inflammatory agents such as salicylates and indomethacin (Indocin) are also useful in milder cases. Dapsone has also been used with excellent response.[98]

References

1. Ellis M: Chronic laryngitis. *In* Ballantyne J, Groves J (eds): Scott-Brown's Diseases of the Ear, Nose and Throat. Vol 4, 3rd ed. London, Butterworth and Co, 1971.
2. Jackson C, Jackson CL: Diseases of the Nose, Throat, and Ear. Philadelphia, WB Saunders Company, 1945.
3. Myerson NC: The Human Larynx. Springfield, Il, CC Thomas, 1964.
4. Kleinsasser O: Microlaryngoscopy and Endolaryngeal Microsurgery. Philadelphia, WB Saunders Company, 1968.
5. Schwartz L et al.: Hypertrophic changes in the interarytenoid space. Arch Otolaryngol 82:287–291, 1965.
6. Gabriel CE, Jones DG: The importance of chronic laryngitis. J Laryngol Otol 74:349–357, 1960.
7. Myerson MC: The smoker's larynx: A clinicopathologic entity. Ann Otol Rhinol Laryngol 59:541–546, 1950.
8. Ryan RF et al.: The pathologic effects of smoking on the larynx. Arch Pathol 60:472–480, 1955.
9. Pang LQ: Allergy of the larynx, trachea, and bronchial tree. Otolaryngol Clin North Am 7(3):719–734, 1974.
10. Williams RI: Allergic laryngitis. Ann Otol Rhinol Laryngol 81:558–565, 1972.
11. Stell PM, McLoughlin MP: The etiology of chronic laryngitis. Clin Otolaryngol 1:265–269, 1976.
12. Donner MW et al.: Acid barium swallow in the radiographic evaluation of clinical esophagitis. Radiology 87:220–225, 1966.
13. Delahunty JE: Acid laryngitis. J Laryngol Otol 86:335–342, 1972.
14. McGavran MH et al.: Isolated laryngeal keratosis: Its relation to carcinoma of the larynx based on a clinicopathologic study of 87 consecutive cases with long-term follow-up. Laryngoscope 70:932–951, 1960.
15. Holbrook A et al.: Treatment of vocal abuse disorders using a vocal intensity controller. J Speech Hear Disord 39:298–303, 1974.
16. Jackson C: Contact ulcers of the larynx. Ann Otol Rhinol Laryngol 37:227–230, 1928.
17. Holinger PH, Johnson KC: Contact ulcer of the larynx. JAMA 172(6):511–515, 1960.
18. Peacher G, Holinger P: Contact ulcer of the larynx. Arch Otolaryngol 46:617–623, 1947.
19. Peacher GM: Voice therapy for contact ulcer of the larynx: A follow-up of 70 cases. Laryngoscope 71:37–47, 1961.
20. Looper EA, Schneider LV: Laryngeal tuberculosis: Study of 500 patients treated at Maryland State Sanatorium from 1923 to 1928. JAMA 91:1012–1018, 1928.
21. Weidman WH, Campbell HB: Laryngeal tuberculosis. Am Rev Tuberc 40:85–98, 1939.
22. Myerson MC: TB of the Ear, Nose and Throat. Springfield, IL, CC Thomas, 1944.
23. Looper EA, Lyons IB: Laryngeal tuberculosis: Observations based on experience of 28 years with laryngeal tuberculosis. Ann Otol Rhinol Laryngol 57:754–768, 1948.
24. Rohwedder JJ: Upper respiratory tract tuberculosis: Sixteen cases in a general hospital. Ann Intern Med 80:708–713, 1974.
25. Auerbach O: Laryngeal tuberculosis. Arch Otolaryngol 44:191–201, 1946.
26. Lell WA: Laryngeal tuberculosis: Diagnosis, incidence, and present day treatment. Arch Otolaryngol 60:350–366, 1954.
27. Wilson G: Diagnosis and treatment of tuberculosis of the larynx and contiguous areas. Arch Otolaryngol 33:145–176, 1941.
28. Acuna RT: Endoscopy of the air passages with special references to scleroma. Ann Otol Rhinol Laryngol 82:765–769, 1973.
29. Friedmann I: The changing pattern of granulomas of the upper respiratory tract. J Laryngol Otol 85:631–682, 1971.
30. Friedmann I: Granulomas of the larynx. *In* Paparella MM, Shumrick DA (eds): Otolaryngology. Vol 3. Head and Neck. Philadelphia, WB Saunders Company, 1973, p 629.
31. Myerson MC: Lymphogranuloma venereum of the hypopharynx and larynx. JAMA 117:1877–1879, 1941.
32. Zinneman HH et al.: Leishmaniasis of the larynx: Report of a case and its confusion with histoplasmosis. Am J Med 31:654–658, 1961.
33. Reddy P et al.: Oral lesions as presenting manifestations of disseminated histoplasmosis: Report of 5 cases. Ann Otol Rhinol Laryngol 79:389–397, 1970.
34. Bennett DE: Histoplasmosis of the oral cavity and larynx: A clincopathologic study. Arch Intern Med 120:417–427, 1967.

35. Gambell EB, Breckenridge RL: Histoplasmosis of the upper respiratory tract. South Med J 59:1134–1138, 1966.
36. King HC, Cline JF: Histoplasmosis involving the larynx. Arch Otolaryngol 67:649–654, 1958.
37. Lyons GD: Mycotic lesions of the larynx. Ann Otol Rhinol Laryngol 75:162–175, 1966.
38. Pickard RE, Kotzen S: Histoplasmosis of the larynx. South Med J 66:1311–1313, 1973.
39. Roberts SE, Forman FS: Histoplasmosis—A deficiency disease: Report of 2 cases with laryngeal involvement. Ann Otol Rhinol Laryngol 58:809:822, 1950.
40. Smith JW, Utz JP: Progressive disseminated histoplasmosis: A prospective study of 26 patients. Ann Intern Med 76:557–565, 1972.
41. Owen RC et al.: Histoplasmosis of the upper respiratory tract. South Med J 59:1134–1138, 1966.
42. Tedeschi LG, Cheren R: Laryngeal hyperkeratosis due to primary monilial infection. Arch Otolaryngol 87:82–84, 1968.
43. Stachowsky L: Primary paracoccidioidomycosis of the larynx. Arch Otolaryngol 78:205–209, 1963.
44. Machado F et al.: Consideracoes relativas a blastomicose Sul-Americana da partipacao laringeia e bronquica em 104 casos-resultados endoscopicos. O Hospital 58:19, 1960.
45. Restrepo A et al.: Paracoccidioidomycosis (South American blastomycosis). Am J Trop Med Hyg 19: 68–76, 1970.
46. Oliver EA: Coccidioidomycosis with cutaneous involvement. Arch Dermatol Syphilol 70:537–538, 1954.
47. Platt MA: Laryngeal coccidioidomycosis. JAMA 237:1234–1235, 1977.
48. Ward PH et al.: Coccidioidomycosis of the larynx in infants and adults. Ann Otol Rhinol Laryngol 86:655–660, 1977.
49. Bennett M: Laryngeal blastomycosis. Laryngoscope 74:498–512, 1964.
50. Ferguson GB: North American blastomycosis: A review of the literature and a report of two cases primary in the larynx. Laryngoscope 61:851–873, 1951.
51. Pillai OS: Rhinosporidiosis of the larynx. J Laryngol Otol 88:277–280, 1974.
52. Ferlito A: Primary aspergillosis of the larynx. J Laryngol Otol 88:1257–1263, 1974.
53. Calcaterra TC: Laryngeal and pharyngeal edema of obscure origin. Arch Otolaryngol 96:341–345, 1972.
54. Michel R et al.: Angioneurotic edema: A review of modern concepts. Arch Otolaryngol 101:544–547, 1975.
55. Johns ME et al.: Hereditary angioneurotic edema: Treatment with epsilon-aminocaproic acid during surgery. Arch Otolaryngol 99:388–389, 1974.
56. Bienstock H et al.: Rheumatoid arthritis of the cricoarytenoid joint: A clinicopathologic study. Arthritis Rheum 6:48–63, 1963.
57. Montgomery W et al.: Arthritis of the cricoarytenoid joint. Ann Otol Rhinol Laryngol 64:1025–1036, 1955.
58. Polisar IA: The cricoarytenoid joint: A diarthrodial articulation subject to rheumatoid arthritic involvement. Laryngoscope 69:1129–1164, 1959.
59. Bienstock H, Lanyi VF: Cricoarytenoid arthritis in a patient with ankylosing spondylitis. Arch Otolaryngol 103:738–739, 1977.
60. Shambrom E, Feher A: Tietze's syndrome: Report of a case with laryngeal involvement. Arch Intern Med 96:697–699, 1955.
61. Bryer D, Rounthwaite FJ: Cricoarytenoid arthritis due to mumps. Laryngoscope 83:372–375, 1973.
62. Grossman A et al.: Rheumatoid arthritis of the cricoarytenoid joint. Proc Canad Otol Soc 14:40–54, 1960.
63. Habib MA: Intra-articular steroid injection in acute rheumatoid arthritis of the larynx. J Laryngol Otol 91:909–910, 1977.
64. Jackson C: Perichondritis of the larynx, traumatic and infective. Trans Am Laryngol Assoc 60:127–143, 1938.
65. Kashima HK, Holliday MJ: Laryngeal chondronecrosis: Clinical variations and comments on recognition and treatment. Trans Am Acad Ophthalmol Otolaryngol ORL 84:878–881, 1977.
66. Stell PM, Morrison MD: Radiation necrosis of the larynx. Arch Otolaryngol 98:111–113, 1973.
67. Bicknell P: Mild hypothyroidism and its effects on the larynx. J Laryngol Otol 87:123–127, 1973.
68. Ritter F: The effects of hypothyroidism on the larynx of the rat. Ann Otol Rhinol Laryngol 73:404–416, 1964.
69. Arnold GE: Disorders of laryngeal function. *In* Paparella MM, Shumrick DA (eds): Otolaryngology, Vol 3. Head and Neck. Philadelphia, WB Saunders Company, 1973.
70. Luchsinger R, Arnold GE: Voice-Speech-Language. Clinical Communicology: Its Physiology and Pathology. Belmont, CA, Wadsworth Publishing Company, Inc, 1965.
71. Jackson C: Acromegaly of the larynx. JAMA 71:1787–1789, 1918.
72. Frable MAS: Hoarseness, a symptom of premenstrual tension. Arch Otolaryngol 75:66–68, 1972.
73. Wendler J: Cyclically dependent variations in efficiency of the voice and its influencing by ovulation inhibitors. Folia Phoniatrica 24:259–277, 1972.
74. Di Benedetto R, Le Frak S: Systemic sarcoidosis with severe involvement of the upper respiratory tract. Am Rev Respir Dis 102:801–807, 1970.
75. Mayock RL et al.: Manifestations of sarcoidosis: Analysis of 145 patients with a review of 9 series selected from the literature. Am J Med 35:67–89, 1963.
76. Carasso B: Sarcoidosis of the larynx causing airway obstruction. Chest 65:693–695, 1974.
77. Raman V: Sarcoidosis of the skin and larynx. Arch Otolaryngol 92:324–326, 1971.
78. Kirschner BS, Holinger PH: Laryngeal obstruction in childhood sarcoidosis. J Pediatr 88:263–265, 1976.
79. Trible W: Sarcoidosis of the larynx. Arch Otolaryngol 68:382–383, 1955.
80. McAlpine JC: Primary amyloidosis of the upper air passages. J Laryngol Otol 77:1–28, 1963.
81. Beasley P: Localized amyloidosis of the larynx. J Laryngol Otol 85:83–88, 1971.
82. Toomey JM et al.: Acute epiglottis due to systemic lupus erythematosus. Laryngoscope 84:522–527, 1974.
83. Sinclair D et al.: Systemic lupus erythematosus with a vocal cord granulomatous nodule. J Otolaryngol 5:337–342, 1976.
84. Lever WF: Pemphigus. Medicine (Baltimore) 32:1–123, 1953.
85. Obregon G: Pemphigus of the larynx. Ann Otol Rhinol Laryngol 66:649–655, 1957.
86. Wallner LJ, Alexander RW: Pemphigus of the larynx. Laryngoscope 74:575–586, 1964.
87. Westein S, Sach A: Pemphigus of the oropharynx and larynx. Arch Otolaryngol 62:214–217, 1955.
88. Shklar G, McCarthy PL: Oral Manifestations of Systemic Disease. Boston, Butterworths, 1976, pp 123–136.

89. Block LJ et al.: Pemphigus of the air and food passages. Ann Otol Rhinol Laryngol 86:584–587, 1977.
90. Friedmann I: The pathology of malignant granuloma of the nose. J Laryngol Otol 63:331–341, 1955.
91. Fahey J et al.: Wegener's granulomatosis. Am J Med 17:168–179, 1954.
92. McDonald TJ et al.: Nasal manifestations of Wegener's granulomatosis. Laryngoscope 84:2101–2112, 1974.
93. McDonald TJ et al.: The protean clinical features of polymorphic reticulosis (lethal midline granuloma). Laryngoscope 86:936–945, 1976.
94. Thomas K: Laryngeal manifestations of Wegener's granuloma. J Laryngol Otol 84:101–106, 1970.
95. Nieberding P et al.: Periarteritis nodosa: Wegener's granuloma type. Arch Otolaryngol 77:512–524, 1963.
96. Eichel BS, Maybery TE: The enigma of lethal midline granuloma. Laryngoscope 78:1367–1386, 1968.
97. Burston HH: Lethal midline granuloma: Is it a pathologic entity? Laryngoscope 69:1–43, 1959.
98. Barranco UP et al.: Treatment of relapsing polychondritis with dapsone. Arch Dermatol 112:1286–1288, 1978.
99. Esdaile J et al.: Vascular involvement in relapsing polychondritis. Can Med Assoc J 116:1019–1022, 1977.

PART III

SURGERY FOR CANCER OF THE LARYNX

14

Management of Carcinoma in Situ and Microinvasive Carcinoma of the Larynx

Byron J. Bailey, M.D.

Laryngologists continue to search for the optimal management techniques for preinvasive and microinvasive carcinoma of the larynx. When the pathologist returns a report indicating the diagnosis of carcinoma in situ or microinvasive carcinoma, the management course to be followed is controversial in that the surgeon cannot turn to the medical literature to find a precise answer to the question, "What is the best treatment for this patient?" The major issues involved in selecting the best plan for therapy include the ease or difficulty of adequate laryngeal examination in each particular patient, the patient's availability for follow-up, the probability that he or she will avoid future exposure to carcinogens (especially cigarette smoking), and the available facilities and training of the management team.

Carcinoma in situ will progress to invasive carcinoma in a significant percentage of patients regardless of the treatment method. We know that the prognosis for progression to invasive carcinoma is worse in cases with more extensive lesions and when multiple areas within the larynx are involved. Carcinoma in situ is particularly ominous when it is located in the supraglottic region, where the epithelial lining consists of respiratory epithelium rather than stratified squamous epithelium. Also, invasive carcinoma has been shown to develop more often when histologic evidence of severe dysplasia of the epithelium is present. We are not always able to recognize those situations in which the problem reflects a "field change" whereby the patient is susceptible to development of malignancy in adjacent areas caused by further exposure to carcinogens.

While some authors believe that every case of carcinoma in situ should be treated by radiotherapy, other equally respected colleagues feel strongly that surgical management is preferable. Many authorities urge that carcinoma in situ not be overtreated, but the published experience indicates that progression of the disease to invasive carcinoma requiring total laryngectomy or resulting in death from disseminated carcinoma appears to be associated with undertreatment or insufficient intensity of patient follow-up. Carcinoma in situ, while preinvasive by definition, must be regarded as a serious "malignant" condition that places the patient at great risk for loss of function or loss of life.

At present, we need more scientific information and more extensive reports of management experience. The need for a standardized system by which to classify carcinoma in situ and microinvasive carcinoma is urgent. The attention of our pathologist colleagues is required to standardize diagnostic terminology and criteria, especially as they relate to categorizing the various stages of epithelial dysplasia and its progression to carcinoma in situ and the earliest stages of invasion into the subepithelial stroma.

HISTOPATHOLOGIC PROGRESSION

Evidence supports the hypothesis that many (or all) neoplasms of the glottic larynx progress through an early phase of dysplastic change to a point where malignant features can be identified, but the neoplasm appears to lack the characteristic of an autonomous growth potential and the capability to invade the deeper structures. Most pathologists agree that glottic carcinoma moves through a spectrum of microscopic changes characterized by the following: (1) hyperplasia and keratosis, (2) keratosis with atypia and dysplasia, (3) carcinoma in situ, and (4) superficial microinvasion. DeSanto[1] proposes that while these four stages may not be distinguishable clinically, the microscopic findings from the initial biopsy may be useful as a guide for selecting patients who can be treated by endoscopic removal with safety and efficacy.

Stutsman and McGavran[2] observed that 13 of 60 patients (21 per cent) who were diagnosed as having T1 invasive carcinoma of the larynx showed no evidence of residual cancer in blocked and step-sectioned (20 slides per specimen) analysis of subsequent hemilaryngectomy surgical specimens. That this same percentage would hold for T1 glottic carcinomas treated by radiation therapy is a reasonable assumption. This observation strengthens the argument for conservative microsurgical laryngoscopic management of a carefully selected group of patients.

If local spread of an autonomous glottic carcinoma follows a period of local containment of the neoplasm by the host, this should generate great interest in the mechanisms by which the invasion of the tumor is prevented. Prevention may involve the following three factors:

1. An early period during which the tumor lacks the virulent characteristics or biological aggressiveness for invasiveness (as demonstrated by transplantation or tissue culture techniques, which show that early carcinomas appear to lack the potential for xenotopic growth).
2. The presence of morphologic defenses in tissue, including the basement membrane layer of mucopolysaccharide substance and reticulum fibers.
3. A variety of host immunologic defenses, currently being intensively investigated.

The defense mechanisms in the larynx have certain parallels with early invasive carcinoma of the cervix, a region that has been more intensively studied for the past four or five decades. We will explore this issue in more detail later in this chapter, discussing the similarities and differences between these two regions.

The primary purpose of this chapter is to propose conservative surgical management of early invasive carcinoma of the larynx in a carefully selected patient population and to share our experience with a specific management protocol for carcinoma in situ and microinvasive carcinoma of the larynx.

"PREMALIGNANT" AND PREINVASIVE CARCINOMA

This section focuses on the histologic features of the spectrum of change from normal epithelium to microinvasive carcinoma in the glottic larynx, the location in 80 per cent to 90 per cent of the cases with which we are confronted. The stratified squamous epithelium of the vocal fold is relatively thin and the interface between the basal cell layer and the underlying stroma is flat and clearly demarcated. Cell maturation progresses normally, and movement toward the surface is characterized by fading and loss of cell nuclei along with progressive flattening of the cells as they approach the surface. No keratin layer is present on the surface of the epithelium.

The earliest stage of change is associated with hyperplasia of the squamous epithelium, apparently a response of the tissue to chronic irritation from vocal abuse or exposure to irritating fumes, such as cigarette smoke or other toxic chemical fumes in the environment. In this stage, the epithelium becomes thicker because of an increased number of squamous cells, and a layer of keratin can be observed on the surface. The progression of cell maturation is not affected in the early stage.

In the second stage of change, epithelial

dysplasia is found in a range from mild to severe. Dysplasia of the epithelial layer is characterized by alterations in the appearance of the cells themselves and in the structural architecture of the entire layer. The cellular changes, called cellular atypia, are characterized by cell nuclei that stain more darkly basophilic (hyperchromatosis) and by polymorphism of the cell nuclei. An increase in the nucleus-to-cytoplasm ratio is observed, along with increased frequency of both normal and atypical mitoses. The alterations in cell arrangement appear as exaggerated deep encroachment of the basal cell layer into the subepithelial stroma. The regular progression of cell maturation between the basal layer and the surface is altered, and nucleated cells are found closer to the surface or, in severe dysplasia, extending all the way to the surface of the epithelium. The superficial layer of keratin is quite thick, and dyskeratotic foci may be found within the epithelium.

Carcinoma in situ is the next stage of change beyond severe dysplasia. For more detailed descriptions of these various stages of histopathologic change, the reader may consult various standard textbooks that deal with laryngeal malignancy.

Historical Review—Carcinoma in Situ. The term *carcinoma in situ,* first introduced by Broders,[3] designates the presence of preinvasive or intraepithelial carcinoma. The diagnosis is made relatively often in the larynx, because the vocal cord is the most common site of origin. Patients with carcinoma in situ arising on the vocal fold develop hoarseness, the complaint that impels them to seek medical attention.

Indirect laryngoscopy reveals changes on the surface of the vocal fold, ranging from patches of white, thickened, plaquelike changes of the epithelium (isolated to multiple) to an inflammatory, red coloration (erythroplasia). The lesions may be discrete or diffuse and may vary in thickness from an almost translucent appearance to thick and fissured plaques. The clinical appearance is difficult to correlate with the severity of the microscopic diagnosis. Large lesions, those that are thick and fissured, those that are multiple, and those appearing in the supraglottic region have been observed to be associated more frequently with carcinoma in situ or microinvasive carcinoma.

The incidence, prevalence, and reversibility of these lesions continue to be uncertain factors. Autopsy studies by Auerbach et al.[4] of the vocal fold epithelium of smokers have demonstrated the presence of cellular atypia in 99 per cent of specimens and carcinoma in situ in 16 per cent of specimens. Similar examinations in nonsmokers and former smokers who had discontinued cigarette smoking at least five years prior to death revealed an incidence of 25 per cent of atypia and no instances of carcinoma in situ. Interestingly, the average age of patients with carcinoma in situ is five to seven years younger than the average age of patients with invasive carcinoma. These observations suggest (1) an extremely high incidence of carcinoma in situ prevails in the population of cigarette-smoking adults in the United States, (2) the time between the development of carcinoma in situ and of invasive carcinoma may be many years, and (3) the local defense mechanisms may contain this malignancy within the epithelium in many individuals. Also, most instances of epithelial dysplasia may be reversed when the carcinogenic exposure ceases. While these views are extremely speculative, they nonetheless indicate a very promising avenue for further investigation.

Most authors advocate either conservative surgical management or radiation therapy for the treatment of carcinoma in situ. Doyle et al.[5] recommend a tumoricidal dose of radiotherapy. They report that 21 of 22 patients were free of disease for at least five years after this treatment. They recommend, however, that radiotherapy should not be given if all of the following conditions exist:

1. The lesion is small, localized, and involves only one vocal cord.
2. Repeat stripping of the vocal cord one month after the original diagnosis reveals no evidence of disease.
3. The patient has stopped smoking.
4. There is no possibility that the patient will be lost to follow-up. These clinicians state that involvement of both vocal cords is an absolute indication for full-course radiotherapy.

Pêne and Fletcher[6] irradiated 79 patients who had carcinoma in situ and reported failure of this treatment in 7 of the 63 patients (11 per cent) in whom the tumor was limited to the glottis. Recurrent cancer was noted in 6 of 23 patients (26 per cent) with extension beyond the cord. Of 11 patients who developed invasive carcinoma, 9 subsequently required total laryngectomy for salvage. This report also indicates that of the 12 failures of radiation therapy treatment, only 2 involved the cord that was affected initially. This raises the question of whether the radiation therapy might be a factor in development of a secondary invasive carcinoma.

Elman et al.[7] reported their experience involving 81 patients with preinvasive carcinoma of the vocal cord. Of these, 67 patients presented with lesions confined to the true cord and 14 patients had preinvasive carcinoma that extended beyond the margins of the true cord. Of the total 81 patients, 69 were treated by radiation therapy and 12 by surgery. In the group receiving radiation therapy, recurrence was observed in 17 per cent of the patients at five years and in 25 per cent of the patients at ten years. Seventeen patients developed recurrence of invasive carcinoma within the larynx; 15 of these patients were salvaged by subsequent therapy. Eleven patients (14 per cent), however, required total laryngectomy for salvage. The recurrences were noted at 7 to 107 months. These observations emphasize the importance of long-term follow-up, as this disease tends to recur many years after initial treatment.

Several surgeons have reported their experience with the surgical management of carcinoma in situ and early invasive carcinoma, describing good results with this approach. Lilli and DeSanto[8] at the Mayo Clinic used endoscopic cordectomy over a ten-year period to treat 33 patients with invasive carcinoma and 8 patients with carcinoma in situ. They report that 40 of these 41 patients are alive and free of disease and that a single patient was lost to follow-up six years after surgical treatment. One patient, who developed carcinoma of the opposite cord, was re-treated transorally and remained free of disease four years after the second operation. None of the patients died of carcinoma, nor did any require total laryngectomy, partial laryngectomy, or radiation therapy. These clinicians treated an additional 24 patients with invasive carcinoma and 33 patients with carcinoma in situ by endoscopic biopsy and surgical diathermy. None of the patients in this second group died from laryngeal cancer (3 died from unrelated causes), but 5 patients had either recurrence of the initial lesion or development of a new laryngeal tumor. Four of these 5 patients were re-treated by endoscopic surgery and a single patient required total laryngectomy eight years after the initial surgery.

The serious nature of carcinoma in situ is emphasized by Miller[9, 10] in his reports of 203 patients with carcinoma in situ managed by surgery and radiation therapy. In the 100 patients treated by direct laryngoscopy and stripping of the epithelium, 25 were failures in the form of recurrent disease, over 50 per cent of these being in the form of invasive carcinoma. Of 60 patients treated by laryngofissure and cordectomy, 4 failures occurred including a patient who developed invasive carcinoma. Of 43 patients treated by radiation therapy only, treatment failed in 22 (51 per cent); more than 80 per cent of these patients developed invasive carcinoma. Miller recommends endoscopic vocal cord stripping as the treatment of choice if the patient can be observed closely for evidence of residual or recurrent disease.

Use of the carbon dioxide laser for surgical endoscopic removal of carcinoma in situ is proposed and described by Vaughan et al.[11] Excisional biopsy of the tumor area is performed using the laser, and the entire specimen is sent to the pathologist for evaluation. Questionable margins are evaluated by frozen-section analysis. The authors feel this technique offers significant advantages to accurate definition and excision of early cancer with preservation of normal laryngeal tissue and minimal postoperative morbidity.

Hellquist et al.[12] have compared the treatment outcome of patients managed by radiation therapy with those managed by surgery, emphasizing the serious nature of severe epithelial dysplasia. The long-term prognosis for the progression of severely dysplastic vocal cord epithelium to invasive carcinoma is almost as serious as that for carcinoma in situ. In a group of 39 patients with severe dysplasia or carcinoma in situ, 16 patients were treated by radiation therapy. Four of these 16 patients developed invasive carcinoma, which was managed by total laryngectomy in 3 and partial laryngectomy in 1 patient. In the remaining group of 23 patients, who were treated by excision or stripping of the vocal cord epithelium, 5 patients developed invasive carcinoma, 2 of whom required total laryngectomy. The authors emphasize that patients with hyperplasia, keratosis, dysplasia, and carcinoma in situ should be followed very carefully because invasive carcinoma may develop many years after the initial diagnosis.

Formerly, a few physicians have advocated less aggressive therapy after a diagnosis of carcinoma in situ and, more recently, Hintz et al.[13] proposed a formal policy of "watchful waiting." This controversial, and generally unaccepted, view was supported by the authors' description of a comparison between 18 patients who received radiation therapy immediately upon diagnosis and 27 patients who were followed by periodic examination. Of the 18 patients treated by radiation therapy, 13 were controlled and the other 5 (28 per cent) developed local recurrence (3 requiring total laryngectomy and 2 requiring partial laryngectomy). Surgical salvage was unsuccessful in 1 of these 5 patients. In the 27 patients followed by periodic examination, 17 (63 per cent) developed invasive carcinoma. Five of these patients required total laryngectomy and 2 died. Patients in the "watchful waiting" management group required total laryngectomy twice as frequently as did patients treated by radiation therapy initially. Mortality was also higher in these patients than in most reported series dealing with carcinoma in situ. These factors support the view that there is no place for a policy of "watchful waiting" in the management of this malignancy.

Management of Carcinoma in Situ at The University of Texas Medical Branch. During the period between 1970 and 1980, physicians in the Department of Otolaryngology at The University of Texas Medical Branch at Galveston diagnosed 25 patients as having carcinoma in situ of the larynx. The usual treatment consisted of microlaryngeal surgical excision or stripping of the mucosa of the involved region, together with instructions to return for follow-up at regular intervals over a period of at least five years. Subsequent direct laryngoscopy and biopsy were performed if the patient developed any deterioration of vocal quality or if indirect laryngoscopy revealed evidence of a suspicious change in the laryngeal epithelium. The number of subsequent direct laryngoscopies performed in the period after the initial diagnosis ranged from none to 8, with an average of 3.2.

The pattern of progression or remission is unpredictable on the basis of our current understanding of histopathologic features that may have prognostic significance. Some patients progressed from carcinoma in situ to microinvasive carcinoma and ultimately to invasive cancer. Other patients were found on subsequent biopsies to have epithelial dysplasia and eventually to regress to biopsy reports that showed only mild atypia.

Of the 25 patients treated during this ten-year period, 3 progressed to microinvasive carcinoma and were managed by radiation therapy. One patient developed invasive carcinoma and required a supraglottic partial laryngectomy; another patient developed invasive carcinoma of the vocal cord, requiring a vertical partial laryngectomy. One patient developed a second primary lesion (adenocarcinoma of the lung) and subsequently died from metastatic lung carcinoma.

MICROINVASIVE CARCINOMA OF THE LARYNX

Evidence supports the hypothesis that squamous cell carcinoma progresses through a series of increasingly ominous stages, beginning with hyperplasia with keratosis, progressing to severe dysplasia and then to carcinoma in situ, with the subsequent stage being microinvasive carcinoma.

Hellquist et al.[14] carefully studied the serious prognostic implications of severe dysplasia in a series of 20 patients. Of 9 patients who received radiotherapy, 3 developed invasive carcinoma, as did 2 of 11 patients in whom minor surgical procedures were performed. The authors emphasize that patients with severe dysplasia should be followed as carefully as those who have been treated for invasive carcinoma.

The stages of transition identified by Friedmann[15] are keratosis (hyperplasia and hyperkeratosis), dysplasia (low grade), dysplasia (high grade), borderline carcinoma in situ, carcinoma in situ, and microinvasive carcinoma. He emphasizes the difficulty in discriminating between these stages and the inconsistency of diagnostic impressions among different pathologists—and even by the same pathologist examining the same section at different times.

Actually, the premalignant potential of various patterns of laryngeal keratosis, atypia, and dysplasia has been studied in relatively few patients, as pointed out by Fechner.[16] Today, while we must be alert to the importance of the more serious histologic changes and suspicious of the potential for progression to invasion and "malignant" biologic behavior, we still await more definitive answers regarding optimal therapy.

Superficially invasive carcinoma of the vocal cord is recognizable.[17] It is suitable for conservative management by sequential endoscopic microlaryngeal stripping procedures.

This section proposes a program of ultraconservative management of early invasive carcinoma of the larynx in a carefully selected patient population. This chapter shares our limited experience with a specific management protocol.

Definition of Microinvasive Carcinoma. Various synonyms—microinvasive carcinoma, superficial carcinoma, and early invasive carcinoma—have been employed to describe the presence of tumor cells in the stroma deep to the basement membrane of the vocal cord epithelium. We still lack standardized terminology or a system for quantifying specifically the amount of invasion in a manner that has prognostic value. Basically, most pathologists use the term *microinvasive carcinoma* to represent more than carcinoma in situ but less than deeply invasive carcinoma involving the vocalis muscle.

Clinically, patients with microinvasive carcinoma present with hoarseness, and indirect examination of the larynx reveals no impairment of vocal cord mobility. The diagnosis could possibly be made in a retrospective manner in 5 per cent to 10 per cent of the carcinomas of the true vocal cord that have been seen in the past. While proposing a separate classification may be premature, microinvasive carcinoma may constitute a distinct subset of laryngeal cancer patients who will be found to deserve a separate category when the system of laryngeal cancer classification is next revised.

Grading System. At The University of Texas Medical Branch in Galveston, we have begun several studies to measure the potential for deeper invasion in patients with microinvasive carcinoma. In the first study, we step-section biopsy specimens and determine the greatest degree of invasion by calculating the extent of tumor invasion in millimeters from the basement membrane.

A second study involves the collection of data regarding the appearance of nests of degenerated epithelial cells surrounded by lymphocytes. We hypothesize that these nests represent areas of invasion that the host defense system has successfully challenged. The presence of these devitalized tumor cell nests may correlate with the earliest period of tumor invasion and may be a favorable prognostic sign (Fig. 14–1).

A third study involves attempts to grow the initial tumor cells in tissue culture. This may provide further information regarding the xenotopic growth potential of these tumors and may correlate with the potential for clinical invasiveness and increase as the tumor becomes more aggressive in some patients. Clearly, these efforts to quantify the degree of invasiveness are essential to the expansion of our understanding of the differences in prognosis and the likelihood of successful management by ultraconservative surgical techniques.

DIAGNOSIS OF MICROINVASIVE CARCINOMA

Patient Accrual. Since we began our attempts to diagnose and treat patients with microinvasive carcinoma prospectively, the accrual of patients for investigation has been limited to one or two cases per year, representing about 5 per cent or less of our laryngeal cancer patient population. At present, the series consists of eight patients who have been followed for five years or longer. We feel the number might increase with aggressive efforts to investigate this problem more intensively, but we urge caution lest a valuable new treatment protocol be used inappropriately and discredited prematurely because of improper patient selection.

Age at Diagnosis. The age of patients in our series ranges from 40 to 60 years, averaging 55 years at the time of initial diagnosis.

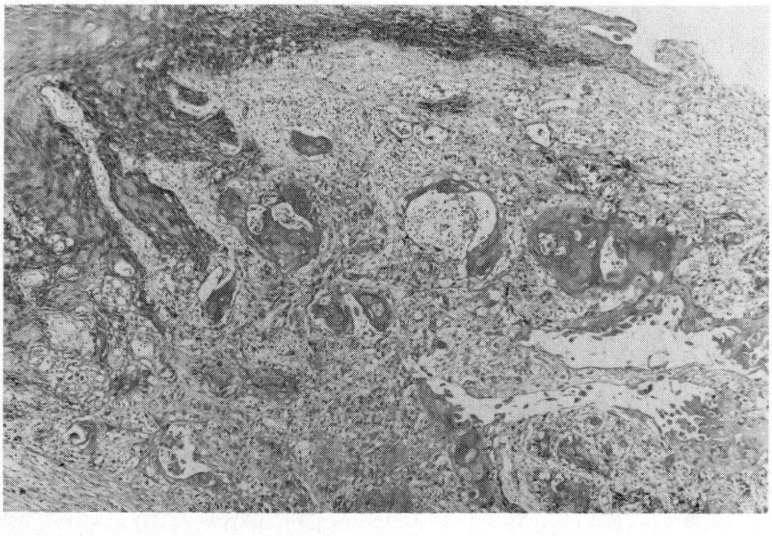

Figure 14–1. Photomicrograph of a tissue specimen obtained from patient with microinvasive carcinoma of the true vocal cord. The fingerlike projections of tumor cells into the subepithelial stroma are surrounded by a rather intense "lymphocyte response" (hematoxylin and eosin [H & E] stain).

Symptoms. Hoarseness is the only symptom we have noted in our patient series. The duration of hoarseness ranges from 2 to 36 months with an average duration of 13 months.

Diagnostic Prerequisites. To be treated by endoscopic sequential excision for superficially invasive carcinoma of the vocal cord, a patient must meet certain specific criteria. The biopsy must be made from a complete sample; partial biopsy specimens are not acceptable.

A thorough search for a second primary must be conducted because of the known multiplicity of primary carcinomas in the region of the head and neck. The clinical picture must suggest and be consistent with a very superficial malignancy. Finally, close and continuing communication must be maintained between the otolaryngologist and the pathologist, not only regarding the initial biopsy specimen but also the interpretation of all subsequent specimens.

MANAGEMENT OF MICROINVASIVE CARCINOMA

Management Prerequisites. The otolaryngologist must be convinced that the patient will return for regular and continuing follow-up. This is the most important factor influencing the decision to utilize this management protocol and is the key to avoiding therapeutic disaster. The otolaryngologist must be able to visualize the larynx without compromise on indirect examination. In the case of an overhanging epiglottis, endoscopic resection of a portion of the tip of the epiglottis would be appropriate to improve the physician's ability to examine the larynx in follow-up.

The operative procedure is performed using microscopic suspension laryngoscopy and standard microsurgical instrumentation. The patient and his family must be educated to monitor the patient's voice for any sign of altered vocal quality; all involved must be trained to watch for other signs and symptoms of cancer of the head and neck to assure proper diagnosis if a second primary carcinoma occurs.

So that the patient can participate in the decision to undertake ultraconservative surgical management, he or she must be informed of the advantages and risks of this approach; the surgeon must avoid overselling the procedure. We suggest that the utilization of endoscopic surgical excision not be pushed to its limits until the surgeon has gained experience with the technique in patients with very early lesions.

Table 14–1. DIAGNOSIS AND MANAGEMENT OF MICROINVASIVE CARCINOMA

1. *Diagnostic prerequisites*
   - Biopsy a complete specimen
   - Search for a second primary carcinoma
   - Lesion apparently superficial
   - Good communication between surgeon and pathologist
2. *Management prerequisites*
   - Larynx visible by indirect examination
   - Patient reliable for follow-up
   - Microlaryngoscopy for suspicious signs and symptoms
   - Patient and family to monitor voice changes
3. *Recommended management pattern*
   - Sequential stripping until two consecutive negative biopsies
   - Indirect laryngeal examination every two months for five years
   - Strong program to discourage smoking
4. *Potential pitfalls*
   - Underdiagnosis
   - Overlooking a second primary
   - Web formation after stripping
   - Loss to follow-up

Proposed Management Pattern. The technique employed in our series involves sequential, endoscopic vocal cord stripping every two months until two negative biopsies are obtained. From that point, repeated indirect laryngoscopy is performed every two months for five years and annually thereafter. Patients who are cigarette smokers participate in an active program of counseling so that they are motivated to discontinue smoking. Continuance of cigarette smoking will increase the likelihood of recurrence or the development of a second primary lesion, regardless of the form of therapy chosen—sequential cord stripping, cordectomy, or radiation therapy. Table 14–1 summarizes the main features of diagnosis and management.

RESULTS OF CONSERVATIVE MANAGEMENT

Case Reports. Summaries describing treatment of four patients present some important features of ultraconservative management and emphasize the need for careful follow-up.

A 54-year-old male with hoarseness for five months underwent direct laryngoscopy and was found to have carcinoma in situ of the left vocal cord (Fig. 14–2). Repeat biopsy three months

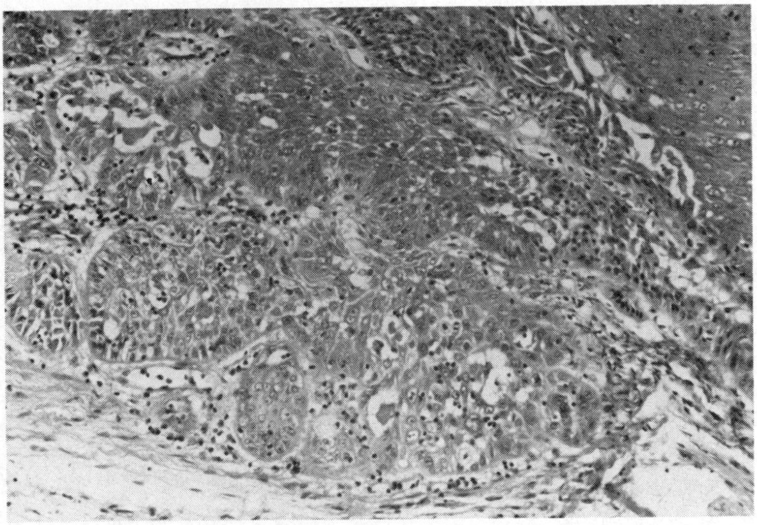

Figure 14–2. Photomicrograph of tissue specimen obtained from patient, showing microinvasive carcinoma of the true vocal cord with a moderate "lymphocyte response" (H & E stain).

later showed microinvasive carcinoma and dysplasia; the next biopsy performed nine months later again showed microinvasive carcinoma and dysplasia. Twenty-six months after that, the biopsy diagnosis was carcinoma in situ; two months later, biopsy showed dysplasia and keratosis; one year after that, a biopsy showed keratosis and atypia. The patient was treated by sequential vocal cord stripping at the time each of the above procedures was performed. He continues to remain free of evidence of laryngeal cancer and has a good voice at this time, now thirteen years after he was first seen. Three years ago, he developed an invasive epidermoid carcinoma of the tongue (T1, N0, M0); since partial glossectomy performed at that time, he has had no recurrence.

A 64-year-old male with a four-month history of intermittent hoarseness underwent direct laryngoscopy; the pathologist reported that the specimen showed carcinoma in situ of the left vocal cord. A question arose regarding microinvasion and, one month later, the patient was referred to The University of Texas Medical Branch in Galveston for a second laryngoscopy. Suspension microlaryngoscopy and stripping of the left true vocal cord revealed microinvasive carcinoma (Fig. 14–3). Similar procedures performed two and five months later revealed mild dysplasia without evidence of carcinoma. After another three months, the pathologist reported that a specimen obtained by stripping showed hyperplasia and keratosis. The patient's larynx was examined indirectly at intervals of two months. Six years later, the patient became hoarse and biopsy of the vocal cord showed carcinoma in situ of both vocal cords. The patient was treated with radiation therapy.

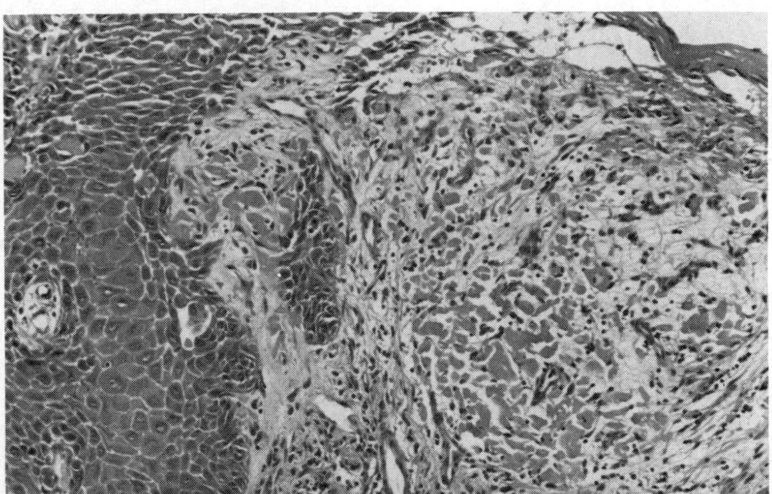

Figure 14–3. Photomicrograph of tissue specimen from patient, showing microinvasive carcinoma with lymphocytes seen within clusters of malignant cells, many of which appear to be undergoing degeneration (H & E stain).

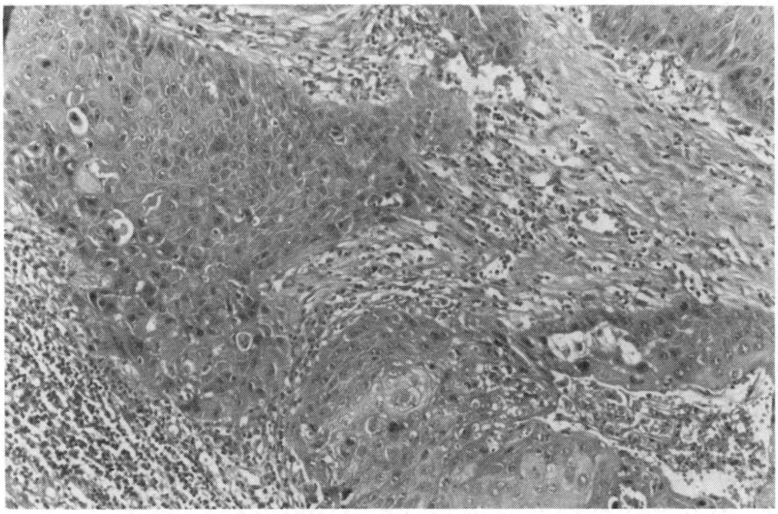

Figure 14–4. Photomicrograph of biopsy specimen, showing microinvasive carcinoma of the true vocal cord (H & E stain).

Twenty-nine months later, there was no evidence of carcinoma.

A 56-year-old male presented with hoarseness of three months' duration associated with a persistent cough. He related a history of smoking three packages of cigarettes per day for about 35 years. Suspension microlaryngoscopy was performed and the pathology specimen showed superficially invasive epidermoid carcinoma (Fig. 14–4). Another suspension microlaryngoscopy two months later revealed dysplasia, parakeratosis, and atypia. Repeat vocal cord stripping three months later disclosed a recurrence of microinvasive carcinoma. The cord stripping was repeated two months later with the finding of epithelial keratosis. A repeat biopsy eight months later revealed mild inflammatory changes. This patient has undergone indirect laryngoscopy every two months for the past two years and has stopped smoking. Laryngeal appearance and the voice are normal. The patient was found to have adenocarcinoma of the lung fourteen months ago and a pneumonectomy was performed. He is now alive and well without evidence of carcinoma in either region.

A 58-year-old male developed hoarseness due to vocal cord polyps 22 years prior to admission. Three endoscopic polyp removals were performed during the next 20 years. Two years before admission, direct laryngoscopy revealed a T1 squamous cell invasive carcinoma of the left true vocal cord and the patient received radiotherapy to 5500 rads. Three months before admission, the patient developed recurrent hoarseness and subsequently

Figure 14–5. Photomicrograph showing microinvasive carcinoma of the true vocal cord. The larynx was irradiated 6 years previously for treatment of invasive epidermoid carcinoma (H & E stain).

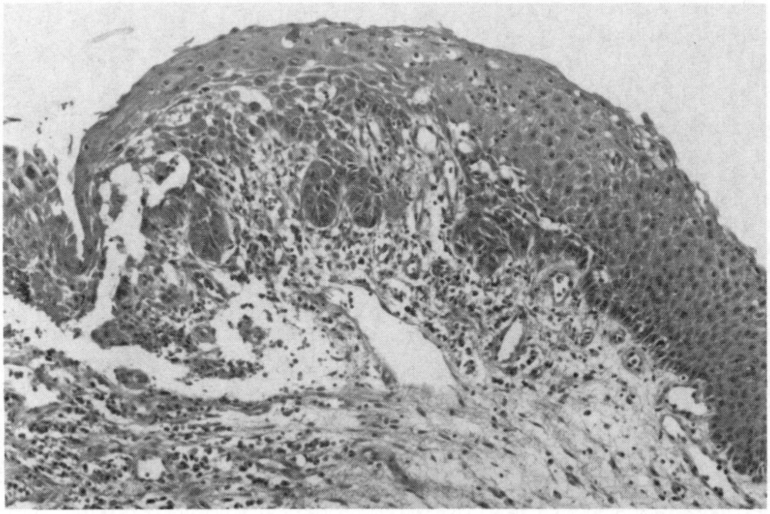

underwent direct laryngoscopy that revealed superficially invasive epidermoid carcinoma of the left true vocal cord (Fig. 14–5). After referral, suspension microlaryngoscopy revealed dysplasia on the first excisional biopsy; six months later, the biopsy specimen showed keratosis. The patient became hoarse three years later and invasive epidermoid carcinoma was diagnosed. Following a vertical partial laryngectomy and laryngoplasty, the patient has been examined indirectly every two months for the past three years. He remains free of any evidence of carcinoma and his voice is of good quality.

Patient Experience. Our series consists of eight patients, all alive and well, with apparently normal laryngeal function. Vocal quality ranges from within normal limits to mild hoarseness. The patients' subjective evaluations of vocal quality are quite favorable. Tracheotomy has not been necessary in any of these patients. Hospitalization has not exceeded two or three days in any case. All eight present no evidence of malignant disease and all are being carefully followed. Fig 14–6 summarizes the pattern of biopsy and sequential stripping and the pathologic findings.

COMPARISON OF EARLY CARCINOMAS OF THE CERVIX AND VOCAL CORD

Carcinomas of both the cervix and the vocal cord almost always go through stages of in situ carcinoma, then to microinvasive carcinoma, and then on to invasive carcinoma. They differ, however, in that hormonal factors such as estrogens may significantly modify the environment in the uterine cervix in a manner that predisposes to cancer progression. This has not been shown in laryngeal carcinoma.

Carcinoma in situ of the uterine cervix is usually found in the transitional zone between squamous and columnar epithelium.[18] Cervical carcinoma in situ progresses to invasive carcinoma in 24 per cent of the patients, according to Fennell.[19] Peterson observed that carcinoma in situ progresses to invasive carcinoma in 22 per cent of women followed for five years and 33 per cent of women followed for nine years.[20] This progression has been reported to be as high as 60 per cent of the patients according to Boys et al.[21]

One reason for the difference in prognosis with carcinoma of the cervix is that the terms

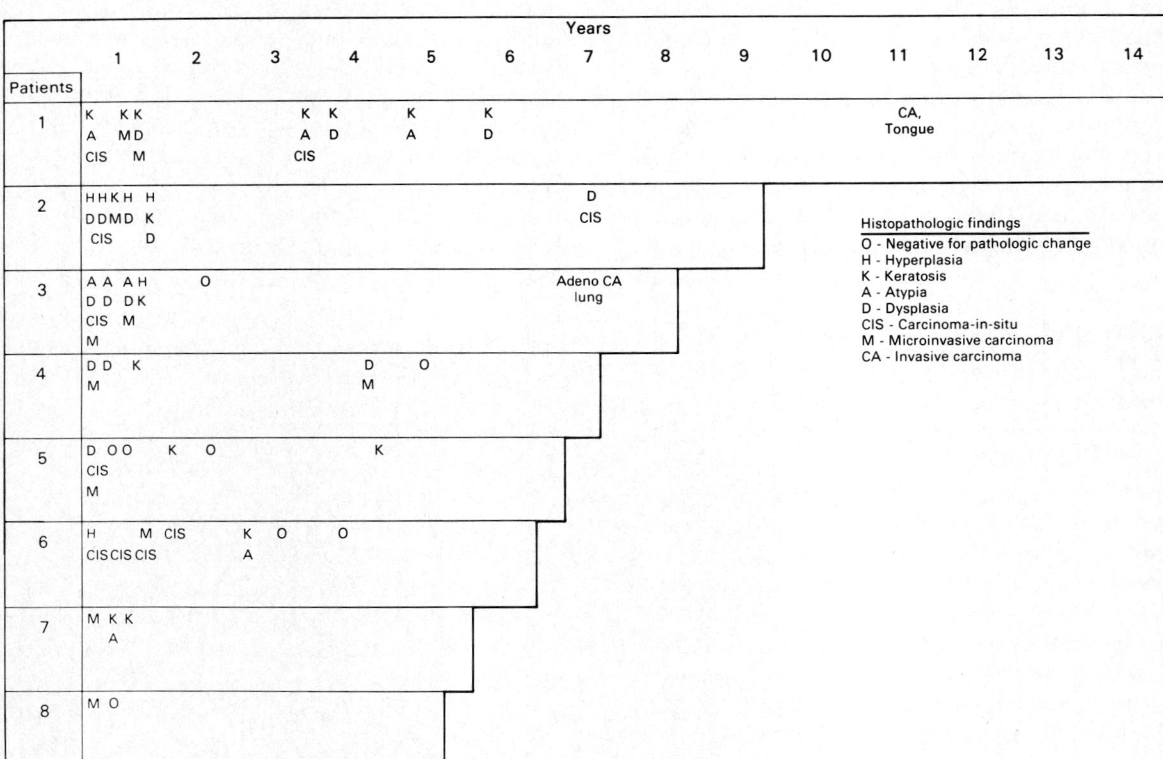

Figure 14–6. Biopsy results in a group of 8 patients with microinvasive carcinoma of the larynx. The time sequence of the laryngeal biopsies, histopathological results, clinical course, and duration of follow-up are illustrated.

carcinoma in situ and *microinvasive carcinoma* are sometimes used to describe the presence of tumor cells in glandular spaces. Observers have noted invasive tumor buds in spaces that are lined with epithelium and thought to be lymphatic channels. Carcinoma in situ and microinvasive carcinoma are also found in some patients in association with metastatic tumor in regional lymph nodes. To date, this observation has not been made in similar tumors of the vocal cord.

Glücksmann and Cherry[18] also observed invasive foci of microcarcinoma of the cervix without a surrounding membrane or basal cell layer. The immediate surrounding cells consisted almost exclusively of lymphocytes; this may be a histopathologic correlate of the host immunologic defense mechanism. They also observed specimens in which the round cell infiltrate had apparently broken up the nest of tumor cells and the appearance of the epithelial neoplastic cells was consistent with impending cell death. They concluded that, at a minimum, the round cell envelope represents an extremely unfavorable environment for the invading cells. They also observed other specimens in which the field was characterized by a complete absence of any lymphocytes surrounding these nests of tumor cells, suggesting diminished host defenses.

The transplantability of animal tumors has been shown to increase in the presence of proven metastasis.[22] This has been quantified by a decrease in the number of innoculated cells required for successful grafting by the intravenous or intramuscular route in the presence of spontaneous distant metastasis. Studies on human subjects also show that millions of tumor cells are needed to graft a tumor into the original host; concomitantly, as the invasiveness of the tumor increases, the ease with which tumor cells can be shown to "take" at distant sites also increases. Something in the nature of the tumor itself appears to change as the tumor becomes more aggressive clinically. This may be comparable to the apparent change in the behavior of bacteria when the colony breaks through its sensitivity to a specific antibiotic and resistant organisms become predominant.

Additional observations on this subject are provided by Woodruff,[23] who carefully studied 196 patients with microinvasive carcinoma of the cervix. He found that when cytopathology, colposcopy, and directed biopsy agree that no more than microinvasive disease is present, no evidence of invasive cancer can be found in specimens removed by conization or hysterectomy. He observed, however, strikingly mature cells in the areas of breakthrough of the basement membrane, differing from flagrant invasion with nests of mixed populations of young and mature cells. Woodruff has developed a grading system using 5 mm of invasion as the cutoff point for safe versus dangerously invasive cancer. True stromal invasion, lymphatic invasion beyond 5 mm, or evidence of tumor cells in lymphatic channels appears to account for the 1 per cent to 2 per cent of patients who eventually succumb to their disease. We recommend more aggressive therapy for this group.

Diagnosing early carcinoma of the cervix presents some unique difficulties. The surgeon must take multiple, repeated biopsies to avoid missing adjacent invasive carcinoma at the time of the initial diagnosis. When multiple biopsies are taken, so-called invasion can be found in 70 per cent of these patients, but the term *invasion* is used to describe the presence of tumor cells within glandular structures rather than referring only to invasion of tumor cells into the stroma deep to the basement membrane.[24]

DISCUSSION AND SUMMARY

Carcinoma in situ is usually seen with invasive carcinoma.[25] Found in 49 per cent of all patients with carcinoma of the larynx, this association was much higher (76 per cent) for those patients with nonkeratinizing invasive carcinoma and rose to 88 per cent for those with nonkeratinizing carcinoma in the region of the glottis. Bauer offers the following definitions:

1. Keratosis—some degree of epithelial hyperplasia with an orderly maturation sequence with normal or hyperplastic cytologic features and some degree of surface keratinization.
2. Keratosis with atypia—some degree of either cellular atypism or disturbance of maturation sequence (may be difficult to differentiate from carcinoma in situ or well-differentiated squamous cell carcinoma).
3. Carcinoma in situ—full-thickness replacement of the epithelium by cells with malignant cytologic features and a disorderly and faulty maturation sequence with minimal differentiation and absence of invasion.
4. Microinvasive carcinoma—extension of malignant epithelial cells deep to the basement membrane into the stroma but without invasion of the vocalis muscle and without clinical evidence of impaired vocal cord mobility.

The foundations for ultraconservative management of microinvasive carcinoma of the larynx have been provided by several investigators. DeSanto[1] has reported the experience at the Mayo Clinic and stresses the importance of conceptualizing a spectrum of microscopic change (keratosis, atypia, in situ carcinoma, and early invasive carcinoma). These changes in severity may not be distinguishable by clinical observation even with microscopic direct laryngoscopy. Keratosis indicates that the epithelial field is at risk. The presence of atypia with keratosis represents progression and a greater risk. In situ carcinoma is dangerous for several reasons. This disease may be multicentric and appears to be capable of progressing to invasion. It is sometimes overtreated or undertreated, and evaluating the role of radiotherapy with this lesion is difficult.

Early invasive carcinoma poses a definite threat to the larynx and to the life of the patient. It can be managed successfully by endoscopic stripping, electrocoagulation, cryosurgery, and laser excision. The results of the experience at the Mayo Clinic involved analysis of 984 patients with carcinoma of the larynx between 1962 and 1972.[1] Invasive carcinoma was diagnosed as T1A in 263 patients and T1B in 96 patients. These lesions were treated by transoral surgery in 48 of the T1A patients (18 per cent) and 5 of the T1B patients (5 per cent). Of the transoral surgery group, none died of the neoplastic disease. Four patients required a total laryngectomy at five years or longer after the original surgery. Of those patients in the same group who were treated by radiotherapy, 84 of 147 required salvage surgery. Remember that this was a highly selected group of patients.

DeSanto concluded that (1) the spectrum of pathological change cannot be recognized clinically and pathologists will disagree among themselves in regard to the specific diagnosis (individual pathologists will also disagree with a previous diagnosis they have made when the slides are reviewed as unknowns after a period of time), (2) carcinoma in situ may be multicentric and progressive, (3) radiotherapy is not predictably successful but is appropriate for some patients, and (4) some patients can be further selected for transoral surgery.

Pêne and Fletcher[6] shed further light on the treatment of early carcinoma by radiotherapy. Reporting their experience with 86 patients, of whom superficially invasive carcinoma was found in 13, they observed that 63 patients had questionable foci of invasion. Cobalt irradiation of the patients with lesions on only one cord resulted in a failure rate of 11 per cent. When lesions had extended beyond the cord, the failure rate was 26 per cent.

A review of other series further emphasizes the significance of laryngeal keratosis. Friedmann[15] notes that the presence of clinically significant keratosis leads to invasive cancer in 1 out of 35 patients according to McGavran et al.[26] and in 1 out of 30 patients according to Norris and Peale.[27] In summarizing the need for more aggressive management with these lesions, Friedmann quotes D. R. Wilson's textbook, *Hall of Mirrors,* stating "a pessimistic pathologist is the best guarantee of surgical success."

Stutsman and McGavran[2] recommend ultraconservative management of superficially invasive epidermoid carcinoma of the true vocal cord. These clinicians emphasize the need to avoid incomplete biopsy sampling and stress the importance of communication among the otolaryngologist, the pathologist, and the patient. They describe the results of treatment in 11 patients successfully managed by endoscopic removal of early glottic carcinoma and estimate that 5 per cent to 10 per cent of superficially invasive carcinoma can be managed by this ultraconservative means.

Microinvasive carcinoma of the true vocal cord appears to be identifiable through close collaboration between the otolaryngologist and pathologist. When the patient is judged to be cooperative and the larynx can be visualized without compromise on indirect examination, the surgeon can safely embark on management by sequential cord stripping and regular office follow-up. Table 14–1 provides the details of the management protocol.

Recent and continuing experience with eight patients is presented. All patients are alive and well without evidence of persistent carcinoma. The vocal quality and other laryngeal functions are preserved.

Further clarification of the behavioral characteristics of early carcinoma of the larynx awaits completion of studies designed to quantify the degree of tumor invasion in relation to patient prognosis, the importance of specific host defense mechanisms, and possible alterations in the xenotopic potential of early neoplasms.

We emphasize awareness of the signs and symptoms of recurrent cancer and stress the avoidance of environmental carcinogens. This conservative management of microinvasive carcinoma offers many advantages for the occasional patient, but failure to appreciate the limitations of microsurgery and the need for close follow-up will increase the risk of undetected residual laryngeal carcinoma or a second primary tumor in an adjacent region.

References

1. DeSanto LW: Selection of treatment for in situ and early invasive carcinoma of the glottis. Can J Otolaryngol 3(4):522, 1974.
2. Stutsman AC, McGavran MH: Ultraconservative management of superficially invasive epidermoid carcinoma of the true vocal cord. Ann Otol Rhinol Laryngol 80:507, 1971.
3. Broders AC: Carcinoma in situ contrasted with benign penetrating epithelium. JAMA 99:1670, 1932.
4. Auerbach O et al.: Histologic changes in the larynx in relation to smoking habits. Cancer 25:92–104, 1970.
5. Doyle PJ et al.: Carcinoma in situ of the larynx. Laryngoscope 87:310–316, 1977.
6. Pêne F, Fletcher GH: Results in irradiation of the in situ carcinomas of the vocal cords. Cancer 37:2586–2590, 1976.
7. Elman AJ et al.: In situ carcinoma of the vocal cords. Cancer 43:2422–2428, 1979.
8. Lillie JC, DeSanto LW: Transoral surgery of early cordal carcinoma. Ann Otol Rhinol Laryngol 77:92–96, 1973.
9. Miller AH, Fisher HR: Symposium of carcinoma of the larynx: Clues to the life history of carcinoma in situ of the larynx. Laryngoscope 81:1475, 1971
10. Miller AH: Carcinoma in situ of the larynx—Clinical appearance and treatment. Can J Otolaryngol 3(4):567–572, 1974.
11. Vaughan CW et al.: Treatment of T_1 and in situ glottic carcinoma: The transoral approach. Otolaryngol Clin North Am 13:509–513, 1980.
12. Hellquist H et al.: Hyperplasia, keratosis, dysplasia and carcinoma in situ of the vocal cords—A followup study. Clin Otolaryngol 7:11–27, 1982.
13. Hintz BL et al.: A 'watchful waiting' policy for in situ carcinoma of the vocal cords. Arch Otolaryngol 107:746–751, 1981.
14. Hellquist H et al.: Carcinoma in situ and severe dysplasia of the vocal cords. Acta Otolaryngol [Stockh] 92:543–555, 1981.
15. Friedmann I: Precancerous lesions of the larynx. Can J Otolaryngol 3(4):528–532, 1974.
16. Fechner RE: Laryngeal keratosis and atypia. Can J Otolaryngol 3(4):516–521, 1974.
17. McGavran MH et al.: Superficially invasive epidermoid carcinoma of the true vocal cord. Can J Otolaryngol 3(4):526–527, 1974.
18. Glücksmann A, Cherry CP: Microinvasive carcinoma of the cervix: Histopathological aspects. *In* Gray L (ed): Dysplasia, Carcinoma in Situ and Micro-invasive Carcinoma of the Cervix Uteri. Springfield, IL, CC Thomas, 1964, pp 351–378.
19. Fennell RH: The histology of carcinoma in situ of the cervix. Ann NY Acad Sci 97:782–791, 1962.
20. Peterson O: Spontaneous course of cervical precancerous conditions. Am J Obstet Gynecol 72:1063, 1956.
21. Boys DA et al.: Significance of in situ carcinoma of the uterine cervix. Br Med J [Clin Res] 1:203–205, 1962.
22. Wallace AC: Metastasis as an aspect of cell behavior. Can Cancer Conf 4:139–166, 1961.
23. Woodruff JO: Carcinoma of the cervix. *In* Novak ER, Woodruff JD (eds): Gynecologic and Obstetric Pathology. Philadelphia, WB Saunders Company, 1974, Chap 5.
24. Galvin GA et al.: Basal cell hyperactivity in cervical biopsies. Am J Obstet Gynecol 70:808, 1955.
25. Bauer WC: Concomitant carcinoma in situ and invasive carcinoma of the larynx. *In* Alberti PW, Bryce DP (eds): Centennial Conference on Laryngeal Cancer. New York, Appleton-Century-Crofts, 1976, p 127.
26. McGavran MH et al.: Isolated laryngeal keratosis. Laryngoscope 70:932, 1960.
27. Norris CM, Peale AR: Keratosis of the larynx. J Laryngol Otol 77:635, 1963.

15

Supraglottic Cancer

William Lawson, M.D., D.D.S.
and Hugh F. Biller, M.D.

ANATOMY AND PATTERNS OF GROWTH

The supraglottic portion of the larynx includes the laryngeal surface of the epiglottis, the aryepiglottic folds, the laryngeal surfaces of the arytenoids, the false cords (ventricular folds), and the ventricle. The superior limit is generally accepted to be the hyoepiglottic ligament and its anterior border, the thyrohyoid membrane, with the hyoid bone itself considered extralaryngeal. While the mucosa of the lingual surface of the epiglottis tip is considered laryngeal, the vallecular mucosa overlying the hyoepiglottic ligament is classified as oropharyngeal. Prior to 1972 the classification[1] of the International Union Against Cancer (UICC) recognized a marginal zone of the larynx comprising the suprahyoid portion of the epiglottis and aryepiglottic folds, also known as the epilarynx. While tumors arising there behave similarly to hypopharyngeal cancers,[2] this region has now been included in the supraglottic larynx. Interpretations vary as to the exact location of the boundary separating the supraglottic and glottic regions through the ventricle.[3] While anatomically the superior arcuate line (where the squamous epithelium of the true cord joins the respiratory mucosa of the ventricle) is the actual boundary, the clinical junction is different. The lateral recess or angle of the ventricle is generally considered to be the boundary, with the floor of the ventricle included in the glottic region and the roof of the ventricle and saccule considered to be supraglottic.[4]

The subdivision of the larynx into three anatomic areas has its basis in its embryologic derivation. The three areas serve as barriers to the vertical spread of tumors and, in addition, the biologic behavior of neoplasms and their pattern of spread at each anatomic site are different. This compartmentalization of the larynx also provides an anatomic basis for partial laryngeal surgery.

While the supraglottic larynx arises from the buccopharyngeal anlage (arches III and IV), the glottic and subglottic portions are derived from the tracheobronchial anlage (arches V and VI).[5] As a consequence of these embryologic partitions, the various portions have independent lymphatic circulations. Dye injection studies in man by Pressman et al.[6] have demonstrated that the submucosal lymphatics of the larynx are also compartmentalized and serve as an important influence in determining the spread of laryngeal neoplasms. Lymphatic flow from the epiglottis is to the false cord and ends abruptly along its inferior border. The ventricle appears to be a compartment isolated from the false cord. The true cord has a sparse lymphatic network and serves as an additional barrier in the vertical lymphatic drainage of the larynx. The left and right sides of the larynx also appear to be independent at all levels. The supraglottic lymphatics drain through the thyrohyoid space to cervical lymph nodes, whereas the infraglottic laryngeal lymphatics drain only to the cervical nodes through the cricothyroid plexus. The anterior neck has no midline partition; lesions that have spread to the prelaryngeal and pretracheal areas should be treated as a block.[7] With advanced supraglottic tumors, anatomic barriers based on embryologic development disappear and tumor dissemination may occur throughout the neck.[8] This is especially true with involvement of the preepiglottic space.[9]

The preepiglottic and paraglottic spaces represent avenues of dissemination of laryngeal carcinoma. The preepiglottic space is particularly important with supraglottic lesions. This space, as classically described by Clerf[10] and by Leroux-Robert,[11] is a funnel-shaped area bounded by the upper thyroid cartilage and thyrohyoid membrane anteriorly, the hyoepiglottic ligament superiorly, and the epiglottis and quadrangular membrane posteriorly. This fat-filled space anterior to the epiglottis can also extend around it posterolaterally in horseshoe fashion. Since this space and the paraglottic space merge, they have been termed collectively the periepiglottic space by Maguire and Dayal.[12] The paraglottic space is that portion of the larynx bounded by the thyroid ala anterolaterally, the conus elasticus inferiorly, the quadrangular membrane medially, and the pyriform mucosa posteriorly.[13] Primary paraglottic tumors can arise from the mucosa of the saccule and ventricle that extend into the paraglottic space; however, most tumors involve it secondarily by extension from the mucosa anywhere in the intrinsic larynx or from the anterior and medial walls of the pyriform sinus. Although extensive supraglottic tumors can spread laterally along the inner face of the thyroid cartilage in this space for great distances, tumor spread inferiorly is limited by the conus elasticus.

The laryngeal cartilages themselves contribute to tumor growth. The epiglottic cartilage has numerous natural dehiscences that facilitate tumor spread into the preepiglottic space. When cartilage invasion occurs, the ossified portion shows the least resistance to tumor spread.[4] Micheau et al.[14] found that the ossified areas were involved in 94 per cent of 70 cases with cartilage invasion studied by organ section. Similar observations were found with serial sections by Kirchner.[15]

That the mucous glands of the larynx influence the spread of carcinoma has been suggested.[16] According to this theory, the absence of mucous glands within the vocal cord, at the anterior commissure, and in the ventricle may explain the tendency of glottic carcinomas to remain localized and the infrequent spread of supraglottic tumors onto the vocal cords. Tumors of the false cord are also believed to extend into the preepiglottic space through such a glandular system, according to Bridger.[17]

Tumors arising in the supraglottic region vary in growth pattern with the site of origin. Lesions of the laryngeal surface of the epiglottis spread superficially and horizontally to the opposite side and also often invade the preepiglottic space through preformed channels, either by cartilaginous destruction or by disruption of thyroepiglottic ligament. Micheau et al.[14] found tumorous destruction of the thyroepiglottic ligament in 15 of 18 epiglottic lesions. They also found the hyoepiglottic ligament an effective barrier to tumor spread from the epiglottis, unless the vallecula or base of the tongue was involved. Epiglottic carcinomas can also invade thyroid cartilage, contraindicating horizontal partial laryngectomy. This should be suspected with lesions extending to the epiglottic petiole or anterior commissure, with poorly differentiated carcinoma, and with ulcerating tumors.[18] Kirchner[15] found on serial section of 10 epiglottic tumors that 8 invaded the epiglottic cartilage, 5 invaded the thyroid cartilage, and 6 invaded the preepiglottic space. Olofsson[4, 19] reported that of 15 epiglottic carcinomas sectioned, 10 invaded the epiglottic cartilage, 2 destroyed the thyroid cartilage, and 10 extended into the preepiglottic space. Tumors arising on the false cords tend to grow upward to the epiglottis, backward to the aryepiglottic folds and arytenoids, and forward to the anterior commissure. Extensive vertical spread of tumors can involve the ventricles indirectly when the paraglottic space is invaded. Carcinoma arising primarily in the ventricle is considered to be rare; however, lesions occurring at this site are capable of extensive supraglottic and transglottic spread. The study by Micheau et al.[14] of 23 laryngectomy specimens from patients with cancer of the ventricle revealed the following: upward spread with destruction of the base of the epiglottis and involvement of the preepiglottic space (11 cases), contralateral spread across the anterior commissure and downward to involve the glottis superficially over the mucosa (9 cases), and deep spread through the paraglottic space with penetration of the conus elasticus (16 cases). While many supraglottic tumors show a pushing pattern of growth and tend to stop at the ventricle, some cross over it onto the glottis.[4] Bocca et al.[20] found that none of 160 supraglottic carcinomas invaded the floor of the ventricle or vocal cord. Olofsson,[4, 19] however, found that of 25 primary supraglottic tumors, 11 remained localized in the supraglottis, 6 spread to the glottis, 6 spread to the vallecula, and 4 spread to the pyriform sinus. Nine tumors were bilateral, generally crossing the midline anteriorly, but the interarytenoid area was involved in 2 cases. Kirchner and Som[21] found that 8 of 30 supraglottic carcinomas extended below the anterior commissure, with 5 invading the thyroid cartilage.

McGavran[22] termed lesions that crossed the ventricle *transglottic*. These lesions often involve the paraglottic space and show an aggressive and infiltrative pattern of growth, cause cord fixation, and carry a poor prognosis.[23] Kirchner and Som[21] found that supraglottic tumors generally extended downward at the level of the anterior commissure ligament to become transglottic, often invading the thyroid cartilage at this point. Kirchner[15] noted on serial section of 19 transglottic lesions that 15 invaded cartilage (thyroid 8, cricoid 5, arytenoid 5) and 16 reached or penetrated the cricothyroid membrane. Vocal cord fixation also indicates an advanced tumor and consequently carries a poor prognosis. With supraglottic lesions, fixation may occur by tumor extension along the paraglottic space, with minimal mucosal findings. Perineural involvement, cartilage invasion, and extralaryngeal extension are seen frequently in patients with vocal cord fixation.[19]

CLASSIFICATION AND STAGING

The system of laryngeal cancer staging and end results reporting published by the American Joint Committee for Cancer Staging and End Results Reporting in 1963 was revised in 1972[24] because of deficiencies that subsequently became apparent. A major objection was the poor survival of patients with fixed cord lesions as compared with bilateral cordal lesions that were reclassified as T3 lesions. Also, T4, N0 M0 tumors were changed from stage IV to stage III lesions. The system underwent further minor modifications in 1977, principally with regard to classification of lymph node metastasis. A further revision, published in 1983,[24] is used in this text. (See Table 4–2 in Chapter 4, Diagnosis of Laryngeal Disease.)

INCIDENCE AND ETIOLOGY

Carcinoma of the supraglottic larynx is generally second to glottic cancer in frequency of occurrence, but wide geographic differences in incidence exist.[25] Of the reported cases of laryngeal carcinoma, supraglottic cancer represents 11 per cent in Sweden,[26] 19.7 per cent in Croatia,[27] 34 per cent in the United States,[28] 49 per cent in Japan,[29] and 67 per cent in Finland.[30] In Finland, supraglottic lesions were seen a decade earlier.[26] Iwamoto[29] found an increased occurrence of supraglottic carcinoma in females in Japan.

Cigarette smoking has been identified as the principal risk factor for the development of supraglottic and glottic carcinoma in epidemiologic studies by Wynder.[31] Heavy alcoholic intake also significantly increased the risk, principally for the supraglottic larynx.[31, 32]

CLINICAL FEATURES

The prominent presenting symptoms with supraglottic carcinoma are hoarseness, throat pain, dysphagia, and the occurrence of a neck mass. Other less common complaints are hemoptysis, ear pain, chronic cough, stridor, and the presence of an oral mass. Hoarseness may result from involvement of the false cord, from extension onto the glottis, or from impaired cord mobility because of involvement of the arytenoid cartilage, cricoarytenoid joint, or paraglottic space. Dysphagia generally represents extension into the hypopharynx or infiltration of the vallecula or base of the tongue. Occasionally, as in lesions of the pyriform sinus, a small or asymptomatic supraglottic tumor may present with palpable cervical lymphadenopathy.

Most lesions arise on the epiglottis; this is followed by the false cords and aryepiglottic folds. Cachin[33] found in his series of 72 early (T1 and T2) supraglottic carcinomas that 56 developed on the infrahyoid epiglottis and false cords, 14 on the epilarynx, and 2 in the ventricle. Among the 221 tumors studied by Coates et al.,[34] 89 per cent involved the epiglottis, 33 per cent the false cords, 20 per cent the aryepiglottic folds, and 7 per cent the ventricles. The lesions were midline in 27 per cent of the cases. Smith et al.[28] reported 552 supraglottic carcinomas distributed between the epiglottis (243), false cords (128), aryepiglottic folds (116), ventricle (38), and arytenoid (27).

Compared with carcinoma of the glottis, carcinoma of the supraglottic larynx results in a significantly reduced five-year survival rate. The prognosis depends on the extent and location of the primary lesion, the presence of cervical lymph node metastasis, and the nature of the primary therapy. Lymph node metastasis appears to be the most important determinant of survival. Development of nodal disease is influenced by the extent and location of the primary lesion. The occurrence of uncontrolled neck metastasis remains a constant source of therapeutic failure with supraglottic carcinoma.

Marginal Zone Lesions. Tumors of the marginal zone or epilarynx, which includes the posterior surface of the suprahyoid portion of the epiglottis and aryepiglottic folds, behave somewhat differently from those in the remainder of the supraglottic larynx. Marginal zone tumors resemble hypopharyngeal cancers in that they spread early to involve the base of the tongue and the pharynx, have an increased incidence of metastatic spread, and less often involve the preepiglottic space.[2] Carcinomas arising on the lingual surface of the epiglottis are considered extralaryngeal and behave as do base-of-tongue tumors. Sessions and Ogura[2] classified these lesions as superior hypopharyngeal tumors. The epilaryngeal region is bounded by the epiglottis posteriorly, a line 1 cm posterior to the circumvallate papillae anteriorly, the glossoepiglottic folds laterally, and the vallecula inferiorly. Analyzing the overall survival (by partial and total laryngectomy) of patients with these tumors, Sessions and Ogura[2] found the rate to be 53 per cent (52 of 97 patients) with marginal lesions, 76 per cent (134 of 177 patients) with supraglottic lesions, and 48 per cent (12 of 25 patients) with lingual epiglottic lesions. Ogura et al.[35] described a 62 per cent survival rate for patients with the more limited lesions that were amenable to treatment by partial laryngopharyngectomy as compared with 28 per cent for those requiring a total laryngectomy. The size of the lesion appeared to be a more important determinant of survival than the presence or absence of lymph node metastasis in this group. Other workers have confirmed this poorer prognosis for tumors of the epilarynx. Taskinen[36] analyzed 932 patients with supraglottic carcinomas, finding a five-year survival rate of 40 per cent for patients with epiglottic and false cord lesions and 25 per cent for those with tumors of the arytenoid and aryepiglottic folds. Similar findings were reported by Cachin (58 per cent to 69 per cent versus 43 per cent).[33]

LYMPH NODE METASTASIS

The extensive lymphatic network of the supraglottis expresses itself in the predilection of supraglottic carcinoma for regional lymph node spread. The incidence of regional metastasis generally reported varies from 25 per cent to 50 per cent. Ogura et al.[37] described a 29 per cent incidence of regional spread; 12 per cent were palpable and 17 per cent were occult lymph nodes. Ogura et al.[35] later reported 23 per cent (41 of 177 cases) had clinically positive lymph nodes. Fayos[38] reported a 25 per cent incidence of lymph node metastasis among their 61 supraglottic tumors. Coates et al.[34] reported that 72 of 221 cases (32 per cent) had palpable nodes. Bocca[39] cited clinical and histologic cervical lymph node metastasis in 35 per cent of 240 cases. Hansen[40] reported clinically positive lymph nodes present in 41 per cent of 511 lesions. Kirchner and Owen[41] reported an incidence of 48 per cent palpable and 40 per cent occult lymph node metastasis among 97 tumors. Smith et al.[28] observed 48 per cent of 546 supraglottic tumors to have metastasized with a high proportion of contralateral, bilateral, and fixed lymph nodes. Shah and Tollefsen[42] described 51 per cent palpable and 34 per cent (22 of 65 cases) occult metastasis in their series of 290 tumors. Som[43] reported lymph node metastasis in 32 per cent of 75 patients, citing a 42 per cent incidence of positive occult contralateral nodes in those patients with a positive palpable ipsilateral node greater than 2 cm in diameter. Kirchner and Som[21] had 60 per cent histologically proven cervical metastasis in 30 cases studied by serial sectioning.

The extent of the primary lesion influences the rate of metastasis. Cachin[33] found palpable lymph nodes in 27 per cent of T1 lesions and 38 per cent of T2 lesions; 6 per cent and 19 per cent, respectively, were fixed. Taskinen[36] reported that 48 per cent of all supraglottic tumors develop metastasis; however, the incidence was only 13 per cent for T1 lesions. Shah and Tollefsen[42] reported incidence of cervical metastasis at 40 per cent for T1, 42 per cent for T2, 55 per cent for T3, and 65 per cent for T4 lesions.

The location of the primary tumor is an additional determinant of metastasis. Tumors of the epilarynx behave similarly to those of the hypopharynx, exhibiting increased regional spread. Jankovic and Merkas[44] reported metastasis in 36.4 per cent of 88 lesions of the suprahyoid epiglottis, arytenoids, and aryepiglottic folds, compared with 15.3 per cent in 391 infrahyoid epiglottic and false cord lesions. Shah and Tollefsen[42] found supraglottic tumors confined to the larynx had a 34 per cent rate of metastasis (66 per cent survival), whereas extension outside the larynx had a 69 per cent spread (37 per cent survival).

The high incidence of clinical and occult cervical lymph node metastasis with these tumors and the direct relationship between nodal disease and prognosis has prompted most surgeons to advocate routine ipsilateral and often contralateral radical neck dissection. Contralateral standard or modified radical neck dissection is often employed when there is histologically proven tumor metastasis in the ipsilateral neck specimen.[21] Coates et al.[34] recommended elective radical neck dissection in all except T1 supraglottic lesions. Bocca[39] attributed the significant improvement in his five-year cure rate for supraglottic carcinoma to the increased use of unilateral and bilateral modified radical neck dissection. Ogura et al.[37] observed an increase in survival from 74 per cent to 78 per cent with elective neck dissection and advocated its application regularly; however, Shah and Tollefsen[42] concluded that routine elective neck dissection was not warranted with supraglottic carcinoma after they observed a five-year survival rate of 32 per cent for patients with occult nodes as opposed to 27 per cent for patients with palpable nodes.

A decrease in the expected recurrence rate presents some evidence that prophylactic radiotherapy to the neck can control occult nodal disease. Fletcher et al.[45] found that only one of 69 N0 patients developed a metastatic node after elective neck irradiation. Goffinet et al.[46] reported that 81 per cent of 31 irradiated patients with supraglottic tumors did not develop cervical metastasis after two years. In five of the six patients who were not cured by radiation therapy, the primary tumor was uncontrolled and presumably reseeded the nodes. Brandenburg and Rutter[47] found that advanced laryngeal tumors (T3 and T4) treated by radiotherapy had a local recurrence rate of 80 per cent and a lymph node metastatic rate of 9 per cent. Similar lesions treated by surgery had a local failure rate of 16 per cent and a regional recurrence rate of 23 per cent, which also suggests that radiation may prevent lymph node metastasis.

MANAGEMENT AND END RESULTS

The treatment of supraglottic carcinoma includes primary radiotherapy,[48] partial or total laryngectomy,[35, 49, 50] and combined therapy.[51] Some clinicians use curative radiation for small tumors and selected advanced lesions, reserving surgery to salvage failures. Other physicians employ conservation surgery for early lesions amenable to partial laryngectomy and use total laryngectomy for advanced tumors. Some surgeons employ total laryngectomy for all operative candidates. Advocates of combined therapy utilize either preoperative or postoperative radiotherapy for patients with advanced primary lesions or for patients with extensive neck metastases. These various therapeutic approaches are considered individually in this chapter because of the differences in reported end results.

Surgery

Partial Laryngectomy. The supraglottic or subtotal horizontal laryngectomy represents a conservation laryngeal procedure in which the upper portion of the larynx is removed without sacrificing the normal functions of the remaining larynx. The basis for this procedure rests in the embryologic derivation and consequent anatomic compartmentalization of the larynx and its lymphatics, which limit tumor spread. That this procedure is oncologically sound is confirmed clinically by series of cases showing identical five-year local control of tumors by supraglottic laryngectomy and by total laryngectomy.[34, 43, 52] An important feature of the procedure is resection of the preepiglottic space, the area involved most frequently by tumor extension.

Historically, selected cases of epiglottic carcinoma have been resected through a lateral pharyngotomy since the early part of this century. In South America during the 1940s, Alonso[53] popularized the "partial horizontal laryngectomy," excising lesions of the epiglottis and false cords along with the preepiglottic space and leaving a pharyngostoma. In 1958 to 1959, Som[54] and Ogura[55] both reported en bloc supraglottic resection and radical neck dissection with primary closure. Som[54] employed direct anastomosis and Ogura[55] used muscle flaps and a skin graft to resurface the pharyngeal defect. Ogura and Biller[52] describe the procedure in its present form. Bocca[39] modified the standard procedure by (1) preserving the hyoid bone, with elevation of the periosteum off its inferior border to permit removal of the preepiglottic space, and (2) closing the pharyngostomy by approximation of the remaining thyroid alae to the hyoid bone with absorbable transfixing sutures. Bocca[39] also considered the cricopharyngeal myotomy unnecessary.

Indications. The horizontal partial laryngectomy (supraglottic resection) is performed for carcinoma involving the epiglottis and false cords.[43, 52, 56] This procedure can be extended to include carcinomas of the aryepiglottic fold and the anterior and lateral walls of the pyriform sinus and selected lesions involving the vallecula and base of the tongue. An elective neck dissection is usually performed because of the high incidence of occult nodes.[37]

Limitations. Certain conditions may limit the degree to which partial laryngectomy succeeds in curing supraglottic carcinoma. These limitations include:

1. Tumor extension onto the cricoid cartilage.
2. Bilateral arytenoid involvement.
3. Arytenoid fixation.
4. Extension onto the glottis or the presence of impaired vocal cord mobility.
5. Thyroid cartilage invasion.
6. Involvement of the apex of the pyriform sinus or postcricoid region.
7. Involvement of the base of the tongue more than 1 cm posteriorly to the circumvallate papillae.

Involvement of the perichondrium or anterior commissure indicates a transglottic lesion; if such a lesion is found at the time of surgery, total laryngectomy should be performed. Subtotal horizontal laryngectomy may also be contraindicated in patients with chronic lung disease or in elderly or debilitated patients in whom postoperative aspiration may be a problem. Failure of swallowing rehabilitation may eventually dictate a total laryngectomy in these patients.

Technique. A transverse incision is made, to which a downward limb may be added if a radical neck dissection is to be performed (Fig. 15–1A). The suprahyoid muscles are severed from the hyoid bone and from the lesser cornu on the contralateral side to the tip of the greater cornu on the involved side (Fig. 15–1B). The hyoid bone is then cut at the contralateral lesser cornu. The strap muscles are severed at the superior border of the thyroid cartilage, exposing the thyroid perichondrium. On the opposite side, the strap muscles are severed only medially, exposing the perichondrium midway from the notch to the posterior aspect. The perichondrium is incised and reflected inferiorly to the lower border of the thyroid ala (Fig. 15–1C). The proposed thyroid cartilage cuts are outlined with methylene blue dye. The anterior cut is made at the junction of the upper one-third with the lower two-thirds, measured from the base of the thyroid notch to the inferior margin of the thyroid cartilage. From this point, on the side of the lesion, the cut is extended straight posteriorly, bisecting the posterior border of the thyroid cartilage approximately midway between the origin of the superior cornu and the inferior cornu. On the contralateral side, the thyroid cartilage cut extends superiorly, bisecting the upper edge of the thyroid ala midway between the notch and the superior cornu (Fig. 15–1D). The pharynx is entered through the vallecula, provided the tumor does not involve the lingual surface of the epiglottis; it is entered through the pyriform sinus if the tumor involves the vallecula, base of the tongue, or lingual surface of the epiglottis. After the pharynx is entered, the epiglottis is grasped with a tenaculum, the patient is paralyzed, and the resection is initiated on the uninvolved side. The aryepiglottic fold is severed above the arytenoid, and then the false cord is sectioned from the true cord at the level of the ventricle. After the anterior commissure is reached, the resected portion of the supraglottis can be rotated so that the side of major tumor involvement is exposed. Assessment at this time determines whether the arytenoid should be resected partially, totally, or not at all. The aryepiglottic fold on the involved side is sectioned, and the resection is completed by traversing the arytenoid to the ventricle and then to the anterior commissure (Fig. 15–1E). The resected supraglottis is removed (Fig. 15–1F). A cricopharyngeal myotomy is then performed, with care taken not to injure the recurrent laryngeal nerve (Fig. 15–1G). If the recurrent laryngeal nerve is not identified, the myotomy should be performed posteriorly to avoid inadvertent injury. If the arytenoid cartilage has been partially or totally removed, the residual cord must be fixed to the midline so as to obtain adequate glottic closure postoperatively. Fixation of the cord in the midline is performed by suturing the vocal process to the cricoid. If the length is insufficient, a piece of cartilage is used to replace the extirpated arytenoid. The vocal cord is then fixed to this cartilage. A small mucosal flap from the pyriform sinus is sutured over the cartilage transplant. The supraglottic resection may be also extended to include the lateral wall of the pyriform sinus and the lateral and posterior pharyngeal walls. These hypopharyngeal mucosal defects may be resurfaced by the use of a split-thickness skin or dermal graft

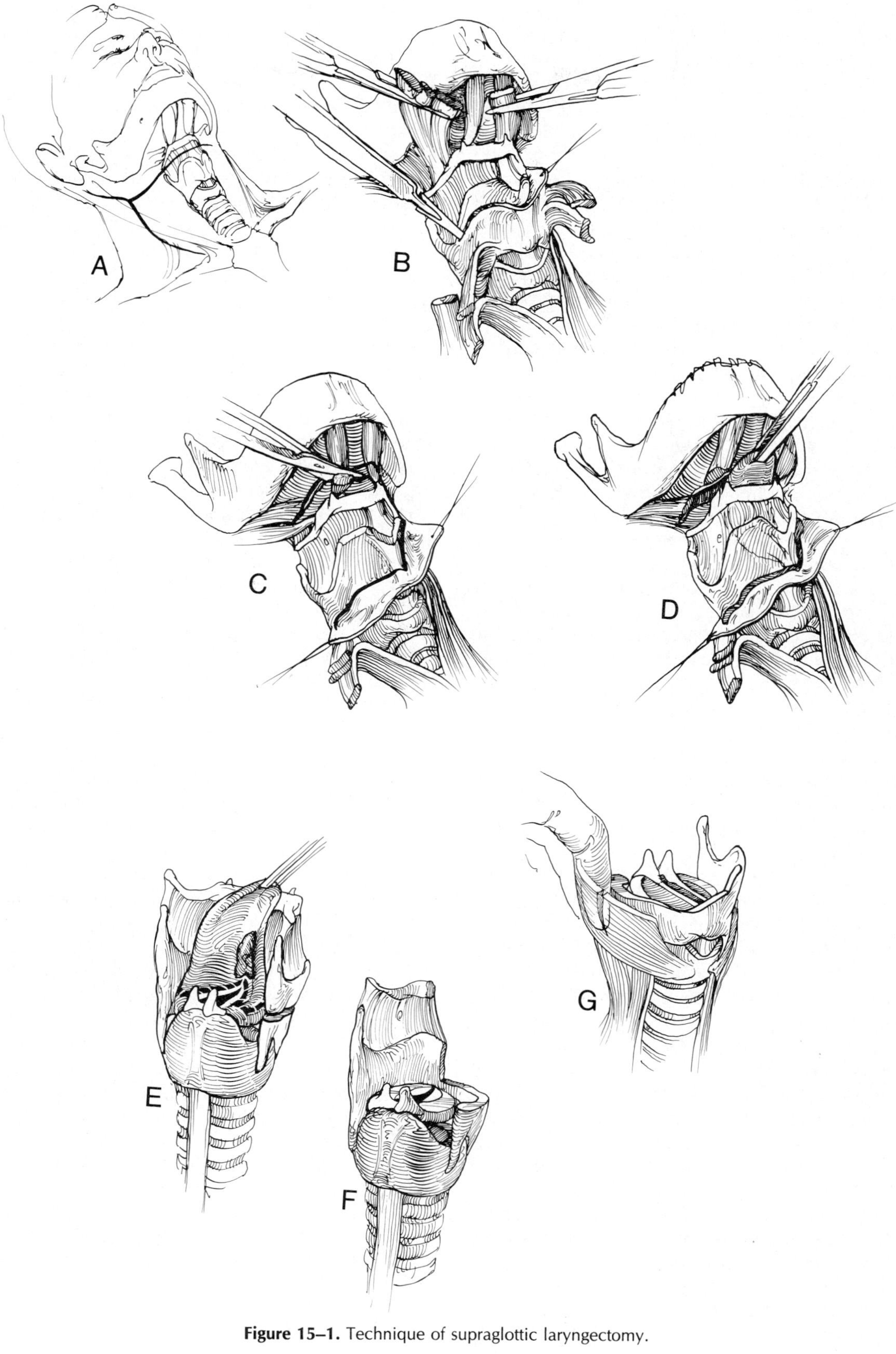

Figure 15–1. Technique of supraglottic laryngectomy.

supported by a Negus stent. In patients who have received high-dose preoperative radiation, the transfer of a regional pedicled flap with the creation of a pharyngostoma is necessary.

Closure is achieved by approximating the perichondrium and strap muscles to the base of the tongue. This closure is performed with nonabsorbable interrupted sutures. Hemovacs (suction catheter drains) are inserted, a dermal graft is utilized to cover the carotid artery, and the skin flaps are reapproximated and sutured. The patient's head is flexed during the postoperative period and he or she is fed by nasogastric tube. The tracheotomy is corked 14 days after surgery and removed the following day if the airway is adequate. The tracheotomy site is allowed to heal and oral feedings are started three weeks after surgery. Initially, the diet consists of pureed foods; after a few days, liquids are introduced. Minimal aspiration occurs during the first few days of oral feedings.

Complications. The complications of supraglottic laryngectomy involve wound healing, the rehabilitation of swallowing, and tracheal decannulation. These are generally related to the extent of the resection, prior radiotherapy, and the patient's age and general medical condition. In elderly patients, in patients with chronic lung disease, or after procedures requiring the removal of an arytenoid or extensive portions of the base of the tongue or pharynx, prolonged aspiration and delayed tracheal decannulation are expected. In these cases, deglutition may be delayed for an additional four to eight weeks. Adequate glottic closure is essential for deglutition without aspiration. Since initiation of normal deglutition requires strenuous activity and since certain patients require additional time to gain weight, nasogastric feedings may be necessary for an additional three to six weeks before successful deglutition is accomplished. Bocca[39] reported only 13 of 250 cases in which dysphagia and dyspnea lasted for several weeks, with spontaneous recovery in all but one case that required total laryngectomy. Bocca[39] also reported only six instances of infection, three of fistula and three of severe pneumonia among 223 cases. Prior high-dose radiotherapy also increases such postoperative complications as infection, hemorrhage, fistula formation, and perichondritis. If fistula formation occurs, closure usually requires the rotation of pedicled flaps.

End Results. Ogura and Biller[52] reported a three-year control rate of 85 per cent (17 of 20 cases) for lesions confined to the epiglottis with supraglottic laryngectomy; the rate dropped to 71 per cent (23 of 32 cases) when the lesion extended onto the false cords. Som[43] described a five-year control rate of 68 per cent (51 of 75 cases) with supraglottic laryngectomy. The same figure was reported by Coates et al.[34] with 30 treated cases.

Ogura et al.[35] reported an overall three-year determinant survival rate of 76 per cent for 177 patients with supraglottic lesions treated by subtotal horizontal laryngectomy and radical neck dissection (some also received preoperative radiotherapy). When clinically positive lymph nodes were noted, survival dropped to a range from 57 per cent to 66 per cent, depending on the size of the primary. Recurrent tumors appeared in 30 patients, of whom 47 per cent could be salvaged by further radiotherapy or surgery. With supraglottic lesions extending onto an arytenoid and requiring its entire removal, Ogura et al.[49] reported a 75 per cent three-year survival rate among 59 patients undergoing extended supraglottic laryngectomy; however, all but 8 patients in this series had received preoperative radiotherapy (50 patients received 2000 to 3000 rads, 2 patients received 4500 rads, and 4 patients were radiotherapy failures after 5000 to 7000 rads). Lymph nodes were occult in 7 of the 20 patients with histologically positive lymph nodes. Analysis revealed that most recurrences appeared within the first year of primary therapy and all within three years. Four of the 12 recurrences were salvaged by surgery, with or without radiotherapy. Among the 4 patients with positive margins, 2 had recurrences. Increased recurrence and diminished survival also correlated well with the presence of positive lymph nodes; however, no correlation was found between the lesion's histopathologic cell type and survival.

Bocca[39] claimed a 75 per cent one-year cure rate for 240 supraglottic tumors treated by supraglottic laryngectomy. He attributed this improved rate over his previous series[20] to both earlier diagnosis and the increased use of radical neck dissection. While Bocca studied a total of 240 cases, 132 cases followed for more than five years showed a 27 per cent failure rate. Most recurrences appeared within the first postoperative year. Analysis of 27 recurrences showed that 17 occurred in the larynx, 2 in the hypopharynx, and 3 in the base of the tongue. In 15 cases with intrinsic laryngeal recurrence, salvage was attempted by radiotherapy in 5 cases and by total laryngectomy in 10. Three of the 5 irradiated patients and 6 of the 10 laryngectomized patients were free of disease from one to seven years.

Total Laryngectomy. Supraglottic carcinomas are not longer candidates for partial subtotal horizontal laryngectomy if they have (1) extended across the ventricle to become transglottic, (2) impaired cord mobility, (3) invaded the thyroid or cricoid cartilage, (4) shown bilateral arytenoid involvement, or (5) spread outside the larynx with extensive invasion of the base of the tongue and hypopharynx. Rather, they are best treated by total laryngectomy. Medical factors (including advanced age, debility, and chronic pulmonary disease) that compromise rehabilitation of deglutition also contraindicate conservation surgery; such patients with supraglottic lesions are best treated by total laryngectomy to eliminate problems with postoperative aspiration.

While disease at the primary site in the earlier lesions is controlled equally well by partial and total laryngectomy, patients with the more advanced lesions requiring total laryngectomy have diminished survival because of extralaryngeal infiltrative growth and lymphatic spread. The increased occult and palpable lymph node disease that accompanies advanced supraglottic lesions requires radical neck dissection in addition to laryngectomy. Ogura et al.[35] reported a three-year determinate survival rate of 66 per cent for 35 patients having supraglottic carcinomas with cord fixation (T3) treated by total laryngectomy and radical neck dissection. Coates et al.[34] had a five-year cure rate of 71 per cent for 117 patients with supraglottic tumors treated by total laryngectomy with a 3 per cent local recurrence rate.

Radiotherapy

Radiotherapy for laryngeal carcinoma presently employs megavoltage radiation with a Cobalt-60 teletherapy unit or a linear accelerator. This permits accurate delivery of a high dosage to a limited area, sparing the surrounding soft tissues and overlying skin. Tumor doses ranging from 6000 to 7000 rads are required for tumor control, with the portal size determined by the location of the tumor.[57] The portals are generally enlarged to include the neck as well as the supraglottis because supraglottic lesions have a high incidence of regional metastases and some evidence suggests that elective neck irradiation decreases the observed lymph node metastases in patients with laryngeal carcinomas and N0 necks.[45–47] Radiation offers little benefit to patients with clinically positive lymph node metastases.

End Results. The overall survival rates reported with radiotherapy for the primary management of supraglottic carcinomas range from 30 per cent to 70 per cent; treatment effectiveness differs markedly with the size and location of the primary tumor and whether cervical lymph node metastases are palpable. Larger primary lesions, tumors of the epilarynx, and the occurrence of regional metastasis all significantly decrease survival. Ogura et al.[35] reported a three-year survival rate of 33 per cent (22 cases) in patients treated by radiotherapy alone. Taskinen[36] found an overall five-year survival rate of 36.1 per cent for 932 patients with supraglottic lesions, most of whom were treated by primary radiotherapy alone. The diminished survival, particularly of those with larger lesions, led Taskinen later to employ combined therapy. Jankovic and Merkas[44] reported a 39.2 per cent five-year survival rate for 439 patients with supraglottic lesions treated primarily by radiotherapy. They claimed that an additional 20 per cent could be salvaged by a second course of radiation. Goffinet et al.[58] described a 46 per cent control rate by radiotherapy alone (52 cases), noting, however, that for advanced primary lesions and positive neck nodes, irradiation provided poor control. Olofsson et al.[59] reported a 47 per cent three-year survival rate for 30 cases (T1 and T2) after primary radiotherapy. Coates et al.[34] reported a 47 per cent control rate for 55 irradiated lesions, the remainder requiring salvage surgery. Hansen[40] also found primary radiotherapy to yield less than a 50 per cent cure rate and treated more advanced lesions with combined therapy. Lederman[60–61A] reported a 53 per cent control rate for T1 tumors and 64 per cent for T2 tumors at five years among 70 cases lacking cervical metastasis. Lauerma[30] claimed cure rates of 69 per cent and 48 per cent respectively for 101 similar cases. Henk[62] reported radical radiotherapy (5000 rads in three weeks) to yield enhanced five-year tumor controls averaging 73 per cent for T1 to T2 lesions and 51 per cent for T3 to T4 tumors. Fletcher et al.[45] claimed 90 per cent of T1 lesions were controlled by radiotherapy.

Analysis by stage shows wide differences in the ability of radiotherapy to control supraglottic carcinomas. Kirchner and Owen[41] found control by radiotherapy to be 64 per cent for T1, 67 per cent for T2, and 5 per cent for T4 tumors. Vermund[63] reported, upon review of 544 supraglottic carcinomas, that radiotherapy controlled 65 per cent of T1, 61 per cent of T2, 36 per cent of T3, and 14 per cent of T4 lesions. These figures for radiotherapy also include salvage surgery. Hansen[40] found that the five-year survival rate of 511 patients with supraglottic carcinomas treated mainly by primary radiotherapy was 68 per cent for stage I, 57 per cent for stage II, 35 per cent for stage III, and 10 per cent for stage IV tumors.

While surgery and radiotherapy appear to yield comparable results in patients with early lesions and N0 necks,[41, 63] the effectiveness of radiotherapy in controlling advanced lesions diminishes markedly. Siirala and Paavolainen[64] reported an overall five-year survival rate of 35 per cent for 64 patients with advanced (stage III, IV) supraglottic lesions. Analysis by treatment modality showed 60 per cent survival for surgery, 34 per cent for combined therapy, and 20 per cent for radiotherapy alone. Henry et al.[65] treated 183 patients with T4 supraglottic tumors (one-third with positive lymph nodes) primarily by radiotherapy and found 42 per cent free of disease at three years. Among 40 cases with recurrence, 22 were operated on and 10 were salvaged. These workers noted no improvement in the cure rate with supervoltage therapy as compared with conventional radiation. Cachin[33] reported a 58 per cent five-year cure rate with radiotherapy (43 cases) for early supraglottic tumors, as opposed to 69 per cent with high-dose radiotherapy combined with partial laryngectomy (13 cases); however, the combined therapy group had greater lymph node disease. Wang et al.[66] reported three-year cure rates of 74 per cent for early (531 T1 and T2 lesions) and 23 per cent for advanced (17 T3 and T4 lesions) supraglottic tumors. The presence of palpable lymph nodes reduced survival from 63 per cent to 22 per cent. These observations led Wang and his associates to employ combined therapy for extensive primary and cervical metastatic disease. Vermund[63] reported a 32 per cent five-year survival after radiotherapy only and a 64 per cent survival after surgery only for 544 patients with T2 to T4 supraglottic carcinomas.

Location of the lesion also appeared to affect survival. Cachin[33] reported that the cure rate for early lesions of the epilarynx (14 cases) treated by radiotherapy, surgery, or a combination fell to 43 per cent from about 60 per cent for lesions located in the remainder of the supraglottic larynx; however, Fletcher et al.[67] reported a control rate of 64 per cent for early infrahyoid and false cord lesions and 69 per cent for suprahyoid and aryepiglottic fold tumors. Fletcher et al.[45] later stated that base-of-tongue and preepiglottic space involvement have continued to fail to respond to radiotherapy.

The findings indicate that primary radiotherapy achieves its greatest success in curing smaller and exophytic supraglottic tumors in patients with N0 necks. In cases with smaller primary tumors and N+ necks, the larynx may be treated by irradiation for cure and a radical neck dissection may be performed. Prophylactic neck irradiation may be given also to the contralateral side as treatment for occult disease. The presence of an advanced tumor with cord fixation or cartilage destruction mandates surgery for cure. In patients with lesions that have infiltrated the pharyngeal wall or the base of the tongue (both of which carry high probability of local recurrence), or in patients with extensive neck metastases, preoperative or postoperative radiotherapy may improve survival. Also, salvage surgery after radiation failure will probably require a total laryngectomy, rather than a conservation procedure, because of the increased incidence of chondritis and the difficulty in assessing the extent of residual or recurrent disease.

Complications. The changes produced in the larynx by therapeutic radiation range from mild soft tissue enlargement[68] to total organ necrosis. Edema of the larynx, particularly of the arytenoids, is a frequent sequela of radiotherapy. Swelling persisting for more than six months should suggest residual or recurrent disease, which may require multiple deep biopsies for diagnosis.[69] Persistent or recurrent hoarseness, ulceration, and alteration of cord mobility all indicate recurrence.[70] While Fayos[38] reported no complications after megavoltage treatment of 192 laryngeal carcinomas, Goffinet et al.[58] described a 9 per cent incidence (19 of 213 cases) that included prolonged and permanent tracheostomy, chondritis, myositis, and extensive cervical and pharyngeal fibrosis. Vermund[63] calculated a 5 per cent incidence of chondronecrosis among 474 cases.

Combined Therapy

Radiotherapy has been used preoperatively or postoperatively in conjunction with surgery to decrease the incidence of local and regional recurrences. Preoperative irradiation may also render patients with fixed neck lesions resectable.

Ogura and Biller[71] postoperatively analyzed 69 patients with supraglottic carcinomas (51 of whom had undergone partial laryngectomy);

one group of these patients received 1500 to 3000 rads preoperative radiation and the other received none. After three years, the two groups exhibited no significant difference in survival. Cachin[33] reviewed 71 cases treated with horizontal partial laryngectomy and 4000 rads preoperatively. The survival was 62 per cent at three years and 53 per cent at five years, comparable to results for nonirradiated cases. Cachin noted a significant increase in complications and suggested that preoperative radiotherapy be eliminated with supraglottic laryngectomy.

Reddi and Mercado[72] reported five-year survival rates of 75 per cent and 50 per cent, respectively, for early and late supraglottic lesions receiving combined therapy. They concluded that low-dose (3000 to 3600 rads) preoperative radiation had limited value in improving prognosis.

Cachin,[33] however, reported increased survival in patients with early lesions treated by combined therapy (69 per cent) as opposed to primary radiotherapy (58 per cent). The poor results using primary radiotherapy for advanced lesions and cases with metastatic disease led Wang et al.[66] to use 4000 rads preoperatively followed by total laryngectomy and radical neck dissection. They reported that the three-year cure rate improved from 23 per cent to 54 per cent for T3 and T4 lesions and from 22 per cent to 55 per cent in patients with lymph node disease. Ogura et al.[35] observed fewer recurrences of disease in patients with supraglottic lesions and clinically positive lymph nodes after treatment with preoperative radiotherapy. For more extensive primary tumors characterized by diminished five-year survival, he recommended preoperative radiation. Hansen[40] and Goldman et al.[51] similarly reported that combined therapy increased cure and decreased recurrence in patients with supraglottic tumors.

Fletcher et al.[67] advocated postoperative radiotherapy in cases of advanced primary lesions with extralaryngeal spread or with extensive neck disease, reporting an increase in the two-year cure rate from 38 per cent to 71 per cent.

RECURRENCE AND SPREAD OF SUPRAGLOTTIC CARCINOMA

Stomal Recurrence. Suggested causes of the development of stomal recurrence following laryngectomy include submucosal extension or lymphatic spread, peritracheal lymph node metastasis, tumor implants at the site of surgery, and origin from a new primary tumor. While stomal recurrences are often found with tumors arising or extending subglotticly,[73, 74] they rarely accompany supraglottic lesions. Whether or not tracheostomy prior to laryngectomy influences stomal recurrence is still controversial. Most surgeons have observed increased stomal recurrence following preliminary tracheostomy[75, 76] whereas others[77] relate it only to the greater size of the obstructive lesions. Radiotherapy generally provides only temporary benefit in management of stomal recurrence. Salvage surgery is employed in patients whose lesions are otherwise resectable and who have limited extension into the mediastinum.[78]

Distant Metastasis. The reported incidence of distant metastasis varies according to the site of the primary lesion and whether calculations are made from clinical or autopsy material. Autopsies in the study by Harrer and Lewis[79] showed diffuse metastases in 16 of 18 patients with carcinoma of the larynx. O'Brien et al.[80] reported that 18 of 29 patients (62 per cent) with laryngeal carcinoma showed distant spread. Abramson et al.[81] found distant metastasis in 34 per cent of 650 patients (75 autopsied) with laryngeal malignancy. The latter two studies showed that supraglottic lesions had the greatest potential for distant spread. Alonso[82] confirmed this, finding that supraglottic tumors comprised 59 per cent and glottic tumors 24 per cent of the series of 107 laryngeal and hypopharyngeal cancers with distant metastasis. Goffinet et al.[58] reported that 18 per cent of 67 supraglottic and 6 per cent of 146 glottic tumors produced distant metastasis. Failure to control the primary tumor or cervical lymph node disease contributes most to the formation of distant metastasis and death.[81, 83] Abramson et al.[81] found that 80 per cent of the patients with distant spread had tumor locally in the neck at the time of autopsy. If the primary tumor is controlled, the initial method of treatment has no influence on distant spread. Alonso[82] found that radiotherapy did not influence the spread rate. Biopsy does not contribute to dissemination; however, tracheostomy and endoscopy carry the risk of seeding into the lower respiratory tract. The size of the primary lesion also does not appear to correlate with the rate of metastasis.[83] Similarly, the patient's age, sex, and physical condition do not seem to influence distant spread. Histologic differentiation also does not affect the ability to disseminate.[84] The commonest site susceptible to spread is the lungs. Abramson et al.[81] found only one of 26 patients with distant spread who lacked pulmonary metastases, which tend to be small and multiple. Other sites of spread in decreasing order of frequency are the mediastinal lymph nodes, skeleton, and liver.[81] Spread may occur to other viscera, including the heart.[79]

References

1. Union Internationale Contre le Cancer and American Joint Committee on Cancer Staging and End Results Reporting: Supplement to TNM Classification of Malignant Tumors. Geneva, AJCC, 1973.
2. Sessions DG, Ogura JH: Classification of laryngeal cancer. *In* Alberti PW, Bryce DP (eds): Workshops from the Centennial Conference on Laryngeal Cancer. New York, Appleton-Century-Crofts, 1976, pp 83–89.
3. Van Nostrand AWP: Classification, anatomy, growth, and spread of laryngeal cancer. *In* Alberti PW, Bryce DP (eds): Workshops from the Centennial Conference on Laryngeal Cancer. New York, Appleton-Century-Crofts, 1976, pp 2–5.
4. Olofsson, J: Growth and spread of laryngeal carcinoma. *In* Alberti PW, Bryce DP (eds): Workshops from the Centennial Conference on Laryngeal Cancer. New York, Appleton-Century-Crofts, 1976, pp 40–53.
5. Hast MH: Applied embryology of the larynx. *In* Alberti PW, Bryce DP (eds): Workshops from the Centennial Conference on Laryngeal Cancer. New York, Appleton-Century-Crofts, 1976, pp 6–10.
6. Pressman JJ et al.: Anatomical studies related to the dissemination of cancer of the larynx. Trans Am Acad Ophthalmol Otolaryngol 64:628–638, 1960.
7. Tucker GF: The anatomy of laryngeal cancer. *In* Alberti PW, Bryce DP (eds): Workshops from the Centennial Conference on Laryngeal Cancer. New York, Appleton-Century-Crofts, 1976, pp 11–25.
8. Sekula J, Horzela T: Studies on the cervical lymph nodes. Arch Otolaryngol 94:118–123, 1971.
9. Kashima HK: The characteristics of laryngeal cancer correlating with cervical lymph node metastasis: Analysis based on 40 total organ sections. *In* Alberti PW, Bryce DP (eds): Workshops from the Centennial Conference on Laryngeal Cancer. New York, Appleton-Century-Crofts, 1976, pp 855–864.
10. Clerf LH: The pre-epiglottic space and its relation to carcinoma in the epiglottis. Arch Otolaryngol 40:177–179, 1944.
11. Leroux-Robert J: Les Epitheliomas Intra-Larynges: Formes Anatomo-Clinques: Voies d'Extension. Thesé Pour le Doctorat en Medicine. Paris, Gaston Dion Cie, 1936.
12. Maguire A, Dayal VS: Supraglottic anatomy: The pre- or the peri-epiglottic space. *In* Alberti PW, Bryce DP (eds): Workshop from the Centennial Conference on Laryngeal Cancer. New York, Appleton-Century-Crofts, 1976, pp 26–39.
13. Tucker GF, Smith HR: A histological demonstration of the development of laryngeal connective tissue compartments. Trans Am Acad Ophthalmol Otolaryngol 66:308–318, 1962.
14. Micheau C et al.: Modes of invasion of cancer of the larynx. Cancer 38:346–360, 1976.
15. Kirchner JA: One hundred laryngeal cancers studied by serial sections. Ann Otol Rhinol Laryngol 78:689–709, 1969.
16. Bridger GP, Nassar VH: Cancer spread in the larynx. Arch Otolaryngol 95:497–505, 1972.
17. Bridger GP: Mucous gland involvement in cancer at the anterior commissure. *In* Alberti PW, Bryce DP (eds): Workshops from the Centennial Conference on Laryngeal Cancer. New York, Appleton-Century-Crofts, 1976, pp 101–105.
18. Kirchner JA: Growth and spread of laryngeal cancer as related to partial laryngectomy. *In* Alberti PW, Bryce DP (eds): Workshops from the Centennial Conference on Laryngeal Cancer. New York, Appleton-Century-Crofts, 1976, pp 54–62.
19. Olofsson J, Van Nostrand AWP: Growth and spread of laryngeal and hypopharyngeal carcinoma with reflections on the effect of preoperative irradiation: 139 cases studied by whole organ serial sectioning. Acta Otolaryngol [Suppl] (Stockh) 308, 1973.
20. Bocca E et al.: Supraglottic surgery of the larynx. Ann Otol Rhinol Laryngol 77:1005–1026, 1968.
21. Kirchner JA, Som ML: Clinical and histological observations on supraglottic cancer. Ann Otol Rhinol Laryngol 80:638–645, 1971.
22. McGavran MH et al.: The incidence of cervical lymph node metastases from epidermoid carcinoma of the larynx and their relationship to certain characteristics of the primary tumor. Cancer 14:55–66, 1961.
23. Kirchner JA et al.: Transglottic cancer. Arch Otolaryngol 99:247–251, 1974.
24. Beahrs OH, Meyers MH (eds): American Joint Committee on Cancer. Manual for Staging of Cancer, 2nd ed. Philadelphia, JB Lippincott Company, 1983.
25. Barclay TH, Rao NN: The incidence and mortality rates for laryngeal cancer from total cancer registries. Laryngoscope 85:254–258, 1975.
26. Martensson B: Epidemiological aspects of laryngeal carcinoma in Scandinavia. Laryngoscope 85:1185–1189, 1975.
27. Krajina Z et al.: Epidemiology of laryngeal cancer. Laryngoscope 85:1155–1161, 1975.
28. Smith RR et al.: Revision of the clinical staging system for cancer of the larynx. Cancer 31:72–80, 1973.
29. Iwamoto H: An epidemiological study of laryngeal cancer in Japan (1960–1969). Laryngoscope 85:1162–1172, 1975.
30. Lauerma S: Treatment of laryngeal cancer: A study of 638 cases. Acta Otolaryngol [Suppl] (Stockh) 225:1–101, 1967.
31. Wynder EL: Toward the prevention of laryngeal cancer. Laryngoscope 85:1190–1196, 1975.
32. Lowry WS: Alcoholism in cancer of the head and neck. Laryngoscope 85:1275–1280, 1975.
33. Cachin Y: Supraglottic carcinomas: The early cases. Laryngoscope 85:1617–1623, 1975.
34. Coates HL et al.: Carcinoma of the supraglottic larynx. Arch Otolaryngol 102:686–689, 1976.
35. Ogura JH et al.: Conservation surgery for epidermoid carcinoma of the supraglottic larynx. Laryngoscope 85:1808–1815, 1975.
36. Taskinen PJ: The early case of supraglottic carcinoma. Laryngoscope 85:1643–1649, 1975.
37. Ogura JH et al.: Elective neck dissection for pharyngeal and laryngeal cancers. Ann Otol Rhinol Laryngol 80:646–651, 1971.
38. Fayos JV: Carcinoma of the endolarynx: Results of irradiation. Cancer 35:1525–1532, 1975.
39. Bocca E: Supraglottic cancer. Laryngoscope 85:1318–1326, 1975.
40. Hansen HS: Supraglottic carcinoma of the aryepiglottic fold. Laryngoscope 85:1667–1681, 1975.
41. Kirchner JA, Owen JR: Five hundred cancers of the larynx and pyriform sinus: Results of treatment by radiation and surgery. Laryngoscope 87:1288–1303, 1977.
42. Shah JP, Tollefsen HR: Epidermoid carcinoma of the

supraglottic larynx: Role of neck dissection in initial surgical management. Am J Surg 128:494–499, 1974.
43. Som ML: Conservative surgery for carcinoma of the supraglottis. J Laryngol Otol 84:655–678, 1970.
44. Jankovic I, Merkas Z: Radiotherapy as the primary approach in the treatment of laryngeal cancer. *In* Alberti PW, Bryce DP (eds): Workshops from the Centennial Conference on Laryngeal Cancer. New York, Appleton-Century-Crofts, 1976, pp 881–888.
45. Fletcher GH et al.: Reasons for irradiation failure in squamous cell carcinoma of the larynx. Laryngoscope 85:987–1003, 1975.
46. Goffinet DR et al.: Irradiation of clinically uninvolved cervical lymph nodes. *In* Alberti PW, Bryce DP (eds): Workshops from the Centennial Conference on Laryngeal Cancer. New York, Appleton-Century-Crofts, 1976, pp 889–895.
47. Brandenburg JH, Rutter SW: Residual carcinoma of the larynx. Laryngoscope 87:224–236, 1977.
48. Ennuyer A, Bataini P: Treatment of supraglottic carcinomas by telecobalt therapy. Br J Radiol 38:661–666, 1965.
49. Ogura JH et al.: Supraglottic carcinoma with extension to the arytenoid. Laryngoscope 85:1327–1331, 1975.
50. Ogura JH et al.: Conservation surgery for epidermoid carcinoma of the marginal area: Aryepiglottic fold extension. Laryngoscope 85:1801–1807, 1975.
51. Goldman JH, Roffman JD: Combined preoperative irradiation and surgery for advanced cancer of the larynx and laryngopharynx. *In* Alberti PW, Bryce DP (eds): Workshops from the Centennial Conference on Laryngeal Cancer. New York, Appleton-Century-Crofts, 1976, pp 365–374.
52. Ogura JH, Biller HF: Conservative surgery in cancer of the head and neck. Otolaryngol Clin North Am 3:641–665, 1969.
53. Alonso JM: Conservative surgery of cancer of the larynx. Trans Am Acad Ophthalmol Otolaryngol 51:633–642, 1947.
54. Som ML: Surgical treatment of carcinoma of the epiglottis by lateral pharyngotomy. Trans Am Acad Ophthalmol Otolaryngol 63:28–49, 1959.
55. Ogura JH: Supraglottic subtotal laryngectomy and radical neck dissection for carcinoma of the epiglottis. Laryngoscope 68:983–1003, 1958.
56. Ogura JH et al.: Roles and limitations of conservation surgical therapy for laryngeal cancer. *In* Alberti PW, Bryce DP (eds): Workshops from the Centennial Conference on Laryngeal Cancer. New York, Appleton-Century-Crofts, 1976, pp 392–394.
57. Wang CC: Treatment of squamous cell carcinoma of the larynx by radiation. Radiol Clin North Am 16:209–218, 1978.
58. Goffinet DR et al.: Carcinoma of the larynx: Results of radiation therapy in 213 patients. Am J Roentgenol 117:553–564, 1973.
59. Olofsson J et al.: Radiotherapy vs conservation surgery in the treatment of selected supraglottic carcinomas. Arch Otolaryngol 95:240–242, 1972.
60. Lederman M: Radiotherapy of cancer of the larynx. J Laryngol Otol 84:867–896, 1970.
61. Lederman M: Cancer of the larynx: I. Natural history in relation to treatment. Br J Radiol 44:569–578, 1971.
61A. Lederman M, Whall MA: Cancer of the larynx: II. The technique of radiation treatment. Br J Radiol 44:578–589, 1971.
62. Henk JM: The influence of oxygen and hypoxia on laryngeal cancer management. Laryngoscope 85:1134–1144, 1975.
63. Vermund H: Role of radiotherapy in cancer of the larynx as related to the TNM system of staging. Cancer 25:485–504, 1970.
64. Siirala U, Paavolainen M: The problem of advanced supraglottic carcinoma. Laryngoscope 85:1633–1642, 1975.
65. Henry J et al.: Radiotherapy in the treatment of T_3–T_4 supraglottic tumors. Laryngoscope 85:1682–1688, 1975.
66. Wang CC et al.: Combined radiation therapy and surgery for carcinoma of supraglottis and pyriform sinus. Am J Surg 124:551–554, 1972.
67. Fletcher GH et al.: The place of radiotherapy in the management of the squamous cell carcinoma of the supraglottic larynx. Am J Roentgenol 108:19–26, 1970.
68. Rideout DF: Appearances of the larynx after radiation therapy. *In* Alberti PW, Bryce DP (eds): Workshops from the Centennial Conference on Laryngeal Cancer. New York, Appleton-Century-Crofts, 1976, pp 266–269.
69. Kagan AR et al.: Significance of edema of the endolarynx following curative irradiation for carcinoma. Am J Roentgenol 120:169–172, 1974.
70. Ballantyne AJ, Fletcher GH: Surgical management of irradiation failures of nonfixed cancers of the glottic region. Am J Roentgenol 120:164–168, 1974.
71. Ogura JH, Biller HF: Preoperative irradiation for laryngeal and laryngopharyngeal cancers. Laryngoscope 80:802–810, 1970.
72. Reddi RP, Mercado R: Low-dose preoperative radiation therapy in carcinoma of the supraglottic larynx. Radiology 130:469–471, 1979.
73. Harris HH, Butler E: Surgical limits in cancers of the subglottic larynx. Arch Otolaryngol 87:490–493, 1968.
74. Norris CM: Causes of failure in surgical treatment of malignant tumors of the larynx. Ann Otol Rhinol Laryngol 68:487–508, 1959.
75. Loewy A, Laker HI: Tracheal stomal problems. Arch Otolaryngol 87:477–483, 1968.
76. Stell PM, Van Den Broeck P: Stomal recurrence after laryngectomy: Aetiology and management. J Laryngol Otol 85:131–140, 1971.
77. Modlin B, Ogura J: Postlaryngectomy tracheal stomal recurrences. Laryngoscope 79:239–250, 1969.
78. Sisson GA: Mediastinal dissection for recurrent cancer after laryngectomy. Trans Am Acad Ophthalmol Otolaryngol 74:767–777, 1970.
79. Harrer WV, Lewis PL: Carcinomas of the larynx with cardiac metastasis. Arch Otolaryngol 91:382–384, 1970.
80. O'Brien PH et al.: Distant metastases in epidermoid cell carcinoma of the head and neck. Cancer 27:304–307, 1971.
81. Abramson AL et al.: Distant metastases from carcinoma of the larynx. Laryngoscope 81:1503–1511, 1971.
82. Alonso JM: Metastasis of laryngeal and hypopharyngeal carcinoma. Acta Otolaryngol (Stockh) 64:353–360, 1967.
83. Probert JC et al.: Patterns of spread of distant metastases in head and neck cancer. Cancer 33:127–133, 1974.
84. Batsakis JH et al.: Laryngeal carcinoma: Stomal recurrences and distant metastases. *In* Alberti PW, Bryce DP (eds): Workshops from the Centennial Conference on Laryngeal Cancer. New York, Appleton-Century-Crofts, 1976, pp 868–876.

16

Glottic Carcinoma

Byron J. Bailey, M.D.

Carcinoma of the larynx arises on the true vocal cords in as much as 75 per cent of the patients presenting for treatment.[1] Hoarseness is usually an early signal of its presence. Properly managed, laryngeal cancer is the most frequently cured malignancy of the aerodigestive tract. Irradiation and surgery provide equally effective treatment for squamous cell carcinoma of the membranous portion of the true cord, but tumors involving the arytenoid area, subglottic region, or anterior commissure have a higher incidence of recurrence when treated either by irradiation therapy alone or by limited hemilaryngectomy (cordectomy) alone.[2]

The technique of partial laryngectomy and laryngoplasty I described in 1966[3] permits maximal resection of extensive glottic carcinoma combined with functional reconstruction, even after removal of both true vocal cords and one arytenoid cartilage. The original technique of vertical partial laryngectomy and laryngoplasty described by J. J. Pressman in 1954[4] effectively controls cancer and preserves the essential laryngeal functions of phonation, respiration, and deglutition. This chapter will report our experience with the modification of this technique in 70 consecutive patients, all managed between 1962 and 1978 with follow-up for at least 5 years.

Therapeutic recommendations for the management of glottic carcinoma must focus upon:

1. Local control.
2. Control of cervical lymph node metastasis.
3. The importance of second primary lesions, observed in 10 per cent to 20 per cent of patients.[5, 6]
4. Maximum preservation of laryngeal function.
5. The morbidity of various therapeutic modalities.

Management of glottic carcinoma has changed dramatically in only three decades. Prior to 1954, surgical options consisted almost exclusively of a choice between thyrotomy (laryngofissure) plus cordectomy for patients with small lesions in the membranous portion of the mobile true cord and total laryngectomy for the remainder of the patients. During the past 30 years, a variety of new surgical techniques have been described and older, previously impractical procedures have been rediscovered.

In this chapter on glottic carcinoma, we shall review important historical developments and present our opinion regarding the indications and contraindications for vertical partial laryngectomy. We shall describe a number of techniques and discuss the complications and results of vertical partial laryngectomy.

HISTORICAL SURVEY

The era of laryngeal cancer surgery opened 120 years ago when Henry B. Sands, a surgeon from New York city, reported the successful excision of a glottic carcinoma by external laryngotomy. Dr. Sands was motivated by the

Table 16–1. LANDMARK EVENTS IN CONSERVATION SURGERY*

100 A.D.	Araeteus	Was first author to write about laryngeal cancer.
1732	Morgagni	Described autopsies of two deaths from laryngeal cancer.
1788	Pelletan	Performed the first external surgical approach to the larynx to remove a foreign body.
1810	Desault	Described the operation "laryngotomy."
1829	H. Albers	Performed experimental partial and total laryngectomies in dogs.
1863	H. B. Sands	Performed the first partial laryngectomy for cancer. The patient, a 30-year-old female, survived two years and died of cancer of the kidney without laryngeal recurrence.
1864	Duncan Gibbs	Removed an epidermoid carcinoma via laryngotomy in a 29-year-old female patient who developed a recurrence one year postoperatively.
1865	Sir Astley Cooper	Removed a malignant tumor of the epiglottis by finger dissection by a transoral approach.
1866	Patrick Heron Watson	Performed the first total laryngectomy on a patient with laryngeal syphilis.
1870	V. Czerny	Was led by interest in Watson's laryngectomy to perform surgical experiments in dogs. He assisted Billroth on the first laryngectomy performed for cancer.
1871	Morell Mackenzie	Was first to advocate preoperative laryngeal biopsies.
1873	T. Billroth	Performed the first total laryngectomy for cancer. The patient, a 36-year-old male, developed local recurrence and died seven months postoperatively.
1875	T. Billroth	Reported a case in which he performed hemilaryngectomy for cancer.
1876	S. Isambert	Reported results in five cases of cancer of the larynx treated by partial laryngectomy. Classified laryngeal tumors using the terms *intrinsic, extrinsic,* and *subglottic.*
1891	J. Hajek	Reported studies of laryngeal lymphatics that supported the concept of partial laryngectomy.
1894	Felix Semon	Published an early series on 12 patients with satisfactory results from partial laryngectomy.
1895	Henry Butlin	Published early results that added impetus to the acceptance of partial laryngectomy.
1903	Felix Semon	Reported a series of 18 cases treated by thyrotomy, 15 of which were cured at one or more years.
1904	P. R. W. de Sancti	Reported studies of laryngeal lymphatics and their importance in regard to cancer.
1904	Chevalier Jackson	Advocated the acceptance of partial laryngectomy in the United States and added many significant refinements to the procedure.
1909	Henry Butlin	Reported a series of 21 patients who had laryngofissure. Only one operative death occurred; 17 patients were alive and well three years postoperatively.
1912	St. Clair Thomson	Reported a series of ten laryngofissures with no operative mortality. One patient died of recurrence, one later required a total laryngectomy, and eight patients were reported cured.
1912	Gluck and Sorensen	Described a standard technique for laryngectomy.
1916	L. H. Lack	Described a technique extending cordectomy to include a portion of the overlying thyroid cartilage.
1922–1930	St. Clair Thomson	Wrote a series of articles simplifying and standardizing the laryngofissure procedure. Reported 70 cases with 76 per cent three-year cure rate.
1930	A. Hautant	Published experience with a modification of the hemilaryngectomy of Gluck and Sorensen, reporting 20 cases with two operative deaths.
1936	Chevalier L. Jackson	Emphasized the importance of radiographic examination of the larynx, including contrast laryngograms.

Table continued on opposite page

same goals that are uppermost in the minds of today's laryngeal surgeons as they evaluate each patient with laryngeal carcinoma for laryngeal conservation surgery. The primary goal continues to be complete removal of all malignant disease; the secondary goal is maximum preservation of the respiratory, phonatory, and sphincteric functions of the larynx.

The fascinating history of this era can be readily divided into thirds, each a 40-year block having its distinctive point of emphasis. During the first third, which may be called the period of "reluctant acceptance of the concept of conservation surgery," innovative surgeons independently devised and employed assorted procedures with varying degrees of success. In different parts of the world, the concept was buried and resurrected on several occasions.

During the second block, the period of "popularization and basic development," a few

Table 16–1. LANDMARK EVENTS IN CONSERVATION SURGERY (*Continued*)

1940	L. H. Clerf	Described modified partial laryngectomy for anterior commissure carcinoma.
1943	E. N. Broyles	Described the histologic features of the anterior commissure tendon and its clinical significance in anterior commissure carcinoma.
1947	J. M. Alonso	Described partial vertical laryngectomy for selected lesions involving the pyriform sinus and partial horizontal laryngectomy for supraglottic malignancy.
1949	H. M. Goodyear	Described the use of acrylic stents after hemilaryngectomy and total laryngectomy to preserve airway patency.
1950	F. A. Figi	Described the use of skin grafts to line the larynx after hemilaryngectomy (this technique had been used previously by others to treat laryngeal stenosis).
1951	M. L. Som	Described the use of sliding mucosal flaps to close the defect after hemilaryngectomy.
1954	J. J. Pressman	Reported a technique for partial laryngectomy. One or both thyroid alae are removed and replaced in a muscular pocket to restore laryngeal support. The lumen of the larynx is lined with perichondrium. Also reported basic observations regarding compartmentation of the laryngeal lymphatics.
1956	J. Leroux-Robert	Described the "extended frontolateral" partial laryngectomy, which allows resection of more extensive malignant lesions.
1956	M. L. Som	Described a technique for partial laryngoesophagectomy.
1958	J. H. Ogura	Modified horizontal partial laryngectomy, eliminating the need for a pharyngostoma.
1960	J. H. Ogura	Refined the technique for partial laryngopharyngectomy with radical neck dissection for pyriform sinus lesions.
1962	J. Miodonski	Reported results with an extended hemilaryngectomy that included partial removal of the cricoid cartilage and the epiglottis.
1965	J. H. Ogura	Reported a technique utilizing a cartilaginous triangle from the superior rim of the thyroid cartilage to reconstruct the glottis after partial laryngectomy.
1967	L. Bernstein and S. Holt	Described the use of the bipedicle sternohyoid muscle flap as a filler in cases of uncompensated unilateral vocal cord paralysis.
1968	A. Maran et al.	Reported experimental results from a variety of laryngoplasty techniques including bipedicle sternohyoid muscle laryngoplasty.
1969	H. Quinn	Described the use of free muscle grafts for glottic reconstruction after partial laryngectomy.
1969	J. E. Delahunty et al.	Reported the results of vocal cord transplantation in dogs.
1969	J. H. Ogura and H. Biller	Reported the use of a monopedicle sternohyoid muscle flap for glottic reconstruction after partial laryngectomy.
1975	J. Kirchner and M. Som	Refined the indications and contraindications for the anterior commissure partial laryngectomy technique.
1975	J. Ogura et al.	Reviewed the role and limitations of conservation surgery in relation to the surgical anatomy of the larynx.
1975	P. Ward et al.	Reported experience regarding the ominous significance of persistent edema and the high incidence of persistent cancer requiring total laryngectomy for salvage.
1979	J. E. Russ et al.	Clarified the role of conservation surgery using whole organ serial sections.
1981	B. W. Pearson	Described subtotal laryngectomy for advanced glottic carcinoma. Phonation was retained.

*Complete references for entries in this table through 1969 may be found in Bailey BJ: Laryngoscope 81:1742–1771, 1971. For more recent references, see: (1) Kirchner JA, Som ML: Laryngoscope 85:1308–1317, 1975; (2) Ogura JH et al.: Can J Otolaryngol 4:400–458, 1975; (3) Ward PH et al.: Laryngoscope 85:522–529, 1975; (4) Pearson BW: Laryngoscope 91:1904–1912, 1981; (5) Russ JE et al.: Am J Surg 138:588–596, 1979.

pioneers collected and reported convincing evidence attesting to the validity of the concept of conservation surgery. Considerable experience was gained in the proper selection of surgical candidates, and the details of a few standardized excisional procedures, known as *hemilaryngectomy* and *laryngofissure,* were broadly disseminated.

The most recent 40 years have been characterized by rapid development in medical science. General advances in antibiotic therapy, blood replacement, and anesthesia set the stage for improvements in the operative and postoperative management of patients with laryngeal cancer. The two latest advances of note have been further clarification of the indications for and the limitations of conservation surgery and emphasis on the reconstructive phase, or *laryngoplasty,* which attempts to enhance postoperative laryngeal function.

To place the current state of surgical management of glottic carcinoma into proper perspective, we retrace the steps of the pioneer physicians who built our present body of knowledge regarding laryngeal cancer surgery. Table 16–1 recounts the landmark events in the evolution, popularization, and investigation of conservation surgery of the larynx.

THE POPULATION AT RISK FOR GLOTTIC CARCINOMA

During 1982, physicians diagnosed 11,000 new cases of glottic carcinoma in the United States.[7] Most of these patients were males older than 40 years who had histories of significant smoking and ethanol intake. Among the patients we have seen, the mean age was 59 years with an average duration of symptoms of 6 months. Two decades ago, males outnumbered females 12 to 1, but at present this ratio has decreased to approximately 6 to 1, probably due to changing patterns of smoking and ethanol intake by women in our society. Recently, several excellent studies have investigated the epidemiology of laryngeal cancer. Silverberg[8] determined that in the United States, one person out of 74 persons diagnosed as having cancer has cancer of the larynx. Wynder et al.[9] reported that the relative risk for development of laryngeal cancer is 7 times greater for patients who smoke 35 or more cigarettes per day than for nonsmokers, and 22 times greater for those who smoke 35 or more cigarettes and drink 7 ounces or more of alcohol per day than for nonsmokers and nondrinkers.

The data from studies dealing with occupational risk factors indicate a convincing association between exposure to asbestos and laryngeal cancer. Other studies indicate that risk for developing laryngeal cancer among workers in nickel refineries ranges from 3.6 to 8 times the risk in the general population.[10, 11] Wynder et al.[9] found that workers exposed to wood dust developed laryngeal cancer 24 times more frequently than the general population. Wada et al.[12] described increased incidence of laryngeal cancer in workers at a Japanese factory manufacturing mustard gas, the risk being approximately 8 times greater than that ordinarily expected.

Correlations between specific occupations and laryngeal cancer have been noted in industries manufacturing isopropyl alcohol,[13] leather, paper, other chemicals, and textiles. Drivers, bartenders, naphthalene cleaners, and barbers[13–19] also appear to be at higher risk for laryngeal carcinoma. Other chemical exposures reported to increase risk include diethyl sulfate,[20] triethanolamine after reaction with sodium nitrite,[21, 22] and styrene.[23, 24]

Outside the continental United States, epidemiologic studies report the highest incidence of laryngeal carcinoma in India,[25] Brazil,[26] Italy and Spain,[27] and Colombia, Israel, Finland, and Hawaii.[28]

Demographic studies in the United States show that incidence of laryngeal carcinoma is 7.5 per 100,000 person-years for white males and 7.9 per 100,000 person-years for black males.[29] Laryngeal cancer is uncommon among American Indians, Japanese-Americans, and Chinese-Americans.[26, 30] The peak incidence for all stages of carcinoma of the larynx in the United States is 38 cases per 100,000 person-years at age 70 for males and approximately 4.5 per 100,000 person-years at age 58 for females.[29]

MANAGEMENT OPTIONS

Preservation of the patient's life commands a higher priority than the preservation of laryngeal function or other secondary considerations. Selecting the most appropriate single modality or combination of treatment options is a complex decision that must take into account the patient's age, occupation, physical and mental health, personal habits, family and occupational environment, and economic needs. The size, extent, and location of the primary tumor and metastatic disease (if any) must be determined. Also, the morbidity of surgery, radiation therapy, and chemotherapy is an extremely important consideration, along with preservation of laryngeal function and provisions for the highest quality of life obtainable after treatment. Unlike carcinoma of the lung, which may routinely warrant an all-out surgical and radiotherapeutic attack, glottic carcinoma will respond successfully to a more conservative approach in 80 per cent to 90 per cent of selected patients.

Conservation surgery generally will cure about 90 per cent of all patients who present with T1 and T2 glottic carcinoma. Radiation therapy is recommended for early cancer of the true vocal cord with normal cord mobility; this treatment almost always results in cure rates equivalent to surgery plus a superior posttreatment voice. DeSanto[6] and others have noted that approximately 25 per cent of patients with glottic carcinoma will present with lesions that are suitable for radiation therapy as the single preferred modality.

Glottic carcinoma associated with a fixed cord or with extension of cancer beyond the interior of the laryngeal skeleton is usually treated by total laryngectomy. Ipsilateral radical neck dissection is recommended in the presence of stage N1, or greater, neck node disease. Important advances in the vocal rehabilitation of patients after total laryngectomy and improved techniques for laryngeal reconstruction after partial laryngectomy have caused us to revise our thinking about the role of surgery. Although removal of the entire larynx no longer means loss of the ability to communicate, these surgical techniques still impose some discomfort and disability upon the patient.

Specific indications for radiation therapy, total laryngectomy, and chemotherapy in more advanced cancer appear in other chapters of this text. The purpose of this chapter is to summarize our current views regarding the management of stage T1 and T2 glottic carcinoma by vertical partial laryngectomy.

Most glottic carcinoma arises on the membranous portion of the true vocal cord and, in about 20 per cent to 25 per cent of patients, the tumor will extend to involve the anterior commissure region at the time of diagnosis. Of patients with glottic carcinoma, 20 per cent will have supraglottic extension onto the inferior one-half of the false vocal cord and another 20 per cent will have subglottic extension in excess of 5 mm from the margin of the true cord.[1, 31] Another 15 per cent to 20 per cent of patients will have posterior extension of the tumor to involve the vocal process or the body of the arytenoid cartilage. Our observations agree with those of Strong[32] that patients whose cancer invades cartilaginous structures will have a higher incidence of postradiotherapy cancer recurrence. In patients who have stage T1 glottic carcinoma involving the anterior commissure or arytenoid cartilage and in patients with superficial T2 glottic carcinoma, surgical excision ranging from laryngofissure and cordectomy[1] to extended frontolateral vertical partial laryngectomy is highly effective.

Biller and Lawson[33] report successful treatment of tumors involving the anterior commissure and both true vocal cords using bilateral vertical partial laryngectomy (frontolateral approach). Their preferred method employs tumor excision with wide margins but preserves adequate function in a series of patients who would otherwise have required total laryngectomy. The patient who presents with diminished cord mobility or apparent cord fixation poses special problems. True fixation of the vocal cord is usually secondary to direct deep extension of cancer invading the vocalis muscle and paraglottic space. Distinguishing this condition from limitation of motion associated with a bulky exophytic tumor may be difficult.[34, 35] Radiographic studies, including computerized tomography, may help in distinguishing deep invasion from involvement of the paraglottic space or thyroid cartilage, as described in Chapter 5 of this volume. Lesinski, Bauer, and Ogura have reported their encouraging experience with conservation surgery in 18 patients with fixation of the true vocal cord;[36] although we have employed vertical partial laryngectomy successfully in patients with markedly diminished cord mobility, we continue to perform total laryngectomy for patients with a completely fixed cord.

Whole-organ histologic serial sections of the larynx provide the opportunity to better understand the biologic behavior of glottic carcinoma. Kirchner[37] observed that true cord fixation reflects deep invasion, noting that a good salvage rate (60 per cent) could be obtained in patients with these lesions when they do not extend below the inferior edge of the thyroid cartilage. He also described the favorable significance of anterior subglottic extension, in contrast to posterior extension encroaching upon the cricoid cartilage.

Kirchner[38] reviewed the patterns of laryngeal cancer spread as studied by serial sections of the larynx and correlated his observations with the use of partial laryngectomy techniques in management. He noted that glottic cancer involving the anterior commissure and both true cords is an indication for the anterofrontal partial laryngectomy (anterior commissure) technique. Extended frontolateral partial laryngectomy is indicated when the tumor involves the entire length of the cord, including the vocal process of the arytenoid. He also reported that subglottic tumor spread is much more ominous when located posteriorly and nearer to the superior margin of the cricoid cartilage. Conservation surgery is indicated for patients with glottic carcinoma that involves either the anterior commissure or the vocal process of the arytenoid. Som[39] manages small surgical defects after hemilaryngectomy by covering the raw surface with an advancement flap of mucosa from the pyriform sinus. He reconstructs defects using a composite flap of inferior constrictor muscle and an attached portion of thyroid cartilage.

The following considerations should help the surgeon to select the proper modality and preoperative plan:

1. Carcinoma limited to the true vocal cord is associated with less than 5 per cent incidence of cervical lymph node metastasis.
2. Vocal cord fixation or tumor extension through the cartilage or otherwise beyond the interior of the endolarynx is associated with a 30 per cent to 40 per cent incidence of cervical lymph node metastasis and with less than 50 per cent five-year survival, free of disease.
3. A second primary lesion will develop in approximately 20 per cent of patients with glottic carcinoma. These lesions will be in the larynx and laryngopharynx in 6 per cent, with the remainder located in other head and neck sites or sites such as lung, gastrointestinal tract, or genitourinary tract. Second primary lesions are reported to occur earlier and twice as frequently following radiation therapy.

Recurrence of glottic carcinoma following radiation therapy can be managed effectively by vertical partial laryngectomy when the patients meet specific criteria for this surgery.[35, 40–43] According to Biller,[44] the following conditions must be met:

1. The contralateral cord must be free of tumor (although the anterior commissure may be involved).
2. The body of the arytenoid cartilage must be free of tumor.
3. The subglottic extension must not exceed 5 mm.
4. Cartilage invasion must be absent.
5. Cord fixation must be absent.
6. The location and extent of the recurrence must correlate closely with the original primary lesion.

Most patients with recurrent carcinoma after radiation therapy require total laryngectomy to be salvaged for cure. This is the strongest argument against the philosophy that all patients with glottic carcinoma should be irradiated first and then observed for recurrence, reserving surgical management for the unfortunate patient who develops recurrent glottic carcinoma. Our experience includes 70 consecutive patients with glottic carcinoma managed by vertical partial laryngectomy. Four of these patients had glottic carcinoma limited to the membranous portion of the true cord, 10 had extension to the vocal process of the arytenoid cartilage, 45 had extension to the anterior commissure, and 11 had transglottic lesions.

Vertical partial laryngectomy and extended frontolateral partial laryngectomy have been highly effective in managing this group of patients, and reconstruction of the surgical defect has been instrumental in preserving laryngeal function. Involvement of the contralateral true vocal cord in 14 of these patients was extensive enough to require reconstruction of the larynx with bilateral bipedicle muscle flaps. The primary lesion was transglottic in 11 patients in whom we judged that the primary carcinoma had originated on the true vocal cord and subsequently extended to involve the laryngeal ventricle and the inferior portion of the ipsilateral false vocal cord. Our preoperative observations found these transglottic lesions were neither bulky nor deeply invasive; nor were they associated with vocal cord fixation.

Indications for a vertical partial laryngectomy and laryngoplasty are:

1. Carcinoma involving the anterior commissure.
2. Carcinoma involving the vocal process or body of the arytenoid cartilage.
3. Selected transglottic carcinoma.
4. Selected patients with recurrent carcinoma following radiation therapy.
5. Verrucous carcinoma that can be totally excised by a conservation surgical procedure.

Five contraindications for these techniques are:

1. Cancer invasion of the posterior commissure.
2. Involvement of both arytenoid regions.
3. Bulky transglottic carcinoma.
4. Thyroid cartilage invasion.
5. Fixation of the vocal cord.

Until four years ago, we considered the presence of a metastatic lymph node a contraindication to vertical partial laryngectomy, but we have now begun to perform hemilaryngectomy and neck dissection for patients with stage N1 neck disease. Because they have been operated on within the past four years, these patients are not included in this analysis of the earlier 70 patients.

Several surgical groups are currently investigating conservation surgery in patients who have true vocal cord fixation. As our experience grows, we may be able to identify a subset of patients in whom vertical partial laryngectomy will be appropriate in the presence of a fixed cord. While we have not pursued this feature in our patient series, we watch with interest the progress being made by other investigators.

Numerous publications document the difficulties of morbidity and tumor recurrence when patients with transglottic carcinoma and with tumors involving the anterior commissure or the arytenoid cartilage are treated with irradiation. Some institutions report results that imply superior radiation therapy resources and personnel. In this era of cancer patient management by an oncology team, specific decisions for management are made appropriately by discussion and continuing analysis of outcome by all members of the team. We hope that placing the efforts to cure cancer as their first priority with preservation of laryngeal function close behind will lead to the proper decision in each case.

SURGICAL TECHNIQUES FOR CORDECTOMY AND HEMILARYNGECTOMY*

Resection of a portion of the larynx for carcinoma has been designated by various names. The main objective is adequate removal of the cancer coupled with conservation of the main laryngeal functions (speech, airway, and prevention of aspiration), hence the overall descriptive term of *conservation surgery.*

The more common surgical procedures performed on the larynx may be organized into the basic classification shown in Table 16–2. Hemilaryngectomy, a true and complete removal of one-half of the entire larynx, is seldom, if ever, performed. This procedure will not be described here. This chapter is concerned with the first two types of partial laryngectomy—cordectomy and vertical or frontolateral laryngectomy. Figure 16–1 outlines the basic portions of the larynx removed in these procedures.

*The material describing surgical changes in this section is adapted from Loré JM Jr.: An Atlas of Head and Neck Surgery, Vol 2, 2nd ed. Philadelphia, WB Saunders Company, 1973, pp 726–743.

Table 16–2. SURGICAL PROCEDURES PERFORMED ON THE LARYNX*

Partial laryngectomy
- A. Cordectomy via laryngofissure
- B. Vertical or frontolateral partial laryngectomy
- C. Horizontal partial laryngectomy
  - 1. Supraglottic procedure
  - 2. Supracricoid procedure
- D. Combinations and extensions of A, B, and C with or without involvement of the ventricle, ventricular bands, aryepiglottic fold, and juxtaposed portion of medial wall of pyriform sinus

Total laryngectomy
- A. Narrow field laryngectomy
- B. Wide field laryngectomy

*Adapted from Loré JM Jr.: An Atlas of Head and Neck Surgery. Vol 2, 2 ed. Philadelphia, WB Saunders Company, 1973.

Simple Cordectomy via Laryngofissure

Surgical Technique for Cordectomy. Details of this operation are shown in Figure 16–1A. The simple cordectomy via a laryngofissure (midline thyrotomy) is limited to a carcinoma of 1 to 5 mm in size on the free edge of the membranous vocal cord at its middle one-third. The resection is carried down to the thyroid cartilage, removing the inner perichondrium. That no cartilage is removed constitutes the main objection by critics of the operation, as invasion of the vocalis muscle may be present. A legitimate difference of opinion exists regarding the treatment of small tumors of the true cord with radiotherapy; the final decision rests on the availability of adequate radiotherapy facilities. This procedure is also useful when the diagnosis is questionable.

Key Points for Cordectomy. When a small carcinoma of the true vocal cord is to be treated by cordectomy, the following points should be kept in mind:

1. Lesion size must not exceed 5 mm.
2. Lesion must be limited to the middle one-third of the vocal cord and must be localized to the free margin of the vocal cord.
3. The vocal cord must have full and complete mobility.
4. Margins must be carefully checked for extension of tumor.

Vertical Partial Laryngectomy

Surgery for vertical or frontolateral laryngectomy may be divided into three basic types of procedure, depending on the extent of the tumor along the edge of the membranous vocal cord. One modification may be applied to any of the three basic types if subglottic extension does not exceed 2 to 3 mm. A second modification may be applied if the vocal process of the arytenoid cartilage is involved.

The delineation of the extent and lines of resection in millimeters has been a point of criticism of partial laryngectomy procedures.

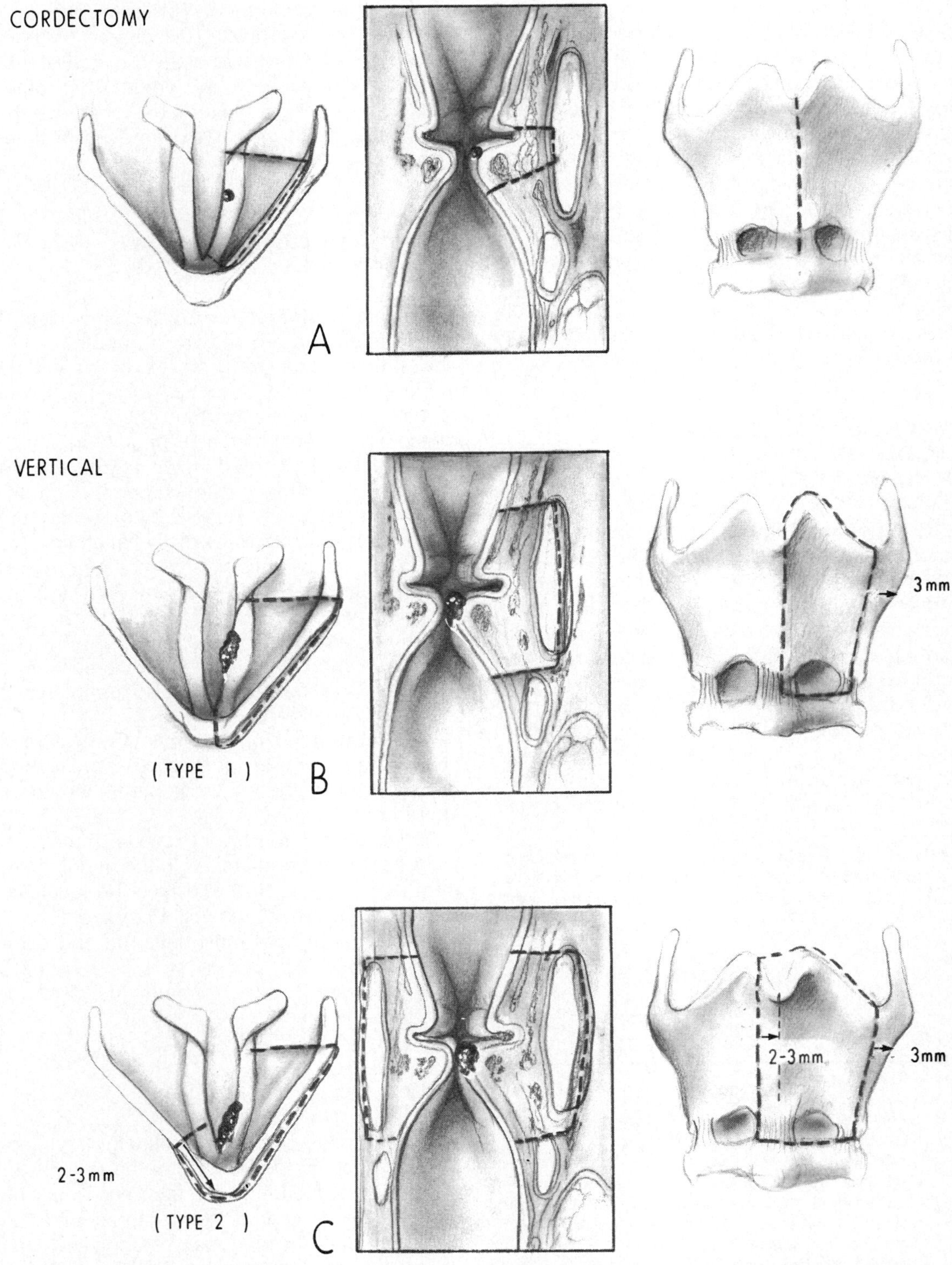

Figure 16–1. Portions of larynx removed in the first two types of partial laryngectomy *A*, Simple cordectomy using a midline thyrotomy approach. *B*, Basic Type 1 vertical partial laryngectomy. *C*, Basic Type 2 vertical partial laryngectomy for anterior commissure carcinoma.

Illustration continued on opposite page

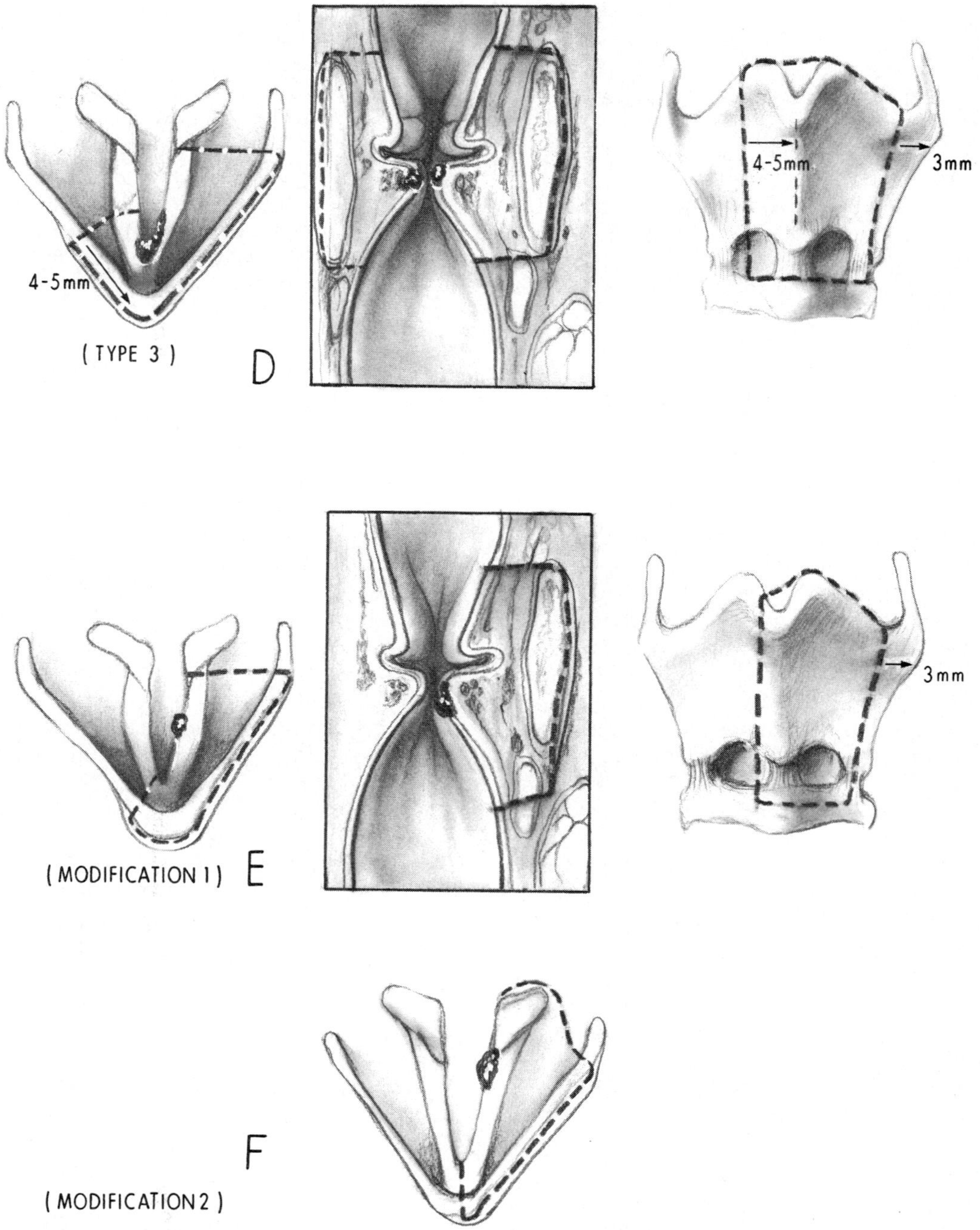

Figure 16–1 *Continued. D,* Basic Type 3 vertical partial laryngectomy for carcinoma extending to the contralateral cord. *E,* Type 3 modified for subglottic extension. *F,* Type 3 modified to include arytenoid resection. (From Loré JM Jr: An Atlas of Head and Neck Surgery, Vol 2, 2nd ed. Philadelphia, WB Saunders Company, 1973, pp 729, 731.)

Over the past two decades, ample evidence has shown that these procedures are safe and effective. Appropriate selection of patients is essential, and all patients undergoing this type of surgery must be given continuous and extremely careful follow-up examinations.

Basic Type 1, Vertical Partial Laryngectomy. Figure 16–1B shows a variation of this technique. Carcinoma must be limited to the membranous vocal cord at its middle one-third. The entire vocal cord, with the vocal process of the arytenoid cartilage and the adjacent thyroid ala, is resected except for a posterior vertical strip of thyroid cartilage 3 mm wide. The anterior line of resection is in the midline. If the lesion extends into the posterior one-third of the vocal cord, the arytenoid cartilage is resected. The subglottic tissue is resected to the superior border of the cricoid cartilage.

Basic Type 2, Vertical Partial Laryngectomy. This procedure is shown in Figure 16–1C. It is appropriate for carcinoma of the membranous vocal cord extending to the anterior commissure. The tissue resected is the same as in Basic Type 1 above, except that 2 to 3 mm of thyroid cartilage and the juxtaposed true and false cords and subglottic soft tissue are resected on the contralateral side. The frontal view of the anterior commissure region (Fig. 16–1C) shows the thyroid ala resected on the contralateral side as well as on the side of the lesion.

Basic Type 3, Vertical Partial Laryngectomy. Figure 16–1D illustrates this procedure, used for carcinoma of the membranous vocal cord extending into the anterior one-third of the opposite (contralateral) vocal cord. The tissue resected is the same as in Basic Type 1, except that 4 to 5 mm of thyroid cartilage and juxtaposed true and false cords and subglottic soft tissue are resected on the contralateral side. The frontal view in Figure 16–1D shows the amount of the thyroid alae resected on both sides.

Modification 1, Vertical Partial Laryngectomy. This procedure is appropriate for carcinoma of the membranous vocal cord with 2 to 3 mm of subglottic extension. The tissue resected intially is the same as in Figure 16–1B, C, or D, depending on the extent of the tumor along the edge of the vocal cord. Next, the upper half of the cricoid cartilage is resected posteriorly to the arytenoid cartilage on the involved side and across the midline on the contralateral side (Fig. 16–1E).

Modification 2, Vertical Partial Laryngectomy. This modification applies to carcinoma of the membranous vocal cord involving a portion of the vocal process of the arytenoid cartilage. The tissue resected is the same as in Figure 16–1F, with the entire arytenoid cartilage resected.

Other Modifications. Since 1971, we have have used partial laryngectomy with laryngoplasty, further modifying the technique for vertical partial laryngectomy. Our preferred technique is described later in this chapter.

Key Points for Vertical or Frontolateral Laryngectomy. When one of the procedures described above is being considered, these points must be observed:

1. Complete evaluation of extent of tumor is accomplished by indirect and direct laryngoscopy, microlaryngoscopy, planograms, and laryngogram. Permission should be obtained for a total laryngectomy.
2. Vocal cords must be mobile. A slightly sluggish vocal cord may not in itself be a contraindication.
3. Lesion must be limited to membranous vocal cord with subglottic extension no more than 2 to 3 mm. Cartilage invasion as demonstrated by an x-ray film or by widening of the thyroid cartilage is a contraindication.
4. Extension into the ventricle may be a limiting factor; however, a primary small neoplasm of the ventricle is usually suitable for this type of resection.
5. Severe to moderate chronic pulmonary disease, e.g., emphysema, is a limiting factor.
6. One arytenoid cartilage along with one-half to two-thirds of its vocal cord must remain on the contralateral side.
7. Regardless of the procedure, entrance into the larynx must be as far away from the tumor as possible, preferably on the contralateral side.
8. A vertical strip of cartilage, 3 mm wide, is preserved along the posterior portion of the thyroid cartilage on the involved side.
9. The resected specimen includes:
   a. true vocal cord.
   b. false vocal cord and walls of ventricle.
   c. either the vocal process or arytenoid cartilage.
   d. thyroid cartilage except for a 3-mm posterior vertical strip on the involved side and a portion of the opposite thyroid ala, depending on the extent of tumor.
   e. anterior and lateral subglottic tissue and, if gross subglottic extension is present, the upper one-half of the cricoid cartilage.
10. Tracheotomy is necessary. A laryngeal keel is usually used when both sides are operated upon. Drains are utilized.
11. The procedure can be performed in patients who are radiation failures; however, extreme care must be exercised

because of difficulty in evaluating the extent of disease.

PREFERRED SURGICAL TECHNIQUES FOR VERTICAL PARTIAL LARYNGECTOMY AND LARYNGOPLASTY

Our preference for the technique employed for vertical partial laryngectomy and laryngoplasty has evolved over the past 20 years. The basic concept as developed by Pressman has undergone several modifications to achieve a more reliable reconstruction in a shorter operating time.

Two different techniques are utilized—one is appropriate for unilateral lesions, the other is suitable for carcinoma involving the anterior commissure or extending to involve a major portion of the contralateral cord. The techniques are identical until the surgeon reaches the step involving incisions of the thyroid cartilage. The unilateral technique and the anterior commissure or bilateral technique will be described separately.

The patient is placed on the operating table in the prone position with the head extended. Endotracheal inhalation anesthesia may be used when the procedure begins and the tube may be changed to the tracheotomy site later. Alternatively, the tracheotomy may be performed under local anesthesia if the surgeon prefers to avoid passing an endotracheal tube through the glottic region. The neck is prepared and draped in a standard manner. A transverse incision passes one finger's breadth below the inferior margin of the cricoid cartilage, curving outward in the natural skin folds of the neck. Just lateral to the anterior jugular veins, it is curved superiorly toward the mastoid tip up to a level just superior to the greater cornua of the hyoid bone (Fig. 16–2). The tracheotomy incision may be

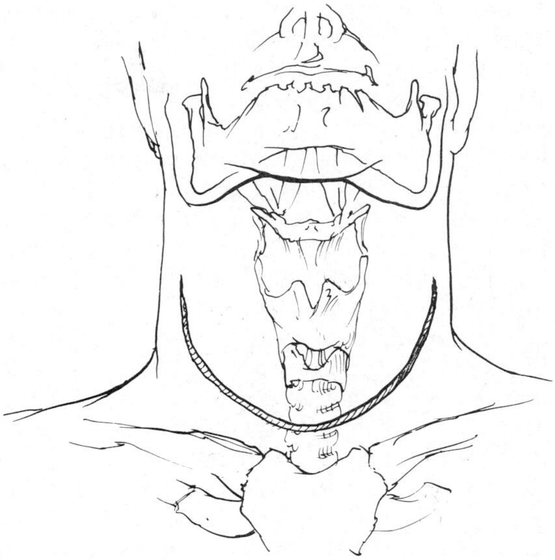

Figure 16–2. Apron incision to expose larynx and anterior neck.

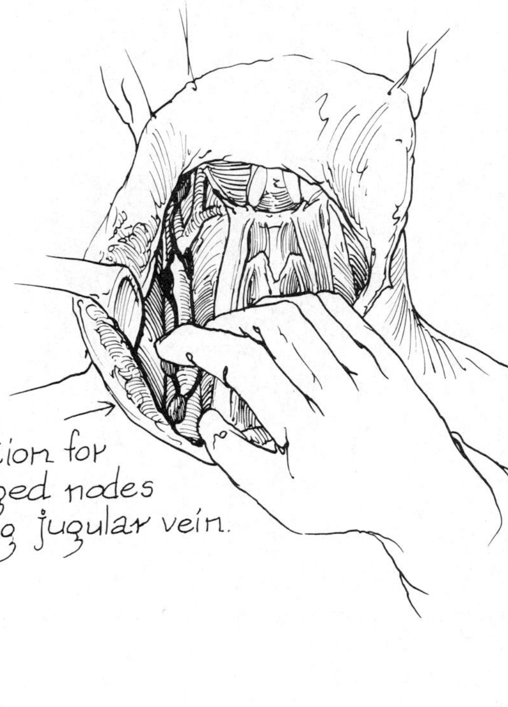

Figure 16–3. Palpation and biopsy of lymph nodes to rule out metastatic carcinoma.

made by dropping a vertical limb approximately 2 cm inferiorly from the midpoint of the skin incision, or it may be made through a separate transverse incision 2 cm inferior to the major neck incision. The anterior cervical flap is elevated deep to the platysma muscle in a superior direction until the entire hyoid bone has been exposed. Care must be taken to avoid injuring the superior laryngeal neurovascular bundle. The inferior flap is elevated laterally for a distance of several centimeters to permit access for direct palpation along the jugular lymphatic chains on each side. The lymph node chains are palpated to confirm the presence or absence of suspicious nodes (Fig. 16–3). Nodes found are examined by frozen-section analysis for metastatic carcinoma. When metastatic disease in the cervical lymph nodes has been ruled out, the operation may continue. During the last four years, we have employed a conservative neck dissection in several cases where we have found cancer in a cervical lymph node.

At this point, the strap muscles (sternohyoid, sternothyroid, and thyrohyoid) and the larynx from the level of the cricoid cartilage to the hyoid bone are clearly visible.

The external perichondrium is elevated and preserved very carefully, using tacking sutures

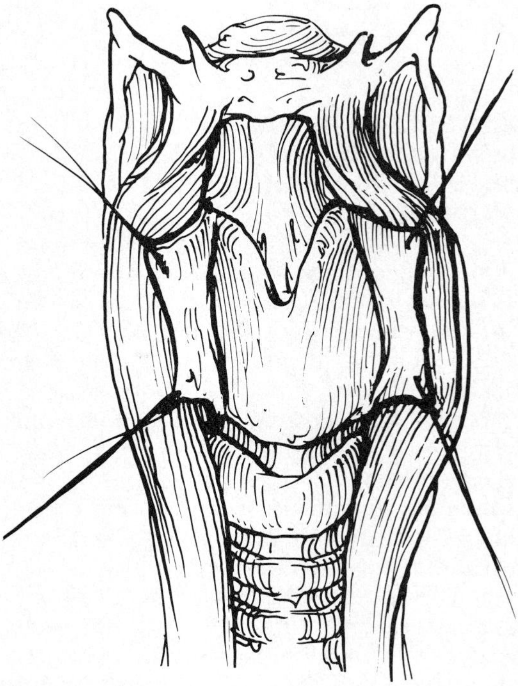

Figure 16–4. External thyroid perichondrium is elevated and preserved carefully.

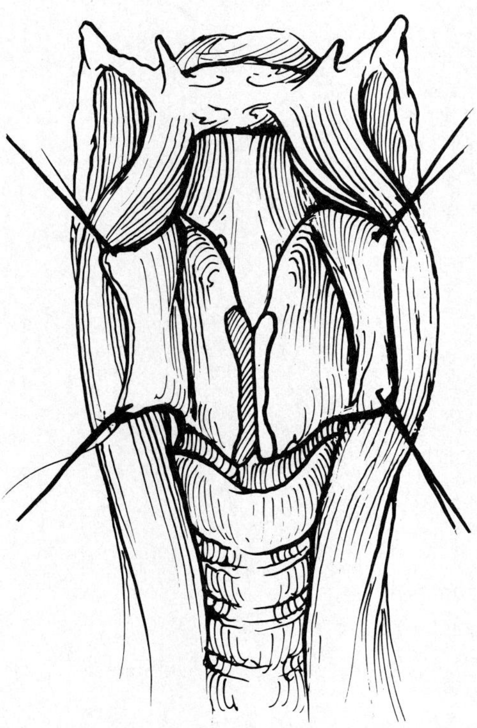

Figure 16–5. Midline thyrotomy to expose the laryngeal lumen.

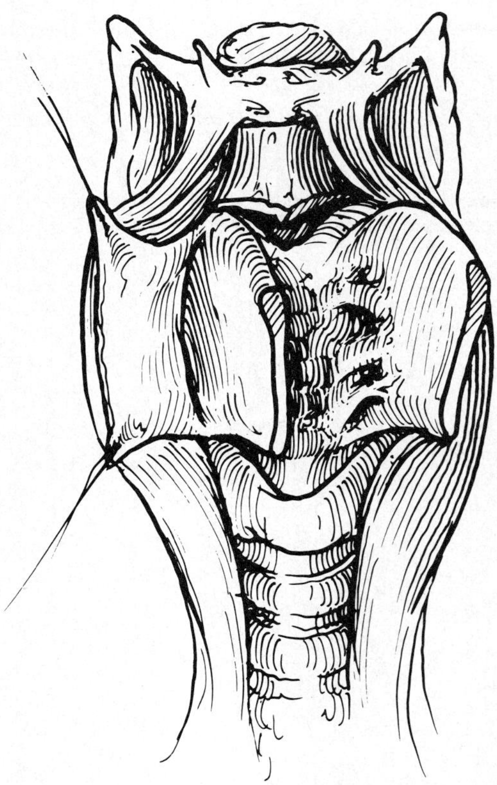

Figure 16–6. Elevation of the internal thyroid perichondrium prior to laryngeal entry.

between the external perichondrium and the overlying sternohyoid muscle complex to prevent shredding and shrinking (Fig. 16–4). No dissection is carried out in the plane between the external thyroid perichondrium and the overlying muscles because the connective tissue in this plane stabilizes the thyroid perichondrial layer and because the perichondrium and muscles form a tissue complex that will be repositioned deep to the thyroid ala as part of the laryngoplasty reconstruction. The external thyroid perichondrium is superior for minimal granulation tissue formation and rapid epithelialization, ultimately becoming an excellent replacement for the laryngeal epithelium.

Unilateral Procedure

In patients who present with a unilateral tumor that does not encroach upon the anterior commissure, a unilateral vertical partial laryngectomy and laryngoplasty is performed. The thyroid cartilage is divided in the midline, using an oscillating surgical saw (Fig. 16–5). The internal thyroid perichondrium on the involved side is elevated carefully away from the thyroid ala, carrying the dissection posteriorly to the level of the superior and inferior cornua (Fig. 16–6). The surgeon enters the subglottic area by an incision just superior to the cricoid cartilage anteriorly and extends this superiorly in the midline to permit visualization of the undersurface of the true vocal cord. With the tumor in sight, the midline soft tissue incision continues until the superior margin of the thyroid cartilage is reached, permitting visualization of the interior of the larynx (Fig. 16–7). Next, the incision is extended anteriorly to posteriorly across the false cord at an appropriate level, well away from the visible tumor margin. The inferior resection line is then carried along the superior margin of the cricoid cartilage as it curves posteriorly and superiorly. The posterior resection line is usually made at the level where the vocal process joins the body of the arytenoid cartilage (Fig. 16–8). Every effort should be made to retain the body

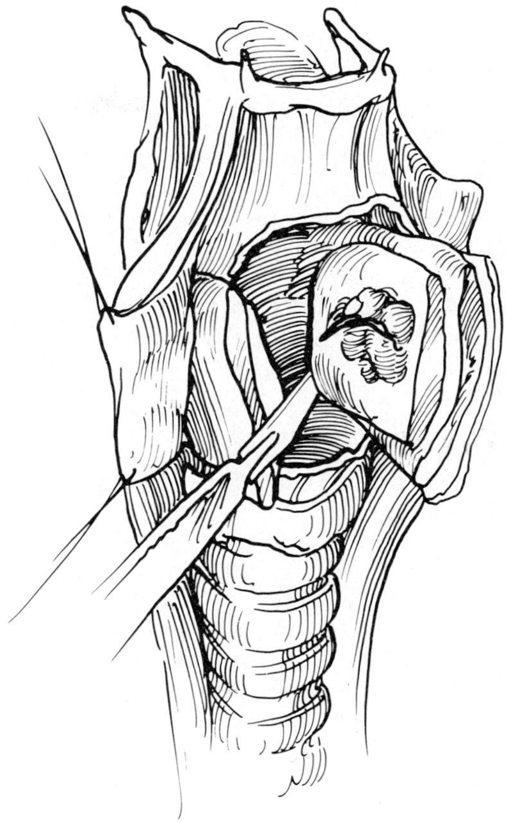

Figure 16–8. Excision of carcinoma with a margin of true cord, ventricle, and false cord but preserving the overlying thyroid cartilage.

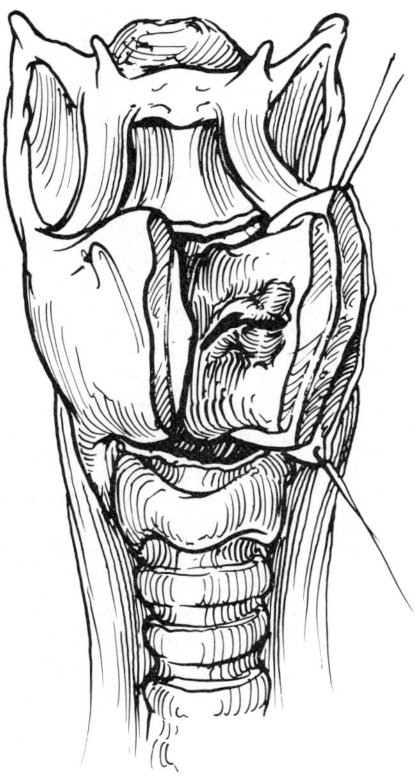

Figure 16–7. Midline laryngeal incision from below or above.

of the arytenoid cartilage to achieve maximum postoperative glottic function.

For the typical unilateral lesion, the specimen will consist of all tissue from the midline anteriorly back to the body of the arytenoid posteriorly. The specimen will extend from the level of the superior margin of the cricoid cartilage inferiorly up to and including the inferior one-half of the false cord superiorly. The deep margin of the tumor specimen will be the internal perichondrium of the thyroid cartilage.

Frozen-section margins are mandatory; they are taken from the "patient side" of the resection rather than from the tumor. Frozen-section margins consist of 2 to 3 mm strips of mucosa from all four epithelial margins. The tumor specimen is analyzed by permanent section techniques.

The surgeon should take care to avoid resection of the epiglottic cartilage, as resection or tethering of the epiglottis would impair postoperative deglutition. The surgical operating microscope may be employed to facilitate visualization, particularly when epithelial changes surround the area of obvious tumor.

Laryngoplasty, the reconstructive stage of the procedure, is accomplished by using a bipedi-

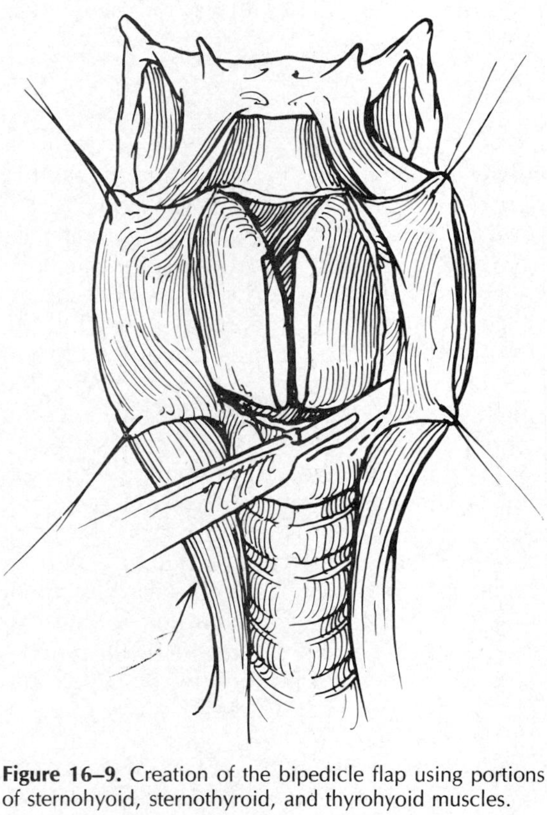

Figure 16–9. Creation of the bipedicle flap using portions of sternohyoid, sternothyroid, and thyrohyoid muscles.

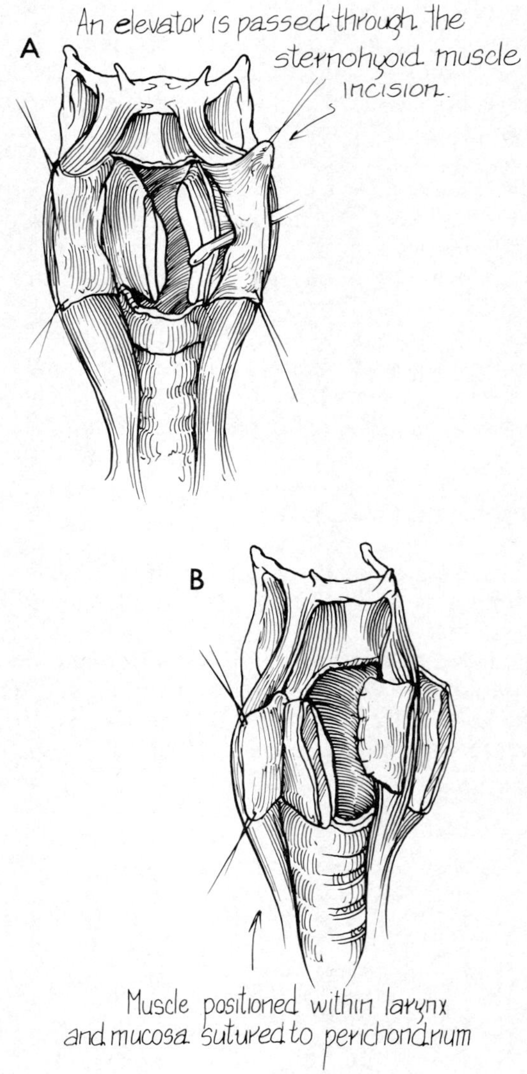

Figure 16–10. Laryngoplasty. *A,* Repositioning the bipedicle flap to lie inside the thyroid cartilage. *B,* Suturing perichondrium-muscle flap to the laryngeal mucosa.

cle muscle flap (sternohyoid, sternothyroid, and thyrohyoid muscles) that is separated from its posterolateral tissue attachments by a vertical incision made from approximately 1 cm above the superior margin of the thyroid cartilage to a point 1 cm below the inferior margin of the thyroid cartilage (Fig. 16–9). This muscle flap complex retains its anatomic attachment to the external thyroid perichrondrium on its deep surface and is left intact superiorly and inferiorly. It is then repositioned to lie deep to the thyroid ala, which is still attached posteriorly (Fig. 16–10, A and B). The external perichondrium now forms the lining of the laryngeal lumen (Fig. 16–11) and is sutured loosely to the adjacent mucosa superiorly, posteriorly, and inferiorly, stabilizing the bipedicle flap prior to careful laryngeal closure. We prefer to use a very abundant muscle flap that appears to contain more tissue than is necessary because of the predictable 30 per cent to 40 per cent postoperative atrophy of the muscle component. Use of a smaller flap can result in a posterior glottic defect when shrinkage is not taken into account. Although muscle flap atrophy has not resulted in postoperative aspiration in our experience, it can leave the patient with a weaker voice than would otherwise be possible. When the contralateral vocal cord has not been resected or biopsied, the thyrotomy is closed by approximation of the two thyroid alae (Fig. 16–12).

We do not consider a postoperative laryngeal stent desirable; however, the use of a silicone rubber (Silastic) keel at the anterior commissure is optional for the unilateral case and highly desirable for the bilateral resection technique to prevent or limit anterior commissure web formation. The keel is sutured in place using 3-0 absorbable suture material and is removed endoscopically three weeks later. The sutures used to retain the keel may also be passed through small drill holes to provide stable closure of the thyroid cartilage incision as will be shown later (see Fig. 16–20).

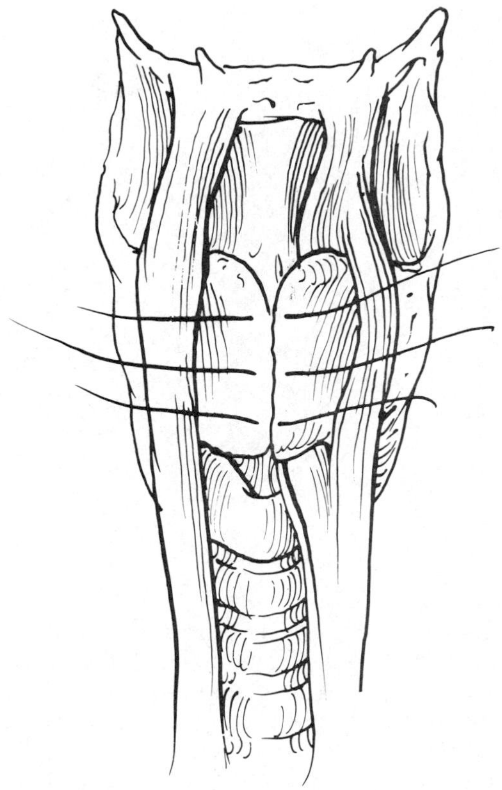

Figure 16–12. Closure of thyroid alae without using a keel.

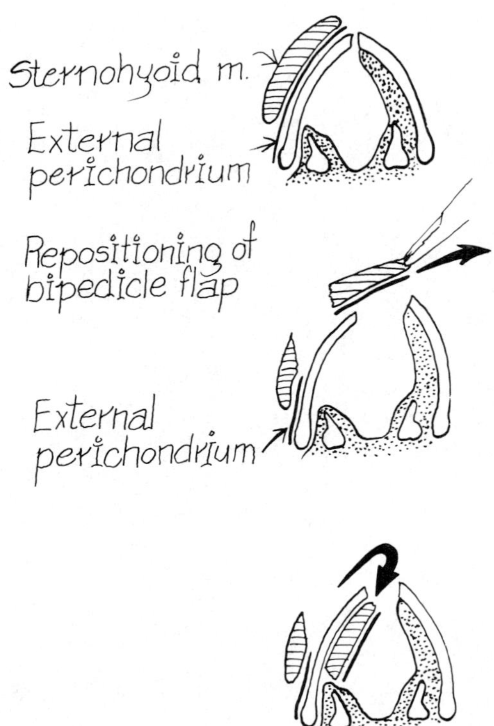

Figure 16–11. Steps in repositioning the bipedicle muscle flap from external to internal position.

The wound is drained by a one-half inch Penrose rubber drain, which passes through the lateral extent of the neck incision on both sides. Recently we have found the Mini flap 10 drain system* adequate for this procedure.

A No. 5 or No. 6 tracheotomy tube replaces the endotracheal tube (Fig. 16–13). A light compression dressing is applied over the skin flap.

Postoperative antibiotics, usually a cephalosporin or penicillin, are used routinely. The patient receives intravenous feeding for three days followed by clear liquids for one week and a soft diet for the next week.

Anterior Commissure or Bilateral Technique

Cancer involving the anterior commissure of the larynx presents special problems for ade-

*McGann Medical Corp., 3-M Co., Santa Barbara, CA 09311

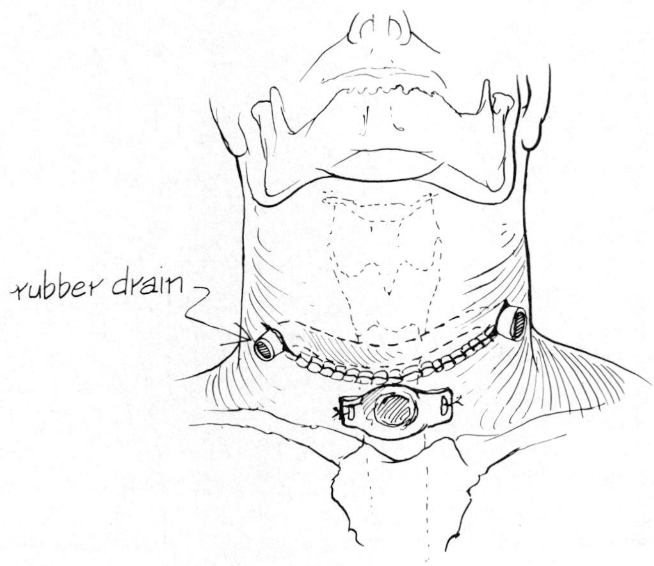

Figure 16–13. Wound closure using a single rubber drain. Tracheotomy tube sutured to the skin.

quate resection and reconstruction. Broyles described the details of the anterior commissure tendon, which attaches anteriorly to the thyroid cartilage along approximately half of its vertical length in the midline. This region has no perichondrial layer and, therefore, has decreased protection against local tumor invasion. This anatomic feature is reported to account for the increased incidence of tumor recurrence (or persistence) after operation as a result of tumor invasion into the thyroid cartilage in the region of the anterior commissure.

The anterior commissure tendon has surgical significance for these reasons:

1. There is no surgical plane inside the larynx in the midline to separate soft tissue from the thyroid cartilage.

2. Midline entry into the larynx will violate the tumor in patients with carcinoma of the anterior commissure.

3. Adequate surgical excision of cancer in this area must include removal of the primary tumor with adjacent areas of likely involvement such as the portion of thyroid cartilage overlying the anterior commissure.

Defining carcinoma of the anterior commissure poses practical problems. Recent studies of serial sections of laryngeal malignancies stressed the high incidence of submucosal spread of tumor beneath a normal-appearing mucosa. For each patient, the surgeon must correlate what he sees grossly with what he may suspect on a microscopic level. For this reason, we consider any lesion within 3 mm of the anterior limit of the cord to carry a high risk of anterior commissure involvement, and we select appropriate surgical management that specifically avoids midline thyrotomy for laryngeal entry.

The technique employed for anterior commissure lesions and for extended frontolateral partial laryngectomy differs in several respects from the procedure used for unilateral carcinoma.

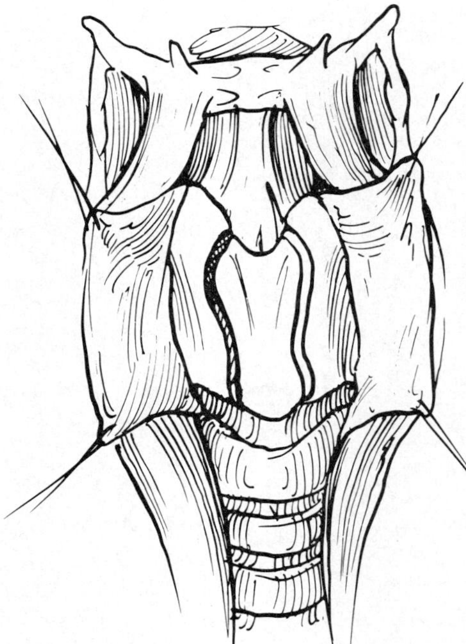

Figure 16–14. Creation of a central cartilage segment in patients with anterior commissure carcinoma.

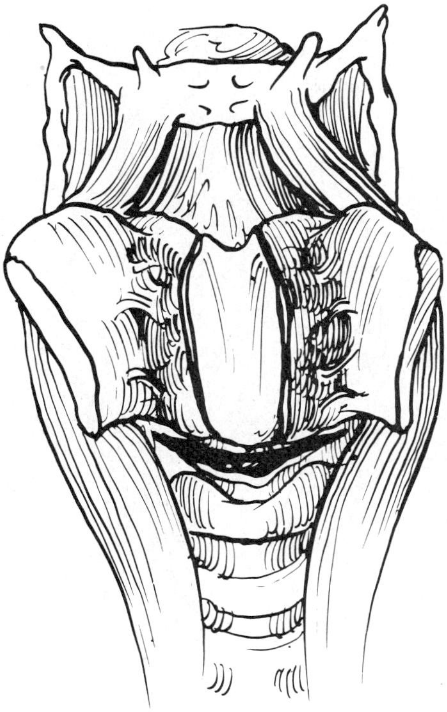

Figure 16–15. Elevation of the internal thyroid perichondrium on both sides.

The external thyroid perichondrium is elevated carefully over both thyroid alae extending posterolaterally to the superior and inferior cornua. The perichondrium is sutured to the overlying muscle complex bilaterally and the thyroid cartilage is divided 5 to 6 mm from the midline on both sides (Fig. 16–14). The internal perichondrium is elevated back to the level of the superior and inferior cornua bilaterally (Fig. 16–15). The cricothyroid ligament is divided, and a vertical incision is made through the thyroid cartilage cut on the side of lesser involvement. This permits visualization of the tumor from below and the superior dissection is continued under direct tumor visualization on the side of lesser involvement to avoid encroaching upon the tumor as this incision opens the larynx (Fig. 16–16). As the entry into the larynx is extended superiorly on the side of lesser involvement, the incision passes around the margin of the tumor and crosses the false cord near its vertical midpoint (Fig. 16–17). Once the superior resection line is completed, the larynx can be opened for direct inspection allowing the superior, posterior, and inferior margins of resection on the side of greater involvement to be completed.

Frozen-section analysis of the patient side of the resection line determines the adequacy of

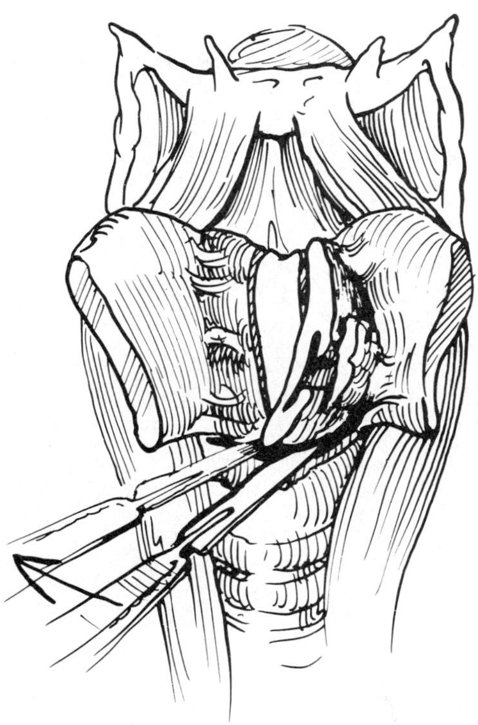

Figure 16–16. Laryngeal entry away from the tumor as first step in resection.

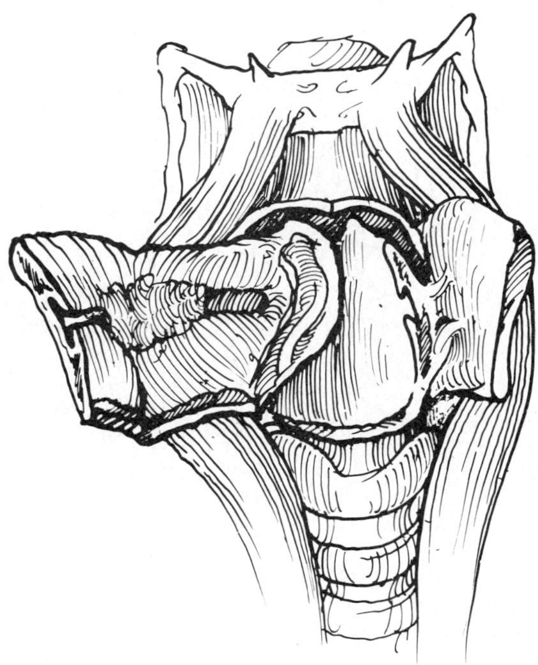

Figure 16–17. Primary resected with adequate margins as exposure is gained.

the resection. It is essential to retain the posterior commissure and one functional arytenoid complex.

The interior of the larynx is then reconstructed bilaterally using the bipedicle muscle-perichondrium flaps on each side, as described previously for unilateral reconstruction (Figs. 16–18 and 16–19).

A Silastic stent is sutured in place through the anterior commissure to avoid anterior web formation (Fig. 16–20). This technique has been described in detail by Blitzer et al.,[45] who report good results in placing a keel at the time of partial laryngectomy and removing it endoscopically two to three weeks later. These authors used this procedure in 12 patients without complications.

The frozen-section tissue diagnosis will differ from the permanent section diagnosis in approximately 15 per cent to 20 per cent of these procedures. These discrepancies most commonly involve a frozen-section report of a clear margin from the "patient side" of the resection and a permanent section report from the specimen indicating that the tumor extends to involve one of the margins. This situation usually results from an artifact produced by the processing of the tumor specimen. It can often be resolved by review of the tumor sections by the surgeons and discussion with the pathologist. Should this not be the case, full-course postoperative radiation therapy is recommended, with particular emphasis on careful postoperative evaluation. If the specimen shows tumor at some point in the deep or lateral extent of

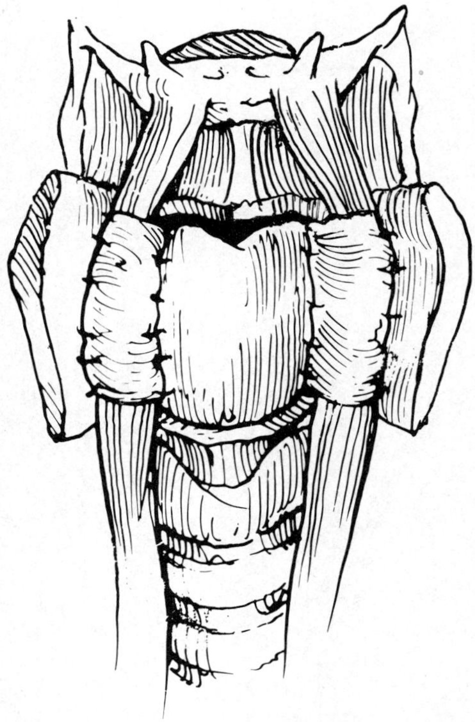

Figure 16–19. Perichondrium sutured to mucosa bilaterally.

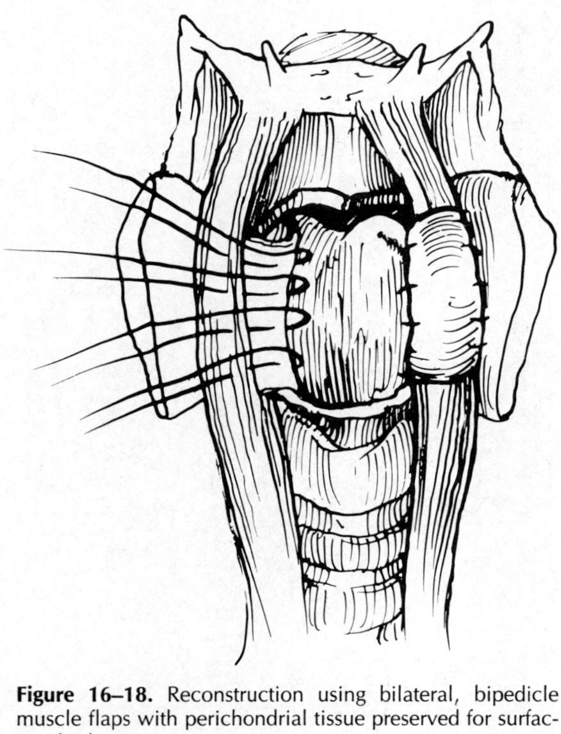

Figure 16–18. Reconstruction using bilateral, bipedicle muscle flaps with perichondrial tissue preserved for surfacing the lumen.

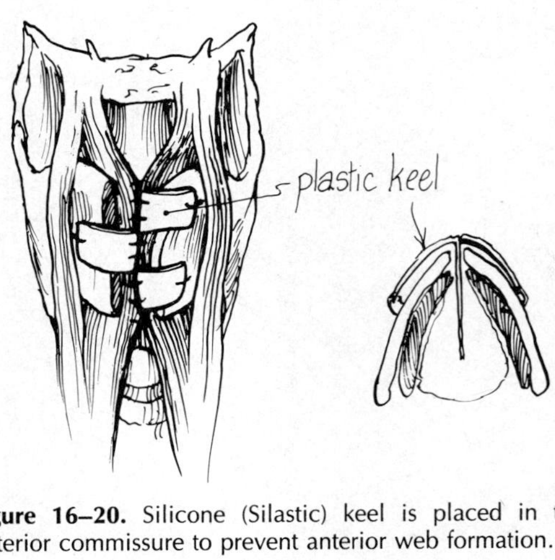

Figure 16–20. Silicone (Silastic) keel is placed in the anterior commissure to prevent anterior web formation.

the specimen, either full-course radiation or total laryngectomy should be considered. No clear evidence exists currently to indicate the superiority of one option over the other. Bauer[46] reports positive margins with examination of the hemilaryngectomy specimen in 39 of 111 patients (35 per cent) undergoing partial laryngectomy. No immediate therapy was instituted in these patients. Seven of the 39 patients with histologically positive margins (18 per cent) subsequently developed recurrent carcinoma. Five patients were treated by total laryngectomy and two by radiation therapy without subsequent recurrence of cancer.

Like Goepfert,[43] we prefer postoperative radiation therapy in this situation for safe and effective control of residual, microscopic disease.

As mentioned previously, we consider stage T3 glottic carcinoma beyond the scope of vertical partial laryngectomy. As other surgeons clarify more details, extended vertical partial laryngectomy followed by full-course radiation therapy will probably become the treatment of choice for many patients with T3 glottic carcinoma.

A small number of patients with primary glottic carcinoma have N1 cervical node metastasis. We believe that vertical partial laryngectomy, combined with conservative neck dissection and followed by postoperative radiation therapy, constitutes adequate treatment for some of those few patients. Extensive observation has substantiated the safety of radiation therapy after vertical partial laryngectomy. Prolonged postoperative edema, slightly diminished postoperative laryngeal function, and occasional problems with postirradiation stenosis or aspiration may occur.

Postoperative Morbidity

The major complications following vertical partial laryngectomy and laryngoplasty include aspiration of saliva and liquids, stenosis, and severe hoarseness.

Aspiration. Postoperative aspiration of saliva and liquids was seen in 4 of the 70 consecutive patients who have undergone vertical partial laryngectomy and have been followed for five years or more. Most patients experience this problem in a mild form during the interval following nasogastric tube feeding but preceding the removal of the tracheotomy tube. Usually quite minor, this problem disappears shortly after decannulation. This mild aspiration is attributed to the presence of the tracheotomy tube and to the discomfort experienced by patients during swallowing after vertical partial laryngectomy and laryngoplasty. Four patients were unable to swallow without significant aspiration of liquids for periods ranging from two weeks to three months postoperatively. No aspiration problems persisted beyond that point. Nutritional problems are easily managed by prolonged nasogastric feeding or, in some instances, by dietary adjustment and exercises comparable to those used in patients who have undergone supraglottic partial laryngectomy. Reassurance and support from the physician and family are essential for these patients during this time.

Two patients developed postoperative stenosis severe enough to prevent decannulation. One underwent a secondary laryngoplasty one year after the initial vertical partial laryngectomy and was successfully decannulated. The other continues to depend upon the wearing of a tracheotomy tube at night. A third patient in the series maintained a psychological dependence upon the tracheotomy tube for many years following vertical partial laryngectomy. She was able to work comfortably as an active salesperson during the day with her tracheotomy tube plugged but preferred to sleep with her tracheotomy tube unplugged during the night.

One patient in the series developed a severe postoperative wound infection. This patient responded to appropriate medical management, but persistent edema delayed decannulation for a period of three months. No long-term sequelae have been noted.

Another patient has severe hoarseness characterized by a very breathy and weak voice. This patient, a young adult male, underwent bilateral tumor resection and bilateral muscle laryngoplasty. While he has no difficulty with aspiration, he cannot approximate the neocords bilaterally (only one arytenoid and the posterior commissure were preserved at the time of surgery) and his voice is little more than a loud whisper. Eleven years after surgery, he does not wish to pursue glottic reconstructive surgery.

Mortality. At present, six of the original patients in the series have died of cancer; three succumbed to recurrent carcinoma in the larynx and three died of carcinoma of the lung. One of the patients who died from lung cancer developed an oat cell carcinoma of the bronchus, while his laryngeal lesion was epidermoid carcinoma. This seems to be an obvious second primary. The relationship of persistent carcinoma versus second primary lesions is unclear in four of the remaining five patients whose fatal malignancies were detected at periods ranging from two years to four and one-half years following the original surgery. The sixth patient developed recurrent carcinoma in the larynx within five months of the original surgery because of inadvertent violation of an anterior commissure carcinoma.

Five patients are known to have died of other causes without evidence of recurrent carcinoma. Four of these patients succumbed to cardiovascular disease, three of them dying after an apparent myocardial infarction. The fourth patient was found to have polycythemia vera and suffered a cerebral vascular accident on the first day after surgery, dying one week later.

One patient died of airway obstruction after being discharged to his home. This patient had an occlusive laryngeal stent in place and had been instructed repeatedly concerning the importance of maintaining a clean and patent tracheotomy tube. After he had been at home approximately one week, he removed the tracheotomy tube in order to shave and apparently was unable to reinsert the tracheotomy tube.

TREATMENT RESULTS WITH VERTICAL PARTIAL LARYNGECTOMY

In our series of seventy consecutive patients followed for longer than five years, six patients died of malignant disease, representing a cancer death rate of 8.6 per cent. As mentioned previously, three patients died of laryngeal cancer and three succumbed to lung cancer. Five patients have died from other causes, adding a raw mortality of 7.1 per cent in terms of raw survival. Death from cardiovascular disease predominates and may reflect the pathology of the cardiovascular system that is often associated with the same etiologic factors considered important in the development of laryngeal cancer.

Eight of the seventy patients (11.4 per cent) developed either a local recurrence or a second primary carcinoma in the larynx. In two of these patients, we also noted cervical lymph node metastases, while the laryngeal recurrence was localized in the remaining six patients. One of the patients who developed recurrent laryngeal carcinoma was salvaged by a second partial laryngectomy and is still alive more than five years later. Three of the patients salvaged by total laryngectomy have remained alive and well for more than five years. Of the remaining four patients, three have died as a result of their laryngeal carcinoma. The fourth patient was salvaged by total laryngectomy for control of the primary and neck disease but died two years later of carcinoma of the lung. Thus, we have a laryngeal recurrence rate of 11.4 per cent for the total series with a salvage rate and five-year survival from this group of 50 per cent.

Analysis of the total group of 70 patients reveals 56 patients alive and well with no evidence of recurrent disease and with adequate laryngeal function from partial laryngectomy. Three additional patients are alive and well with no evidence of disease after total laryngectomy for salvage of a local recurrence. The death rate from cancer in this series of patients is 8.6 per cent (6 of 70) and the death rate from noncancer causes is 7.1 per cent (5 of 70).

In our experience, vertical partial laryngectomy has provided a five-year cure rate of 87 per cent; the salvage of three additional patients by total laryngectomy has raised the surgical cure rate to 91.4 per cent. These results compare favorably with other reports from major institutions and we continue to recommend the specific technique of vertical partial laryngectomy and laryngoplasty described in this chapter. The versatility and effectiveness of this technique in managing more extensive laryngeal carcinoma and the advantages of the reconstructive element in preserving and enhancing the postoperative laryngeal functions of phonation, respiration, and deglutition have been documented sufficiently to warrant routine use.

To successfully manage glottic carcinoma, the surgeon must adhere strictly to the basic principles of initial treatment described by DeSanto and Pearson.[47] We have modified these slightly as follows:

1. Glottic carcinoma is a very curable disease.
2. Glottic cancer behavior varies widely at different sites.
3. The classification does not dictate the treatment.

4. Great responsibility rests with the physician prescribing the first treatment.

5. The first treatment anticipates later problems.

6. The use of combined therapy must be justified.

7. Careful case selection is a key factor.

8. Reconstruction after resection is very important.

9. Frequent, regular follow-up is critical.

10. Life is more important than the larynx.

In summary, we have reviewed the historical evolution of the surgical management of glottic carcinoma and described the epidemiologic and etiologic factors known at this time. The indications and contraindications for vertical partial laryngectomy have been presented and several specific techniques described.

References

1. Neel HB III et al.: Laryngofissure and cordectomy for early cordal carcinoma: Outcome in 182 patients. Otolaryngol Head Neck Surg 88:79–84, 1980.
2. Biller H et al.: Hemilaryngectomy for T2 glottic cancers. Arch Otolaryngol 93:238, 1971.
3. Bailey BJ: Partial laryngectomy and laryngoplasty: A technique and review. Trans Am Acad Ophthalmol Otolaryngol 70:559–574, 1966.
4. Pressman JJ: Cancer of the larynx: Laryngoplasty to avoid laryngectomy. Arch Otolaryngol 59:395–412, 1954.
5. Daly CJ, Strong EW: Carcinoma of the glottic larynx. Am J Surg 130:489–492, 1975.
6. DeSanto LW: Current concepts in otolaryngology: The options in early laryngeal carcinoma. N Engl J Med 306:15, 910–912, 1982.
7. Silverberg E: Cancer statistics. CA 33:9–25, 1983.
8. Silverberg E: Cancer statistics. CA 29:6–21, 1979.
9. Wynder EL et al.: Environmental factors in cancer of the larynx: A second look. Cancer 38:1591–1601, 1976.
10. Rothman KJ et al.: Epidemiology of laryngeal cancer. Epidemiol Rev 2:195–209, 1980.
11. Pedersen E et al.: Cancer of respiratory organs among workers at a nickel refinery in Norway. Int J Cancer 12:32–41, 1973.
12. Wada S et al.: Mustard gas as a cause of respiratory neoplasia in man. Lancet 1:1161–1163, 1968.
13. Public Health Service, Centers for Disease Control, National Institute of Occupational Safety and Health: Occupational Exposure to Isopropyl Alcohol: Criteria for a Recommended Standard. DHEW publ [NIOSH] 76-142, Washington DC, GPO, 1976.
14. Decoufle P et al.: A Retrospective Survey of Cancer in Relation to Occupation. NIOSH Research Report. DHEW publ [NIOSH] 77-178. Washington DC, GPO, 1977.
15. Versluys JJ: Cancer and occupation in the Netherlands. Br J Cancer 3:161–185, 1949.
16. Blot WJ et al.: Patterns of laryngeal cancer in the United States. Lancet 2:674–675, 1978.
17. Milham S Jr: Occupational Mortality in Washington State, 1950–1971 Vol I–III. DHEW publ [NIOSH] 76-175, A, B and C. Washington DC, GPO, 1976.
18. Registrar General's Decennial Supplement, England and Wales, 1951. Occupational Mortality. London, HMSO, 1958.
19. Wolf O: Carcinoma of the larynx among naphthalene cleaners. Z Gesamte Hyg 24:737–739, 1978.
20. Lynch J et al.: An association of upper respiratory cancer with exposure to diethyl sulfate. J Occup Med 21:333–341, 1979.
21. Hoshino H, Tanook H: Carcinogenicity of triethanolamine in mice and its mutagenicity after reaction with sodium nitrite in bacteria. Cancer Res 38:3918–3921, 1978.
22. Inone K et al.: Mutagenicity tests and in vitro transformation assays on triethanolamine. Mutat Res 101:305–313, 1982.
23. Meretora T et al.: Clastogenic activity of styrene in occupational exposure (meeting abstract). Mutat Res 53:229, 1978.
24. Ponomerkov V, Tomatis L: Effects of long-term oral administration of styrene to mice and rats. Scand J Work Environ Health 4(1978):(suppl 2) 127–135, 1978.
25. Jussawalla DJ et al.: Cancer incidence in greater Bombay: Assessment of the cancer risk by age. Br J Cancer 22:623–636, 1968.
26. Waterhouse J et al. (eds): Cancer Incidence in Five Continents. Vol 3. Lyon, IARC Scientific Publications No 15, 1976.
27. Terracini B et al.: Descriptive epidemiology of cancer of the larynx in the province of Torino, Italy. Tumori 64:445–456, 1978.
28. Doll R: The geographical distribution of cancer. Br J Cancer 23:1–8, 1969.
29. National Institutes of Health, Public Health Service: Third National Cancer Survey: Incidence Data. National Cancer Institute Monograph 41. DHEW publ [NIH] 75-787. Washington DC, GPO, 1975.
30. New Mexico Tumor Registry: Cancer in New Mexico 1969–1972. Albuquerque NM, 1974.
31. Woodhouse RJ et al.: Treatment of carcinoma of the vocal cord: A review of 20 years experience. Laryngoscope 91:1155–1162, 1981.
32. Strong EW: Operative management of carcinoma of the larynx. *In* Najarian JS, Delaney JP (eds): Advances in Cancer Surgery. New York, Stratton Intercontinental Medical Book Corp, 1976, pp 211–220.
33. Biller HF, Lawson W: Bilateral vertical partial laryngectomy for bilateral vocal cord carcinoma. Ann Otol Rhinol Laryngol 90:489–491, 1981.
34. Guerrier Y: Difficult indications for partial laryngectomy. ORL 41:262–272, 1979.
35. Wagenfeld JH, Bryce DP: Some aspects of the management of laryngeal carcinoma: J Otolaryngol 8:3, 274–283, 1979.
36. Lesinski SG et al.: Hemilaryngectomy for T3 (fixed cord) epidermoid carcinoma of larynx. Laryngoscope 86:1563–1571, 1976.
37. Kirchner JA: Staging as seen in serial sections. Laryngoscope 85:1816–1821, 1975.
38. Kirchner JA: Growth and spread of laryngeal cancer as related to partial laryngectomy. Laryngoscope 85:1516–1521, 1975.
39. Som ML: Cordal cancer with extension to vocal process. Laryngoscope 84:1298–1307, 1974.
40. Burns HP et al.: Verrucous carcinoma of the larynx:

Management by radiotherapy and surgery. Ann Otol Rhinol Laryngol 85:538–543, 1976.
41. Nichols RD et al.: Partial laryngectomy after radiation failure. Laryngoscope 90:571–575, 1980.
42. Burns H et al.: Conservation surgery in laryngeal cancer and its role following failed radiotherapy. Arch Otolaryngol 105:234–239, 1979.
43. Goepfert H et al.: Treatment of laryngeal carcinoma with conservative surgery and postoperative radiation therapy. Arch Otolaryngol 104:576–578, 1978.
44. Biller HF et al.: Hemilaryngectomy following radiation failure for carcinoma of the vocal cords. Laryngoscope 80:249–253, 1970.
45. Blitzer A et al.: Modification of the anterior commissure technique of partial laryngectomy. Arch Otolaryngol 106:503–504, 1980.
46. Bauer WC et al.: The significance of positive margins in hemilaryngectomy specimens. Laryngoscope 85:1–13, 1975.
47. DeSanto LW, Pearson BW: Initial treatment of laryngeal cancer. Minn Med 64:691–698, 1981.

17

Glottic Reconstruction

Byron J. Bailey, M.D.

The complex structure and function of the larynx are altered dramatically by trauma and surgical resection for carcinoma. This topic has received a great deal of attention in other chapters of this book and elsewhere in the medical literature during the past twenty years. The purpose of this chapter is to review and bring together the reported observations and results of innovative techniques designed to deal with this set of problems.

Historically, partial laryngectomy was a multistage technique. The surgical wound usually included the creation of a laryngocutaneous fistula (laryngostoma). This feature provided a measure of safety and assisted in rehabilitation of the larynx by subsequent, staged surgical procedures. As the trend shifted to the concept of a single-stage procedure, the focus of attention shifted away from the fine points of functional rehabilitation and toward the adequate excision of laryngeal carcinoma.[1]

During the past two decades, various procedures have been devised to reconstruct the larynx after trauma or partial resection for cancer; they are designed to restore the interrelated and complex functions of phonation, respiration, and deglutition. These techniques are grouped into those performed as primary steps at the initial surgery and others done later to achieve one or more of the following goals:

1. Vocal enhancement.
2. Prevention of aspiration.
3. Correction of impaired respiration by restoring the patency of the laryngeal lumen.
4. Prevention of infection, granulation tissue formation, and chondritis by covering the exposed cartilage and tissue in the area of surgical resection.

The voice may be unacceptably harsh after a severe injury or surgical resection. This may be secondary to fibrosis, arytenoid dysfunction, or neural injury. After a partial laryngectomy without reconstruction, the defect usually results in a hoarse but relatively audible voice. Uncommonly, the voice may be extremely weak and breathy.

Aspiration of at least a minor degree usually follows hemilaryngectomy when reconstructive procedures are not employed.[2] A small but significant percentage of patients have serious aspiration that results in pneumonia and nutritional complications and that, in rare instances, may be fatal or require total laryngectomy. Procedures that replace bulk in the area of tumor resection are helpful after limited resections and are critical after extended frontolateral and bilateral tumor excision, particularly when one arytenoid cartilage is removed.

Respiratory function is compromised by an inadequate laryngeal lumen following partial laryngectomy in some patients.[3] When the raw operative surface is left to heal by granulation, the duration of the healing process and the degree of tissue replacement is unpredictable.

When the granulation tissue and fibrosis is excessive, postoperative stenosis results. Conversely, aspiration may persist if the new tissue growth is insufficient. The surgeon must always remember that respiration requires laryngeal patency, while voice production and avoidance of aspiration require a competent glottic sphincter. These mutually competitive requirements for airway dimensions consisting of only a few millimeters place a high premium on predictably reliable reconstructive techniques; this has led to the development of a number of innovative primary and secondary reconstructive surgical procedures.

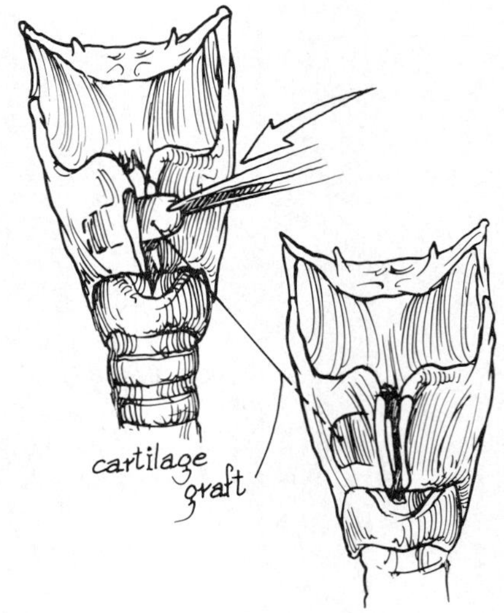

Figure 17–1. Medial displacement of paralyzed or partially resected vocal cord by implantation of a cartilage graft.

HISTORICAL BACKGROUND

The earliest effort to restore laryngeal function is attributed to Professor Ottokar Chiari[4] of Vienna. He described a procedure in which cervical skin was transposed into the laryngeal lumen for functional rehabilitation. Unfortunately, both his technique and the underlying principles remained unrecognized for almost forty years, during which time the surgical wound was left to heal by second intention.

The surgical management of glottic insufficiency secondary to vocal cord paralysis received considerable attention from laryngeal surgeons during the 1940s and early 1950s. Procedures devised to provide for vocal enhancement and to alleviate aspiration were subsequently incorporated in the repair of surgical defects following partial laryngectomy.

In 1942, Meurman of Helsinki published the details of operative mediofixation of the vocal cord for patients with unilateral paralysis. His technique[5] resulted in displacement of the paralyzed vocal cord toward the midline after implantation of costal cartilage in a pocket created between the internal perichondrium and the thyroid cartilage at the level of the vocal cord (Fig. 17–1). He demonstrated his postoperative results with motion pictures and recordings at a meeting of the Swedish Medical Society and ultimately reported on the results in fifteen patients, in whom only one complication was observed—a result of the loss of the cartilage implant secondary to infection.

Morrison[6] published a description in 1948 of a surgical procedure designed to accomplish mediofixation of the arytenoid cartilage by disarticulating this cartilage from its joint and fixing it near the midline on the superior surface of the cricoid cartilage. This medial repositioning of the vocal cord corrected glottic insufficiency in patients with unilateral vocal cord paralysis.

In 1952, Libersa[7] described a modification of Meurman's technique for medial relocation of the vocal cord. Libersa was the first to utilize an acrylic implant in a lateral laryngeal pocket, and he succeeded in eliminating problems of glottic insufficiency by this means.

Professor Opheim of Oslo[8] described a triangular thyroid cartilage implant placed in a horizontal pocket at the level of the vocal cord to reposition the cord medially. This technique had the advantage of utilizing a smaller implant, making possible more precise placement of a cartilaginous segment obtained from a local donor site, thus eliminating the need for a second operative field.

Reconstructive procedures designed specifically to restore function following partial laryngectomy began slightly later but overlapped the evolution of techniques employed for vocal cord paralysis. Goodyear[9] approached the problem of reliable control of the healing phase of the operative site after partial laryngectomy by using various obturators that were placed in the laryngeal lumen. Figi[10] advocated the immediate use of skin grafts for repair of the surgical defect to cover the raw surface after hemilaryngectomy. This was particularly important during this time since efforts were being made simultaneously to extend the scope of the operation and to prevent problems with postoperative stenosis. Som[11] was the first surgeon to propose covering the raw surface with a mucosal advancement flap from the posterior arytenoid and pyriform sinus regions.

The term *laryngoplasty* was introduced by Pressman[12] in 1954. This was the first description of the use of tissue bulk (muscle) to provide a controlled and reliable replacement to fill the defect created by the cancer excision. The thyroid cartilage was divided in the midline anteriorly and each half was carefully removed by a subperichondrial dissection. After excision of the tumor, a pocket was created in the strap muscle group on each side, and the cartilage segments were inserted with closure of the wound around a plastic stent that was placed in the lumen of the larynx. The technique also had the advantage that the lumen was lined by the external thyroid perichondrium, a tissue that undergoes rapid epithelialization without developing excessive granulation tissue. The subsequent modification of this technique has been described in detail in Chapter 16 of this volume, Glottic Carcinoma.

In 1958, Waltner[13] described the use of a costal cartilage implant, in a manner similar to that described by Meurman, to accomplish vocal improvement in a patient who had undergone laryngofissure and cordectomy two years previously. The surgery was accomplished using local anesthesia and following a tracheotomy. The subperichondrial pocket was carefully created to be the same size as the cartilage implant, and the patient's voice was used as an intraoperative guide to obtain the best vocal result.

Conley[14] published his experience using a transposition mucosal flap to resurface the area of tumor excision. This pharyngoepiglottic flap was employed in 18 patients over a five-year period. Three patients in this series experienced aspiration and required a feeding tube for an extended period, and a single patient developed postoperative stenosis.

Two years later, Conley[15] reported his experience with a unilateral, pedicled skin flap that was designed to create a "new cord." He advocated this technique because of its advantages in resurfacing and filling the tissue defect. He noted that it was very successful in forming a replacement for the vocal cord that provided a superior postoperative voice. He also emphasized the great value of this technique in extending the scope of partial laryngectomy surgery. His results in the five patients reported were excellent in regard to function and cancer control.

In 1961, Harpman[16] was the first to describe the use of a free mucosal graft in the reconstruction and resurfacing of the laryngeal surgical defect.

While many of these techniques have been displaced by subsequent modifications and improvements, the pioneering surgeons who introduced these procedures served the specialty of laryngology well and set the stage for the techniques more widely used today.

ADJUNCTIVE OPERATIVE PROCEDURES FOR GLOTTIC RECONSTRUCTION

Vocal Enhancement and Prevention of Aspiration. Various surgical procedures are available for glottic reconstruction following the adequate excision of glottic carcinoma by vertical partial laryngectomy (hemilaryngectomy), frontolateral partial laryngectomy, or extended frontolateral partial laryngectomy. Surgical techniques to replace tissue that has been surgically excised serve to reconstitute the competence of the glottic sphincter mechanism. This section reviews some of the reconstructive procedures used more commonly for immediate repair at the time of the initial surgery.

A controversy remains concerning the need for removing the ipsilateral thyroid cartilage along with glottic carcinoma. Some surgeons sacrifice this tissue routinely in the course of performing hemilaryngectomy, but many others have observed that tumor excision that includes the internal perichondrium of the thyroid cartilage constitutes adequate tumor removal. Some of these reconstructive procedures rely on the presence of the ipsilateral thyroid cartilage, while others may be performed after its removal.

After partial laryngectomy, replacement of the excised tumor bulk provides a cushion for the remaining cord to meet, resulting in improved phonation. Maran et al.[17] compared hemilaryngectomy with and without the repositioning of the strap muscles into the interior of the larynx to replace the excised tissue. Postoperative measurements of the fundamental frequency and subglottic pulmonary pressure showed that the muscle transposition provided superior functional results with regard to voice, respiration, and the avoidance of aspiration by providing a more competent sphincter mechanism. The ability to achieve glottic closure and to increase the subglottic pulmonary pressure is an important factor in restoring an efficient pulmonary air-driving force for voice production.

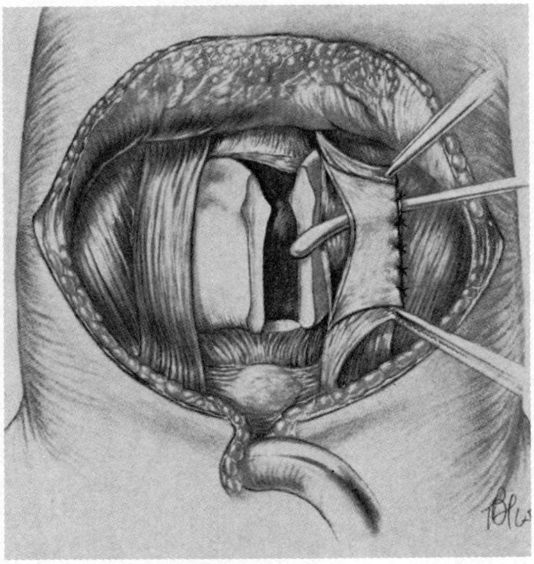

Figure 17–2

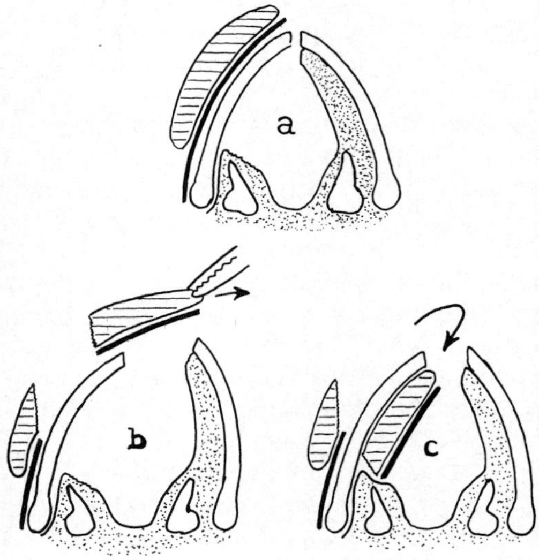

Figure 17–3

Figure 17–2. An elevator is passed through the sternohyoid muscle incision to facilitate placing the bipedicle muscle flap inside the denuded thyroid ala. (From Bailey BJ: Laryngoscope 85:967, 1975.)

Figure 17–3. Repositioning of a bipedicle flap of sternohyoid muscle *(horizontal lines)* and external perichondrium of thyroid cartilage *(heavy line)* so that it is internal to the thyroid cartilage. (From Bailey BJ: Laryngoscope 85:968, 1975.)

This concept is fundamental to our preferred technique for laryngoplasty, which has been described in detail in Chapter 16 of this volume. We use a bipedicle muscle flap for bulk and perichondrium to line the laryngeal lumen, as shown in Figures 17–2 and 17–3.

Quinn[18] uses a free graft of thyrohyoid muscle to reconstruct the glottic defect after vertical partial laryngectomy. He sutures a free muscle graft (1 by 2 by 3 cm) into the defect and then covers it by a mucosal advancement flap from the pyriform sinus (Fig. 17–4). He found it necessary to augment the technique with polytetraflouroethylene (Teflon) injection into the muscle graft in two patients but reported achieving good phonation in ten of eleven patients in whom the technique was used successfully.

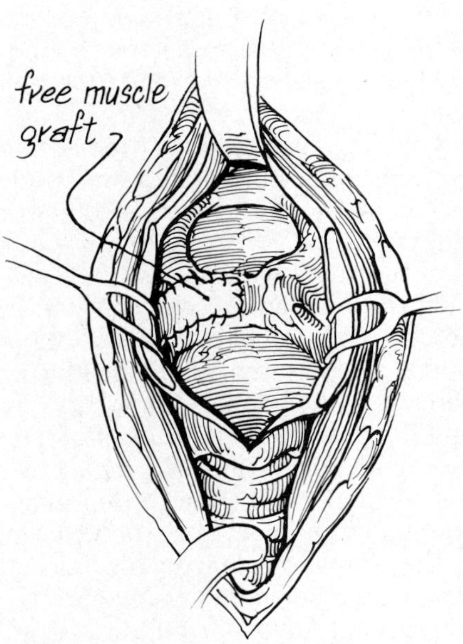

Figure 17–4. Free graft of the thyrohyoid muscle is sewn into the surgical defect after vertical partial laryngectomy.

Removal of the arytenoid cartilage is a necessary step in vertical partial laryngectomy when the glottic tumor extends posteriorly. According to Blaugrund and Kurland[19], arytenoid cartilage removal often results in a degree of glottic incompetence and is frequently associated with some aspiration on swallowing after hemilaryngectomy when no laryngoplasty technique is employed. These authors recommend the use of a local pedicle flap consisting of the lateral and posterior portion of the thyroid cartilage to reconstruct the surgical defect (Fig. 17–5). This cartilage segment is left attached to an inferior constrictor muscle pedicle, and the tissue bulk may be augmented by suturing an additional cartilage graft to the primary myochondral pedicle flap. The area is then covered by a regional advancement mucosal flap. Blaugrund reported excellent graft take and postoperative healing in five of six dogs that

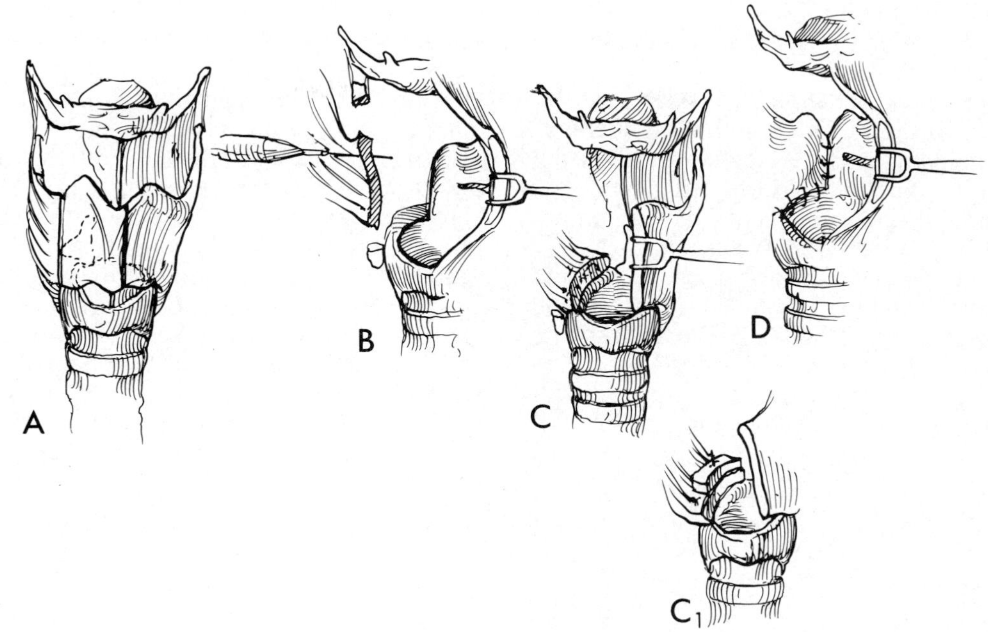

Figure 17–5. Laryngoplasty using a local pedicle flap composed of the lateral and posterior portions of the thyroid cartilage and retaining the anatomic attachment to the adjacent inferior constrictor muscle.

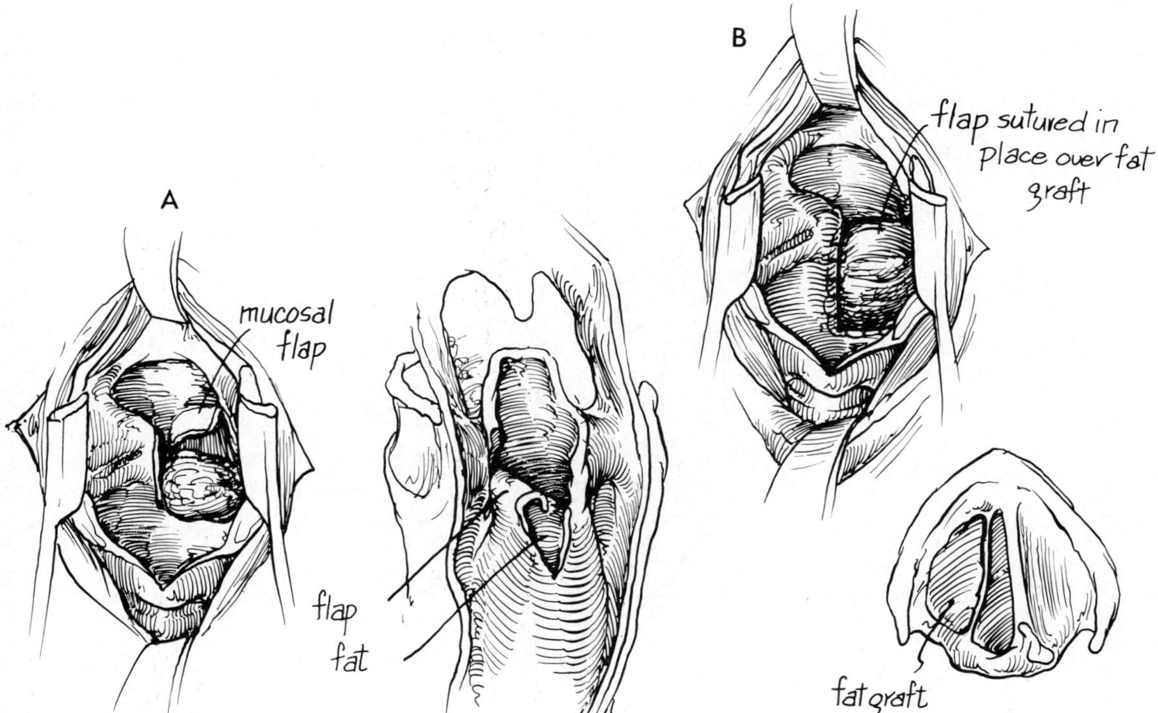

Figure 17–6. Free fat graft augmenting the glottic region after vertical partial laryngectomy.

were studied initially. Excellent functional results were obtained with this procedure in four of five patients.

Postoperative aspiration has been noted by Dedo[20] to be the major complication after vertical hemilaryngectomy. He recommends the use of a free fat graft to fill the surgical defect at the time of surgery to restore glottic competence. The fat graft employed is approximately the size of the distal phalanx of the thumb and is obtained from the subcutaneous tissue in the region of the hyoid bone. It is placed in the surgical defect, with more bulk posteriorly than anteriorly, and is then covered by an advancement mucosal flap from the region of the pyriform sinus (Fig. 17–6). If the fat graft is too small or undergoes atrophy, Dedo also describes the successful injection of Teflon as a later procedure to augment the tissue bulk in this area and to correct minor degrees of glottic insufficiency. He has also observed that use of the regional mucosal advancement flap has eliminated the problem of glottic stenosis following vertical partial laryngectomy. He had observed this complication previously when he was employing a split-thickness skin graft to reconstruct the surgical defect.

Transposition of cervical skin flaps into the laryngeal lumen to accomplish laryngoplasty has been recommended by Conley.[21] He has

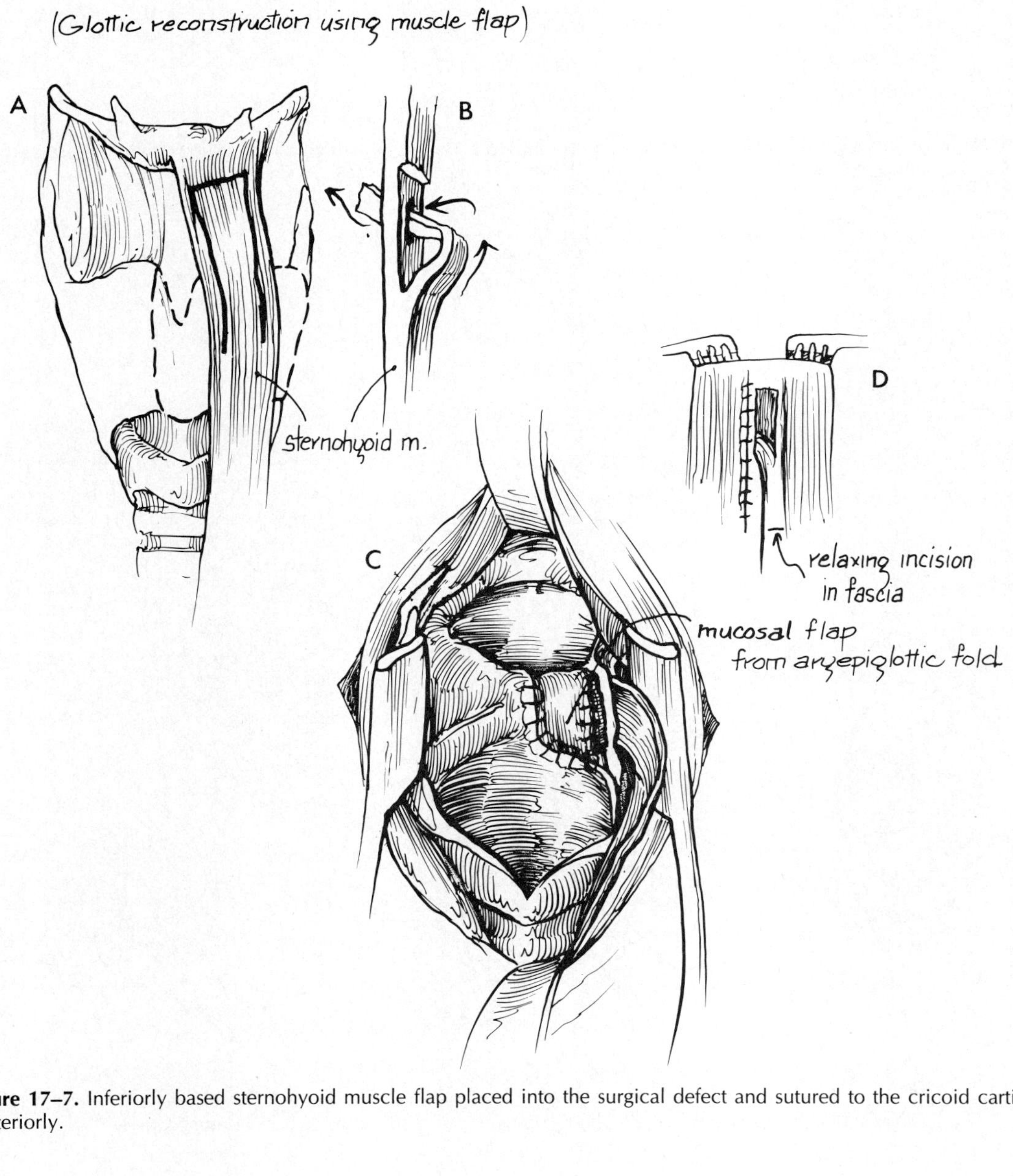

Figure 17–7. Inferiorly based sternohyoid muscle flap placed into the surgical defect and sutured to the cricoid cartilage posteriorly.

described using this technique as a single-stage procedure in 16 patients who have undergone unilateral "hemireconstruction" and 44 patients who have been managed by a two-stage bilateral reconstruction, called "augmented hemilaryngectomy." Some postoperative problems were noted with granuloma formation, growth of hair in the region of the glottis, and (infrequently) infection. The resultant voice is described as low pitched, soft, and of limited range. Apparently, aspiration and stenosis were not encountered with these procedures.

Sessions et al.[22] have described the prevention of aspiration after vertical partial laryngectomy with arytenoid cartilage removal by transposing an inferiorly based sternohyoid muscle flap that is placed in the surgical defect and sutured to the cricoid cartilage posteriorly. Sessions also emphasizes the importance of suturing the epiglottic remnant to the hyoid bone and attaching the contralateral cord remnants anteriorly to the remaining thyroid cartilage. The area of reconstruction is covered with mucosa from the aryepiglottic fold or pyriform fossa region (Fig. 17–7). When bilateral resection is performed (anterior commissure technique), he advises placing an anterior commissure keel until epithelialization has been completed so as to prevent webbing from scar tissue at the anterior commissure. Great emphasis is placed on the details of the postoperative diet with progression from nasogastric tube feedings for seven to ten days to thick liquids, carbonated beverages, and pureed vegetables, fruits, and desserts. In the immediate postoperative period, the surgeon must address the issue of adequate nutritional intake for proper wound healing.

A similar approach in which the glottic area is reconstructed with a digastric tendon graft is proposed by Park et al.[23] A 2 cm section of the ipsilateral digastric tendon is sutured posteriorly in the arytenoid region and anteriorly to the thyroid cartilage. The tendon is then covered with an advancement mucosal flap. Good results were obtained in a series of five patients in whom this technique was employed, but granulation tissue in two of these patients required excision.

The concept of "imbrication laryngoplasty" has been proposed by Pleet et al.[24] This technique consists of a through-and-through resection of the region of the glottic carcinoma, excising the adjacent thyroid cartilage along with the specimen. The defect is then closed by suturing the superior resection margin (ventricular fold) to the inferior resection margin (immediate subglottic region). This reconstitutes the tissue bulk on the involved side and provides a cushion for the opposite cord to meet

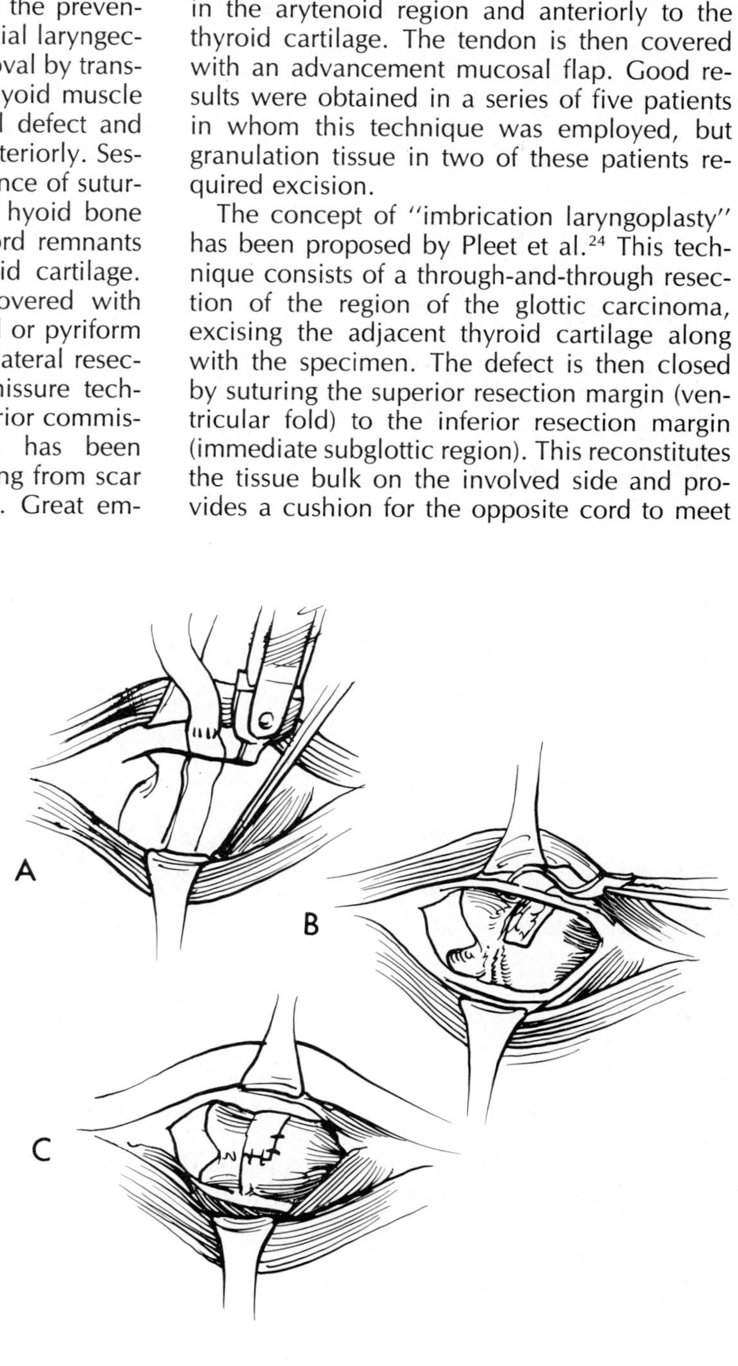

Figure 17–8. Horizontal external thyroid perichondrial flap based on the ipsilateral side is turned into the larynx and sutured posteriorly.

during phonation and deglutition. Good results are reported in a series of four patients, but one of these patients developed severe postoperative infection with granulation tissue and resistant *Pseudomonas* organisms, delaying decannulation for about six months.

Reconstruction of the glottic defect after partial laryngectomy using a perichondrial transposition flap has been described by Zollinger et al.[25] The perichondrial flap is based on the ipsilateral side but is elevated from the external surface of the thyroid cartilage on the side contralateral to the surgical resection. The transposition flap is turned into the surgical defect and sutured to the cricoarytenoid area posteriorly in the larynx; during the postoperative healing phase, it provides tissue for the development of a neocord (Fig. 17–8).

The use of a free flap is advocated by Nagahara et al.[26] The donor sites for the free flap tissue are the groin and deltopectoral areas; the flaps are sewn into place to reconstruct the laryngeal defect after extensive partial laryngectomy.

Primary Reconstruction for Glottic Competence After Supraglottic Partial Laryngectomy. Resection of a portion of the glottic region in continuity with supraglottic partial laryngectomy poses a dual challenge in restoration of glottic competence. The surgical extirpation of the supraglottic larynx removes the protective anatomic structures that are important in glottic closure during deglutition—specifically, the epiglottis and ventricular folds. Ogura and Dedo[27] reported a technique in which a pseudocord is created by dividing the upper portion of the ipsilateral thyroid ala and folding it medially to fill the tissue defect. This repositioned cartilage is secured by two mattress sutures, and the arytenoid cartilage is sutured to the cricoid cartilage in the midline with a heavy silk suture. The area is then covered with a mucosal flap from the pyriform fossa (Fig. 17–9). Good results were reported in four patients who were free of aspiration and whose voices were described as normal to slightly hoarse.

When it is necessary to extend the thyroid cartilage resection associated with supraglottic partial laryngectomy or when there is deep invasion of tumor into the vocalis muscle, the technique described by Ogura and Dedo would not be appropriate or possible. Mobilization and fracture of the superior cornu of the contralateral thyroid cartilage can be used to reconstruct the surgical defect in these circumstances, according to Friedman et al.[28] This

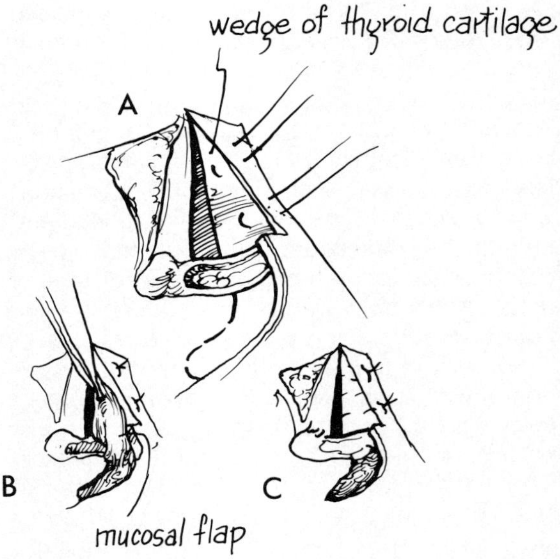

Figure 17–9. Creating a pseudocord by folding the superior portion of the thyroid cartilage medially to fill the defect after an extended supraglottic partial laryngectomy.

myochondral pedicle flap provides sufficient bulk posteriorly to restore the competence of the glottic sphincter. A mucosal advancement flap from the hypopharynx and pyriform sinus region is used to cover the myochondral flap. Good functional results were obtained in the eight patients who underwent this procedure. Two of the eight later developed recurrent carcinoma and required total laryngectomy; one patient is presumed to have residual cancer. This emphasizes the difficulties encountered when the indications for partial laryngectomy are extended to include supraglottic carcinoma with significant glottic extension. Sessions[29] has described using a free sternocleidomastoid muscle graft to reconstruct a large glottic defect following a supraglottic partial laryngectomy with excision of one true vocal cord and the ipsilateral thyroid and cricoid cartilage. The free muscle graft was sewn into place and the pharyngeal defect was closed by suturing the thyroid perichondrium to the base of the tongue and the lateral pharyngeal wall. The patient did well for almost a year before problems with aspiration developed, presumably due to atrophy of the muscle graft. A gastrostomy was subsequently required for feeding, but the patient has been decannulated and the voice is described as strong. The use of postoperative radiation therapy may have been a factor in producing the fibrosis and atrophy noted in this patient.

Modifications of the procedure for supraglot-

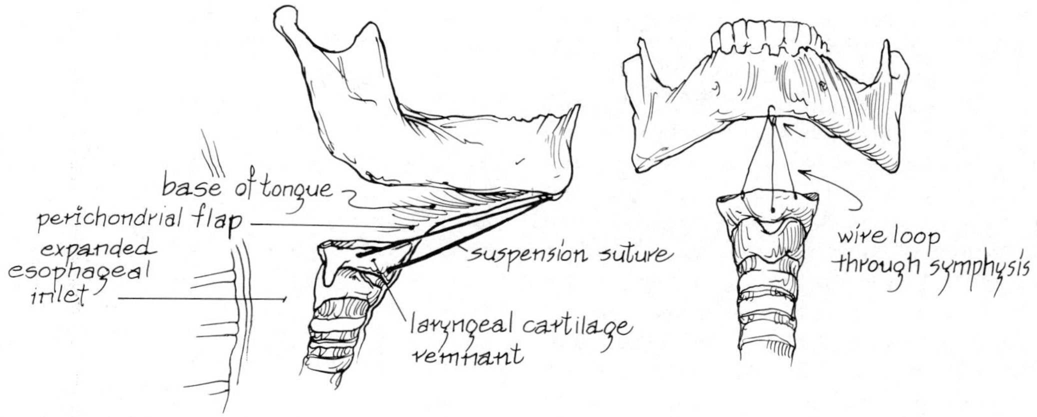

Figure 17–10. Suturing the laryngeal remnant to the mandible so that the postoperative glottic position will be placed as far superiorly and anteriorly as possible.

tic partial laryngectomy have been introduced by various authors, who suggest that these procedures are helpful in terms of early restoration of adequate swallowing. Calcaterra[30] emphasizes the importance of assuring that the laryngeal remnant is positioned as far superiorly and anteriorly as possible after surgery. He advises suspending the thyroid cartilage remnant from the mandible to bring the glottis to a higher and more anterior position and to utilize the shelflike protection afforded by the base of the tongue (Fig. 17–10). A similar step is recommended by Goode, who suspends the thyroid cartilage remnant from the digastric muscles after a standard supraglottic partial laryngectomy. He also recommends lateral laryngeal suspension to prevent aspiration after extensive resection of the mandible, pharynx, and base of the tongue (Fig. 17–11).[31]

Factors that have been noted to increase the problems of aspiration following supraglottic partial laryngectomy include the following:

1. More extensive resection.
2. Excision that involves removal of an arytenoid cartilage.
3. Persistence of postoperative edema (a factor that must also concern the surgeon in regard to persistence of carcinoma).
4. Persistent edema following radiation therapy.
5. Improper healing with the formation of granulation tissue and postoperative fibrosis.
6. Inadequate reconstruction of the surgical defect.

Nerve paralysis subsequent to surgical injury to the recurrent laryngeal nerve or to the superior laryngeal nerve will impair postoperative function and may result in aspiration during swallowing. This important factor is emphasized by Ward et al.,[2] who recommend that there be no unnecessary dissection in the region of these important neural structures during the course of the surgical procedure. This potential complication is particularlarly important in the case of vertical partial laryngectomy and is the basis for our recommendation that there be no

Figure 17–11. Frontal and lateral views showing the location of the laterally suspended larynx and the final placement of the suspension sutures. (From Hillel AD, Goode RL: Laryngoscope 93:27, 1983.)

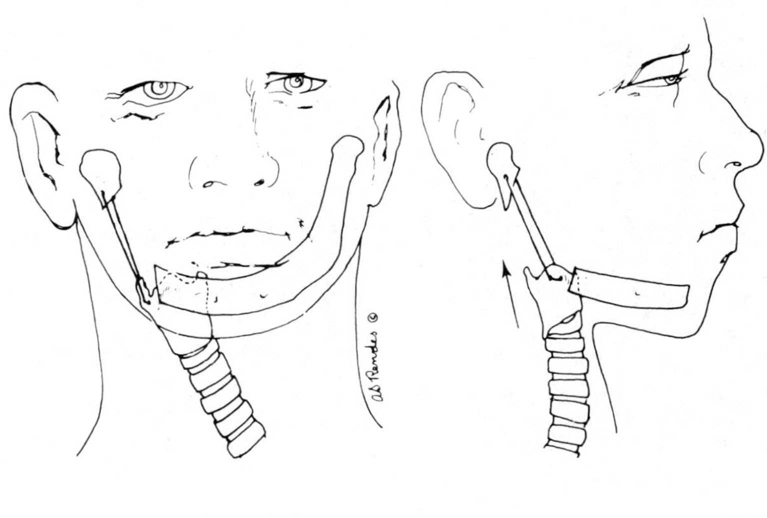

unneccessary dissection between the strap muscles and the external thyroid perichondrium during the elevation of reconstructive muscle flaps. In the case of the bipedicle muscle flap laryngoplasty, we emphasize that the muscle-splitting incision should not be carried more than 1 cm above and below the limits of the thyroid cartilage and should be accomplished far posteriorly, where it is well away from the superior laryngeal nerve and its branches. Careful attention to this detail has avoided problems with postoperative aspiration after vertical partial laryngectomy in our series, and total laryngectomy for relief from aspiration has not been necessary.

A different approach has been recommended by Silva and Loré,[32] who utilize a transposition flap of cervical skin to cover the raw surface of the base of the tongue rather than suturing it to the perichondrium after supraglottic partial laryngectomy. An epidermal shave is performed over the base of the skin flap to permit the lower margin of the incision to be sutured to the de-epithelized area, so that this procedure can be accomplished in one stage.

Vertical partial laryngectomy for tumors involving both vocal cords presents a reconstruction challenge in regard to the restoration of glottic function. Biller and Lawson[33] have reported the use of the posterior one-third of both thyroid alae to reconstruct the glottic region. The superior cornua are excised and the constrictor muscle is separated from the superior aspect of the thyroid alae. This permits a 90 degree forward rotation of the cartilage on each side toward the anterior midline (Fig. 17–12). Transposition cervical skin flaps are then rotated to the interior of the larynx in the manner described by Conley. Four of five patients who have undergone this procedure have developed good airways, adequate glottic closure, and satisfactory voice production.

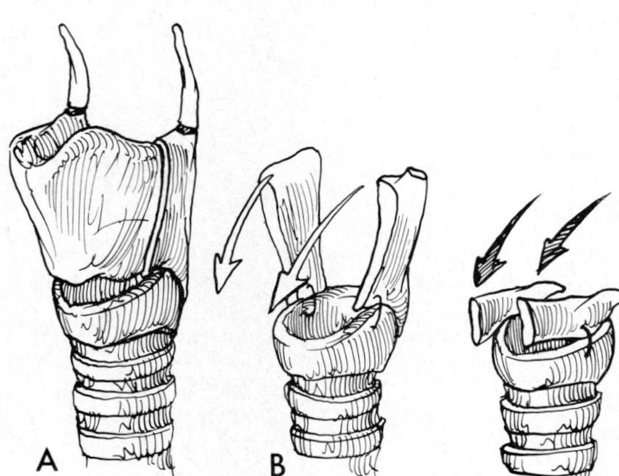

Figure 17–12. Posterior one-third of each thyroid cartilage is rotated anteriorly to reconstruct the glottic region after an extended bilateral resection.

Very extensive carcinoma in the glottic region may be managed by surgical procedures designated as *near-total laryngectomy.* This concept is developed more completely in Chapter 20 of this volume, but also deserves mention here. Tucker[34] cites the preliminary work by Bouche et al. of France, Sedlaček of Czechoslovakia, and Kambič of Yugoslavia. This technique permits removal of all of the glottic region except for one arytenoid and one-half of the posterior commissure area. The posterior one-fourth of the thyroid cartilage is preserved on each side. The surgical defect is reconstructed by mobilizing the epiglottis along its anterior surface and displacing it inferiorly into the laryngeal defect, where it is retained by suturing to the cricothyroid membrane (Fig. 17–13). Flaps of external thyroid perichondrium are then sutured together in the midline as an additional layer of closure. Tucker reports excellent results in a series of ten patients in regard to early decannulation and excellent laryngeal function with this one-stage reconstruction procedure. The indications for this technique are said to be as follows:

1. The tumor must spare one arytenoid and the posterior commissure.
2. The epiglottis must be preserved.
3. Ventricular involvement must be minimal.
4. Subglottic extension must be 1 cm or less.
5. Fixation of the cord or cords must be absent.

This technique has also been employed for reconstruction of the glottis secondary to severe trauma. Kennedy[35] reports the use of epiglottic reconstruction in a patient with total loss of laryngeal function secondary to scarring that resulted from a high tracheotomy. He left a laryngeal stent in place for eight weeks; the patient was decannulated four weeks after its removal and was noted to have an excellent airway and a good-to-excellent voice. Schechter[36] has also reported good results using a similar procedure for epiglottic reconstruction following partial laryngectomy for malignancy involving the anterior commissure region.

Glottic carcinoma with extension into the posterior subglottic region has been regarded by most surgeons as a contraindication for partial laryngectomy procedures. The proximity to the cricoid cartilage and the difficulty in reconstituting the competence of the glottic region have been addressed by Biller and

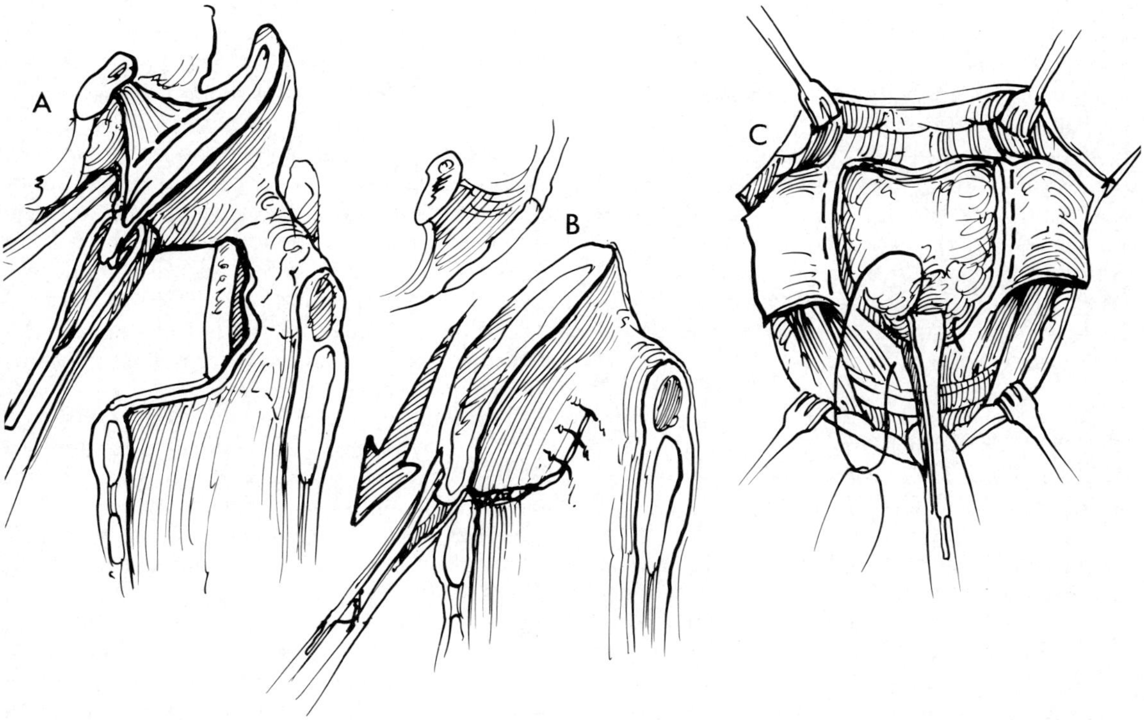

Figure 17–13. Laryngoplasty accomplished by mobilizing the epiglottis and displacing it inferiorly to reconstruct a large anterior glottic defect.

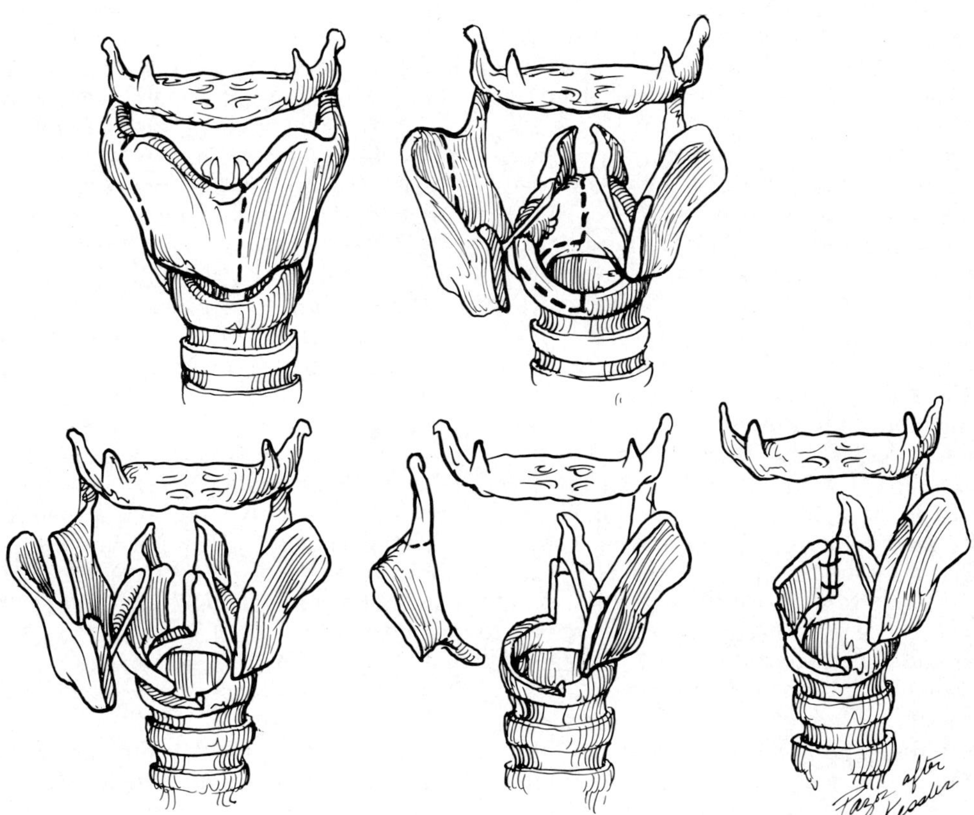

Figure 17–14. After resection of most of the ipsilateral cricoid cartilage, the defect is reconstructed using a pedicled myochondral flap (inferior constrictor muscle and thyroid cartilage).

Som.[37] To avoid total laryngectomy for these patients, the surgeon must excise most of the cricoid cartilage on the ipsilateral side to adequately excise the tumor. These authors propose repair of the surgical defect with a pedicled portion of thyroid cartilage in a manner that extends the laryngoplasty reported by Blaugrund and Kurland (Fig. 17–14). Utilizing careful case selection, they have employed this technique in a series of five patients, with excellent results in three and postoperative stenosis in one. A supraglottic recurrence developed in one other patient.

ADJUNCTIVE SURGICAL PROCEDURES FOR DELAYED GLOTTIC RECONSTRUCTION

Secondary Reconstruction After Vertical Partial Laryngectomy for Glottic Cancer. Secondary surgical procedures are essential to correct severe glottic insufficiency or significant respiratory obstruction following vertical partial laryngectomy. Secondary operation for vocal enhancement is less urgent but may be important for certain patients who rely heavily upon their ability to communicate.

Sessions et al.[3] defined glottic insufficiency as "glottic function either active or passive which is inadequate for physiological function either normal or adaptive. Glottic insufficiency may refer to a glottic chink which is too open (incompetent) or too closed (stenotic) for adequate function. Incompetent glottic insufficiency primarily affects deglutition and phonation, while respiration is usually adequate. Stenotic glottic insufficiency primarily affects the respiratory function and may occur with adequate phonation and deglutition. Late glottic insufficiency is defined as post-surgical glottic insufficiency still present for more than six months after partial laryngectomy."

Sessions et al.[3] have reviewed their experience in the surgical treatment of functional disability after partial laryngectomy in 55 patients. The technique employed most frequently is Teflon injection to reconstitute glottic insufficiency; this was employed in 8 of 21 patients after hemilaryngectomy and in 16 of 34 patients after supraglottic partial laryngectomy. Glottic insufficiency secondary to a large amount of tissue loss requires surgical reconstruction of a pseudocord. The technique for glottic reconstruction that these authors describe employs an inferiorly based sternohyoid muscle pedicle flap, which is sutured to the cricoid-arytenoid area posteriorly and covered with an advancement flap from the pyriform fossa region. The authors point out that it is not the size of the primary lesion and its subsequent excision that predispose the patient to postoperative glottic insufficiency but rather the specific region requiring excision. The areas of greatest functional significance are the arytenoid cartilage and the base of the tongue; patients who require extensive resection in these areas can be expected to have postoperative difficulty. Surgical excision or damage involving the vagus or the recurrent laryngeal nerve will result in problems with deglutition.

Implantation of a free fat graft to restore glottic competence has been advocated by Dedo[20] and described earlier in this chapter. He usually employs this as a primary reconstructive technique, but he also utilizes it to accomplish a secondary reconstruction to eliminate aspiration and enhance the quality of the voice. Variability in the amount of resorption of the fat graft implant has generated some criticism concerning the complete predictability of this technique; however, it is noted that even partial retention of the fat graft results in a tissue bed that is more receptive to Teflon injection than is the case with extensive fibrosis.

Total laryngectomy has been employed by many surgeons as a lifesaving measure in patients with recurrent pneumonia secondary to aspiration. Montgomery[38] has described a technique for glottic closure in patients with life-threatening aspiration. This procedure avoids the morbidity of total laryngectomy while closing the glottis to the possibility of further aspiration.

Our personal experience with secondary glottic reconstruction has been less extensive than that reported by Sessions.[3] We have attempted to restore glottic competence by the injection of Teflon according to the method described by Arnold.[39] In a group of five patients with aspiration after classic hemilaryngectomy, we found that it was impossible to accomplish glottic closure because of extensive fibrosis in the region of the surgical defect. We have achieved a satisfactory result in the management of this problem by transposing a sternohyoid muscle flap in three cases and by implantating cartilage grafts in four other patients.

Surgical Procedures for the Repair of Glottic Stenosis After Partial Laryngectomy. Stenosis after vertical partial laryngectomy has been reported as an uncommon complication, but it appears in almost every reported series of

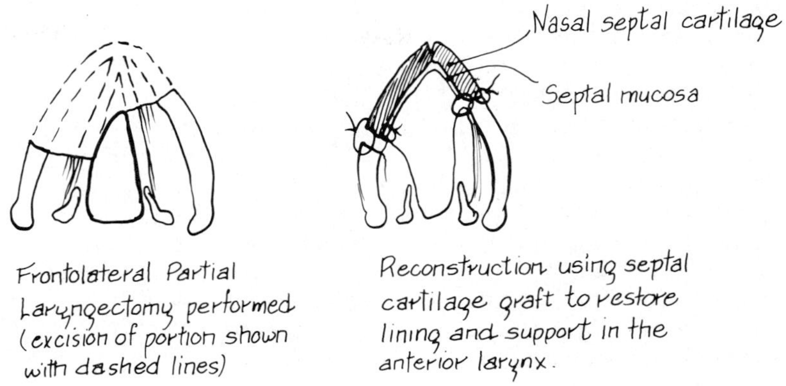

Figure 17–15. Nasal mucoseptal graft to reconstruct the anterior one-half of the larynx following resection of anterior glottic stenosis.

appreciable size. Stenosis is more commonly encountered with extended vertical partial laryngectomy procedures and following postoperative infection or radiation. When the postoperative glottic aperture is inadequate for good respiratory function, including function during moderate exercise, the tentative diagnosis of stenosis is made. It is essential that the possibility of residual carcinoma be entertained at this point. In fact, every case of postoperative laryngeal stenosis should be considered to arise from residual tumor until this possibility has been ruled out.

The management of stenosis secondary to excessive fibrosis begins with an emphasis on prevention. Postoperative stents and anterior commissure keels are advised when the surgical excision encroaches upon the anterior commissure region. Postoperative granulation tissue within the laryngeal lumen should be excised to avoid the transition to fibrosis with restriction of the airway. Endoscopic dilatation has only limited value in most cases of severe glottic stenosis. Laser excision of glottic scar tissue may be successful, but reports concerning the efficacy of this technique are contradictory.

Duncavage et al.[40] have investigated the use of a composite nasal septal graft to reconstruct the stenosis produced in dogs that had undergone vertical partial laryngectomy. Laurian and Zohar[41] reported excellent results in managing ten patients with glottic stenosis by the introduction of nasal mucoseptal grafts in the anterior commissure region (Fig. 17–15). Decannulation was possible in all ten patients at four to six days postoperatively. The functional results are described as good in eight of the ten patients in this series, but the follow-up period is somewhat brief, ranging from a few months to three years.

ADJUNCTIVE PROCEDURES FOR SECONDARY RECONSTRUCTION FOLLOWING SUPRAGLOTTIC PARTIAL LARYNGECTOMY

Supraglottic partial laryngectomy for lesions extending to the base of the tongue or to one arytenoid cartilage are more likely to be associated with postoperative aspiration secondary to glottic insufficiency. Aspiration is the predominant functional disability following supraglottic laryngectomy, and a variety of surgical methods have been employed for correction of glottic incompetence.

According to Sessions,[3] Teflon injection is successful in eliminating aspiration in many patients. When Teflon injection is insufficient, the most popular alternatives are muscle flap reconstruction or the implantation of cartilage or fat grafts. Nasogastric tube feeding is quite helpful in maintaining the patient's nutritional status during the interim period before successful correction has been accomplished. For long-term problems, gastrostomy is the logical solution for maintenance of feeding requirements. In rare cases of severe aspiration, glottic closure techniques or total laryngectomy must be considered. The sternohyoid muscle transposition reconstruction via thyrotomy and suturing is advocated by Sessions, who has obtained good results with this technique. Of 34 patients with functional disability after supraglottic laryngectomy, various forms of surgical treatment were effective in all but 5 patients with persistent moderate aspiration, 2 patients with a poor voice, 1 patient with a permanent gastrostomy, and 1 patient who succumbed from inanition.

Posterior glottic insufficiency after supraglottic partial laryngectomy may result in significant persistent aspiration. Biller et al.[42] advocate a technique for correction of posterior glottic insufficiency by remedial repositioning of the arytenoid cartilage. They utilize an extralaryngeal approach similar to that employed for arytenoidectomy as described by Woodman. The cricothyroid articulation is separated and the dissection is carried to the cricoarytenoid joint. A cartilage graft is introduced into the region of the posterior glottic insufficiency to fill the tissue defect. The technique was completely successful in eliminating aspiration in four patients and partially successful in a fifth patient in whom the procedure was performed. One patient had extensive granuloma formation at the time of surgery and the procedure was unsuccessful for technical reasons.

References

1. Conley JJ: Glottic reconstruction and wound rehabilitation. Arch Otolaryngol 74:239–242, 1961.
2. Ward PH et al.: New insights into the causes of postoperative aspiration following conservation surgery of the larynx. Ann Otol Rhinol Laryngol 86:724–736, 1977.
3. Sessions DG et al.: Late glottic insufficiency. Laryngoscope 85:950–959, 1975.
4. Chiari O: Chirurgie des kehlkopfes und der luftrohre. Neue Deutsche Chirurgie Vol 19. Stuttgart, Enke, 1916.
5. Meurman Y: Operative mediofixation of the vocal cord in complete unilateral paralysis. Arch Otolaryngol 55:544–553, 1952.
6. Morrison LF: The reverse king operation. Ann Otol Rhinol Laryngol 57:945, 1948.
7. Libersa C: Traitement chirurgical de la paralysie laryngée en abduction. J Fr Oto-Rhino-Laryng 1:480, 1952.
8. Opheim O: Unilateral paralysis of the vocal cord: Operative treatment. Acta Otolaryngol 45:226–230, 1955.
9. Goodyear H: Hemilaryngectomy: Method of maintaining a satisfactory airway and voice. Ann Otol Rhinol Laryngol 58:581–585, 1949.
10. Figi F: Removal of carcinoma of the larynx with immediate skin graft for repair. Ann Otol Rhinol Laryngol 59:474–486, 1950.
11. Som ML: Hemilaryngectomy: A modified technique for cordal carcinoma with extension posteriorly. Arch Otolaryngol 54:524–533, 1951.
12. Pressman JJ: Cancer of the larynx: Laryngoplasty to avoid laryngectomy. Arch Otolaryngol 59:395, 1954.
13. Waltner JG: Surgical rehabilitation of voice following laryngofissure. Arch Otolaryngol 67:99–101, 1958.
14. Conley JJ: The use of mucosal flaps for wound rehabilitation in partial laryngectomy. Arch Otolaryngol 69:700–703, 1959.
15. Conley J: Glottic reconstruction and wound rehabilitation. Arch Otolaryngol 74:239–242, 1961.
16. Harpman JA: Management of raw areas in the larynx. Arch Otolaryngol 73:678–680, 1961.
17. Maran AGD et al.: Reconstructive surgery for improved glottic closure and voice following partial laryngectomy. Laryngoscope 78:1916–1936, 1968.
18. Quinn, HJ Jr: A new technique for glottic reconstruction after partial laryngectomy. Laryngoscope 79:1980–2011, 1969.
19. Blaugrund SM, Kurland SR: Replacement of the arytenoid following vertical hemilaryngectomy. Laryngoscope 85:935–941, 1975.
20. Dedo HH: A technique for vertical hemilaryngectomy to prevent stenosis and aspiration. Laryngoscope 85:978–984, 1975.
21. Conley J: Regional skin flaps in partial laryngectomy. Laryngoscope 85:942–949, 1975.
22. Sessions DG et al.: Deglutition after conservation surgery for cancer of the larynx and hypopharynx. Otolaryngol Head Neck Surg 87:779–796, 1979.
23. Park NH et al.: Hemilaryngectomy and vocal cord reconstruction with digastric tendon graft. Surg Gynecol Obstetr 155:253–256, 1982.
24. Pleet L et al.: Partial laryngectomy with imbrication reconstruction. Ann Otol Rhinol Laryngol 84:882–889, 1977.
25. Zollinger WK et al.: Perichondrium flap reconstruction of the larynx. Trans Am Acad Ophthalmol Otolaryngol 82:167, 1976.
26. Nagahara K et al.: Laryngeal reconstruction by free flap transfer. Plast Reconstr Surg 57:604, 1976.
27. Ogura JH, Dedo HH: Glottic reconstruction following subtotal glottic-supraglottic laryngectomy. Laryngoscope 75:865–878, 1965.
28. Friedman WH et al.: Contralateral laryngoplasty after supraglottic laryngectomy with vertical extension. Arch Otolaryngol 107:742–745, 1981.
29. Sessions DG: Extended partial laryngectomy. Ann Otol Rhinol Laryngol 89:556–557, 1980.
30. Calcaterra T: Laryngeal suspension after supraglottic laryngectomy. Arch Otolaryngol 102:716, 1976.
31. Hillel AD, Goode RL: Lateral laryngeal suspension. Laryngoscope 93:26–31, 1983.
32. Silva N, Loré JM Jr: Partial horizontal supraglottic laryngectomy: A method of reconstruction. Laryngoscope 87:1165–1168, 1977.
33. Biller HF, Lawson W: Bilateral vertical partial laryngectomy for bilateral vocal cord carcinoma. Ann Otol Rhinol Laryngol 90:489–491, 1981.
34. Tucker HM et al.: Glottic reconstruction after near-total laryngectomy. Laryngoscope 89:609–618, 1979.
35. Kennedy TL: Epiglottic reconstruction of laryngeal stenosis secondary to cricothyroidostomy. Laryngoscope 90:1130–1136, 1980.
36. Schechter GL: Epiglottic reconstruction and subtotal laryngectomy. Laryngoscope 93:729–734, 1983.
37. Biller HF, Som ML: Vertical partial laryngectomy for glottic carcinoma with posterior subglottic extension. Ann Otol Rhinol Laryngol 86:715–718, 1977.
38. Montgomery WW: Surgery to prevent aspiration. Arch Otolaryngol 101:679, 1975.
39. Arnold G: Vocal rehabilitation of paralytic dysphonia: Technique of intracordal injection. Arch Otolaryngol 76:358–368, 1962.
40. Duncavage JA et al.: Composite nasal septal graft reconstruction of the partial laryngectomized canine. Ann Otol Rhinol Laryngol 86:285–290, 1978.
41. Laurian N, Zohar Y: Laryngeal reconstruction by composite nasal mucoseptal graft after partial laryngectomy: Three years follow-up. Laryngoscope 91:609–615, 1981.
42. Biller HF et al.: Correction of posterior glottic incompetence following horizontal partial laryngectomy. Ann Otol Rhinol Laryngol 91:448–449, 1982.

18

Surgery of Laryngopharyngeal and Subglottic Cancer

Harlan Muntz, M.D., and Donald G. Sessions, M.D.

Early detection plays a major role in reducing cancer deaths, particularly in malignancies of the head and neck in areas where small tumors may present symptoms of hoarseness, pain, or dysphagia. Tumors of the laryngopharynx, on the other hand, are notorious for presenting no symptoms until very late in their courses. Rarely do small cancers compromise the upper aerodigestive path. This characteristic, coupled with the high incidence of early metastases to regional lymph nodes, leads to a poor prognosis for laryngopharyngeal cancers. Despite the development of new treatment regimens, cure rates remain disappointing. Recent advances in techniques of surgical ablation and reconstruction have produced some increase in survival and, of more importance, improved quality of life. The therapeutic combination of surgery and irradiation has also increased cure rates.

This chapter will discuss the anatomy, staging, incidence, survival, and surgical treatment of cancers of the laryngopharynx and subglottic area.

ANATOMY

Hypopharynx. The hypopharynx is the anatomic region contiguous with the nasopharynx and oropharynx superiorly and the cervical esophagus inferiorly; it is bounded anteriorly by the posterior larynx and posteriorly by the prevertebral fascia. It extends from the plane of the hyoid bone to the plane of the inferior aspect of the cricoid cartilage (Fig. 18–1).

The principal divisions of this space are the pyriform fossa or sinus, the postcricoid area, the posterior and lateral hypopharyngeal wall, and the marginal area. The hypopharyngeal region is a skeletal muscular tube used in the reflex propulsion of food from the mouth and oropharynx into the cervical esophagus by means of coordinated mechanical action. Involved in the muscular activity in this region are both the hypopharyngeal portion of the inferior constrictor and the inferior-most portion of the middle constrictors. The vagus nerve innervates these constrictors.

Other anatomic features in this area include the larynx anteriorly, the carotid sheath laterally, and the prevertebral space overlying the fourth through the sixth cervical vertebrae posteriorly.

Cervical Esophagus. The cervical esophagus is a continuation of the gullet beneath the inferior aspect of the plane of the cricoid cartilage. Its function is to move the food bolus by peristalsis towards the stomach. Its muscular

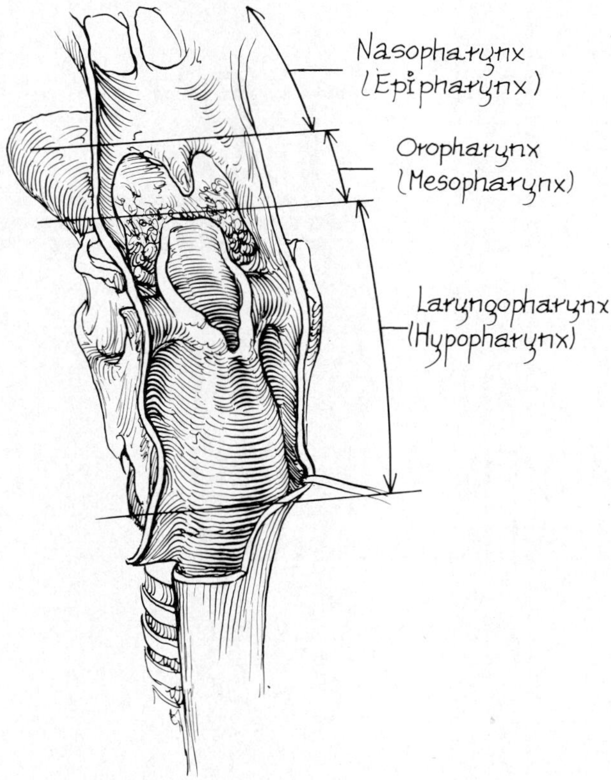

Figure 18–1. Posterior view of the three pharyngeal regions.

layer consists of predominantly striated muscle invested in a loose coat of connective tissue. The mucosal lining consists primarily of stratified squamous epithelium.

Anatomically, the cervical esophagus is intimately related to the trachea anteriorly, the lateral lobes of the thyroid laterally, and the connective tissue of the prevertebral fascia posteriorly. The inferior boundary of the cervical esophagus is at the level of the innominate artery.

Marginal Area. The supraglottic larynx contains several distinct anatomic sites including the epiglottis, false vocal cords, ventricles, and petiole. Tumors that originate on the aryepiglottic folds, although traditionally described as supraglottic, are included in this chapter and considered later under Natural History of Tumors.[1]

The aryepiglottic fold is a mucosa-covered ridge of muscle between the epiglottis and the arytenoid cartilage. The aryepiglottic muscle fibers arise from the anterior border and apex of the arytenoid cartilage and insert into the mucosa superiorly and into the lateral edge of the epiglottic cartilage.

Tumors of the aryepiglottic fold may extend into the larynx or into the hypopharynx, but the characteristics of their growth are like those of hypopharyngeal or pyriform sinus cancers. Tumors of the marginal area are very aggressive, with local spread to the pyriform sinus, lateral pharyngeal wall, and supraglottic larynx and with early metastasis to the regional cervical lymph nodes.

Pyriform Sinus. The pyriform sinus (fossa) is the largest area of the region of the hypopharynx. Anatomically, it is an inverted three-sided pyramid bounded superiorly by the glossoepiglottic folds, medially by the aryepiglottic folds, laterally by the lateral pharyngeal wall, and inferiorly by an apex lateral to the cricopharyngeus muscle.

No natural barrier inhibits the spread of pyriform sinus tumors and only thin connective tissue separates the pyriform sinus from the neck. Local spread is aggressive and regional lymph node metastasis occurs very early.

NATURAL HISTORY OF TUMORS

Pyriform Sinus. Pyriform sinus tumors account for about two-thirds of all hypopharyngeal tumors. Between 50 per cent and 70 per cent of these lesions have already metastasized

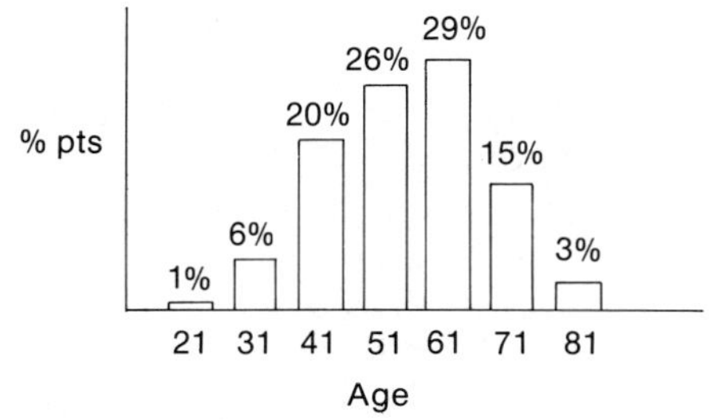

Figure 18–2. Incidence of hypopharyngeal cancer, grouped by patient age in decades.

Table 18–1. STAGING OF PYRIFORM SINUS CANCER

T1	One site of pyriform sinus only (e.g., aryepiglottic fold, anterior, medial, or lateral wall only)
T2	Two sites involved (e.g., aryepiglottic fold and medial wall or medial and anterior walls)
T3	Three sites involved (e.g., aryepiglottic fold, medial wall, and a third site such as apex)
T4	Tumor outside of inferior hypopharynx (e.g., postcricoid, larynx, or base of tongue)

to the regional cervical lymph nodes by the time the primary tumor is detected. Figure 18–2 indicates the incidence of cancer of the hypopharynx with age. Sixty-seven per cent of patients have their cancers diagnosed between the ages of 50 and 70. Males with pyriform sinus cancer outnumber females almost 6:1.

Pyriform sinus cancers are diagnosed most often late in their courses, when the tumor has become extensive. More than 60 per cent involve three or more sites and almost 30 per cent have extended beyond the hypopharynx (Table 18–1 and Fig. 18–3).[2]

Local infiltration occurs rapidly because no anatomic barrier exists to prevent tumor spread from the pyriform sinus and because the region is rich in lymphatic vessels. Of those patients exhibiting metastasis to the cervical lymph nodes, more than half are stage N1 (i.e., the node is mobile, ipsilateral, and less than 3 cm in size).

Treatment of cancers of the pyriform fossa should include the combined efforts of the surgeon and radiotherapist. Survival remains limited despite advances in both surgical technique and radiation oncology. Net five-year survival is about 25 per cent.[3] Survival figures at three years are somewhat better but still disappointing. As in most tumors, better survival can be documented with small lesions and less extensive neck disease. Less than one-quarter of patients with cancer of the pyriform fossa survive three years if extensive neck disease is found. If no adenopathy is detected clinically, nearly one-half survive three years (Fig. 18–4).

Marginal Area. Tumors of the marginal area (aryepiglottic fold) have a natural history similar to tumors of the pyriform fossa. No natural barrier prevents tumor spread, particularly after the tumor has extended into the pyriform fossa laterally or the base of the tongue superiorly.

Marginal tumors generally present late because symptoms of dysphagia or hoarseness occur only when the tumor is large or deeply invasive. Only about 10 per cent of these tumors are localized to the aryepiglottic fold at the time of presentation. Most of these tumors have extended to the supraglottic larynx, to the apex of the pyriform sinus, or even beyond the region. Lymphatic spread is somewhat less aggressive than it is in tumors of the pyriform fossa, even though the primary tumor is generally more advanced (Table 18–2). More than half of the marginal tumors have no clinically palpable nodes at the time of presentation. Fewer patients with marginal tumors have extensive neck disease at the time of presentation

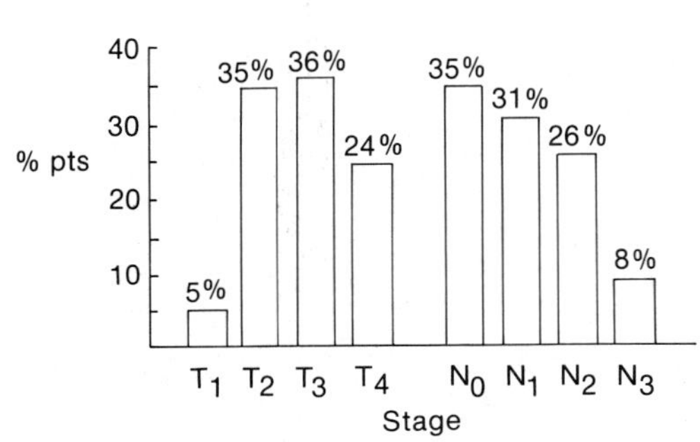

Figure 18–3

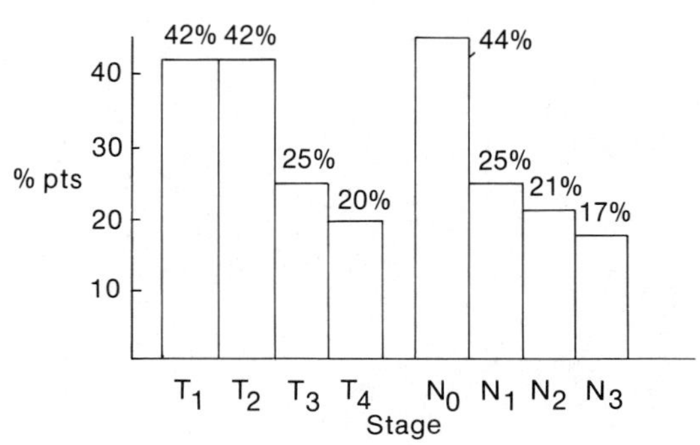

Figure 18–4

Figure 18–3. Incidence of pyriform sinus cancer, grouped by T and N staging.

Figure 18–4. Three-year survival with no evidence of disease in pyriform fossa cancer, grouped by T and N staging.

Table 18–2. STAGING CRITERIA FOR MARGINAL LESIONS*

T1	Tumor limited to the aryepiglottic fold with normal mobility
T2	Tumor of the aryepiglottic and one of the following: ventricular bands, or medial wall of the pyriform sinus, or epiglottis (with normal mobility)
T3	Tumor of the aryepiglottic fold with vocal cord fixation and/or with two of the following: tumor of medial or anterior walls of the pyriform sinus, tumor of ventricular bands, extension down to but not involving the pyriform apex of the pyriform sinus
T4	Tumor of the aryepiglottic fold with involvement of all three walls of the pyriform sinus and/or extension beyond the larynx

*Marginal lesion staging from Ogura JH et al.: Laryngoscope 85:1801–1807, 1975. Nodal staging from Beahrs OH, Myers MH (eds.): American Joint Committee on Cancer: Manual for Staging of Cancer, 2nd ed. Philadelphia, JB Lippincott Company, 1983, p 35.

compared to patients with carcinoma of the pyriform sinus (Fig. 18–5).[1] Survival rates are much higher for marginal lesions than for pyriform sinus lesions (Fig. 18–6).

Postcricoid and Posterior Hypopharyngeal Wall. Tumors of the postcricoid area and the posterior hypopharyngeal wall are less common. Their clinical manifestations include the following symptoms: sensation of a foreign body in the throat, pain on swallowing, difficulty in swallowing, and bleeding. About 30 per cent of hypopharyngeal tumors present on the postcricoid or on the posterior pharyngeal wall.[4] These tumors are aggressive and their presentation is accompanied by nodal disease in the neck in more than half of the patients. At the time of diagnosis, most postcricoid cancers are circumferential at the cricopharyngeal sphincter.

Postcricoid lesions, because of their location, negate the possibility for conservation laryngeal surgery. Total laryngectomy or total laryngopharyngectomy is required even for small lesions when surgery is part of the therapy. Cancers of the posterior hypopharyngeal wall are difficult to treat, and they exhibit high local and regional recurrence rates. About 15 per cent will have distant metastasis. Risk of perioperative mortality and morbidity is great. Postoperative complications leading to death occurred in 5 per cent of those patients receiving radiation followed by surgical ablation.[5, 6] Although treatment with full-course radiation therapy may be more immediately palliative, survival has been increased only for those patients who had surgical treatment with or without combined radiotherapy.

PREOPERATIVE EVALUATION

Presentation. Cancers of the laryngopharynx usually present late in the course of the disease. Typical complaints include dysphagia, odynophagia, hoarseness, persistent sore throat, and referred otalgia. Some patients present with hemoptysis or airway obstruction. One of the more common presenting complaints, however, is a mass in the neck. Occasionally, the cervical mass is a direct extension of the tumor into the soft tissue of the neck.

Diagnostic Steps. Complete evaluation of the head and neck including otoscopy and indirect mirror laryngoscopy should be done on any patient presenting such complaints. Pay partic-

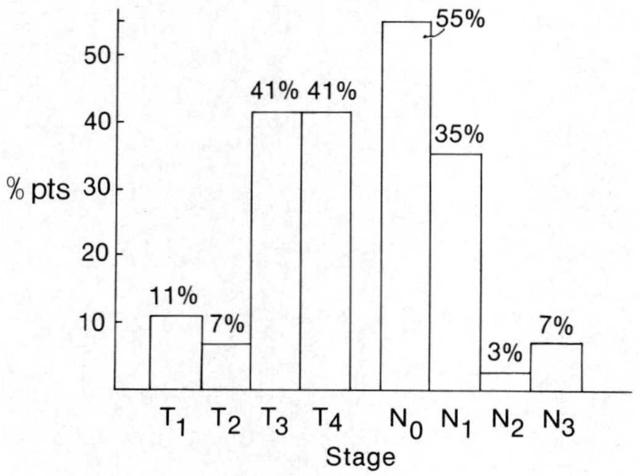

Figure 18–5

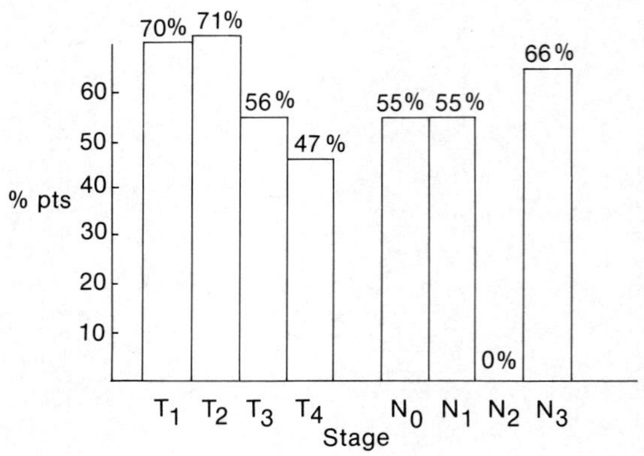

Figure 18–6

Figure 18–5. Incidence of marginal cancer, grouped by T and N staging.

Figure 18–6. Incidence of three-year survival with no evidence of disease in marginal cancer, grouped by T and N staging.

ular attention to the base of the tongue, the pyriform fossa including the apex, the pharyngeal walls, the postcricoid area, and the endolarynx. Use the flexible fiberoptic laryngoscope when mirror examination is inadequate.

Radiologic examination precedes biopsy to avoid the abnormal swelling in the area caused by the biopsy. Techniques available include plain films, polytomes, contrast laryngograms, and computed tomogram (CT) scans. Plain films and polytomes yield information regarding cartilage destruction and soft tissue masses. Contrast laryngograms evaluate the pyriform fossa and provide information regarding vocal cord mobility, the laryngeal ventricles, the anterior commissure, and the subglottic area.[7]

At present, high-resolution computed axial tomograms result in excellent delineation of laryngopharyngeal tumors and can be used for pretreatment measurement and mapping of these cancers. Computed tomograms give suggestive information regarding preepiglottic space involvement, but their value in determining presence or absence of cartilage invasion remains questionable.[8]

The most important part of the preoperative evaluation is direct laryngoscopy. This procedure may be done under local or general anesthesia. Complete and precise mapping of the lesion is carried out and biopsy is performed for tissue diagnosis. Tumor mapping allows for staging, treatment planning, and prognostication.

Standardized pulmonary function tests are employed when conservation surgery is anticipated. Although they are not absolute, guidelines regarding pulmonary function test results assist the clinician in making safe preoperative decisions regarding the appropriateness of conservation surgery.

Staging. For selection of the proper therapy for laryngopharyngeal cancers, the pathologic type of tumor should be described, and the exact locations and extent of the primary tumor and the metastases should be classified according to a staging system. Pretreatment staging of laryngopharyngeal tumors represents an amalgamation of the physical examination, radiologic tests, direct laryngoscopy, and the biopsy results. Table 18–3 indicates the general T (tumor) staging for the hypopharynx.

Table 18–3. T STAGING OF CANCER OF THE HYPOPHARYNX*

Tis	Carcinoma in situ
T1	Tumor confined to one site
T2	Extension of tumor to adjacent region or site without fixation of hemilarynx**
T3	Extension of tumor to adjacent region or site with fixation of hemilarynx
T4	Massive tumor invading bone or soft tissues of neck

*From Beahrs OH, Myers MH (eds.): American Joint Committee on Cancer: Manual for Staging of Cancer, 2nd ed. Philadelphia, JB Lippincott Company, 1983, p 35.

**Fixation here means fixation of the hypopharyngeal tumor to the hemilarynx and implies nonmobility of the hemilarynx. It does not refer to fixation of the vocal cords.

Treatment. Laryngopharyngeal cancer is highly aggressive, presenting with advanced local and regional disease. A combination of surgery and irradiation has increased survival in these patients. High-dose preoperative radiotherapy (5000 rads total tumor dose) combined with surgery can decrease the local recurrence rate in laryngopharyngeal cancers.[1, 3, 9–11] Recently, in an effort to decrease postoperative morbidity, surgical excision has been followed by postoperative irradiation. The postoperative irradiation begins within three to four weeks after the surgery. Because of the high incidence of cervical metastasis, both the ipsilateral and contralateral neck are irradiated.

Table 18–4 indicates the appropriate surgical treatment of cancer of the hypopharynx by T stage. The surgical approach to the primary includes a wide excision of the primary cancer

Table 18–4. SURGICAL TREATMENT OF CANCER OF THE HYPOPHARYNX

Primary Site	T1	T2	T3	T4
Pyriform sinus	PLP + ND	PLP + ND	PLP + ND or TLP + ND + PER	TLP + ND + PER
Postcricoid	TL + ND + LTA	TLP + ND + LTA	TLP + ND + PER	TLP + ND + PER
Posterior wall	PP + ND	PP + ND	PP + ND	TLP + ND
Pharynx		TL + PER	TL + PER	TL + PER

Key: LTA = laryngotracheal autograft; ND = neck dissection; PER = pharyngoesophageal reconstruction; PLP = partial laryngopharyngectomy; PP = partial pharyngectomy; TL = total laryngectomy; TLP = total laryngopharynectomy en bloc with a radical neck dissection. Where appropriate, functional laryngeal structures are preserved, resulting in satisfactory deglutition, respiration, and phonation. About 42 per cent of patients with laryngopharyngeal cancer are eligible for conservation surgery.[2] For lesions involving the pyriform sinus or the lateral and posterior hypopharyngeal walls, an oblique partial laryngopharyngectomy is performed. This operation is not applicable to lesions that involve the pyriform apex, invade cartilage, extend beyond the laryngopharynx, involve the glottic or subglottic larynx, or extend beyond the paralaryngeal space. These larger lesions require a total laryngopharyngectomy.

Role of Additional Treatment Modalities. Interest in pretreatment chemotherapy for laryngeal cancers has increased recently. Early results indicate good preoperative tumor response without any increase in surgical morbidity. Whether this will effect an improvement in survival remains to be established.

SURGICAL PROCEDURES

Presurgical Preparation.

When cancer of the laryngopharynx is diagnosed, the most important part of the presurgical preparation is informing the patient. The patient's cooperation is encouraged both preoperatively and postoperatively for the best results. Without this cooperation, even the best of surgical techniques may be wasted.

Presurgical preparation includes complete, informed consent. This allows for latitude in making intraoperative decisions concerning partial or total removal of the larynx and in reconstructing with pedicle flaps when necessary. Patients must understand that factors present at the time of surgery may prevent conservation surgical procedures. Alternative procedures for reconstruction must be discussed in detail before the surgery. Informed consent includes thorough discussion of all possible postoperative complications including loss of voice, difficulty with swallowing, bleeding, infection, pharyngocutaneous fistula, prolonged hospitalization, and even death. Patients must understand the need for a temporary or permanent tracheostomy, nasogastric feeding tube, urinary catheter, and intensive care unit admission postoperatively.

Stabilization of medical problems including chronic lung disease, cardiovascular disease, and diabetes is vital. Patients with pulmonary problems require intensive preoperative respiratory therapy. Nutritional status is assessed and enteral or parenteral hyperalimentation is instituted to achieve positive nitrogen balance.

Prophylactic antibiotics are begun prior to surgery. The patient is taken to the operating room with a nasogastric tube and a urinary catheter in place. The nasogastric tube is used for decompression and placed on drainage for 24 to 48 hours postoperatively. After this period, tube feedings are begun and continue until peroral alimentation can be resumed. The catheter is used to monitor the patient's fluid status and is ordinarily removed the morning after surgery.

Surgical Excision

History. In 1877, Czerny first described an attempt at resection.[12] The evolution of the surgical treatment of laryngopharyngeal carcinoma since that time has been disappointing. Many factors contribute to this. Tumors are often large and resections may be quite debilitating. Major compromise of both gullet and airway are necessary and, with the risk of severe infection and high recurrence rate, surgery of this area continues to be difficult. By 1908, VonHacker quoted a 48 per cent mortality rate for ablative surgery of this area.[13]

In 1920, Trotter described a lateral transhyoid pharyngotomy for pharyngeal cancers.[14] This was a reasonable approach, but some surgeons were less aggressive in resecting the tumors because they wished to facilitate reconstruction. This resulted in very early recurrence and death from tumor. Others at that time were intent on radical procedures that would be oncologically sound. The resections were immense[15] and the prevailing attitude maintained that primary reconstruction was not part of the surgeon's role.

Complete excision cured a small number of patients but involved total laryngectomy with loss of voice and pharyngeal fistula that required daily dressings and nasogastric alimentation. This cure was sometimes considered worse than the disease. Only as new techniques in reconstruction became available was there renewed enthusiasm for surgical treatment of these lesions.

In 1947, Alonso reported a series of patients from Uruguay in whom cancers of the larynx and hypopharynx were excised with preservation of voice.[10] These procedures included a temporary pharyngostoma that was closed secondarily.[16] In the United States, these procedures did not gain much attention until Ogura[17] clearly defined the soundness of the oncologic principles and described one-stage excision with immediate reconstruction.

The goals of ablative surgery are twofold. First and foremost, the tumor and regional lymphatics must be removed so that the patient may have the best chance for cure. Second, when clinically feasible, the larynx should be spared to allow normal phonation, respiration, and deglutition.

Partial Laryngopharyngectomy. Partial laryngopharyngectomy is performed for those laryngopharyngeal tumors that can be excised while sparing the tissues of the larynx and hypopharynx sufficiently to result in satisfactory function.

Indications. General indications for partial laryngopharyngectomy include the following conditions:

1. The contralateral vocal cord must be tumor free and mobile.
2. The ipsilateral arytenoid may be involved.
3. The ipsilateral vocal cord should be mobile but may be superficially involved.
4. The apex of the pyriform sinus, the cricopharyngeal sphincter, and the postcricoid area must be tumor free.
5. There must be no invasion of thyroid cartilage by tumor.

A neck dissection is always performed in patients satisfying these criteria. In patients in whom the anterior or lateral wall of the pyriform sinus exhibits tumor involvement, pedicle flap reconstruction is planned preoperatively.

Procedure. After the patient is intubated under general anesthesia, a horizontal curvilinear neck incision is employed and the skin flap raised. A low tracheostomy is made and the endotracheal tube is placed below. An ipsilateral neck dissection is performed. The ipsilateral hemithyroid is removed with the neck dissection, which is based on the thyrohyoid membrane. The suprahyoid muscles are separated from the hyoid bone superiorly. The hyoid bone is divided and retracted downward to gain access to the vallecula above the tumor. The strap muscles are divided at the superior aspect of the thyroid ala to allow elevation of the perichondrial flap, exposing the portion of the thyroid cartilage to be excised. Precise cuts are made in the thyroid cartilage alae by an oscillating electric saw. The site of the tumor,

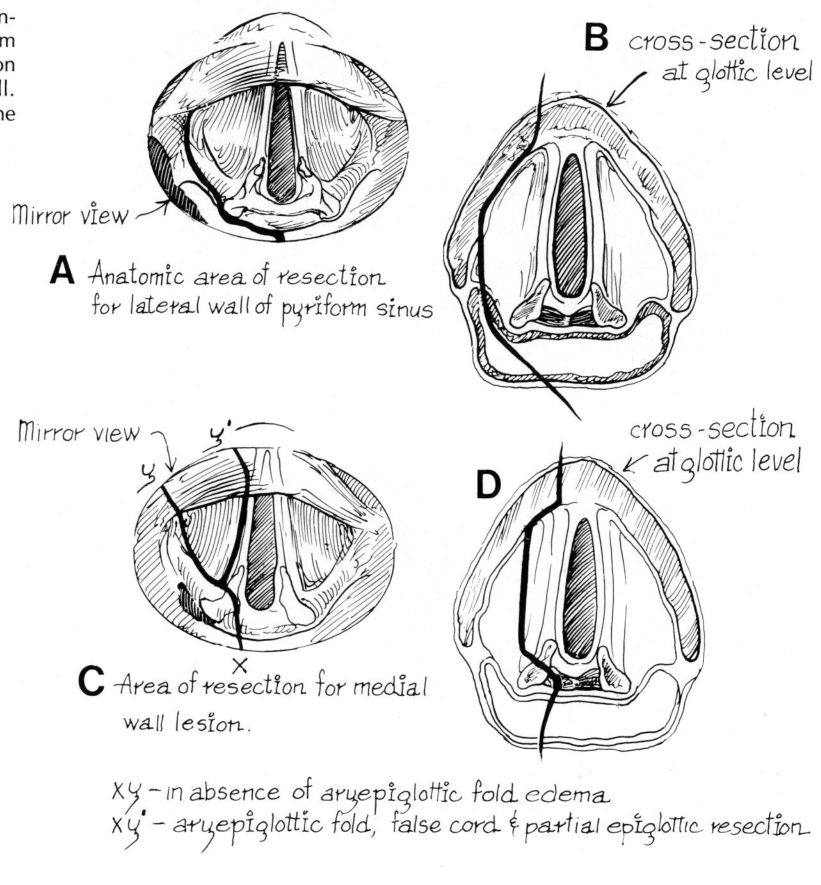

Figure 18–7. Partial laryngopharyngectomy procedure for pyriform sinus carcinoma. *A* and *B*, Resection for cancer arising on the lateral wall. *C* and *D*, Resection for cancer of the medial wall.

which has been fully evaluated preoperatively, determines the position of the cut. If the lesion involves only the pyriform sinus anterior and lateral walls, then the cartilage cut goes laterally and inferiorly from the midline, superior to the insertion of the inferior cornu (Fig. 18–7).

If the lesion involves the supraglottic larynx, the aryepiglottic fold, or the medial wall of the pyriform sinus, the cut must go from just contralateral to the midline just superior to the vocal cord level at the midline, and then inferior and lateral to the insertion of the ipsilateral inferior cornu of the thyroid cartilage (Fig. 18–8).

With the patient paralyzed, the pharynx is entered through the contralateral vallecula. The tumor is excised under direct vision. If at this point the criteria for partial surgery are not met, then the procedure is converted to a total laryngopharyngectomy.

The form of laryngeal reconstruction depends upon the presence or absence of the ipsilateral arytenoid cartilage after excision of the tumor. If the arytenoid is excised during the resection, then the remaining vocal cord remnant is sutured and fixed to the cricoid cartilage in the midline posteriorly.

Primary closure of the lateral pharyngeal wall is possible only with lesions that do not extend beyond the medial wall of the pyriform sinus. Lesions that are larger and that encompass areas including the anterior and lateral walls of the hypopharynx require split-thickness skin grafts or pedicle flaps for closure. Deltopectoral or pectoralis major myocutaneous flap closure of these defects produces rapid primary healing and improved functional results.

Total Laryngopharyngectomy. Total laryngopharyngectomy is the required excisional procedure for patients with larger laryngophar-

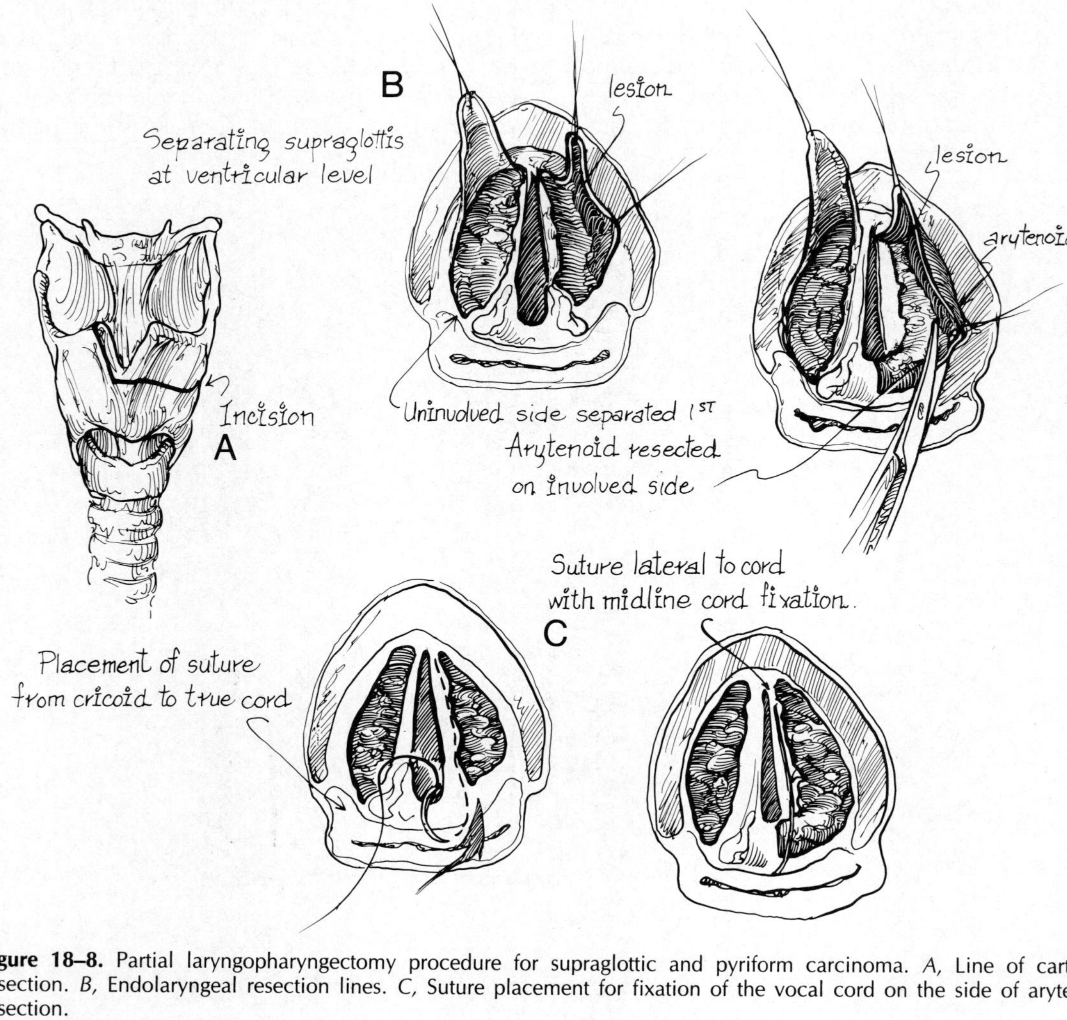

Figure 18–8. Partial laryngopharyngectomy procedure for supraglottic and pyriform carcinoma. *A,* Line of cartilage resection. *B,* Endolaryngeal resection lines. *C,* Suture placement for fixation of the vocal cord on the side of arytenoid resection.

yngeal tumors that require removal of the entire larynx and part or all of the pharynx for cure. This procedure is indicated for patients with laryngopharyngeal cancer involving the thyroid cartilage, the postcricoid area, the pyriform apex, or the cricopharyngeal sphincter, and for patients with vocal cord fixation.

Technical considerations are similar to those in partial laryngopharyngectomy except that an en bloc total laryngectomy is performed. The pharynx is entered through the vallecula or the contralateral pyriform sinus. Reconstruction after total laryngopharyngectomy requires pedicle flap rotation. A permanent tracheostoma is created.

When possible, enough mucosa may be left to close the neopharynx, but usually such closure risks severe stenosis of the gullet and increases the chance for wound breakdown. In very large lesions, tumor removal with an adequate surgical margin necessitates removal of an entire segment of the gullet, leaving superiorly a pharyngeal opening and inferiorly the proximal esophageal opening without intervening tissue. In both cases, reconstruction of the gullet is accomplished by bringing in distant tissue either by pedicled flap or free graft.

Laryngotracheal Autograft—Postcricoid Cancer. Excision of a postcricoid cancer requires total laryngectomy. The required removal of the postcricoid plate precludes safe separation of the digestive system and the airway. In 1952, Asherson described an excision technique that allows for reconstruction of the defect using the uninvolved anterior portion of the larynx.[18]

Technically, this reconstruction is performed through a low collar incision. After elevation of the neck flap, the superior laryngeal and thyroid vessels are identified and preserved to provide adequate blood supply to the autograft. Dissection in the plane of the prevertebral space permits palpation of the area to determine the possibility of resection. If the tumor is found to be resectable, a horizontal tracheostomy is done and the endotracheal tube is sutured into position. The lower trachea is dissected free along the party wall to mobilize it enough to allow fashioning of the permanent tracheostoma.

A segmental resection of the postcricoid tumor is then performed. The larynx is entered inferiorly on the contralateral or least involved side. The dissection is carried vertically, from inferior and lateral up just anterior to the vocal process, which is left attached to the specimen. A vertical cut is then made on the ipsilateral side up through the thyroid cartilage. This allows the postcricoid cancer to be excised under direct vision.

The laryngotracheal autograft is used to reconstruct the anterior pharyngoesophageal wall. Stiffness is reduced by carefully removing the thyroid cartilage in a subperichondrial plane (Fig. 18–9).

In patients with small postcricoid cancers, autograft of the anterior larynx is sutured to the remaining posterior pharyngeal wall. The epiglottic tip may be excised and mucosa closed over the defect. In patients with a circumferential cancer of the postcricoid area, the entire pharynx and cricopharyngeal sphincter must be removed. A laryngotracheal autograft cannot reconstruct a 360-degree loss, so a pedicle flap is necessary for reconstruction.

Survival has improved very little over the years. At present, the overall five-year survival rate is 20 per cent to 36 per cent with combined treatment, and three-year survival is only 20 per cent to 47 per cent. Failure at the primary site is 10 per cent to 15 per cent, but the rate of regional nodal failure is exceptionally high, even when neck dissection and radiation therapy are combined. More than one-third of the cases developed distant metastasis.

As stated earlier in this chapter, treatment of these aggressive tumors is at best disappointing. Increased awareness by medical personnel of the symptoms of laryngopharyngeal cancers and earlier discovery of tumors may lead to improvement. The institution of chemotherapeutic protocols in the future offers hope of fewer failures in treatment of the many patients with distant metastases.

Reconstructive Surgery

Surgery for tumors of the laryngopharynx poses a reconstructive problem of the highest magnitude. Early efforts at reconstruction resulted in an operative mortality approaching 75 per cent, with three-fourths of those who survived the operation succumbing to recurrent tumor.[19] Excision of tumors of the larynx and hypopharynx creates a defect of both the airway and the digestive tract. Reconstruction of the permanent tracheostoma has controlled the airway problem after total laryngectomy. Recreation of the gullet has been the major problem.

History. As early as 1908, surgeons in Germany attempted to reconstruct the cervical esophagus using laterally based rectangular skin flaps.[13] Inadequate excision of the tumor re-

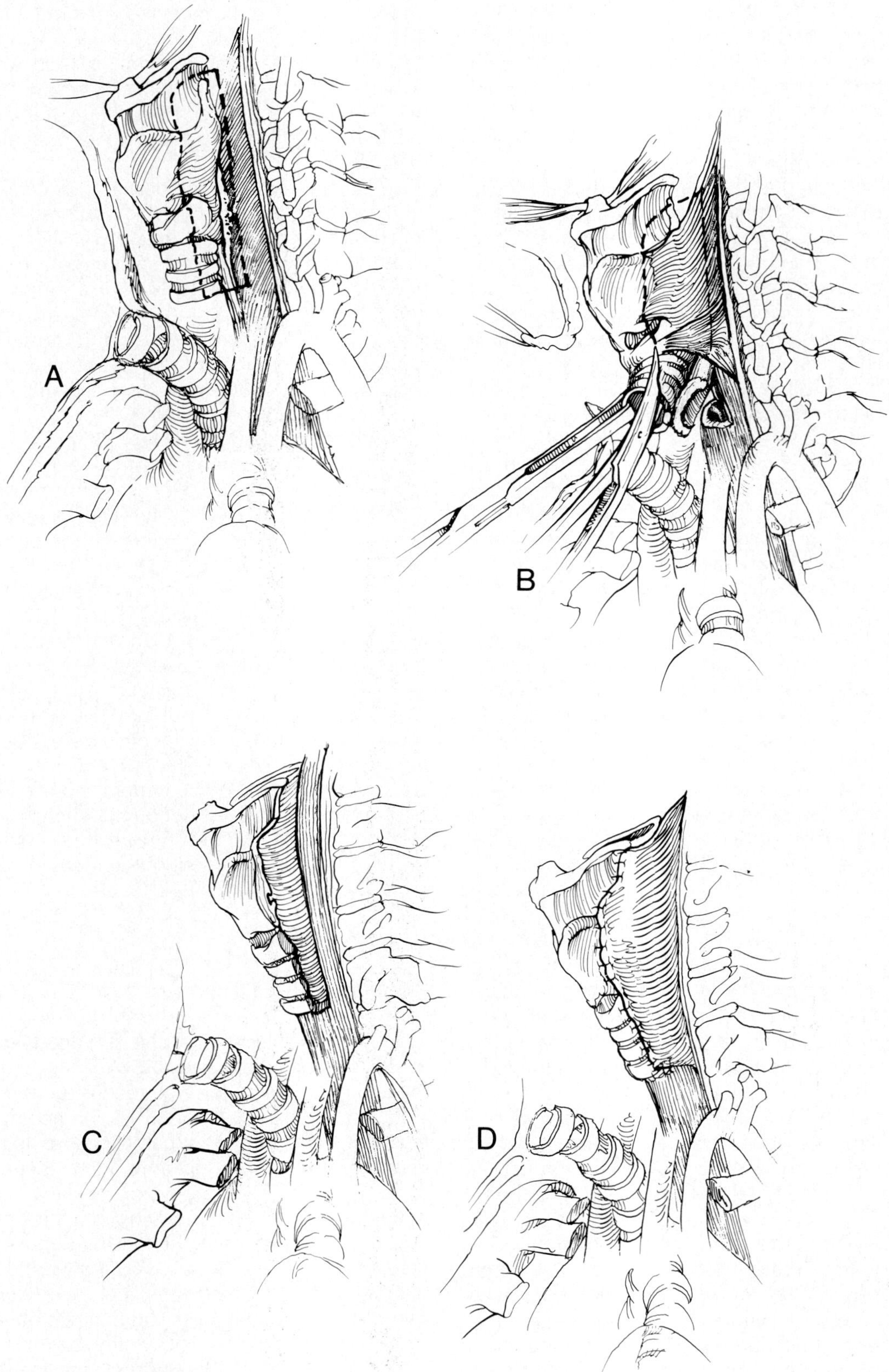

Figure 18–9. Laryngotracheal autograft for postcricoid cancer. *A* and *B,* Area of resection. *C* and *D,* Reconstruction using the laryngotracheal autograft anteriorly and a regional pedicle flap posteriorly.

sulted in a high incidence of local failure. In 1949, Rob and Bateman began using fascia lata grafts with a tantalum gauze stent.[20] Later, split-thickness skin was sutured around tanatalum mesh or a plastic stent.[21] This was sewn in place to preserve the lumen of the gullet. The complication rate following this form of reconstruction was unacceptably high and included infection, necrosis, and fistula formation.

In 1948, Wookey used laterally based neck flaps to reconstruct the cervical esophagus after total laryngopharyngectomy.[22] This procedure necessitated a pharyngostoma that was closed at a second stage. Although a satisfactory gullet resulted, wound infection and fistula formation were common, and the procedure was inappropriate in patients who had undergone preoperative radiotherapy.

In 1965, Ogura and Dedo described the use of bilateral nondelayed acromiopectoral flaps for the reconstruction of large defects of the pharyngoesophagus. This method proved adequate for reconstruction but required a minimum of three stages; although functionally satisfactory, it was deforming from a cosmetic standpoint.[23]

In 1965, Bakamjian reported a two-stage method for pharyngoesophageal reconstruction using a nondelayed medially based pectoral skin flap.[24] The deltopectoral skin flap has been an extremely successful two-stage technique in creating a neoesophagus. Complications are minimal and the functional result is highly satisfactory.

A significant surgical advance in this area has been the use of pectoralis major myocutaneous flaps for pharyngoesophageal reconstruction. These flaps are based on the thoracoacromial artery and large defects of the pharyngoesophagus can be closed as a one-stage or two-stage procedure.[25]

Immediate reconstruction of the cervical esophagus by a revascularized free jejunal graft was reported by Sidenberg et al. in 1959.[26] Recent interest in the development of microsurgery for small vessels has permitted the more successful use of this technique.

Deltopectoral Flap in Reconstruction of Pharyngoesophageal Defects. The medially based chest flap combines the advantages of satisfactory tissue length and ease of use. Also, it is outside the area of the radiation port. The

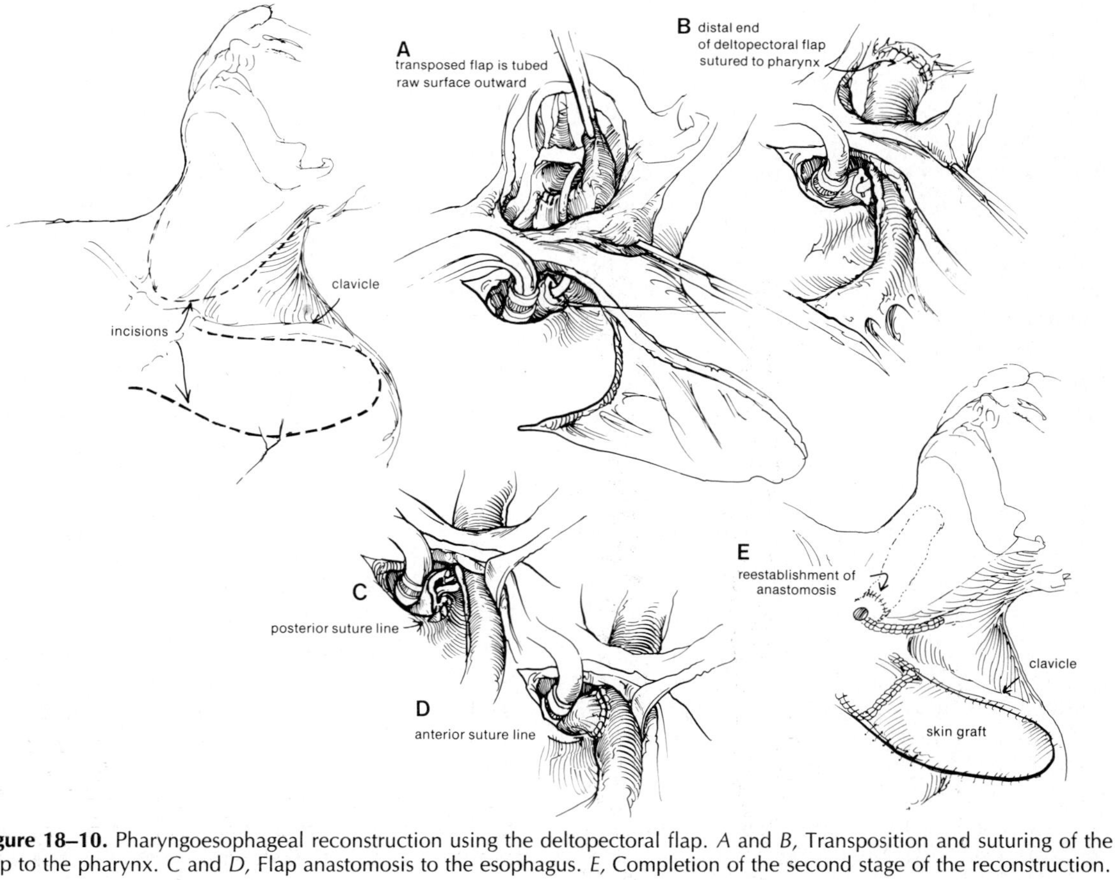

Figure 18–10. Pharyngoesophageal reconstruction using the deltopectoral flap. *A* and *B,* Transposition and suturing of the flap to the pharynx. *C* and *D,* Flap anastomosis to the esophagus. *E,* Completion of the second stage of the reconstruction.

flap is used for the staged reconstruction of part or all of the pharynx after resection for laryngopharyngeal cancer.

Technique. With the patient in the supine position, the full-thickness pedicle of the deltopectoral flap is based parasternally, straddling the first four intercostal spaces, with the blood supply derived from the first four perforating branches of the internal mammary artery. The superior margin lies near the level of the clavicle and the inferior margin is parallel to it, beginning at the fifth intercostal space and terminating at the apex of the anterior axillary fold. The deltoid portion may be extended to suit the reconstructive need.

In general, the width and length of the flap are those of an unfolded standard 4-inch by 4-inch surgical sponge, which is sometimes useful in flap design. The defect being reconstructed determines the ultimate length and shape of the flap. This flap can be used unstaged, but staging achieves a greater margin of safety (Fig. 18–10). Initial staging of the flap includes incision of the parallel length lines and elevation of the flap down through the pectoral fascia. The distal end of the flap skin is not incised at the first stage. The flap is then sutured back in place, drained, and a bulky, nonpressure dressing applied.

After an interval of three weeks, the second stage is performed. The flap is raised again, and the distal portion is elevated and divided. To assure good flap viability, the patient's nutritional status and hemoglobin must be maintained at satisfactory levels. The best clinical indicator of flap viability appears to be a venous filling time of less than 5 s after the distal skin attachment is divided. If the compressed area of the distal skin of the flap does not regain its precompression color by 8 to 10 s, then the flap should be resutured into place. If the venous filling time is 5 s or less, the flap is utilized at this time.

To reconstruct the pharyngoesophagus, the distal end of the flap is sutured to the base of the tongue. The proximal edge of the flap is sutured to the esophageal remnant circumferentially for a full 360 degrees. The remainder of the flap is tubed and sutured on itself. The flap suture line is closed distal to proximal, externalizing the inferior pharyngostoma. The controlled fistula thus created manages the oral secretions and directs them away from the tracheostoma. The exposed muscle over the chest and shoulder is covered with a split-thickness skin graft for more rapid healing and reduction of fluid loss.

Three weeks after this stage, the flap is divided just lateral to the esophageal suture line and closed on itself. The remainder of the deltopectoral flap is replaced on the chest.

This technique is reliable and carries little morbidity. Incidence of fistula formation is low. Patients ordinarily swallow within one month after the initial resection. Deglutition is performed successfully and some patients have been able to produce neoesophageal speech.

Pectoralis Major Myocutaneous Flap in Reconstruction of Pharyngoesophageal Defects. The blood supply to the skin overlying a muscle is derived predominantly from perforating vessels from the muscle itself.[27] The pectoralis major myocutaneous flap derives its blood supply from the pectoral branch of the thoracoacromial artery, which pierces the clavicopectoral fascia inferior to the clavicle on a line from the acromion to the xiphoid process. In addition to this artery, the neurovascular bundle is composed of the pectoral vein and the lateral pectoral nerve (Fig. 18–11). Blood is supplied to the flap skin by the pectoralis major muscle directly underlying the skin paddle. For greater length, the flap can safely be extended several centimeters inferiorly and medially.

Following the outline of the necessary skin paddle, the incision is carried down through the pectoral muscle. The skin is sutured to the muscle in several areas to prevent inadvertent removal of the skin paddle. A horizontal incision is made along the line of the standard inferior incision for a deltopectoral flap. The skin and subcutaneous tissue superior to the flap paddle are elevated off the pectoral muscle superiorly to the level of the clavicle and an incision is made to afford a generous opening into the neck.

The flap paddle is then elevated on the pectoralis major base at the clavicle in the well-defined plane deep to the muscle. The plane of dissection is carried over the pectoralis minor and a hand is inserted under the pectoralis major. Palpation reveals the pulsatile pectoral artery. Medially, the muscle is divided at its insertions. Laterally, the tendon is divided toward the identified pectoral artery (Fig. 18–11C).

The paddle of skin in the pectoral pedicle is tunneled over the clavicle and under the overlying skin in the previously dissected layer. The skin paddle is sutured to the base of tongue, pharynx remnant, and esophagus and tubed on itself (Fig. 18–11D). The neck skin flap is closed as indicated.

The flap is placed under no tension. A bulky

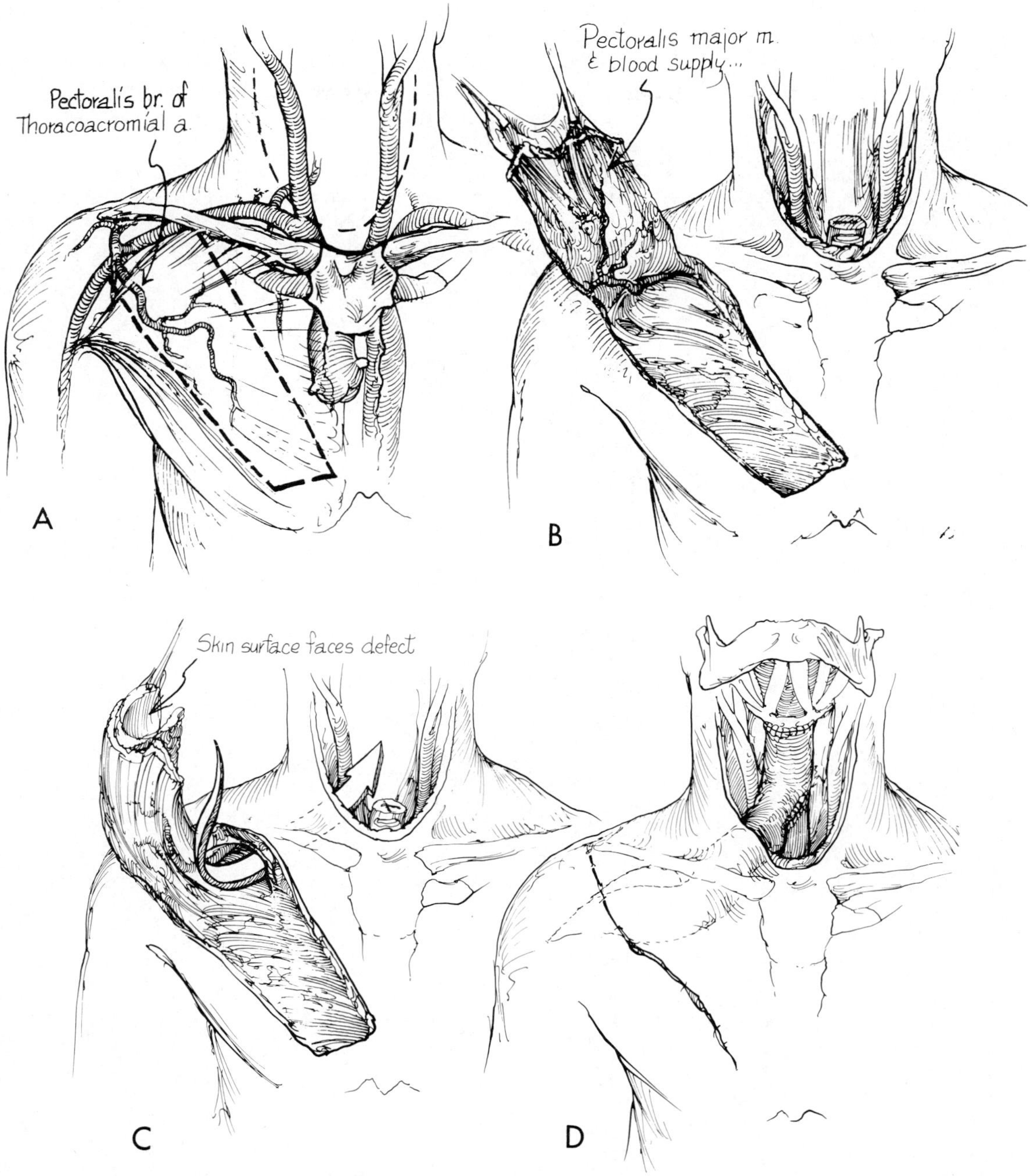

Figure 18–11. Pharyngoesophageal reconstruction using the pectoralis major myocutaneous flap. *A* and *B*, Elevation of the flap. *C* and *D*, Transposition of the flap through a skin tunnel and anastomosis with the pharynx.

nonpressure dressing is applied and suction drainage is employed for both the neck and the chest.

Less extensive reconstruction can be performed in a one-stage procedure. Experience has shown that extensive laryngopharyngeal reconstruction with the pectoralis major myocutaneous flap results in fewer complications if a controlled pharyngostoma is employed.

The chest defect is closed primarily by extensive undermining. Occasionally, split-thickness skin grafting is required.

Intestinal Autograft in Laryngopharyngeal Reconstruction. Recent developments in microvascular surgical techniques have allowed the use of free intestinal autografts in reconstruction of the cervical esophagus. Vigorous preoperative bowel preparation with antibiotics is necessary. After the resection of the laryngopharyngoesophageal tumor, a second team of physicians harvests the intestinal autograft through a midline abdominal incision. The ileocolic segment is advantageous in that its vessels are well defined and exhibit little anatomic variation. The caliber of these vessels allows ease in handling; however, most surgeons today prefer an isolated segment of jejunum. The vessels may be palpated and seen easily when the mesenteric apron is transilluminated by the operating room lights. The segmental vein and artery are identified and divided (Fig. 18–12A). As the reanastomosis of the distal and proximal bowel is accomplished, the harvested segment is perfused with iced heparinized saline until the venous return is clear (Fig. 18–12B).

The anastomosis of the segmental artery to the external carotid is end-to-side using 7-0 Tevdec suture in a running simple stitch. The clamp is opened; if no significant blood leakage is noted, the clamp is replaced and the jejunal vein is anastomosed to the internal jugular vein

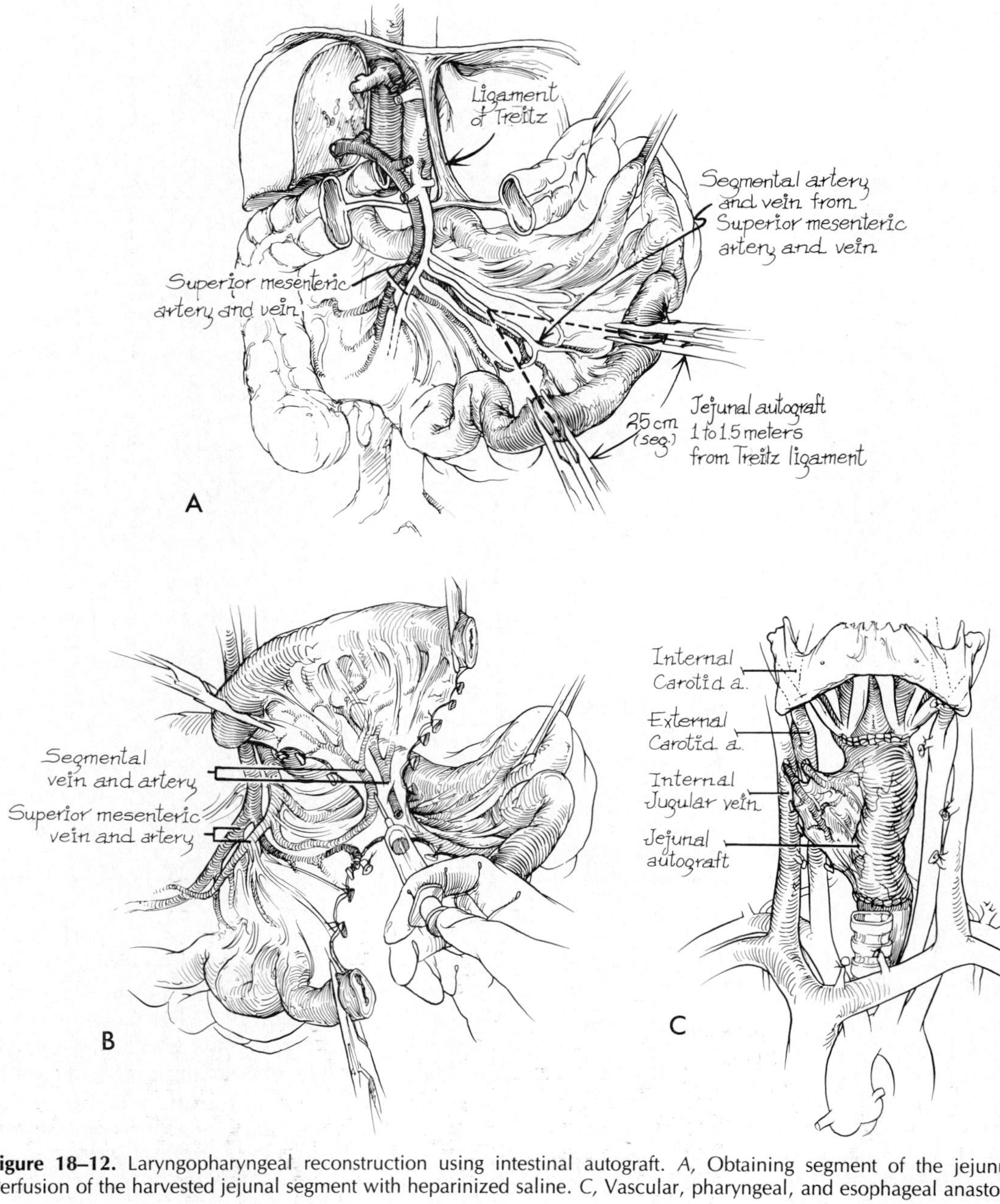

Figure 18–12. Laryngopharyngeal reconstruction using intestinal autograft. *A,* Obtaining segment of the jejunum. *B,* Perfusion of the harvested jejunal segment with heparinized saline. *C,* Vascular, pharyngeal, and esophageal anastomoses.

in the same end-to-side technique. Releasing the clamps allows for vascularization. The jejunal segment becomes pink and peristalsis may be noted.

The graft is trimmed to size and anastomosed to the pharynx and esophagus in two layers (Fig. 18–12C). The nasogastric tube traverses the reconstructed area and is used initially for decompression and later for tube feedings. Care is taken not to put pressure on the reconstruction. A Gastrografin swallow is performed before oral feedings are resumed about two weeks postoperatively.

This technique requires the availability of an experienced microvascular surgeon. Operative morbidity is directly related to surgical technique.

Disadvantages of the technique include increased operating time and postoperative cardiopulmonary complications. Use of the jejunum may affect the amount of postoperative radiation that can be given. Improved techniques and better patient selection have reduced morbidity and mortality following this procedure.

Gastric Transposition (Pull-up) Operation. Since 1960, methods for reconstructing the gullet following total laryngopharyngectomy have been described by which the stomach is mobilized and advanced through the posterior mediastinum into the neck to allow primary closure of the surgical defect.[28] This operation consists of four parts:[29] (1) the laryngopharyngectomy (Fig. 18–13A), (2) the mobilization of the stomach (Fig. 18–13B), (3) the mobilization of the esophagus and the "pull up" of the esophagus and stomach into the neck (Fig. 18–13C), and (4) the division of the esophagus from the stomach with its anastomosis to the remaining pharynx (Fig. 18–13, D to F). Preoperatively, these patients should be given adequate bowel preparation and otherwise managed in the same way as patients undergoing any other form of reconstuction. The separation of the surgical fields permits a two-team approach, using a head and neck surgical team for the total laryngopharyngectomy, with an abdominal surgical team concomitantly mobilizing the stomach. This approach significantly reduces the anesthesia time.

During the laryngopharyngectomy or immediately thereafter, a midline incision is used to enter the abdomen. The liver is divided to afford access to the gastroesophageal junction. The stomach is freed by a dissection of the outer anastomotic arcade of both the greater and lesser curvature. Only the right gastric and right gastroepiploic vessels are preserved. Mobilization should continue down to the duodenum and include the head of the pancreas. The surgeon must pay attention to the venous drainage from this area because without adequate drainage the transposed tissue will engorge and die. The stomach is also mobilized by division of the gastrohepatic omentum.

The stomach and esophagus are freed through the chest from inferiorly as far as possible under direct vision. The right crus must be divided to gain easier access to the mediastinum. Using blind finger dissection, the abdominal surgeon releases the esophagus throughout its thoracic course. At the same time, the head and neck team frees the upper thoracic esophagus by a similar dissection from above. Once the esophagus is completely freed, gentle traction is used to draw the stomach into the neck. The abdominal surgeon reflects the duodenum and pancreas up toward the hiatus to give added length. The pylorus should lie just above the hiatus and the cardia of the stomach near the manubrium sterni.

The esophagus is removed to the gastroesophageal junction and the pharynx is anastomosed to the stomach under no tension. This may be done in an interrupted bowel suture technique or with an EEA (end-to-end anastomosis) stapler. The neck wound is irrigated with copious amounts of normal saline and closed routinely, as is the abdominal wound.

The importance of the anastomosis should be reemphasized. Tension at the pharyngogastric anastomosis will cause it to break down. Because of the complexity and nonstandard nature of the stomach mobilization, this procedure should be performed by an experienced abdominal surgeon who is a member of the head and neck reconstruction team. This will enable him to become more familiar with the intricacies of adequate mobilization of the stomach.

Because of the excellent blood supply of the stomach and the relative ease of its mobilization, the gastric pull-up operation is a safe and reliable technique for reconstruction. Another advantage is early feeding. Most patients who require total laryngopharyngectomy have a poor prognosis for prolonged survival. Early return to normal deglutition and early discharge from the hospital are essential for true palliation. Usually normal bowel sounds are heard and the gastropharyngeal anastomosis has healed in seven to ten days. The patient can then begin to eat.

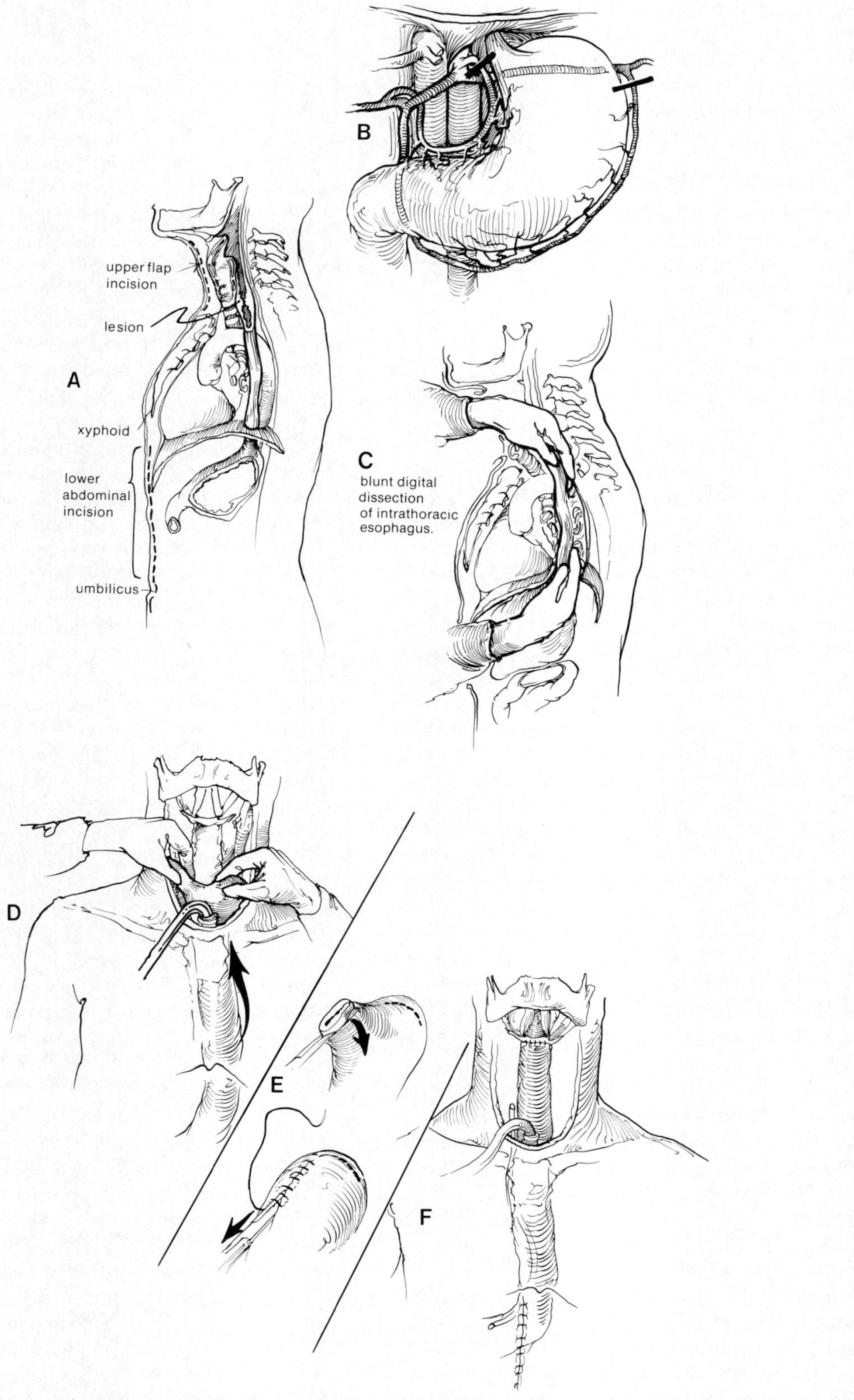

Figure 18–13. Laryngopharyngeal reconstruction using gastric transposition (pull-up). *A,* Lateral view of the operative areas. *B* and *C,* Mobilization of the stomach and intrathoracic esophagus. *D, E,* and *F,* Division of the esophagus from the stomach followed by pharyngeal anastomosis.

Postsurgical Considerations

Complications. Treatment of laryngopharyngeal carcinoma can be associated with significant morbidity.[30] Table 18–5 indicates the complications of primary treatment for tumor originating in the pyriform sinus in a series of patients with or without low-dose preoperative radiation therapy. The most common complications include wound slough (4.2 per cent) and carotid catastrophe (6.7 per cent).

Wound slough (4.2 per cent overall) varies from a superficial area of skin loss at the site of flap trifurcation to complete flap necrosis. Management includes conservative débridement followed by local wound care with or without flap reconstruction, depending on the site and size of the tissue loss and the overall clinical setting.

Salivary fistulas may develop after breakdown of the internal suture lines. Fistulas that expose the carotid artery system pose a serious management problem. Prophylactic treatment in the high-risk patient occasionally includes the construction of a controlled pharyngostoma.[31] Following primary closure, much of the postoperative management of the patient is performed with the possibility of fistula in mind. To prevent fistulas and encourage wound healing in high-risk patients, decannulation and oral intake are delayed for three weeks postoperatively. In addition, any patient who postoperatively displays abnormal wound healing, such as cellulititis or edema, is placed on a high dose of intravenous antibiotics until the complication is resolved. Decannulation and peroral feeding are similarly delayed.[31] Salivary fistulas most commonly occur seven to ten days after surgery. When a fistula is diagnosed, it is rerouted to form a direct fistula at the shortest possible distance from the dehiscent suture line to the outside through the overlying skin. The direct fistula thus created is medial to the carotid artery. A pressure dressing is applied to decrease dead space and facilitate sealing down of the flaps. The wound is cultured and appropriate antibiotics are instituted. Twice daily, local wound care is given. Concomitantly, an attempt is made to place the patient in an optimal metabolic state. This may require enteral or parenteral hyperalimentation. When the skin flaps are seated down and the fistula tract has matured, the defect is closed on itself and covered with a reconstructive local flap if there is spontaneous closure.

The fistula rate following partial laryngopharyngectomy with radical neck dissection (9.8 per cent) is significantly higher than that following partial pharyngectomy and total laryngectomy with radical neck dissection (5.6 per cent).

When necrosis of the skin flaps or salivary fistulas has exposed the carotid artery, its resistance to infection is decreased, its blood supply is diminished, and it is unable to withstand the constant systolic thrust of the blood passing through it. Factors associated with increased incidence of carotid catastrophe include wound infection, fistula, previous irradiation, positive resection margins, and persistent tumor.

Following major laryngopharyngeal resection, any oozing of blood in the early postoperative period, especially after the first 24 hours, should be considered as bleeding from

Table 18–5. COMPLICATIONS AFTER SURGERY WITH AND WITHOUT PREOPERATIVE RADIOTHERAPY—LARYNGOPHARYNGEAL CANCER ORIGINATING IN PYRIFORM SINUS*

	Total Laryngectomy		Partial Laryngopharyngectomy	
	Without Radiotherapy	*With Radiotherapy*	*Without Radiotherapy*	*With Radiotherapy*
No complications	20 (46.5%)**	17 (60.7%)	19 (48.7%)	40 (47.6%)
Infection	1 (2.3%)	0	0	1 (1.2%)
Wound slough	2 (4.7%)	2 (7.1%)	4 (10.3%)	7 (8.3%)
Fistula	3 (7%)	1 (3.6%)	3 (7.7%)	9 (10.7%)
Hemorrhage	1(2.3%)	0	0	1 (1.2%)
Carotid artery exposure and/or blowout	4 (9.3%)	3 (10.7%)	2 (5.1%)	4 (4.8%)
Operative death	0	2 (7.1%)	0	2 (2.4%)
Fatal complication	2 (4.7%)	1 (3.6%)	2 (5.1%)	3 (3.6%)
Other	10 3.3%)	2 (7.1%)	9 (23%)	17 (20.2%)
Totals	43	28	39	84
	χ^2 = 13.568	v = 13.34 P 0.50	χ^2 = 3.441	v = 11.14 P 0.99

*Adapted from Gall A et al.: Cancer 39:624–630, 1977.
**Values given as number of patients (per cent of total).

Table 18–6. THREE-YEAR SURVIVAL—LARYNGOPHARYNGEAL CANCER

	N0	N1	N2
T1			
Tumor free	7 (58%)*	4 (57%)	—
Death from	5 (42%)	3 (43%)	—
T2			
Tumor free	5 (50%)	6 (46%)	—
Death from	0 (0%)	6 (46%)	—
T3			
Tumor free	4 (16%)	5 (20%)	11 (17%)
Death from	16 (46%)	16 (64%)	5 (83%)
T4			
Tumor free	8 (42%)	11 (28%)	0 (0%)
Death from	10 (53%)	26 (67%)	8 (100%)

*Values given as surviving patients (per cent of total).

the carotid or innominate artery, and immediate steps should be taken for wound exploration and elective ligation. The prodromal sign of a small fresh bleed from under the flap frequently precedes major vessel rupture.

Patients with exposure of the carotid artery following wound necrosis or fistula are transferred to the intensive care unit and treated as impending carotid blowout problems. Blood is made available, large bore intravenous infusion is begun, cuffed tracheostomy tube is placed, and resuscitation equipment is kept nearby. Wet dressings are maintained over the vessel and coverage pedicle flaps are staged.

In the event of carotid rupture, the hemorrhage is treated with pressure and the patient is stabilized and taken to the operating room for ligation of the vessel. Hypotension has been the only common factor present in those patients who had major cerebral complications but absent in those patients surviving with no neurological deficit.[32, 33] Emergency carotid ligation results in mortality as high as 50 per cent, while elective ligation of a necrosing artery is associated with mortality of 12 per cent and a probable neurologic deficit of 33 per cent.[8, 34–36]

Results. Length of survival of patients treated for laryngopharyngeal cancer correlates with the extent of the primary tumor and the amount of spread to the cervical lymph nodes. Table 18–6 shows three-year survival rates by stage in a series of treated laryngopharyngeal cancers. Early cancers of the pyriform sinus and larynx area are rare, and treatment of these smaller tumors (T1, T2) results in a satisfactory survival rate, with approximately 50 per cent of patients showing a three-year cure. Treatment of larger tumors of the pyriform fossa (T3, T4) results in a significant decrease in survival (16 per cent to 42 per cent). Lymph node metastasis decreases three-year survival to 20 per cent to 28 per cent.

Partial laryngopharyngectomy is as effective as total laryngopharyngectomy in properly selected patients. Table 18–7 shows that partial laryngopharyngectomy controls the primary site as well as the total procedure, and the local failure rate for both sets of patients was 14 per cent. The table also shows that if the primary tumor is larger (indicated by the need for the total procedure), then treatment failure increases both in the neck (18 per cent vs. 32 per cent) and in the distant areas (15 per cent vs. 37 per cent). Other reported studies have confirmed the value of conservation surgery in treating these tumors.[3]

Combination of surgery and radiotherapy has increased survival (Tables 18–8 and 18–9) probably because of a decrease in local and neck recurrence of carcinoma.[3, 5] As survival of this group increases, failure secondary to distant disease also increases.

Follow-up Considerations. Because of the high frequency with which laryngopharyngeal cancers recur at both the neck and primary sites, these patients should be carefully fol-

Table 18–7. FAILURE BASED ON SURGICAL APPROACH TO THE PRIMARY SITE*

	Partial Laryngo-pharyn-gectomy (per cent)	Total Laryngo-pharyn-gectomy (per cent)
Local	14	14
Regional	18	32
Distant	15	37

*Adapted from Marks J et al.: Cancer 41:1008–1015, 1978.

Table 18–8. SURVIVAL AND FAILURE RATES—SURGERY ALONE OR SURGERY PLUS RADIOTHERAPY*

	Surgery Only (per cent)	Surgery, Radio-therapy (per cent)
NED, five years	22	33
Local recurrence	15	10
Neck recurrence	15	4
Distant metastasis	22	27

*Adapted from Jesse RH et al.: Cancer 35:1163–1166, 1975.

lowed. Monthly follow-up for indirect examination of the larynx and neck is essential. Every six months, chest x-rays should be obtained to rule out metastasis to the hilar or mediastinal nodes, pulmonary metastasis, or a second primary. Accurate assessment of nutritional status is important for patient well-being. Professional and nonprofessional support to help the patient deal with the emotional and financial pressures of the prolonged hospital stay, fear of cancer, and possible loss of voice is encouraged. Voice rehabilitation training is instituted one month after surgery.

SUBGLOTTIC CARCINOMA

Carcinoma of the subglottic region occurs rarely.[37] The subglottic region of the larynx is defined as an anatomic region that is cylindrical in shape; its inferior margin is the inferior border of the cricoid cartilage, and it is limited superiorly by an imaginary circle 5 mm below the free margin of the vocal cords.[37] Tumors of the subglottic region may be primary or secondary. Primary subglottic tumors originate in the region more than 5 mm below the free margin of the true vocal cord. Tumors that originate at the glottic level and extend more than 5 mm below the free margin of the true vocal cord are described as glottic tumors with subglottic extension (secondary).

Primary Subglottic Cancer. Primary subglottic cancer is extremely rare, presenting no symptoms until the tumor is advanced in size. Patients then present with shortness of breath, stridor, pain, or hoarseness. Examination reveals a large subglottic mass that can usually be seen without difficulty beneath the vocal cords with a largyngeal mirror. Vocal cord paralysis, usually unilateral, may be present. More than 40 per cent of these patients will exhibit a cervical node metastasis at the time of initial examination. Work-up includes xerogram, contrast laryngogram, barium swallow, high-resolution CT scan, direct laryngoscopy, and biopsy.

Primary subglottic cancer is usually epidermoid cancer (55 per cent). Adenoid cystic cancer is the most common form of glandular cancer of the subglottic area. The other common pathology is chondrosarcoma.

The classification system for subglottic cancer is shown in Table 18–10. Most of the primary subglottic tumors are T2 or larger at the time of diagnosis. Surgical treatment of primary subglottic cancer is total laryngectomy. With large tumors involving the cricoid cartilage, no way exists at present to maintain a satisfactory func-

Table 18–10. TNM CLASSIFICATION—CANCER OF SUBGLOTTIS

Tis	Carcinoma in situ
T1	Tumor confined to subglottic region
T2	Tumor extension to vocal cords with normal or impaired mobility
T3	Tumor confined to larynx with cord fixation
T4	Massive tumor with cartilage destruction or extension beyond the confines of the larynx or both

Table 18–9. SURVIVAL AS RELATED TO TREATMENT—HYPOPHARYNGEAL CANCER*

Treatment	Three-Year Survival (per cent)	Five-Year Survival (per cent)
Surgery		
Alone	37	30
Preop. radiotherapy	47	36
Postop. radiotherapy	20	20
Radiotherapy		
Alone	28	19
Surgical salvage	55	25
Palliative	0	0

*Adapted from Inoue T et al.: Cancer 31:649–655, 1973.

Table 18–11. INCIDENCE—GLOTTIC-SUBGLOTTIC TUMORS

Tumor Site	Number of Cases	Per Cent
True cord, unilateral	392	67
True cord, bilateral	14	2
Anterior com. primary	5	1
True cord, unilat., with ant. com.	78	13
True cord, bilat., with ant. com.	97	16
Subglottic primary	5	1
Totals, glottic	591	100
True cord with subglottic	132	22

Table 18–12. TUMOR EXTENSION (132 PATIENTS)

Stage	Number of Patients	Subglottic Extension 5–9 mm	10–14 mm	15–19 mm	20 mm	Totals
Stage II						
T2N0	85	46 (35%)	26 (20%)	13 (10%)		85 (65%)
Stage III						
T2N1	2					
T3N0	16					
T4N0	26					
T3N1	1	6 (4%)	11 (8%)	4 (3%)	26 (20%)	47 (35%)
T3N2	1					
T4N2	1					
Totals	132	52 (39%)	37 (28%)	17 (13%)	26 (20%)	132 (100%)

Table 18–13. TUMOR EXTENSION (127 PATIENTS)

Primary Site	Subglottic Extension 5–9 mm	10–14 mm	15–19 mm	20 mm	Totals
True cord, unilateral	32 (25%)*	16 (13%)	9 (7%)	13 (10%)	70 (55%)
True cord, bilateral	0	2 (2%)	0	0	2 (2%)
Anterior commissure	0	0	0	1 (1%)	1 (1%)
True cord, unilat., with ant. com.	9 (7%)	7 (5%)	3 (2%)	2 (2%)	21 (16%)
True cord, bilat., with ant. com.	9 (7%)	8 (6%)	5 (4%)	9 (7%)	31 (24%)
Other	1 (1%)	0	0	1 (1%)	2 (2%)
Totals	51 (40%)	33 (26%)	17 (13%)	26 (21%)	

*Values given as number of cases (per cent of total).

Table 18–14. PRIMARY TREATMENT—SUBGLOTTIC EXTENSION TUMORS (125 PATIENTS)

Stage	Total Laryngectomy	Hemilaryngectomy	Radiotherapy	Totals
II	18 (15%)	52 (42%)	11 (8%)	81 (65%)
III	28 (23%)	11(8%)	5 (4%)	44 (35%)
Totals	46 (38%)	63 (50%)	16 (12%)	

Table 18–15. THREE-YEAR SURVIVAL BY SITE AND PROCEDURE—SUBGLOTTIC EXTENSION TUMORS (125 PATIENTS)

Site	Total Laryngectomy	Hemilaryngectomy	Radiotherapy	Totals
True cord, unilateral	11/17 (65%)*	35/41 (85%)	6/10 (60%)	52/68 (76%)
True cord, bilateral	—	0/1 (0%)	0/1 (0%)	0/2 (0%)
Ant. com. primary	0/1 (0%)	—	—	0/1 (0%)
True cord, unilat., with ant. com.	7/8 (88%)	9/12 (75%)	1/1 (100%)	17/21 (81%)
True cord, bilat., with ant. com.	11/19 (58%)	7/8 (88%)	3/4 (75%)	21/31 (68%)
Other	0/1 (0%)	1/1 (100%)	—	1/2 (50%)
Totals	29/46 (63%)	52/63 (83%)	10/16 (63%)	91/125 (73%)

*Values given as surviving patients/total cases (per cent surviving).

Table 18–16. OVERALL SURVIVAL BY STAGE—SUBGLOTTIC EXTENSION TUMOR (132 PATIENTS)

	Subglottic Extension				
Stage	***5–9 mm***	***10–14 mm***	***15–19 mm***	***20 mm***	**Total**
II	43/46 (93%)*	15/26 (58%)	8/13 (62%)	—	66/85 (78%)
III	3/6 (50%)	8/11 (73%)	2/4 (50%)	16/26 (62%)	29/47 (62%)
Totals	46/52 (88%)	23/37 (62%)	10/17 (59%)	16/26 (62%)	95/132 (72%)

*Values given as surviving patients/total cases (per cent surviving).

tional aerodigestive interface when a major portion of the posterior cricoid cartilage is removed. Treatment of these patients with total laryngectomy with or without radical neck dissection resulted in a three-year survival rate of 66 per cent. Failure to control tumor at the primary site was the most common cause for treatment failure and subsequent death.

Secondary Subglottic Cancer. Table 18–11 presents the relative incidence of subglottic primaries and of glottic primaries with extension to the subglottic area as compared to the incidence of other glottic primaries. Less than 1 per cent of patients have primary subglottic epidermoid carcinoma, while 22 per cent have a glottic primary with subglottic extension.

Table 18–12 shows the staging and amount of subglottic extension in 132 patients with primary glottic cancer. No T1 (stage I) lesions appear since, by definition, any glottic tumor with subglottic extension is T2 or greater.

Sixty-five per cent of patients are stage II and 35 per cent are stage III. Five patients have nodal metastasis. Fifty-two patients (39 per cent) have 5 mm to 9 mm subglottic extension; twenty-six (20 per cent) have subglottic extension greater than 20 mm. Subglottic extension by primary glottic site is shown in Table 18–13. Fifty-five per cent of these lesions arose from one vocal cord; most are T2 lesions. Forty per cent of these subglottic lesions involve one or both true cords and the anterior commissure.

Treatment of patients with subglottic extension of a primary glottic carcinoma includes hemilaryngectomy, total laryngectomy with or without radical neck dissection, and therapeutic irradiation (Table 18–14). The choice of therapy depends on the stage of the tumor. Hemilaryngectomy is reserved for patients whose tumors have not resulted in vocal cord fixation despite extension to the subglottic region and for patients who are radiation failures and had small transglottic tumors with subglottic extension without vocal cord fixation. Total laryngectomy with or without radical neck dissection is used for patients with more advanced lesions and vocal cord fixation. Therapeutic irradiation is used for patients with surface cancer from the glottis into the subglottic region. Most of these patients have first been treated surgically, either with hemilaryngectomy or total laryngectomy. Survival by primary site and therapeutic modality appears in Table 18–15. Three-year survival (no evidence of disease) for hemilaryngectomy (all sites) is 52 of 63 patients (83 per cent); for total laryngectomy, 29 of 46 patients (63 per cent); and for therapeutic irradiation, 10 of 16 patients (63 per cent). Survival by stage in patients with subglottic extension is shown in Table 18–16. Survival with stage II lesions with less than 10 mm subglottic extension is 43 of 46 patients (93 per cent). Patients with stage II and III lesions with subglottic extension greater than 10 mm have significantly decreased survival rates (50 per cent to 72 per cent). Patients with unilateral lesions limited to the vocal cords or anterior commissure involvement with less than 10 mm subglottic extension do better (90 per cent survival) than patients with greater subglottic extension.

Nineteen per cent of patients with secondary subglottic cancer from a glottic primary have tumor recurrence. Recurrence is most often

Table 18–17. RECURRENCE—SUBGLOTTIC EXTENSION TUMORS

Subglottic Extension	Number of Patients	Number of Recurrences	Per Cent of Total
5–9 mm	52	5	10
10–14 mm	37	4	11
15–19 mm	17	5	29
20 mm	26	11	42
Totals	132	25	19

Table 18–18. CAUSE OF DEATH—SUBGLOTTIC EXTENSION TUMORS (35 PATIENTS)

	Primary Uncontr.	Neck Uncontr.	Distant Met.	Compl. of Treatment	Second Primary	Intercurrent Disease	Total of Stage
Stage II	2 (6%)	2 (6%)	4 (11%)	1 (3%)	5 (14%)	5 (14%)	19/85 (22%)*
Stage III	4 (11%)	2 (6%)	3 (9%)	1 (3%)	—	6 (17%)	16/47 (34%)
Totals	6 (17%)	4 (12%)	7 (20%)	2 (6%)	5 (14%)	11 (31%)	

*Values given as number of deaths/total number of cases (per cent deaths).

local, regardless of treatment modality. Table 18–17 shows recurrence in relation to the extent of subglottic extension. Subglottic extension greater than 15 mm shows an increase in tumor recurrence regardless of treatment modality. Tumors with greater than 26 mm subglottic extension show a more frequent recurrence rate (92 per cent) than other tumors with less subglottic extension.

The cause of death in patients with secondary glottic cancer appears in Table 18–18. Almost half of the deaths are caused by intercurrent disease or a second primary cancer. Patients with stage III tumors and with more than 20 mm subglottic extension show decreased survival. Secondary involvement of the subglottic area by a glottic primary carries a poorer prognosis than other primary glottic lesions. Stage II glottic cancers that involve less than 10 mm of the subglottic carry a significantly better prognosis than the remainder of stage II or stage III tumors. Patients with T3 lesions with vocal cord fixation with subglottic extension show a decreased survival rate.

References

1. Ogura JH et al.: Conservation surgery for epidermoid carcinoma of the marginal area (aryepiglottic fold extension). Laryngoscope 85:1801–1807, 1975.
2. Marks J et al.: Carcinoma of the pyriform sinus—An analysis of treatment results and patterns of failure. Cancer 41:1008–1015, 1978.
3. Inoue T et al.: Treatment of carcinoma of the hypopharynx. Cancer 31:649–655, 1973.
4. Lederman M: Role of irradiation in the treatment of cancer of the hypopharynx, postcricoid, and cervical esophagus. *In* J Conley (ed): Proc the Int Workshop Cancer Head Neck. Washington, Butterworths, 1967, pp 347–356.
5. Jesse RH et al.: The efficacy of combining radiation therapy with a surgical procedure in patients with cervical metastasis from squamous cancer of the oropharynx and hypopharynx. Cancer 35:1163–1166, 1975.
6. Marks J: Pharyngeal wall cancer: An analysis of treatment results, complications and patterns of failure. Int J Radiat Oncol Biol Phys 4:587–593, 1978.
7. Ogura JH et al.: Laryngograms: Their value in the diagnosis and treatment of laryngeal lesions. Laryngoscope 70:780, 1960.
8. MacComb WS: Carotid body tumors. Ann Surg 127:269, 1948.
9. Lederman M: Radiotherapy of cancer of the larynx. J Laryngol Otol 84:867–896, 1970.
10. Alonso JM: Conservative surgery of cancer of the larynx. Trans Am Acad Ophthalmol Otolaryngol 51:633–642, 1947.
11. Leroux-Robert J: Indications for radical surgery, partial surgery, radiotherapy, and combined surgery and radiotherapy for cancer of the larynx and hypopharynx. Ann Otol Rhinol Laryngol 65:137–153, 1956.
12. Czerny H: Nerve operationen. Zentralbl Chir 433–434, 1877.
13. VonHacker V: Operationen. Verh Dtsch Ges Chir 37:359–425, 1908.
14. Trotter W. Method of lateral pharyngotomy for exposure of large growth in epilaryngeal region. J Laryngol Otol 35:289–291, 1980.
15. Eggers L: Carcinoma of the upper esophagus and pharynx. Ann Surg 81:695–698, 1925.
16. Ogura JH et al.: Partial laryngopharyngectomy and neck dissection for pyriform sinus cancer. Laryngoscope 70:1399–1417, 1960.
17. Ogura JH et al.: Conservation surgery for epidermoid carcinoma of the supraglottic larynx. Laryngoscope 85:1808–1815, 1975.
18. Asherson N: Pharyngectomy for postcricoid carcinoma: One stage operation with reconstruction of the pharynx using the larynx as an autograft. J Laryngol Otol 68:550, 1954.
19. Richards LG: A half century of triological transactions. Laryngoscope 64:595–625, 1954.
20. Rob LG, Bateman GH: Reconstruction of the trachea and cervical oesophagus: Preliminary report. Br J Surg 37:202–205, 1949.
21. Negus VE: Reconstruction of pharynx after pharyngolaryngectomy. Br J Plast Surg 6:99, 1953.
22. Wookey H: The surgical treatment of carcinoma of the hypopharynx and oesophagus. Br J Surg 35:249–266, 1948.
23. Ogura JH, Dedo HH: Repair of large pharyngostoma utilizing bilateral non-delayed regional pedicle flaps. Laryngoscope 75:588–600, 1965.
24. Bakamjian VY: A two-stage method for pharyngoesophageal reconstruction with a primary pectoral skin flap. Plast Reconstr Surg 36:173–183, 1965.
25. Theogaroj SD et al.: The pectoralis major musculocutaneous island flap in single stage reconstruction of the pharyngoesophageal region. Plast Reconstr Surg 65 (3):267–276, 1980.
26. Sidenberg B et al.: Immediate reconstruction of the cervical esophagus by a revascularized isolated jejunal segment. Ann Surg 149:162–171, 1959.
27. Owens N: A compound neck pedicle designed for repair of massive facial defects: Formation, development, and application. Plast Reconstr Surg 15:369, 1955.
28. Ong GB, Lee TC: Pharyngogastric anastomosis after esophageal-pharyngectomy for carcinoma of the hypopharynx and cercival esophagus. Br J Surg 48:193–200, 1960.

29. LeQuesne LP, Ranger D: Pharyngolaryngectomy with immediate pharyngogastric anastomosis. Br J Surg 53:105–109, 1966.
30. Gall A et al.: Complications following surgery for cancer of the larynx and hypopharynx. Cancer 39:624–630, 1977.
31. Dedo DD et al.: Incidence, predisposing factors, and outcome of pharyngocutaneous fistulas complicating head and neck cancer surgery. Ann Otol Rhinol Laryngol 84:833, 1975.
32. Moore OS, Baker HW: Carotid artery ligation in surgery of the head and neck. Cancer 8:712, 1955.
33. Moore OS et al.: Factors influencing the safety of carotid artery ligation. Am J Surg 118:666, 1969.
34. Borsanyi ST: Rupture of the carotids following radical neck surgery in radiated patients. Eye, Ear, Nose, Throat Monthly 41:531–533, 1962.
35. Follette WJ: Management of complications of head and neck surgery. Laryngoscope 76:1949–1970, 1966.
36. Martin H et al.: Neck dissection. Cancer 4:441, 1951.
37. Sessions DG et al.: Carcinoma of the subglottic area. Laryngoscope 85:1417–1423, 1975.

Suggested Readings

1. Chrysopathis P: The contribution of vascular surgery to esophageal replacement. Br J Surg 53:122–126, 1966.
2. Garage T et al.: The use of revascularized and ileocolic autografts for primary repair after pharyngolaryngoesophagectomy. Am J Surg 136:477–485, 1978.
3. Jesse RH et al.: Vocal cord cancer with anterior commissure extension—Choice of treatment. Am J Surg 122:437–439, 1971.
4. Orton H: Lateral transhyoid pharyngectomy. Trotter's operation for malignant conditions of the laryngopharynx. Arch Otolaryngol 12:320–330, 1930.
5. Sasaki TM et al.: Free jejunal graft reconstruction after extensive head and neck surgery. Am J Surg 139:650–653, 1980.
6. Shah J et al.: Carcinoma of the hypopharynx. Am J Surg 132:434–444, 1976.
7. Sisson G et al.: Reconstruction of the hypopharynx and cervical esophagus after radical surgery. Laryngoscope 66:1268–1290, 1956.
8. Som ML: Laryngectomy, primary closure with laryngotracheal autograft. Arch Otolaryngol 63:474, 1956.
9. Wang U et al.: Combined radiation therapy and surgery for carcinoma of the supraglottic and pyriform sinus. Laryngoscope 82:1883–1890, 1972.
10. Wang CC, Schulz MD: Treatment of cancer of the larynx by irradiation. Ann Otol Rhinol Laryngol 72:637–646, 1963.
11. Ward PC et al.: Evaluation of computerized tomography, cinelaryngoscopy and laryngography in determining the extent of laryngeal disease. Ann Otol Rhinol Laryngol 88:454–462, 1979.

19

Transglottic Carcinoma and Total Laryngectomy

Charles M. Stiernberg, M.D.
and Byron J. Bailey, M.D.

Laryngeal carcinoma with cord fixation or transglottic growth usually requires aggressive management. Preoperative or postoperative radiotherapy, combined with total laryngectomy and neck dissection, is most often the treatment of choice. Conservation laryngeal procedures for transglottic carcinomas are indicated only in the case of limited and superficial tumors. Throughout this chapter, we will use the term *advanced glottic carcinoma* to refer to glottic tumors that are associated with cord fixation, cartilage invasion, or extralaryngeal spread.

In their 1961 study of cervical lymph node metastases from epidermoid carcinoma of the larynx, McGavran et al. classified laryngeal tumors into glottic, infraglottic, supraglottic, and transglottic groups, based upon anatomic sites of involvement. They coined the term *transglottic* to describe tumors that cross the laryngeal ventricle in a vertical plane.[1] These tumors involve the supraglottic and glottic regions of the larynx, while the subglottis may or may not be involved. Posterior laryngeal neoplasms, which spread vertically, are not transglottic if the ventricle of Morgagni is not involved. Transglottic is thus a descriptive term. It does not indicate the site of origin of a laryngeal neoplasm as do the terms used by the currently popular classification system of the American Joint Committee on Cancer (AJCC).[2] Accordingly, McGavran and associates identified a group of laryngeal tumors, the transglottic group, that yields a high incidence of both clinically apparent and occult regional metastases.[1]

A quarter century prior to McGavran's study, LeRoux-Robert first reported serial sectioning of entire larynges to study laryngeal carcinoma. Though he did not use the term, his report was probably the first to characterize transglottic tumors histologically.[3] Tucker also demonstrated a technique of whole organ serial sectioning[4] that various authors have used in their studies of laryngeal cancer. Many have found that transglottic carcinoma has a locally aggressive biologic nature, as well as a tendency towards regional metastasis.

Laryngeal anatomy has been covered in Chapter 2 of this volume and will not be repeated here, but review of laryngeal regions and spaces is helpful. Understanding these areas is central to a discussion of transglottic and advanced glottic carcinomas and their clinical presentations. Particular attention should be given to the boundaries between laryngeal regions and surrounding laryngeal spaces. The paraglottic space has special importance in the spread of laryngeal cancer, particularly deeply infiltrating glottic carcinomas.[5]

CLINICAL PRESENTATION AND EVALUATION

Management of advanced laryngeal carcinoma is based on the anticipation of extensive spread and aggressive biologic behavior. A thorough history, careful physical examination, radiographic studies, endoscopy, and biopsies are indicated.

Symptoms. The symptoms of patients with transglottic carcinoma differ little from those of patients with strictly glottic tumors. Hoarseness is the most common symptom; it has been present for many months in most instances. If true cord fixation is present, dysphagia and aspiration may be associated symptoms. McGavran[1] and others[6] have found most transglottic carcinomas to be larger than 2 cm. Patients with larger tumors may present with dypsnea as the chief complaint. Extensive lesions causing moderate to severe compromise of the airway will frequently warrant emergency treatment.

Referred ear pain is often noted in patients with advanced glottic and transglottic carcinomas. Pittam and Carter found referred otalgia in 18 of 50 patients in their clinicopathologic study of randomly selected laryngectomies for squamous carcinoma.[6] They concluded that the presence of referred ear pain is highly significant and observed tumor invasion of the laryngeal cartilages in 11 of 12 patients. Transglottic carcinoma accounted for 78 per cent of the tumors with cartilage invasion. Bilateral tumors sometimes produced bilateral otalgia. Coughing or swallowing increased this pain in a few patients. These investigators proposed that this symptom is secondary to distortion or disruption of sensory fibers of the vagus nerve, although the pain did not correlate with histologic evidence of perineural invasion.[6]

Regional Metastases. Patients with advanced glottic and transglottic carcinomas may present with cervical nodal metastases. Though the overall incidence of regional metastasis for all patients with glottic carcinoma has been variously reported to range from 1 to 7 per cent,[7,8] this is not the case for transglottic carcinomas. In McGavran's important study of the correlation between cervical metastasis and the characteristics of laryngeal carcinoma, he found cervical node metastases in 13 of 25 transglottic carcinoma patients. Thirty-one per cent of patients with clinically negative findings revealed positive occult nodes when they underwent elective neck dissection. None of the patients in this series had posterior triangle metastases and very few metastases were found in the submaxillary areas; however, a high incidence of contralateral metastases was noted in the supraglottic and transglottic carcinoma groups, especially among those patients with positive ipsilateral nodes.[1] Other authors have confirmed these findings in patients with transglottic carcinoma.[9]

Studying 500 patients with cancer of the larynx and pyriform sinus, Kirchner and Owen found a 20 per cent incidence of palpable cervical node metastasis in patients with transglottic carcinoma. A 46 per cent rate of occult cervical nodes was found in 26 patients who had elective neck dissection. Only pyriform sinus and supraglottic cancer groups approached this high incidence.[8] Earlier, Kirchner et al. reported 50 patients with transglottic cancer, among whom 15 (30 per cent) had cervical node metastases. They found a high correlation between regional metastasis and the size and cellular differentiation of the primary.[9]

Ogura et al. reported 411 cases of laryngeal and laryngopharyngeal cancers, of which 63 were transglottic.[10] All of these patients were treated by surgery. In the transglottic group, the overall rate of cervical metastasis was 26 per cent. Palpable nodes were present in 11 of 63 patients (17 per cent) and positive occult nodes in 6 of 52 patients (11 per cent). Though their figures are lower than those reported in other studies, these investigators did show a significantly higher incidence of metastasis in the transglottic group than in patients with other advanced glottic cancers. For example, in the group of patients with fixed cord glottic cancers, only 13 per cent had cervical metastases. This study emphasizes the tendency of transglottic carcinoma to metastasize.[10]

Biller et al. studied the incidence of delayed contralateral cervical metastasis in laryngeal and laryngopharyngeal cancers. Of 67 patients with transglottic carcinoma, 21 (31 per cent) had ipsilateral neck metastases and 4 (6 per cent) had contralateral metastases. They showed that the probability for patients with ipsilateral metastasis to develop contralateral metastasis is 14 per cent. Only the supraglottic and base of tongue carcinoma groups had higher rates.[11]

Physical Examination. The clinician should conduct a thorough head and neck examination giving special attention to indirect laryngoscopy and neck palpation. Indirect laryngoscopy will often be more informative than direct laryngoscopy. The examiner should document the extent of the lesion and cord mobility as seen indirectly. Assessing the degree of airway compromise is crucial in those patients with dyspnea. The lesion should be drawn or outlined on standard printed diagrams. Indirect laryngoscopy will provide information about the anteroposterior and superior extent of the tumor, but evaluation of the ventricle and subglottis may not be possible because of tumor bulk, cord fixation, or both. Neck palpation for cervical metastasis carries equal importance in the preoperative evaluation. This is especially true in view of the high rate of cervical metastasis for these advanced cancers.

Radiographic Evaluation. The primary value of preoperative radiographic examination is to reveal the local extent of the malignancy. Chapter 5 of this volume covers this well. Both mucosal spread and deep infiltration of laryngeal cancer can be accurately quantified by radiographic assessment when the proper modality is used.[12] Several radiographic procedures for evaluating advanced glottic and transglottic carcinoma are available. These include soft tissue x-rays of the neck, cineradiography, tomography, contrast laryngography, and computerized tomographic (CT) scanning. Each procedure offers different but valuable information, except, perhaps, for soft tissue x-rays of the neck. These are sometimes useful for supraglottic tumors but are less useful for glottic and subglottic tumors. Cineradiography may confirm limitations of movement or fixation of a vocal cord as seen by indirect or direct laryngoscopy, but subglottic extension is probably best demonstrated by tomography or contrast laryngography.[13] The CT scan can yield information on both deep infiltration and mucosal spread, and has become the most popular modality used for overall assessment of local invasion. Xeroradiography, formerly quite popular for assessing invasion of laryngeal cartilage, is now being replaced by the newest generation of CT scanners.

Pittam et al. compared radiographic detection of transglottic carcinomas to detection by direct laryngoscopy. Ten of fourteen transglottic tumors were correctly identified by laryngeal tomograms. Radiographically, the laryngeal ventricle was usually noted to be obliterated, but the clinical value of this finding was decreased by a high false positive rate (7 of 17). Also, subglottic extension was correctly identified radiographically in only 9 of 17 cases.[6]

Endoscopy. Many authors have commented on the difficulty in diagnosing transglottic carcinoma and obtaining an accurate biopsy. In fact, many of these tumors are understaged following direct laryngoscopy. Pillsbury serially sectioned 114 laryngeal specimens and found a 50 per cent error rate in the staging of transglottic carcinomas. In this report, 89 per cent of the laryngeal cancers that were inaccurately staged were underestimated. The high rate of error in staging resulted mainly from a failure to predict extension of cancer outside of the larynx. The study showed that there should have been more T4 and fewer T3 lesions in the original clinical staging.[14]

The presence of adjacent carcinoma makes it more difficult to examine such areas as the anterior commissure, laryngeal ventricle, and subglottis. The ventricle is seen at direct laryngoscopy by using the tip of the laryngoscope to push the lower edge of the ventricular band laterally or by pulling it upward with a laryngeal hook. In most transglottic carcinomas, the laryngeal ventricle is obliterated, with the tumor spreading extensively beneath the mucosa of the ventricular band and vocal folds. Upon direct laryngoscopy, only a small area of ulceration may be seen. The tendency of the carcinoma to invade deeply into the paraglottic space, without spreading extensively on the surface, causes difficulty in obtaining a positive biopsy specimen.[9] Vermund reports that residual tumor may remain below the mucosa after irradiation, particularly if the tumor infiltrated deeply and involved muscle or cartilage. He states that persistent or recurrent tumor may become difficult to diagnose as ulcerations heal and no gross tumor is visible on laryngoscopy.[15] Therefore, the surgeon must cut deeply to obtain an adequate biopsy specimen for transglottic carcinoma.

Histopathology of specimens obtained preoperatively has been compared to that of specimens removed at the time of surgical treatment. Cellular differentiation of the biopsy does not always correlate with tumor differentiation, but major discrepancies are rare.[1]

STAGING

A valid staging and classification system for laryngeal cancer is of paramount importance, not only in planning treatment, but also in comparing results of various series. Numerous systems have been proposed and revised over the past two decades.[2, 14] Each differs from the others, but most recognize the significance of a fixed hemilarynx. The present authors use the most current edition of the classification for laryngeal cancer by the American Joint Committee on Cancer.[2] This system classifies a tumor as T1 when it is confined to one or both vocal cords with normal mobility, and T2 when a glottic lesion with normal or impaired cord mobility extends to the supraglottic or subglottic areas, or both. Carcinoma confined to the larynx that fixes one or both vocal cords is classified as T3, and thyroid cartilage invasion or extension beyond the confines of the larynx (or both) is designated T4. The AJCC system for classifying laryngeal tumors frequently forces the physician to make decisions regarding the origin of the tumor and cord fixation versus impaired cord mobility. These judgments are frequently not easily made. Transglottic carcinoma may arise from the superior surface of the true vocal cord, the ventricle, or the false cord.

The reader is referred to the Manual for Staging of Cancer (1983) for a description of cervical node classification and stage groupings.[2] Inaccurate staging of laryngeal cancer can lead to inappropriate treatment.

The prognosis differs for fixed cord glottic and transglottic cancers. Fixation reflects deep invasion, but T3 glottic tumors that have not extended below the inferior margin of the thyroid cartilage have a better prognosis than do similarly staged transglottic tumors.

Most transglottic carcinomas are T3 or T4 tumors. In their study of 500 patients with cancer of the larynx and pyriform sinus, Kirchner and Owen found 64 transglottic lesions with 4 staged as T4, 57 as T3, and 3 as T2.[8] The current classification systems fail to use the term *transglottic,* thereby omitting important information concerning propensity for local spread and cervical metastasis. Furthermore, neoplasms that are predominantly supraglottic but that cross the anterior commissure may be classified as transglottic, although they do not behave as glottic-transglottic tumors do. Nevertheless, the use of an accepted staging system should be a routine step for all surgeons. Only by such use will we be able to compare the results of various treatment regimens and to perfect classification and staging systems.

PATHOLOGY

Squamous cell carcinoma is the most common type of glottic and transglottic malignancy. The term *transglottic* may be applied to neoplasms of other histologic types, but it must be remembered that this term was coined in a review of epidermoid carcinomas.[1] In this chapter, *transglottic* and *glottic* will refer specifically to squamous cell carcinoma, unless otherwise specified.

Histologic characteristics of primary laryngeal malignancies have been correlated with the clinical course of patients. McGavran et al. found that poorly differentiated neoplasms show a higher incidence of cervical nodal metastasis.[1] Kirchner found that 63 per cent of patients with poorly differentiated transglottic carcinomas developed regional metastases versus 23 per cent of those with well-differentiated or moderately well-differentiated tumors.[9] Poorly differentiated tumors are also associated with infiltrating margins. Peripheral growth of transglottic carcinoma occurs usually by infiltration; however, differentiation has not been shown to correlate with tumor size or a tendency for cartilage invasion.[1, 9]

Larger glottic neoplasms tend to spread deeply and extralaryngeally. Kirchner found metastases in 55 per cent of the patients with transglottic carcinoma larger than 4 cm.[9] McGavran observed a 40 per cent metastatic rate for tumors greater than 2 cm, but this study included laryngeal tumors involving various regions, rather than only transglottic neoplasms.[1] Although Pillsbury found no invasion of laryngeal cartilage with transglottic tumors under 2 cm, he found such invasion in 75 per cent of the patients with lesions greater than 3 cm.[14]

Much has been learned from the study of serially sectioned laryngeal tumors, but the precise pathophysiology of this disease warrants further investigation. LeRoux-Robert[3] and Baclesse[16] proposed the laryngeal ventricle as the origin for transglottic carcinoma. Bryce points out that, while this seems logical, squamous metaplasia of the ventricular mucosa is rarely seen in the nonirradiated patient. Also, no small ventricular tumors have been found among the large number of larynges that have been serially sectioned in many laboratories. He believes that transglottic carcinoma arises from the superior surface of the true vocal cord and spreads laterally to invade deeply into the paraglottic space.[17]

Invasion of laryngeal cartilages occurs commonly with transglottic and advanced glottic carcinoma, but less frequently with the latter. Kirchner found cartilage invasion in 75 per cent of patients with transglottic tumors.[9] Of 28 serially sectioned larynges from patients with fixed cord lesions, Olofsson found that 18

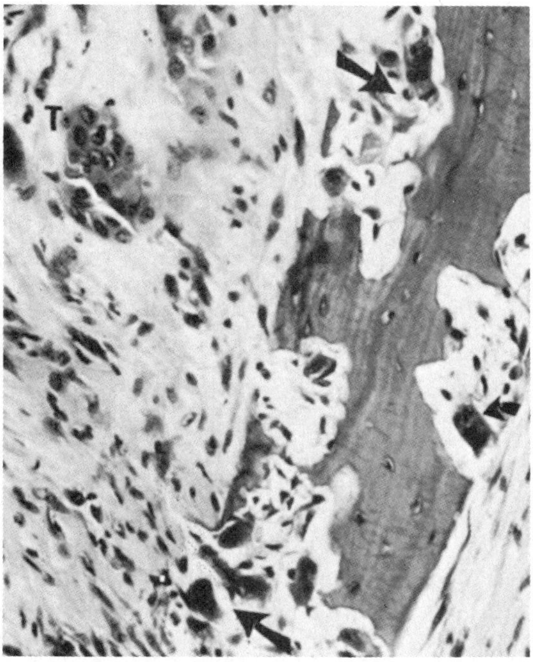

Figure 19–1. Multinucleate osteoclasts *(arrows)* erode focus of metaplastic bone in thyroid cartilage in front of the advancing tumor (T). (Hematoxylin and eosin stain, × 240.) (From Pittam MR, Carter RL: Head Neck Surg 4 (3):204, 1982. Copyright 1982, John Wiley & Sons, Inc.)

showed spread outside the larynx, and 15 invaded the thyroid cartilage.[18] Cricoid and arytenoid cartilages are invaded less frequently. Cartilage invasion occurs in areas of calcification and is found most often in the lower one-third of the thyroid cartilage. Destruction of ossified laryngeal cartilage by tumor occurs in a biphasic pattern. Ossified cartilage, which is essentially well-formed metaplastic bone, contains osteoclasts, which are noted to cluster about infiltrating carcinoma and serve to resorb this metaplastic bone. After the initial osteoclastic response, the tumor cells encroach upon the bone (Fig. 19–1).[6] This same two-phase process occurs when squamous cell carcinoma invades skeletal bone.[19] Prostaglandins and various nonprostaglandin stimulants released by squamous cell carcinoma may promote this osteoclastic activity.[20]

In addition to destroying cartilage, neoplastic disease invading the paraglottic space can exit inferiorly through the cricothyroid membrane or posteriorly into the pyriform sinus. The paraglottic space is bounded by the thyroid cartilage anterolaterally, the conus elasticus inferomedially, the ventricle and quadrangular membrane medially, and the pyriform sinus mucosa posteriorly. The spread of glottic cancer may be restrained by the conus elasticus medially and the thyroid cartilage laterally, but it commonly spreads through the cricothyroid membrane (Fig. 19–2). Kirchner found 16 of 19 transglottic tumors to reach or penetrate this membrane.[21] Among tumors spreading beyond the larynx, Olofsson noted 3 of 18 fixed-cord tumors to do so between the cricoid and thyroid cartilages.[18]

Invasion of the intrinsic laryngeal muscles is the primary cause of vocal cord fixation. The thyroarytenoid muscle is involved most frequently. Tumor cells seem to advance subepithelially along the axis of muscle fibers, presumably taking the path of least resistance. In the review of 28 serially sectioned larynges with fixed cords, Olofsson noted that the thyroarytenoid muscle was involved by tumor in every specimen. Nests of viable cancer cells were observed infiltrating the muscle. The lateral cricoarytenoid muscle was involved in 19 of 28 specimens; it was followed by the interarytenoid (11 of 28) and posterior cricoarytenoid (7 of 28) muscles.[18] It is important to

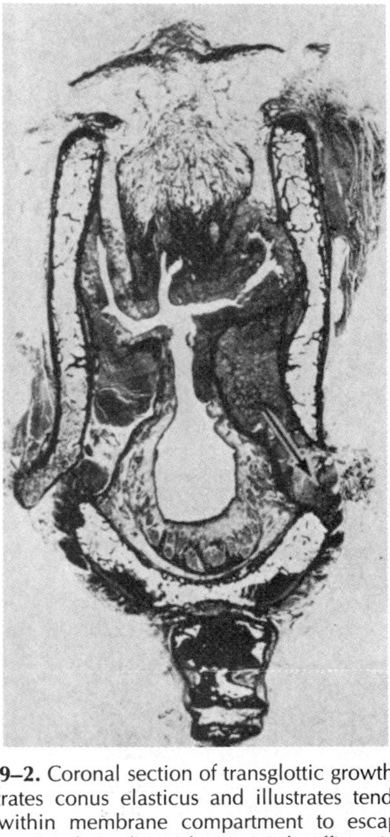

Figure 19–2. Coronal section of transglottic growth *(arrow)* demonstrates conus elasticus and illustrates tendency of cancer within membrane compartment to escape from larynx via cricothyroid membrane (Verhoeff's stain, × 1). (From Pillsbury HRC, Kirchner JA: Arch Otolaryngol 105:159, 1979. Copyright 1979, American Medical Association.)

recognize when tumor invades the interarytenoid or posterior cricoarytenoid muscles, because tumor in these areas could be inadequately excised at the time of surgery. With reference to this Harrison noted, "If undetected, carcinoma will be left in the margins of the pharyngeal repair and the recurrence will be placed above the stoma."[22]

TREATMENT

Transglottic carcinoma or glottic carcinoma with a fixed cord usually requires total laryngectomy and neck dissection. Some authors advocate vertical frontolateral hemilaryngectomy for selected T3 glottic carcinomas and for superficial transglottic carcinomas. Others argue that deep local invasion and the high rate of cervical metastasis contraindicate this operation, noting that advanced glottic and transglottic tumors can insidiously invade thyroid cartilage and spread extralaryngeally. Olofsson concluded that cord fixation contraindicates conservation surgery.[18] Skolnik et al. have also stated that total laryngectomy, with or without neck dissection, should be the treatment for all T3 glottic carcinomas.[23] Considering the high rate of regional metastasis, preoperative or postoperative radiotherapy plays a significant role in the treatment of these tumors. The type of neck dissection performed will vary with the presence of palpable nodes and their location. Our policy at the University of Texas Medical Branch is to treat advanced glottic and transglottic carcinomas with wide-field laryngectomy and radical neck dissection, usually sparing the eleventh cranial nerve, and postoperative radiotherapy.

Laryngectomy and Neck Dissection

History. In 1873, Bilroth performed the first total laryngectomy for cancer of the larynx. His patient was a 36-year-old religious instructor who survived seven months before succumbing to recurrent tumor.[24] In the ensuing years, the operation was not generally accepted because of high morbidity and mortality; however, in 1892, Solis-Cohen improved the procedure by devising the technique of diverting the tracheal stump to the skin.[25] Later, in the first part of this century, Gluck and his colleague, Sorenson, refined the laryngectomy operation.[25] They had performed 160 total laryngectomies by 1922, at which time the operation became less popular as radiotherapy for laryngeal cancer was introduced. Improved surgical techniques and reduced postoperative infection rates followed the introduction of antibiotic therapy, and the operation regained popularity. The present-day laryngectomy is based on the wide-field operation first described by Jackson and Babcock in 1931, but their technique included resecting only portions of the hyoid bone, the epiglottis, and the cricoid cartilage.[26] Modern laryngectomy includes resection of all these structures as well as the strap muscles and perilaryngeal tissue, including the ipsilateral lobe of the thyroid gland.

In 1906, Crile[27] first described resection of regional lymph nodes for cancer of the head and neck; this technique was called *neck dissection*. Based upon the observation that most head and neck cancers spread first to regional lymph nodes, this operation has increased patient survival when performed in conjunction with total laryngectomy for transglottic and advanced glottic carcinomas.

Technique. The technique involves a wide-field total laryngectomy with en bloc radical neck dissection, sparing the accessory nerve, when possible. The neck dissection is performed first and the specimen remains attached to the lateral aspect of the larynx from the hyoid bone superiorly to the lower edge of the cricoid cartilage inferiorly. This connection assures that the lymphatics coming from the larynx through the thyrohyoid and cricothyroid membranes are not violated intraoperatively.

Various skin incisions have been proposed for operations in the neck. The choice for total laryngectomy and neck dissection depends upon several factors. The incision should be low enough in the neck to permit good exposure of the larynx. If a previous tracheostomy has been performed, an elliptical excision of the surrounding area is necessary. In addition, the surgeon should have adequate exposure to perform an ipsilateral neck dissection and to extend the incision for a contralateral neck dissection if this is indicated. The skin incision should cross the carotid artery only once on each side of the neck, preferably in the lower half of the neck at a maximum distance from the carotid bifurcation. Previous radiation to the neck is also a factor. The MacFee incision is commonly used when the neck has been irradiated.[28]

We prefer a low apron flap with the tracheostoma incorporated into the midline of the incision. On the ipsilateral side, the incision

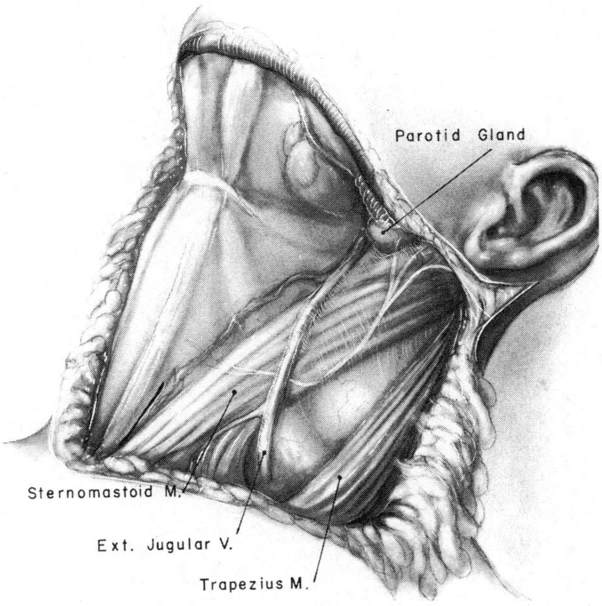

Figure 19–3. Extent of the skin flap elevation is the anterior border of the trapezius muscle posteriorly, the mandible superiorly, the clavicle inferiorly, and the contralateral sternocleidomastoid muscle medially. The plane of dissection is between the platysma muscle and superficial layer of the deep cervical fascia. (From Loré JM Jr: An Atlas of Head and Neck Surgery, Vol 2, 2nd ed. Philadelphia, WB Saunders Company, 1973, p 765.)

starts at the mastoid tip and drops inferiorly along the posterior border of the sternocleidomastoid muscle until a natural skin crease permits the incision to curve across the neck horizontally at the level of the third tracheal ring. The incision is extended superiorly in a symmetric manner on the contralateral side but only to the level of the hyoid bone. On the side of the neck dissection, an S-shaped incision is made from the lower portion of the apron flap down to the midportion of the clavicle.

The skin flaps are elevated and include the platysma muscle. We prefer to use a thermal knife, which reduces blood loss during the procedure.[29] The apron flap is elevated superiorly up to the inferior edge of the mandible. The flap elevation extends to the anterior border of the trapezius muscle posteriorly, to the clavicle inferiorly, and to the contralateral sternocleidomastoid muscle medially (Fig. 19–3).

The contralateral neck is explored for metastases. The fascia is divided along the anterior border of the sternocleidomastoid muscle, permitting exploration of the anterior cervical triangle and palpation for nodal metastases.

Technique—Neck Dissection. The neck dissection is begun inferiorly by transecting the sternocleidomastoid muscle approximately 2 cm above its attachment to the clavicle. The internal jugular vein is identified and doubly ligated using 3-0 silk suture ligatures (Fig. 19–4). After the vein is transected, blunt dissection is carried down to the deep layer of the deep cervical fascia, where the phrenic nerve is identified. The carotid artery and vagus nerve are also identified at this time. They are retracted medially as the internal jugular vein and paratracheal nodes are dissected superiorly (Fig. 19–5). Cervical fascia overlying the phrenic nerve, brachial plexus, and scalene muscles represents the deep plane of the neck dissection. As the dissection progresses from medial to lateral just superior to the clavicle, the transverse cervical vessels are encountered. These are suture-ligated and cut, unless a trapezius myocutaneous flap is planned. The thoracic duct and subclavian vein are carefully avoided when dissecting in this area of the neck. If either the thoracic duct on the left or the accessory duct on the right is cut, it must be ligated.

The spinal accessory nerve may be spared if there is no evidence of metastatic disease in the spinal accessory node chain or in the upper

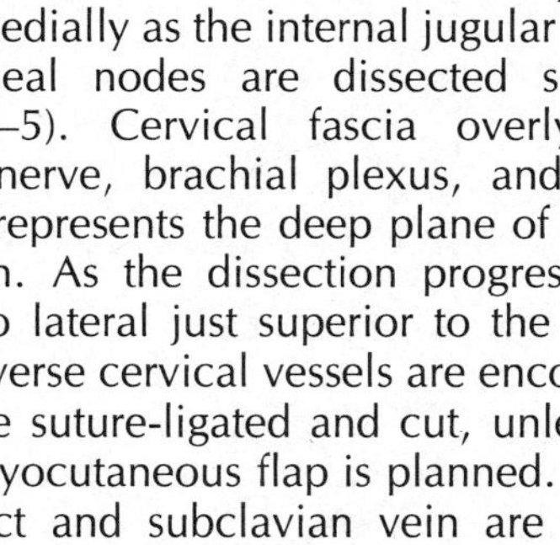

Figure 19–4. The internal jugular chain is identified beneath the transected and retracted sternocleidomastoid muscle. It is doubly ligated with 3-0 silk suture ligatures. (From Loré JM Jr: An Atlas of Head and Neck Surgery, Vol 2, 2nd ed. Philadelphia, WB Saunders Company, 1973, p 547.)

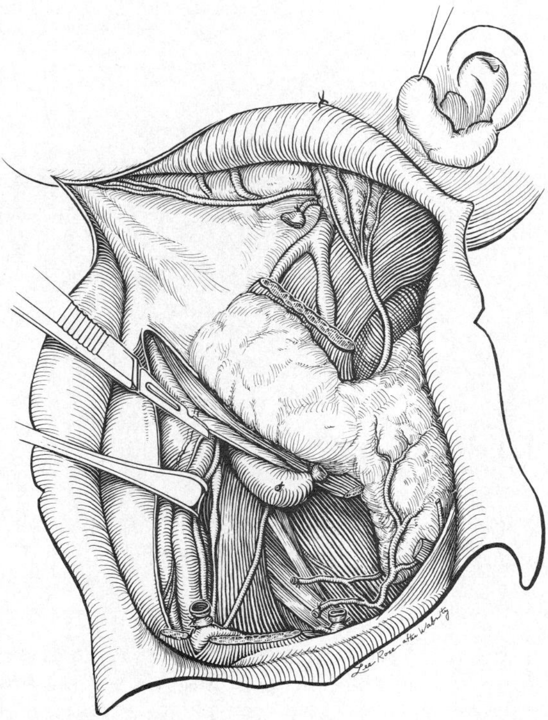

Figure 19–5. The common carotid artery and vagus nerve are identified and retracted as the internal jugular vein, paratracheal nodes, and fascia are dissected superiorly. The phrenic nerve, scalene muscles, and brachial plexus are in view. (Adapted from Loré JM Jr: An Atlas of Head and Neck Surgery, Vol 2, 2nd ed. Philadelphia, WB Saunders Company, 1973, p 549.)

jugular chain. Neither McGavran nor Pittam found positive cervical nodes in the posterior triangles of the neck in his series.[1, 6] Careful sharp and blunt dissection exposes the nerve in the posterior triangle of the neck. Dissection continues beneath the sternocleidomastoid muscle, but completion of the nerve dissection superiorly is not possible until the neck dissection has been carried up to this area.

The anterior border of the trapezius muscle serves as the posterior limit of the neck dissection. The neck specimen is dissected inferiorly to superiorly and posteriorly to anteriorly. Cutaneous plexus nerves are sacrificed as they are encountered.

The superior portion of the neck dissection crosses the upper attachment of the sternocleidomastoid muscle and the tail of the parotid gland, continuing anteriorly along the lower border of the mandible to the submental triangle. Nodes, fascia, and adipose tissue are dissected out of this triangle and reflected downward; they remain attached to the hyoid bone. Transection of the sternocleidomastoid muscle superiorly will reveal the posterior belly of the digastric muscle. The tail of the parotid gland is transected at a level approximated by an imaginary line drawn from the tip of the mastoid to the angle of the mandible. The posterior facial vein is ligated at this time, as are other smaller veins in the area. Retraction of the posterior belly of the digastric muscle exposes the upper internal jugular vein, which is doubly ligated and divided in a fashion similar to the technique used on the inferior portion of the vein. Care should be taken to avoid injuring the 10th, 11th, and 12th cranial nerves (Fig. 19–6).

As the dissection continues anteriorly, the submaxillary gland is encountered. The facial vein and artery are identified and ligated. The prevascular and postvascular lymph nodes are

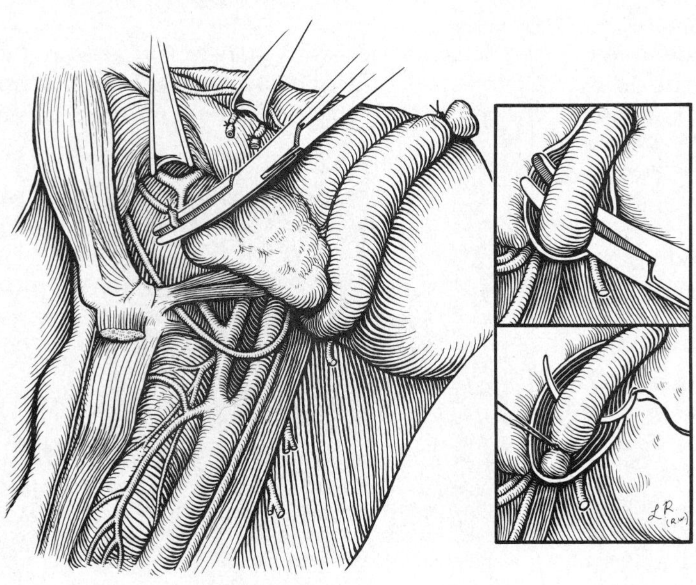

Figure 19–6. Superiorly, important landmarks include bifurcation of the carotid artery, hypoglossal and lingual nerves, and Wharton's duct, which is ligated and cut after the submaxillary gland has been dissected. The upper internal jugular vein is isolated, ligated, and cut (see inserts) in a fashion similar to that done inferiorly. (Adapted from Loré JM Jr: An Atlas of Head and Neck Surgery, Vol 2, 2nd ed. Philadelphia, WB Saunders Company, 1973, p 549.)

included in the dissection. The mandibular branch of the facial nerve, initially identified when the skin flap is raised, is preserved unless metastatic disease is close to it. The deep limit of dissection in the submandibular triangle is the hyoglossus muscle. The hypoglossal nerve is identified as it crosses the bifurcation of the carotid artery and is dissected anteriorly as it passes under the digastric tendon. Wharton's duct and tributaries of the lingual vein are also ligated and cut. Chorda tympani nerve fibers branching from the lingual nerve to innervate the gland are transected (Fig. 19–6). If no gross disease is present in the upper neck, the digastric and stylohyoid muscles are preserved.

When the neck dissection is complete, the specimen is attached to the larynx from the hyoid bone superiorly to the cricoid cartilage inferiorly, and includes the ipsilateral lobe and isthmus of the thyroid gland. Retraction of the carotid artery laterally facilitates dissection of the lobe from the anterior cervical triangle, exposing the tracheoesophageal groove and the inferior constrictor muscle. The superior thyroid artery is suture-ligated and cut as it branches from the external carotid artery.

Technique—Total Laryngectomy. The laryngectomy begins with transection of the strap muscles inferiorly, just below the level at which the tracheostoma will be created. The sternohyoid and sternothyroid muscles are transected carefully to avoid injury to the thyroid gland beneath the latter. The omohyoid muscle is cut on the contralateral side; the thyroid isthmus is dissected away from the anterior tracheal wall. The isthmus is divided and included with the ipsilateral lobe as part of the specimen. The contralateral thyroid lobe is detached from the tracheal wall, reflected laterally, and sutured beneath the contralateral sternocleidomastoid muscle (Fig. 19–7). The trachea is incised, and the original endotracheal tube is replaced by an armored, sterile tube that passes across the chest field and is secured by a silk suture to the skin. The entry site, determined by the degree of subglottic extension of the tumor, is usually between the third and fourth tracheal rings. The tracheal transection is beveled posteriorly and superiorly to permit construction of a large tracheostoma.

Once the armored tube is placed and secured, attention turns to removing the larynx. The pharynx is entered by sharp dissection through the suprahyoid muscles. The greater cornua of the hyoid bone are dissected from the underlying tissue. The epiglottis is visualized and grasped with noncrushing forceps;

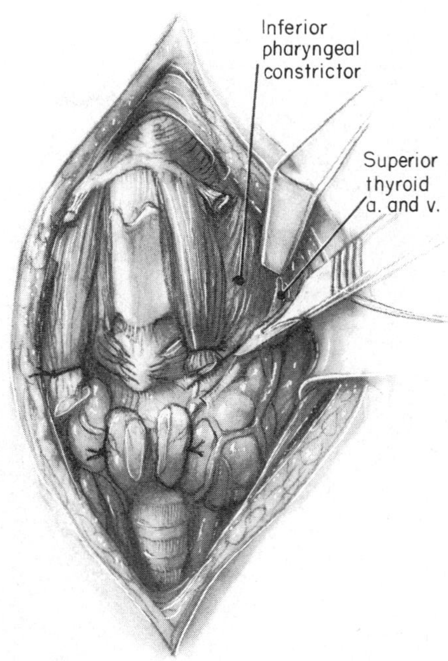

Figure 19–7. The laryngectomy is begun by transection of the strap muscles (sternohyoid and sternothyroid muscles) inferiorly and dissection of the thyroid gland isthmus off the trachea. The isthmus is ligated, cut, and resected with the ipsilateral thyroid lobe as part of the surgical specimen. (From Loré JM Jr.: An Atlas of Head and Neck Surgery, Vol 2, 2nd ed. Philadelphia, WB Saunders Company, 1973, p 753.)

anterior traction facilitates the scissor dissection inferiorly to the greater cornua of the thyroid cartilages. The superior laryngeal vessels are ligated and cut. The inferior constrictor muscles are divided on each side as the dissection proceeds inferiorly to the cricoid cartilage. The two lateral incisions are joined by cutting across the postcricoid pharyngeal mucosa, and the last few centimeters of dissection cross the common wall between the esophagus and the trachea (Fig. 19–8).

The field is then inspected for bleeding vessels, which are ligated or electrocoagulated. Copious irrigation with an antibiotic solution is performed before closing the pharynx. When possible, the pharynx is closed in a single vertical line, using a 4-0 chromic catgut suture and Connell-type mattress stitch. Special attention is given to inverting the mucosal edges. Two more layers are sutured in an interrupted stitch fashion, using the inferior constrictor muscles as one layer. Occasionally, the surgeon must close the pharynx in a T-shaped fashion. This technique has a higher incidence of fistula, presumably at the trifurcation formed in the closure.

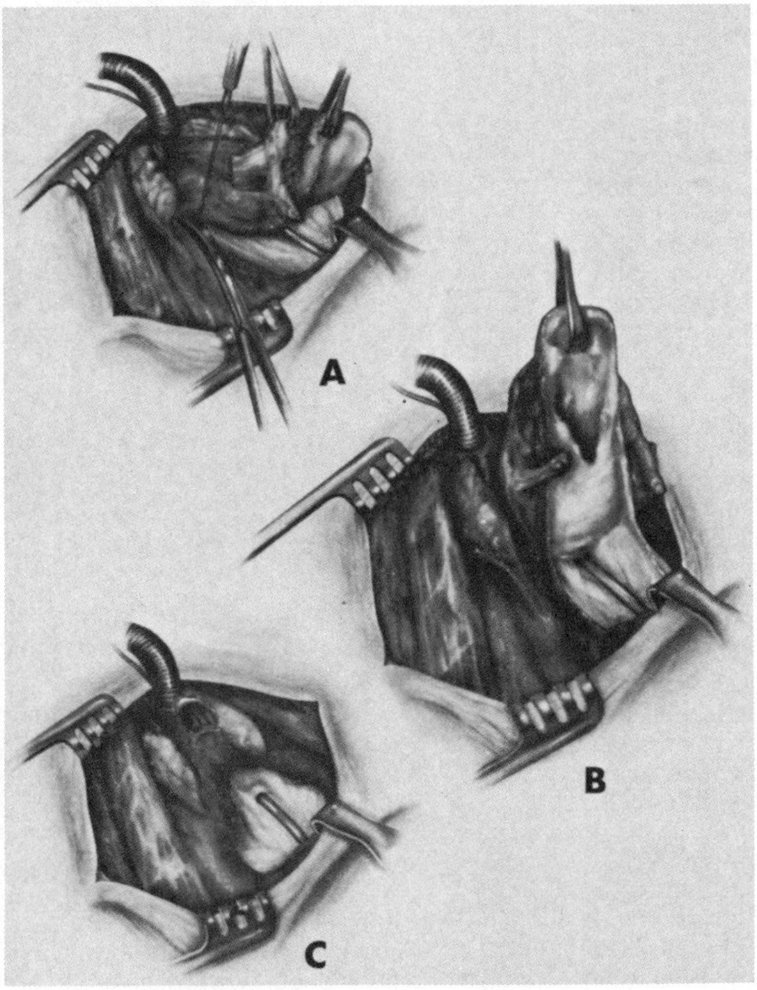

Figure 19–8. The pharynx is entered sharply through the suprahyoid musculature *(A)*. The epiglottis is grasped and retracted anteriorly and inferiorly as the larynx is removed *(B)*. The last few centimeters of the dissection is down through the common wall of the esophagus and trachea *(C)*. (From Ogura JH, Thawley SE: Surgery of the Larynx. *In* Paparella MM, Shumrick DA (eds): Otolaryngology Vol 3: Head and Neck. Philadelphia, WB Saunders Company, 1980, p 2544.)

The final steps of the operation include harvesting and suturing a dermal graft to protect the carotid, fashioning the tracheostoma, and closing the skin incision. A dermal graft is used routinely to cover the carotid artery from several centimeters above the bifurcation to just above the clavicle. The skin flaps are closed using a 3-0 or 4-0 absorbable synthetic suture for the platysma muscle and subcutaneous tissue and staples for the skin. The tracheostoma is constructed by suturing the skin edges to the trachea with 3-0 nylon or silk sutures. The closure must be meticulous so that mucosal and skin edges are well approximated and no tension exists. We recommend placing the stoma in the original flap incision after taking an ellipse of skin from each flap to create a circular margin for anastomosis with the trachea. Some surgeons prefer placing the stoma in a separate incision in the inferior flap, feeling that this is less likely to result in postoperative stomal stenosis.[30]

Results of Treatment

Many reports of treatment results for laryngeal cancer have been published in the last decade. The various studies are difficult to compare because most are retrospective and contain many variables within each patient series. Even the tumor classification systems differ among studies. Laryngeal cancer patients diagnosed after the 1977 modifications in the AJCC classification system will be staged differently than those diagnosed by the 1972 version. While prospective studies are preferable, some of the larger retrospective series in the literature clearly show trends that indicate the superiority of certain treatment modalities for advanced glottic carcinoma.

Skolnik et al. retrospectively reviewed 264 cases of glottic carcinoma and found an overall five-year determinate survival rate of 55 per cent. Among these patients, 85 were classified as T3 N0 M0 (AJCC, 1972) with one-year and five-year survival rates of 86 per cent and 55 per cent, respectively. For the stage III patients as a group, the results showed improved five-year survival rates for those treated primarily by surgery rather than radiotherapy (49 per cent versus 30 per cent).[23]

Woodhouse et al. reviewed 323 patients with carcinoma of the vocal cord and compared the control of their primary lesions by types of treatment. They found that radiotherapy controlled only 50 per cent of the primary lesions for T3 and T4 patients as a group; however, one patient in this small group was salvaged by total laryngectomy, bringing the overall control of the primary lesions by radiotherapy with salvage surgery to 57 per cent. On the other hand, control of lesions by surgery as the primary treatment was 81 per cent for patients with a fixed vocal cord and 78 per cent for the T4 patients. These investigators concluded that total laryngectomy is the treatment of choice for all T3 and T4 laryngeal glottic carcinomas, with radiotherapy alone reserved for a few carefully selected patients who have favorable T3 lesions.[7]

Miller examined the results of radiotherapy for two groups of glottic carcinoma patients, one with partially impaired cord mobility and the other with cord fixation. Patients with partially impaired cord mobility had a three-year recurrence-free rate of 63 per cent, while the group with cord fixation had only a 23 per cent three-year recurrence-free rate. Furthermore, transglottic carcinoma patients had even worse treatment results, with no patient with cord fixation in this group living for three years without tumor recurrence. Miller does not recommend radiotherapy as the primary treatment for carcinoma of the glottis when cord fixation is present.[31]

In 1969, Vermund observed that only 29 per cent of patients with complete cord fixation who were treated with radiotherapy alone survived for five years, as compared with 47 per cent of patients with impaired cord mobility. Surgery produced better results, with five-year survival in 55 per cent of patients with complete cord fixation and 74 per cent in those with impaired cord mobility. When he combined results from five institutions, he noted that the overall rate of five-year survival for patients with fixation of a vocal cord was 42 per cent when treated initially with radiotherapy as compared to 61 per cent when treated initially with surgery.[15]

Ogura et al. reported 63 cases of transglottic carcinoma and 37 cases of glottic carcinoma with cord fixation. All cases were treated by resection of the primary lesion and a neck dissection. The transglottic group had a three-year absolute survival rate of 64 per cent, and the T3 glottic carcinoma group had a three-year survival rate of 60 per cent. Some patients in each group did receive preoperative low-dose radiotherapy (1500 to 3000 rads).[10]

Some surgeons advocate hemilaryngectomy as an acceptable procedure in selected cases of glottic carcinoma with a fixed vocal cord. Kirchner details the indications for such cases. He found that a 60 per cent cure rate can be achieved.[13] Som agrees, stating that his cure rate was 58 per cent for T3 lesions.[32] Transglottic carcinomas are a different matter, however. Radiotherapy as the primary mode is not ordinarily indicated but is advised for patients who refuse surgery or who have medical problems that introduce excessive operative risks.

To achieve the best possible results in treating patients with transglottic and advanced glottic carcinomas, we advocate surgery followed by radiation therapy. Except for an occasional T3 glottic carcinoma and superficial, early transglottic carcinoma treated with hemilaryngectomy, the procedure of choice should be total laryngectomy and neck dissection, followed by postoperative radiotherapy. We believe these methods can achieve a five-year survival rate near 60 per cent with these very aggressive tumors.

COMPLICATIONS

As with most surgery, the best safeguard against complications following laryngectomy is to recognize causal factors and to prevent potential problems. The fundamental principle is selection of the correct procedure for each patient. Intraoperatively, attention to the fundamentals of good surgical technique and attention to obtaining adequate margins for tumor resection will enhance the patient's chances for a smooth postoperative course. Preoperative evaluation of the patient's nutritional status and any systemic disease (e.g., diabetes mellitus or peripheral vascular disease) is very important. Previous treatment, especially preoperative radiotherapy, has a significant bearing on the outcome of the surgery.

Preoperative Considerations. Recent interest in the nutritional status of patients with head and neck cancer has led to the development of numerous assessment batteries. Bassett et al. used anthropometric measurements, skin tests, questionnaires, and laboratory assessments to characterize the nutritional status of 50 consecutive new head and neck cancer patients. They found an expected positive relationship between tumor stage and nutritional impairment, and noted that the best predictor of impaired nutritional status was the patient's description of his recent diet.[33] Hooley et al. used a prognostic nutritional index (PNI) as a predictor of major postoperative complications for patients undergoing head and neck surgery. The PNI (in per cent) was calculated using the following formula:

$$\text{PNI} = 158 - 16.6(\text{ALB}) - 0.78(\text{TSF}) - 0.2(\text{TFN}) - 5.8(\text{DH})$$

where ALB is serum albumin (gm/dl); TSF, triceps skin fold thickness (mm); TFN, serum transferrin (mg/dl); and DH, delayed hypersensitivity skin tests (number of positive responses). They found that the higher the PNI, the greater the chance of a major postoperative complication, especially in patients with advanced disease. They suggested using the PNI as a routine preoperative screening device.[34]

The advantages and disadvantages of preoperative and postoperative radiotherapy have been debated at length. Thawley reviewed 554 patients in a study of complications of combined radiation therapy and surgery for carcinoma of the larynx and hypopharynx. Within the total laryngectomy group (which included patients with tumors not of glottic origin), he found no significant difference between complication rates when either preoperative or postoperative radiation was employed. Among the patients with glottic cancer who underwent total laryngectomy, the complication rate was 16 per cent for patients who received preoperative radiation and 12.8 per cent for those who received postoperative radiation.[35]

Wide discrepancies are apparent among reported rates of surgical complications following preoperative radiation. Comparisons in the literature are difficult because patient populations and radiation dosages differ among studies; however, complication rates and the amount of radiation given appear to correlate. Many authors note significant delay in wound healing and increased length of hospital stay among surgical patients who have undergone preoperative radiation. Trible noted this in his discussion of wound healing following curative radiation (7000 rads), and Habel found that wound healing required twice as much time in the laryngectomy group with preoperative radiation compared to a nonirradiated group of patients.[36, 37] Among those patients undergoing radical neck dissection in addition to total laryngectomy, the preoperative radiotherapy patients had a 74 per cent overall complication rate compared with 39 per cent for the postoperative radiotherapy patients.[37] On the other hand, Gall et al. reported no significant difference in complication rates between patients who did or did not receive preoperative radiation (3000 to 4500 rads). This study compared patients undergoing total laryngectomy alone with those undergoing total laryngectomy combined with preoperative radiation.[38]

A reduction in the number of complications has been described following the use of protective muscle flaps and dermal grafts for the carotid artery, better placement of skin incisions, and other protective surgical techniques.[37, 39]

Infection. Wound infections resulting in large areas of necrosis following total laryngectomy and radical neck dissection occur rarely, but when they do, the results are devastating. Superficial wound infections can be treated by appropriate antibiotics, draining the wound, and meticulous local care. If infection only causes suture line dehiscence or a small area of skin loss, good local care followed by split-thickness skin grafting will suffice. Prophylactic antibiotics given to patients undergoing total laryngectomy will reduce the incidence of postoperative infections. Brand et al. reported a prospective, double-blind, randomized study of patients with cancer who underwent major head and neck surgery. They found a statistically significant ($P = 0.05$) higher rate of infection with the perioperative use of cefazolin as compared to gentamicin plus clindamycin. Also, they indicated that a longer duration of therapy decreased the infection rate.[40] We begin prophylactic antibiotics six to eight hours prior to surgery.

Salivary Fistula. A salivary fistula may develop following any surgical procedure in the neck that involves entering the pharynx or esophagus. In the patient who has had a total laryngectomy, the fistula usually appears seven to ten days after surgery and is recognized by purulent saliva collecting beneath the skin flap, or exiting through a suture line or drain site. Also, it is suspected when saliva continues to be seen in sump drains in the neck. Direct fistulas are those in which the skin opening is over the mucosal defect, allowing an epithelialized communication to form. More common are the indirect fistulas, in which the openings are several centimeters apart and the tract is not epithelialized.[41] The incidence of fistulization following total laryngectomy in nonirradiated patients is less than 10 per cent. Kornblut and Shumrick state that this rate can be much higher in patients who have received preoperative radiation.[42]

Most indirect salivary fistulas heal with proper treatment. The patient is given nothing by mouth and a nasogastric tube is used for feeding. Appropriate antibiotic therapy, wound drainage, débridement of necrotic areas, and meticulous local wound care with frequent changes of pressure dressings are essential elements in fistula management.[42] We have noted that a sump drain may continue to collect large amounts of saliva because the tip of the drain has been dislodged and is keeping open the area of mucosal dehiscence. When the measures described above fail, an indirect type of fistula must be converted to a direct type and closed surgically with a local or regional flap from a nonirradiated area. Nutrition is an important factor in treatment, and persistent fistulas may not close until the patient is in positive nitrogen balance.

Vascular Rupture. Delayed arterial hemorrhage occurring several days to weeks after total laryngectomy and radical neck dissection is usually secondary to carotid artery rupture. This is the most dreaded postoperative complication of head and neck surgery, and some authors have suggested autogenous tissue coverage of the vessel following radical neck dissection. Levator scapulae muscle flaps and dermal grafts have been the most popular methods in recent years. Other techniques that have been proposed are: (1) rotation of the carotid bulb into a muscle pocket,[43] (2) rotation of prevertebral fascia over the vessel,[44] and (3) transposed omentum.[45] When possible, muscle coverage is the best technique for providing carotid protection. In appropriately selected cases, the conservative neck dissection in which the sternocleidomastoid muscle is spared reduces the risk of arterial rupture. Also, when reconstruction necessitates usage of a pectoralis myocutaneous flap, the carotid is better protected.

Preoperative radiotherapy and its temporal relation to surgery are recognized as factors contributing to wound breakdown and carotid rupture.[46, 47] Other factors include the choice of skin incision and thickness of the skin flaps.

A major postoperative complication such as skin necrosis or salivary fistula usually precedes carotid artery rupture; Heller and Strong found these in two-thirds of patients who suffered carotid rupture.[48] A fistula that develops near the carotid artery bathes the vessel in contaminated saliva. Infection and necrosis then ensue, causing the platysma-skin flap to dehisce or elevate and expose the underlying vessel. The patient often has a minor prodromal or sentinel hemorrhage prior to the carotid rupture. Bleeding may come from the oral cavity, from a dehiscent suture line, or from the trachea.

When carotid rupture is suspected, immediate wound exploration is required. Proximal and distal control and ligation of the vessel will usually be necessary.[30] This is done as far from the area of infection as possible. The carotid bulb is a weak area and a common site for rupture.

Early attention to skin necrosis or dehiscence over the carotid artery may prevent rupture. The area is cleaned of necrotic tissue and the involved region is resurfaced using nonirradiated, healthy tissue, ideally a myocutaneous flap. Though the routine use of dermal grafts to cover the carotid artery at the time of a radical neck dissection is controversial,[46] we advocate its utilization, whether or not the patient has had previous radiotherapy.

Tracheostomal Stenosis. Tracheostomal stenosis can occur from three weeks to one year

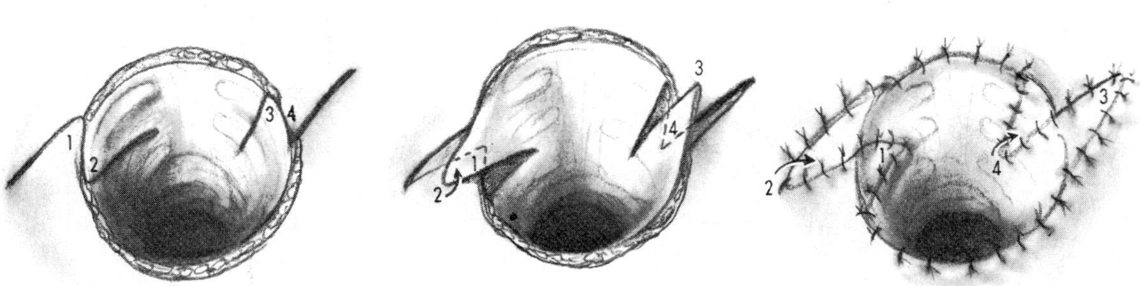

Figure 19–9. Following the excision of scar tissue, Z-plasties can be used to revise the stoma. (From Loré JM Jr: An Atlas of Head and Neck Surgery, Vol 2, 2nd ed. Philadelphia, WB Saunders Company, 1973, p 761.)

following total laryngectomy. The patient may have respiratory distress or other symptoms of hypoxia. In a study of 107 patients who had undergone total laryngectomy, Yonkers and Mercurio reported that 46 required stomal revision procedures.[49] Though higher than rates in some other reports,[50, 51] this rate does reflect that benign stomal stenosis poses a common problem for the head and neck surgeon. The complication appears more often in women (perhaps because of the smaller tracheal diameter) and in black patients, who are predisposed

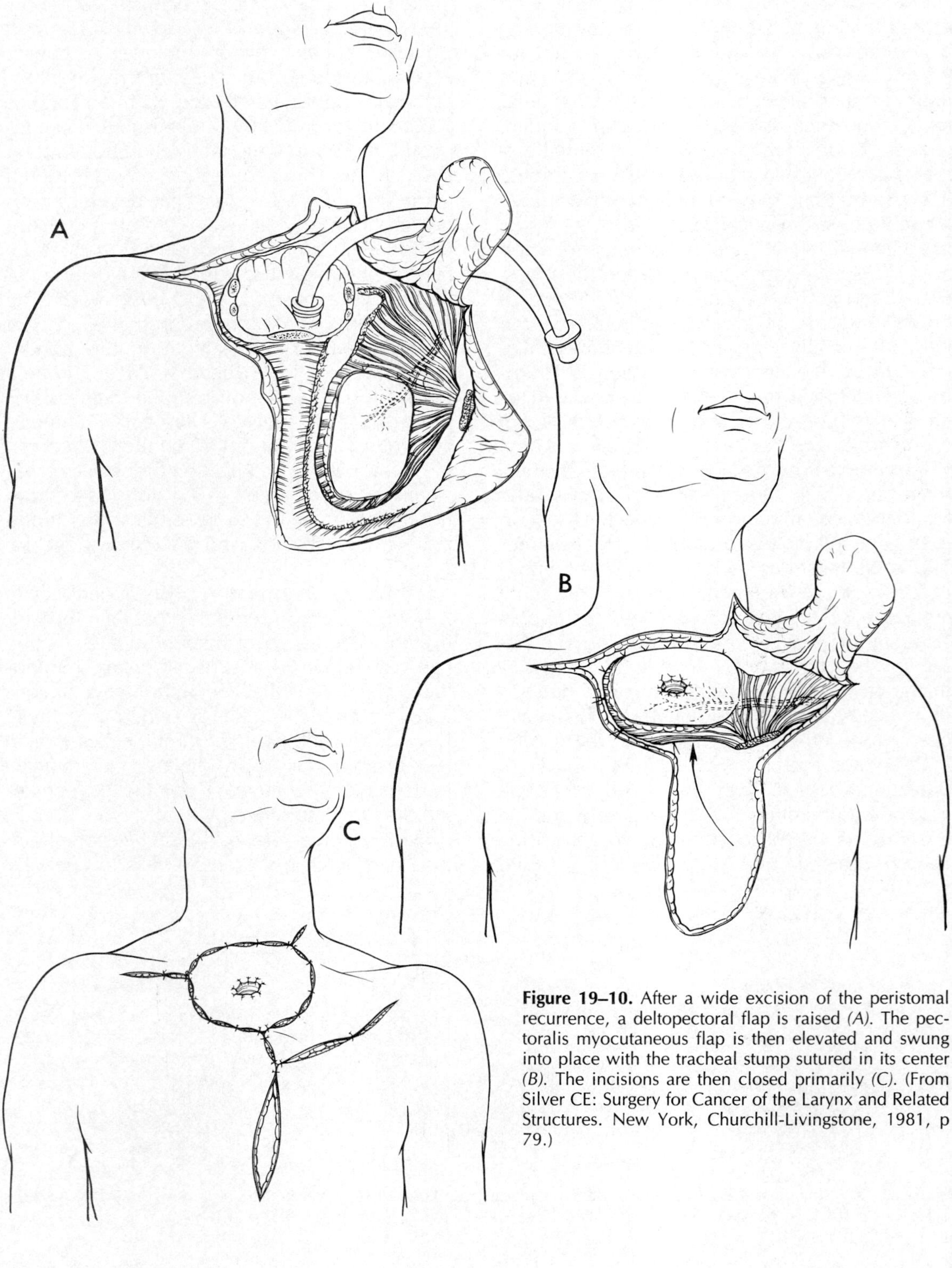

Figure 19–10. After a wide excision of the peristomal recurrence, a deltopectoral flap is raised *(A)*. The pectoralis myocutaneous flap is then elevated and swung into place with the tracheal stump sutured in its center *(B)*. The incisions are then closed primarily *(C)*. (From Silver CE: Surgery for Cancer of the Larynx and Related Structures. New York, Churchill-Livingstone, 1981, p 79.)

to form keloids.[52] Yonkers and Mercurio identified three basic types of stenosis: (1) the vertical slit, (2) the superior shelf, and (3) the concentric stenosis. Concentric stenosis was the most common type and appeared to be related to various postoperative wound infections, to the use of radiotherapy, and to errors in technique, timing, or management.[49] Dilations, using progressively larger laryngectomy tubes, and steroid injections have been proposed for treatment of mild stenosis;[30] however, laryngectomy tubes and stomal buttons cause discomfort and crusting. Dilation frequently fails and is used only as a temporary measure. There are several methods for surgical revision of a stoma. The scar can be excised and local skin flaps, such as Z-plasty transposition flaps, can be used to gain length and avoid an unbroken suture line or tension. Meticulous technique is used in approximating the edges (Fig. 19–9).

Stomal Recurrence. Recurrent cancer is an ominous postoperative complication of total laryngectomy. In patients with advanced glottic and transglottic carcinomas, the tracheostoma is a common site for recurrence. The incidence varies from 1.7 per cent to 14.7 per cent.[30] Predisposing factors are inadequate tracheal resection margins, previous tracheostomy, and residual disease in the paratracheal nodes or thyroid gland. Subglottic extension also increases the risk of stomal recurrence.

Implantation of tumor cells at the time of surgery has been proposed as a cause of stomal recurrence by several authors.[51] Kiem et al. studied what he called preoperative tracheostomy (performed two or more days prior to laryngectomy) and operative tracheostomy (done at the time of laryngectomy). In a series of 116 laryngectomy patients, the incidence of peristomal recurrence was 41 per cent in the former group and 14 per cent in the latter group. These authors suggested "emergency laryngectomy" for patients with airway obstruction secondary to laryngeal cancer.[53] More recently, tumor debulking with the CO_2 laser is advocated to avoid preoperative tracheostomy and emergency laryngectomy.

Patients with laryngeal carcinoma who have subglottic extension greater than 2 cm require more than standard laryngectomy and radical neck dissection. Adequate exposure inferiorly during the laryngectomy is mandatory to achieve a tumor-free margin and to resect paratracheal lymph nodes. Removal of the manubrium sterni permits dissection along the trachea 3 cm lower than is usually possible;[22] however, careful dissection to avoid pneumothorax or injury to major vessels is essential.

Stomal recurrence is easier to prevent than to treat. Though preoperative or postoperative radiotherapy will decrease the probability of stomal recurrence in high-risk patients, it offers little as a treatment for this problem once it has occurred. The highest cure rate will be achieved by an aggressive surgical approach with wide excision of skin and resection of the manubrium, trachea, and mediastinal lymphatics. Silver describes this procedure, using a pectoralis myocutaneous flap for reconstruction of the defect. The rich vascular supply of this flap permits the surgeon to bring the trachea through the center of the flap and to suture to the skin with highly predictable success (Fig. 19–10).[30]

References

1. McGavran MH et al.: The incidence of cervical lymph node metastases from epidermoid carcinoma of the larynx and their relationship to certain characteristics of the primary tumor. Cancer 14:55–66, 1961.
2. Beahrs OH, Myers MH (eds): American Joint Committee on Cancer. Manual for Staging of Cancer, 2nd ed. Philadelphia, JB Lippincott Company, 1983.
3. LeRoux-Robert J: Les Epitheliomes Intra-Larynges. Thesis. Paris, Gaston Doin et Cie, 1936.
4. Tucker GF Jr: A histological method for the study of spread of carcinoma within the larynx. Ann Otol Rhinol Laryngol 70:910, 1961.
5. Tucker GF Jr: Some clinical inferences from the study of serial laryngeal sections. Laryngoscope 73: 728–748, 1963.
6. Pittam MR, Carter RL: Framework invasion by laryngeal carcinomas. Head and Neck Surg 4(3):200–208, 1982.
7. Woodhouse RJ et al.: Treatment of carcinoma of the vocal cord. Laryngoscope 91:1155–1162, 1981.
8. Kirchner JA, Owen JR: Five hundred cancers of the larynx and pyriform sinus: Results of treatment by radiation and surgery. Laryngoscope 87:1288–1303, 1977.
9. Kirchner JA et al: Transglottic carcinoma: Its growth and spread within the larynx. Arch Otolaryngol 99:247–251, 1974.
10. Ogura JH et al.: Elective neck dissection for pharyngeal and laryngeal cancers: An evaluation. Ann Otol Rhinol Laryngol 80:646–653, 1971.
11. Biller HF et al.: Delayed contralateral cervical metastases with laryngeal and laryngopharyngeal cancers. Laryngoscope 81:1499–1502, 1971.
12. Noyek AM et al.: The radiologic diagnosis of malignant tumors of the larynx. J Otolaryngol 6:368–373, 1977.
13. Kirchner JA, Som ML: Clinical significance of fixed vocal cord. Laryngoscope 81:1029–1044, 1971.
14. Pillsbury HRC, Kirchner JA: Clinical versus histopathologic staging in laryngeal cancer. Arch Otolaryngol 105:157–159, 1979.
15. Vermund H: Role of radiotherapy in cancer of the larynx as related to the TNM system of staging. Cancer 25:485–504, 1970.
16. Baclesse F: Carcinoma of the larynx. Br J Radiol [Suppl 3]:1–62, 1949.
17. Bryce DP: The management of laryngeal cancer. J Otolaryngol 8:105–126, 1979.

18. Olofsson J et al.: Vocal cord fixation in laryngeal carcinoma. Acta Otolaryngol (Stockh) 75:496, 1973.
19. Carter RL et al.: Direct bone invasion in squamous carcinomas of the head and neck: Pathological and clinical implications. Clin Otolaryngol 5:107–116, 1980.
20. Tsao S-W et al.: Some mechanisms of local bone destruction by squamous carcinomas of the head and neck. Br J Cancer 43:392–401, 1981.
21. Kirchner JA: One hundred laryngeal cancers studied by serial section. Ann Otol Rhinol Laryngol 78:689–709, 1969.
22. Harrison DFN: The pathology and management of subglottic cancer. Ann Otol Rhinol Laryngol 80:6–12, 1971.
23. Skolnik EM et al.: Carcinoma of the laryngeal glottis. Therapy and end results. Laryngoscope 85:1453–1466, 1975.
24. Billroth T, Gussenbauer C: Ulber die Erste durch T. Billroth am Menschen ausgefuhrte Kehldopf-Extirpation und die Auswendig eines Kunstlichen Kehlkopfes. Arch Klin Chir 17:343, 1874.
25. Holinger PH: A century of progress of laryngectomies in the northern hemisphere. Laryngoscope 85:322, 1975.
26. Jackson C, Babcock W: Laryngectomy for carcinoma of the larynx. Surg Clin North Am 11:1207, 1931.
27. Crile G: Excision of cancer of the head and neck. JAMA 47:1780–1786, 1906.
28. MacFee W: Transverse incisions for neck dissections. Ann Surg 151:279–284, 1960.
29. Fee WE: Use of the Shaw scalpel in head and neck surgery. Otolaryngol Head Neck Surg 89:515–519, 1981.
30. Silver CE: Surgery for Cancer of the Larynx and Related Structures. New York, Churchill-Livingston, 1981, pp 55–81.
31. Miller D: Management of glottic carcinoma. Laryngoscope 85:1435–1439, 1975.
32. Som ML: Cordal cancer with extension to vocal process. Laryngoscope 85:1298–1307, 1975.
33. Bassett MR, Dobie RA: Patterns of nutritional deficiency in head and neck cancer. Otolaryngol Head Neck Surg 91:119–125, 1983.
34. Hooley R et al.: Predicting postoperative head and neck complications using nutritional assessment. Arch Otolaryngol 109:83–85, 1983.
35. Thawley SE: Complications of combined radiation therapy and surgery for carcinoma of the larynx and inferior hypopharynx. Laryngoscope 91:677–700, 1981.
36. Trible W: The effect of preoperative radiation or subsequent surgery in carcinoma of the larynx. Ann Otol Rhinol Laryngol 66:953–962, 1957.
37. Habel DW: Surgical complications in irradiated patients. Arch Otolaryngol 82:382–386, 1965.
38. Gall AM et al.: Complications following surgery for cancer of the larynx and hypopharynx. Cancer 39:624–631, 1977.
39. Follette WJ: Management of complications of head and neck surgery. Laryngoscope 76:1949–1970, 1966.
40. Brand B et al.: Prophylactic perioperative antibiotics in contaminated head and neck surgery. Otolaryngol Head Neck Surg 90:315–318, 1982.
41. Shumrick DA: Neck dissection. *In* Paparella MM, Shumrick DA (eds): Otolaryngology Vol 3: Head and Neck, 2nd ed. Philadelphia, WB Saunders Company, 1980, pp 2966–2986.
42. Kornblut A, Shumrick DA: Complications of head and neck surgery. Arch Otolaryngol 94:246–254, 1971.
43. Conley JJ: Carotid artery protection. Arch Otolaryngol 75:530–535, 1962.
44. Cheek HB, Rise EN: Carotid artery protection and a new technique. Arch Otolaryngol 86:73–76, 1967.
45. Goldsmith HA, Beattie EJ: Carotid artery protection by pedicle omental wrapping. Surg Gynecol Obstet 130:57–60, 1970.
46. Hillerman BL, Kennedy TL: Carotid rupture and tissue coverage. Laryngoscope 92:985–988, 1982.
47. Loré JM Jr: An Atlas of Head and Neck Surgery, Vol 2, 2nd ed. Philadelphia, WB Saunders Company, 1973.
48. Heller KS, Strong EW: Carotid arterial hemorrhage after radical head and neck surgery. Am J Surg 138:607–610, 1979.
49. Yonkers AJ, Mercurio GA: Tracheostomal stenosis following total laryngectomy. Otolaryngol Clin North Am 16:391–405, 1983.
50. Langenbrunner DJ, Chandler JR: Tracheal stoma stenosis: Causes and correction. Southern Med J 61:838–842, 1968.
51. Loewy A, Laker HI: Tracheal stomal problems. Arch Otolaryngol 87:477–483, 1968.
52. Doyle PJ, Dubeta KR: Post-laryngectomy tracheostome stenosis: Etiology and treatment. J Otolaryngol 6:284–289, 1977.
53. Keim WF et al.: Study of post laryngectomy stomal recurrences. Arch Otolaryngol 81:183–186, 1965.

20

The Theory and Technique of Near-Total Laryngectomy

Bruce W. Pearson, M.D.

Several basic principles apply to near-total laryngectomy. The patient is a candidate if a predominantly unilateral laryngeal or pyriform cancer causes one vocal cord to be fixed. The anterior portion of the opposite cord may be involved, but it must move normally and its arytenoid must be free of tumor. The laryngotomy, or entry, which is usually made through the contralateral ventricle, must be planned with precise knowledge of the extent of the cancer and the anatomy of the laryngeal muscles. The operation is designed to ablate all of the cancer but not all of the larynx. A mucosal bridge will be preserved, connecting the trachea with the pharynx over the uninvolved arytenoid. The recurrent laryngeal nerve on the nontumor side must be spared to innervate a dynamic shunt, capable of contraction on swallowing. Adequacy of the resection must be confirmed with negative histopathologic margins while the patient is on the operating table and before reconstruction. The object of the reconstruction is to build a primitive tracheopharyngeal sphincter with the laryngeal leftovers and to augment its diameter (if necessary) with a flap of mucosa from the pharynx.

Near-total laryngectomy produces a biologic prosthesis-free method of obtaining shunt speech in patients who formerly would have undergone total laryngectomy. It can be performed only at the time of the excision. It does not avoid the need for a permanent tracheotomy. There are still some laryngeal and pharyngeal cancers too large and indistinct to lend themselves to this method of surgical management. The principal advantages of near-total laryngectomy over previous surgical attempts to produce the same result are its freedom from aspiration and stenosis and the very high percentage of successful voices achieved.[1]

PREOPERATIVE CONSIDERATIONS

Near-total laryngectomy is an alternative to total laryngectomy only as long as it is onocologically safe to preserve a narrow myomucosal strip of larynx. This strip connects the trachea and the pharynx over the single uninvolved arytenoid. For this chapter, we have chosen to illustrate the operation by a case of invasive transglottic carcinoma originating in the right vocal cord.

For our example, clinical examination shows

the entire right half of the larynx to be infiltrated. The cancer is too large to be encompassed by a conventional hemilaryngectomy. Hemilaryngectomies spare the cricoid. The subglottic extension in this case is such that the cricoid cannot be preserved.

Both the right arytenoid and the anterior commissure are involved; so is the anterior aspect of the opposite vocal cord, at least superficially. Because of the extensive infiltration of the right ventricle and in view of the fixation of the right cord, the right paraglottic space is probably involved. The paraglottic space underlies the thyroid cartilage and the floor of the pyriform sinus. Therefore, a safe resection must encompass the right thyroid cartilage and the right pyriform mucosa, at least medially.

A near-total laryngectomy is designed to ablate the entire right hemilarynx, including the necessary parts of the cricoid and the anterior commissure and the front of the opposite cord. Posteriorly, it extends beyond the arytenoid to the posterior commissure. Below, it includes some trachea and the thyroid gland. Above, it includes the whole preepiglottic space, the hyoid, and the vallecula.

A careful preliminary laryngoscopy must show the posterior commissure, the left arytenoid, and the left ventricle to be free of tumor. This is important because the proposed resection would otherwise be unsafe. The posterior commissure and the left ventricle will be the margins of the resection. The mucosa over the left arytenoid, vital to the speaking shunt, will be preserved.

At the conclusion of the resection, the operator will fashion a shunt to connect the airway and the foodway. The tissues to do this must be preserved in continuity. The function of the shunt is to convey pulmonary air into the pharynx when the patient attempts exhalation

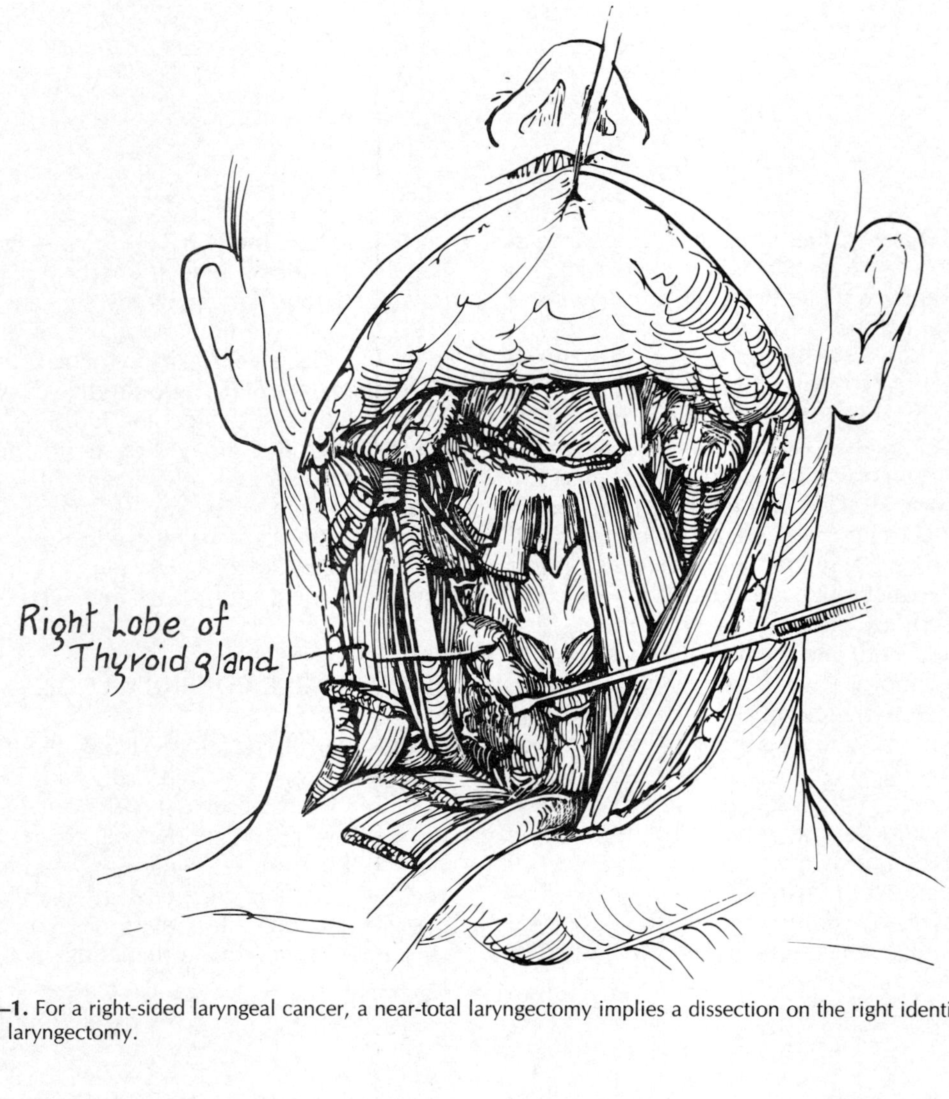

Figure 20–1. For a right-sided laryngeal cancer, a near-total laryngectomy implies a dissection on the right identical to that for a total laryngectomy.

against a closed tracheostomy. For this to occur at physiologic pressures (10 to 40 cm H_2O), a minimum diameter of 6 mm is required.[2] Sound (voice) will be automatic. It derives from passive oscillations of the shunt walls when air is forced through. This is not unlike voice production in the larynx. The sound enters the pharynx at a physiologic level, not the esophagus as in alaryngeal or puncture speech. It is punctuated by normal breaths, unlike the continuous tones of the electrolarynx. Since it is not required to rise through the esophagus and the operated pharyngoesophageal segment, as it would be in a tracheoesophageal puncture fistula, it is relatively independent of pharyngeal stenosis or substitution by a flap, for example.

Before dealing with the larynx directly, the surgeon completes adequate biopsies through the laryngoscope and obtains an unequivocal frozen-section diagnosis of invasive carcinoma. Then a tracheotomy is fashioned in the anterior tracheal wall, immediately below the thyroid isthmus. A flexible wire-spiral endotracheal tube is inserted and sutured in place.

An apron flap is raised to the mandible to expose the larynx and the right neck. Whenever cervical metastases are suspected, a neck dissection is performed. Usually the neck specimen may be detached from the field before the laryngeal surgery begins.

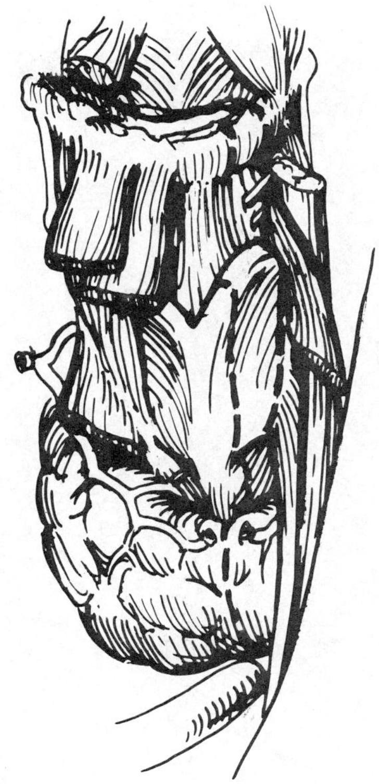

Figure 20–2. Removing segments of the hyoid bone and thyroid cartilage on the left prepares the larynx for opening. The thyroid gland is divided at this time. To expose the cricoid, the surgeon reflects left cricothyroid muscle.

TECHNIQUE OF NEAR-TOTAL LARYNGECTOMY

On the side with the cancer, the full height of the larynx is isolated (Fig. 20–1). The cricoid level is not spared. On the right (for this example), the near-total laryngectomy is anatomically identical to a wide-field total laryngectomy.

The structures divided on the right side (Fig. 20–1) include, from above downwards:

1. The suprahyoid muscles.
2. The superior laryngeal nerve.
3. The superior thyroid artery and vein.
4. The inferior pharyngeal constrictor muscle.
5. The middle thyroid vein and inferior thyroid artery.
6. The recurrent laryngeal nerve.
7. The strap muscles over the right thyroid lobe.

The technical steps that characterize near-total laryngectomy occur on the side opposite the cancer (in this case, the left) (Fig. 20–2). These steps address the following questions:

1. How should we handle the strap muscles?
2. Where should we interrupt the hyoid bone and thyroid cartilage, which inhibit access to the soft tissues of this side?
3. What should be done with the cricothyroid muscle?
4. Where can we penetrate the laryngeal lumen safely? The surgeon must jeopardize neither the tumor nor the shunt-to-be.
5. How can we obtain good visual identification of the tumor early in the sequence?

The left strap muscle layer is preserved by detaching it from the hyoid. First, the prelaryngeal fascia is opened vertically at the medial edge of the sternohyoid muscle. All median prelaryngeal soft tissues, including fascia and lymph nodes, remain with the specimen. The sternohyoid and thyrohyoid muscles are reflected to the oblique line, exposing the anterior half of the left thyroid ala. The thyroid lobe is separated from the isthmus, so that the right lobe and isthmus will also accompany the surgical specimen.

The left cricothyroid muscle should be clearly delineated. A valuable landmark to note, the cricothyroid triangle should be defined by its three borders. These are the anterior edge of

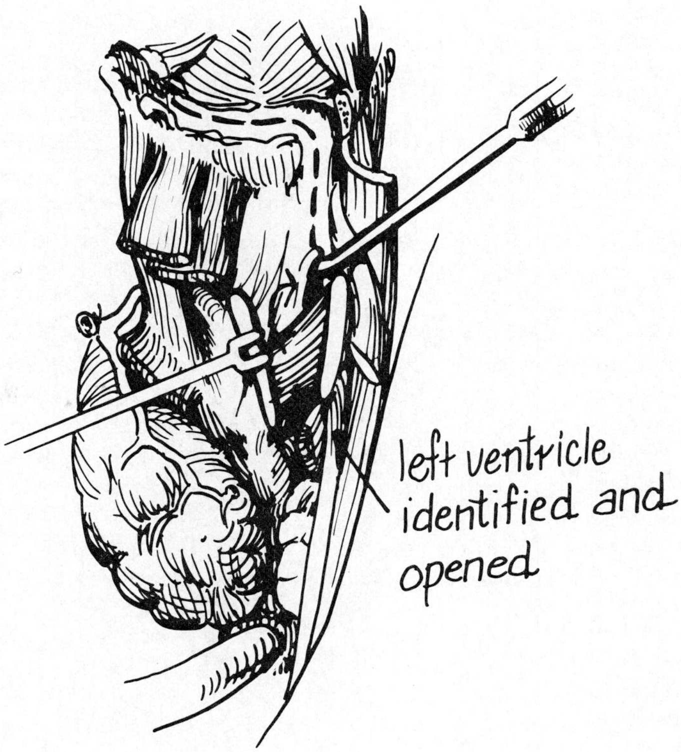

Figure 20–3. A safe left lateral laryngotomy depends on the surgeon's ability to identify and open the laryngeal saccule. The preliminary laryngoscopy has shown this to be free of cancer.

the cricothyroid muscle, the lateral edge of the cricothyroid ligament, and the inferior edge of the thyroid cartilage. At one corner is the inferior thyroid tubercle, the lower termination of the oblique line. Emanating from the triangle are several small vessels that need cautery. They join the internal laryngeal circulation to the cricothyroid vascular arcade. The left cricothyroid muscle should be freed with a scalpel and elevated clear of the cricoid.

A lateral laryngotomy is performed on the left to break the protective encasement of the hyoid bone and the thyroid cartilage (Fig. 20–3). The goal is to identify and enter the left ventricle. First, to break the hyoid arch, the anterior end of the left greater horn of the hyoid is removed with a rongeur (without breaching the preepiglottic space).

A wedge of lateral thyroid ala is removed—approximately its middle third. The lower apex of the wedge is the cricothyroid triangle. The upper base of the wedge is the thyrohyoid membrane. The cartilage of the upper third of the wedge is easily elevated and resected. The middle third is a little more difficult to elevate because some ventricular glands and thyroepiglottic muscle wisps adhere to it. The lower third is the hardest to elevate of all because it is bony and closely approximated by the main glottic musculature, the thyroarytenoid. It is important to remove the cartilage without disturbing the soft tissues in the larynx so that the deep anatomy can be recognized as soon as the wedge is removed. A curved nasal elevator, the Kazanjian forceps, and an air-driven saw are useful tools.

Now, the stage is set for opening the left ventricle. But why open here? First, the safety of the left ventricle as a site of entry into the laryngeal lumen was decided at laryngoscopy. It is known to be free of disease. Second, its anatomic reliability, based on its constant position deep to the thyroid ala and immediately superior to the thyroarytenoid muscle, maintains orientation. Third, its distensibility, once it is perforated, permits the greatest vision for the least dissection. Finally, its dispensability is known. The ventricle is never needed for reconstruction.

The outer aspect of the ventricle is vascularized by the ventral branch of the superior laryngeal artery.[3] Close inspection usually reveals a few fibers of thyroepiglottic muscle also. These fibers sweep up lateral to the saccular glands, and the periosteum is thickened where these took origin from inside the resected ala.

The anatomy of a ventricular entry should be reviewed on a cadaver before the entry is performed on a patient. Otherwise, the surgeon is tempted to enter through more familiar territory, such as the pyriform or the vallecula, or the conus elasticus. The ventricle is usually the best site of entry. It is far enough away from the cancer to be safe, yet it lies close enough to the cancer so that the elements of the shunt will not be ruined. Rarely, the vallecula may be chosen, to accommodate the case in which a supraglottic laryngectomy is still under consideration. Pyriform entries hurt the shunt and are not recommended. Conus elasticus entries limit visibility of the true cords. They may breach cancer or, more likely, sacrifice some subglottic mucosa that would best be kept for the shunt.

As soon as the ventricle is opened, the very mobile margins of this window should be distended with hooks. The inferior margin of the ventricular band, which looks like the undersurface of a miniature turbinate, should be visualized. Now, with the cut thyroid and hyoid margins also distracted with hooks, the left false cord can be divided with scissors. This is accomplished by inserting one blade through the ventriculotomy and laying the other on the lateral thyrohyoid membrane. Feeling the false cord with the inner blade, cut upwards and through it, in an upward and outward direction, trying to stay between the epiglottic and the cuneiform cartilages. As the false cord parts, the epiglottis and the lateral margins of the vallecula can be visualized. The hyoid is already cut and freed from its supraglottic musculature, so it is relatively easy to continue across the vallecula with the scissors (Fig. 20–4).

Once the false cord and vallecula are incised, the supraglottic complex is free to be drawn forward. The tumor will now be apparent, and the surgeon can study its margins under direct vision. An excellent view of the intact glottis is also obtained. Retraction places the "good side" left vocal cord on the stretch and permits the selection of a rational line of transection down through the glottis and the cricoid (Fig. 20–5).

To accomplish the division of the left cord, the tongue base is retracted with a Deaver and the epiglottis is drawn forward with an Allis. Hooks are used to help separate the remnants of the left thyroid ala. The anterior commissure and the front of the left cord are evaluated, and the body of the left true cord is divided with scissors. This division is directed down through the full height of the thyroarytenoid muscle. It continues into the conus and to the upper margin of the cricoid. From here, it continues through the cricoid arch, always maintaining an appropriate distance from the cancer. It may

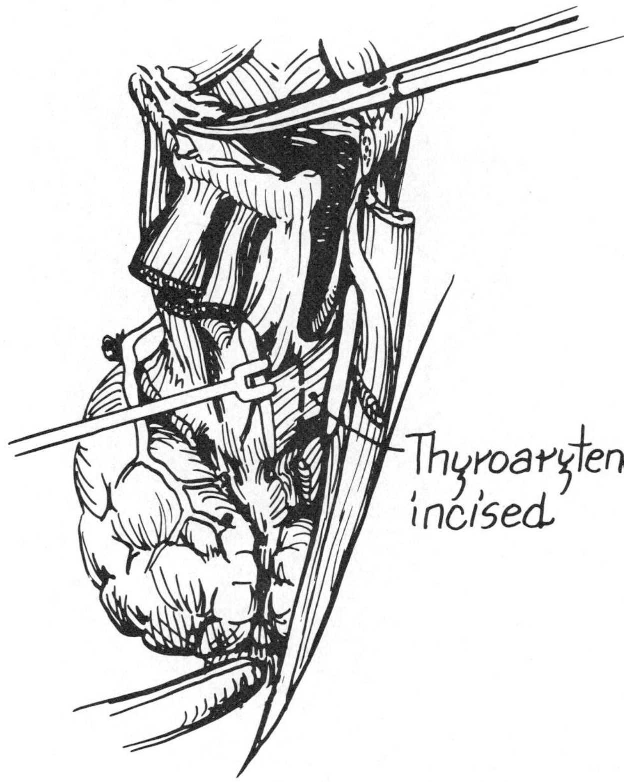

Figure 20–4. The supraglottic larynx is isolated by cutting up through the left false cord, then across the vallecula. The glottic and subglottic tissues are incised next, cutting down through the left cord and the thyroarytenoid muscle to the cricoid.

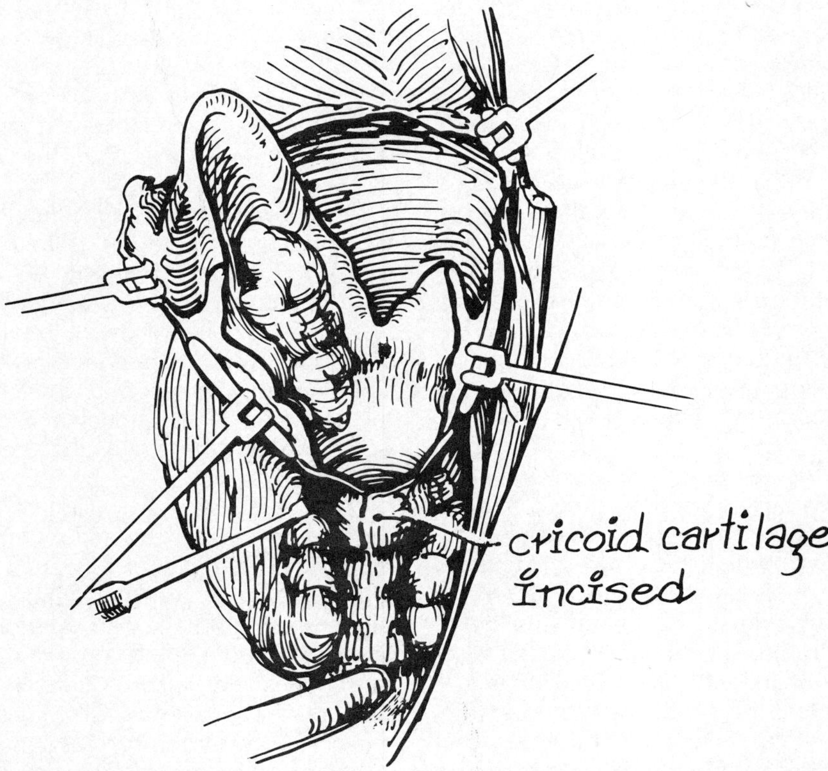

Figure 20–5. The tumor is visible, obliterating the right vocal cord, ventricle, and false cord. The laryngeal incision continues down through the cricoid and swings around through the right upper trachea, deep to the thyroid gland.

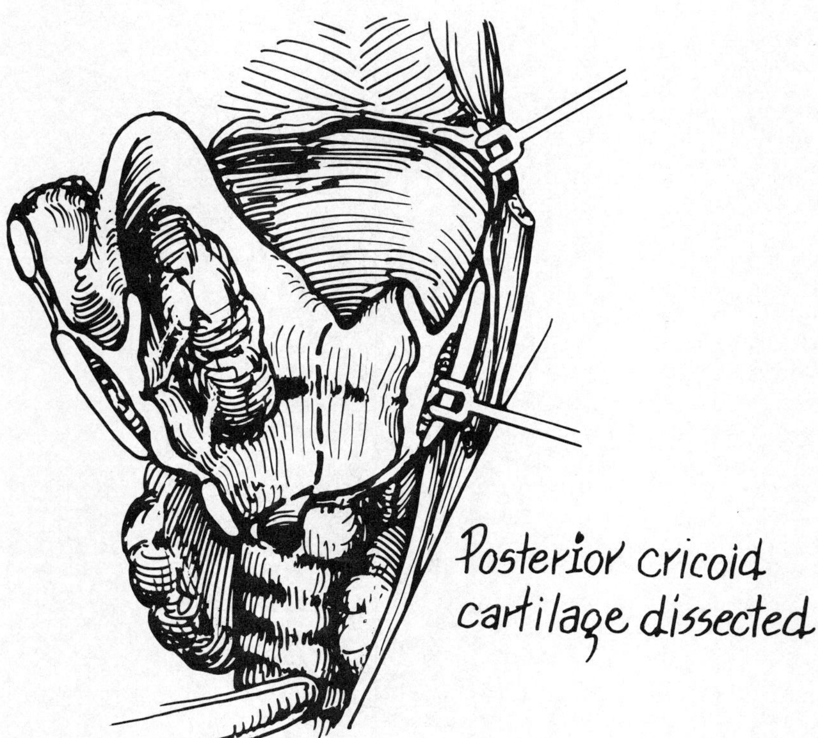

Figure 20–6. The incision is continued around inside the trachea and up the posterior cricoid plate and is kept an appropriate distance from the subglottic extension of the tumor.

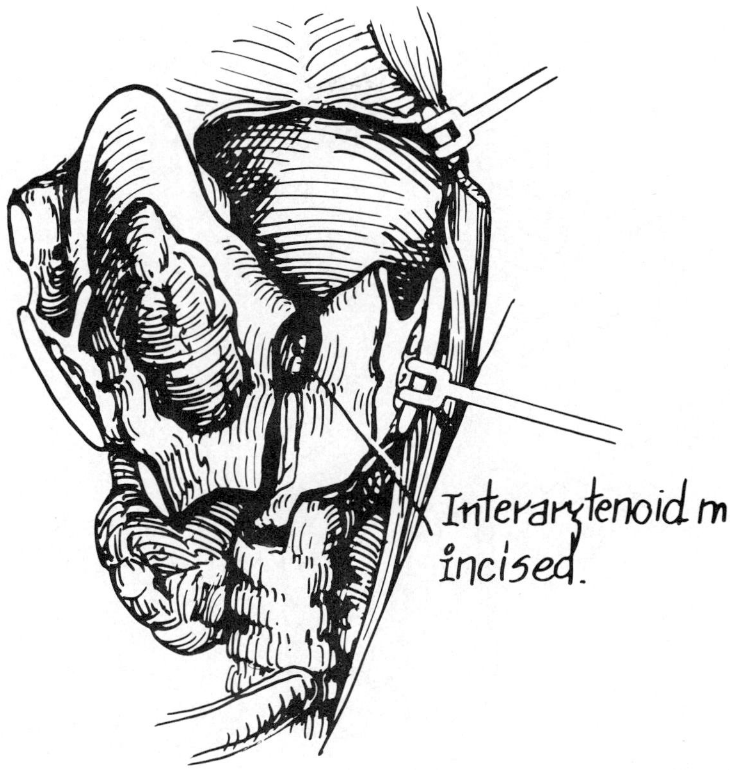

Figure 20–7. The interarytenoid muscle is cut in the midline.

even proceed into the upper trachea, if the cancer requires it. In most cases, the cricoid arch is divided obliquely in approximately the midline (Fig. 20–6).

The cricoid cartilage is a complete ring, and the incision through the anterior arch, which breaks the ring in only one place, does not allow it to be freely opened. Enough exposure can be created with hooks so that the posterior plate of the cricoid can be split with a scalpel (Fig. 20–7). The division of the posterior plate is usually made in the midline. The anterior and posterior cricoid cuts are connected through the first tracheal ring, well below cancer on the right side.

When the posterior incision passes through the anterior lamina of the posterior cricoid plate, the rest of the cricoid, which is brittle, breaks through its cancellous interior. This allows the two vertical columns of larynx (the specimen and the remnant) to be fully rotated apart. A finger is placed in the hypopharynx to elevate the posterior larynx, and the interarytenoid muscle, which is quite distinctive, is divided on the stretch. Any remnants of posterior cricoid plate are cleanly divided, and the near-total laryngectomy specimen is ready to be separated from the pharynx.

Separation between the laryngeal specimen and the pharynx is accomplished under direct vision (Fig. 20–8). All of the medial pyriform wall and as much of the lateral pyriform mucosa as is necessary will be taken with the specimen. Final delivery is achieved by dividing the right posterior cricoarytenoid fibers, the pyriform mucosa, and any remnants of the right inferior constrictor or pharyngeal wall that might still be attached to the specimen.

The tissue removed by near-total laryngectomy encompasses the entire right half of the larynx and more (Fig. 20–9). The preepiglottic space, the anterior commissure, the true and false cords and the arytenoid on the right, the prelaryngeal fascia, the right strap muscles, and the right thyroid lobe and isthmus are always included for a right-sided tumor. As much of the right hypopharynx is included as the tumor dictates. On the left (the good side), the anterior half of the membranous true cord was included with the specimen, but the left arytenoid must stay with the patient. Attached to it must be enough innervated muscle and mucosa to build a dynamic tracheopharyngeal shunt.

The basic surgical goal of near-total laryngectomy is radical excision of the tumor. This is not a conservative operation. It is designed to anticipate that the thyroid cartilage and the paraglottic space are invaded. Extralaryngeal metastases are not contraindications, of course; they are within the scope of the neck dissection

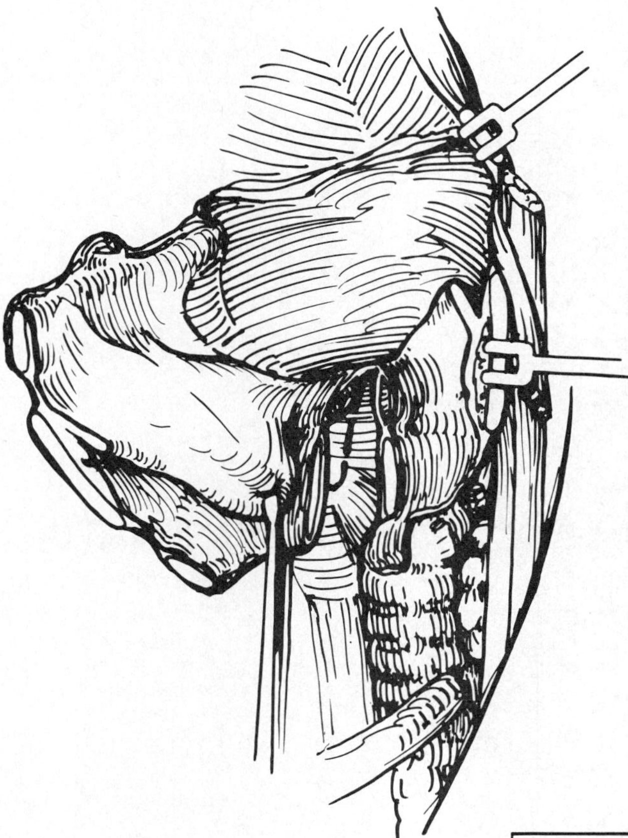

Figure 20–8. Here the epiglottis is retracted downward to permit a better view. A laryngeal specimen is cut free of the pharynx; as much right pyriform is taken as the cancer requires.

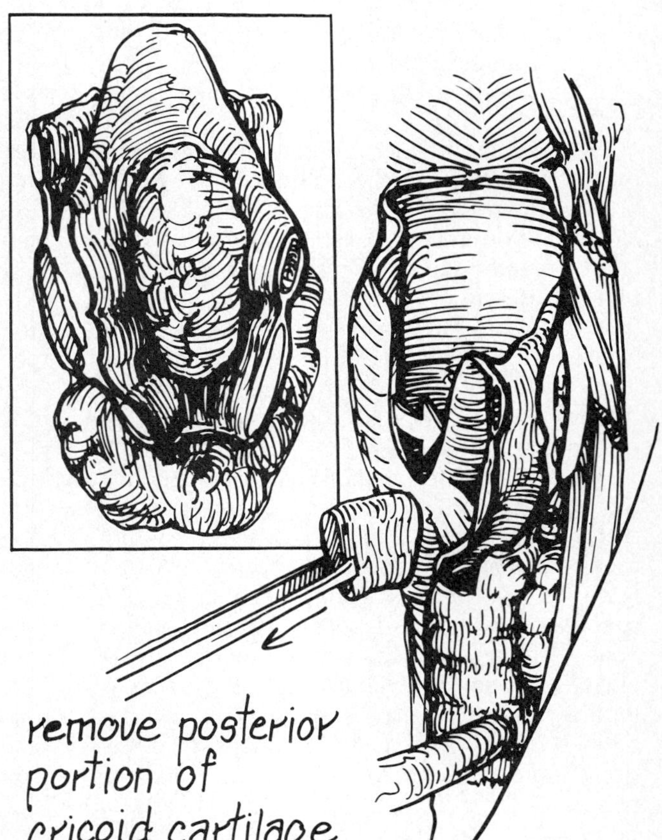

Figure 20–9. To prepare for the reconstruction, the pyriform defect is repaired. The left laryngeal remnant is rendered flaccid by removing most of its remaining cricoid cartilage. The left recurrent nerve must not be damaged.

that usually accompanies near-total laryngectomy. In practice, the near-total operation provides a surgical option that exceeds extended conventional partial operations in terms of cancer removal. On the other hand, it avoids the principal debility of total laryngectomy, which is loss of the voice. The fact that a voice is reliably attained rests on preservation of the mucosal continuity between the airway and the foodway over the uninvolved arytenoid.

To maintain this mucosal continuity free of aspiration requires the construction of a primitive sphincter. This begins while the pathologist confirms the specimen margins. To construct an effective speaking shunt, the surgeon wants a flaccid laryngeal remnant, which can be rolled into a tube. But the strip of tissue connecting the trachea and the pharynx (i.e., the residual left larynx) is too rigid.

Flaccidity is achieved by submucosal resection of the residual cricoid cartilage (Fig. 20–9). Anteriorly, cartilage is removed piecemeal, leaving the subglottic mucosa inside and the cricothyroid muscle outside. The removal is carried back as far as the cricothyroid joint. It is not necessary to proceed further, and it is probably unwise to do so because of the danger to the left recurrent laryngeal nerve. Posteriorly, in the midline, an additional strip of cricoid plate should be resected between the laryngeal subglottis and the pharyngeal postcricoid tissues. At the conclusion of these resections, the only portion of cricoid remaining is a small remnant adjacent to the left cricothyroid joint in the vicinity of the recurrent laryngeal nerve. The remaining arytenoid sits atop this remnant.

Once flaccidity is achieved and the margins are reported negative, the all-important diameter of the speaking shunt is adjusted.[4] A small flap of mucosa from the hypopharynx is usually employed (Fig. 20–10). The projected diameter of the speaking shunt is 6 mm. If the larynx is that of a large man or if the tumor is pyriform and none of the left vocal cord has been taken, a 6 mm diameter may be achievable without pharyngeal flap augmentation. In most cases, however, there is not enough larynx remaining and augmentation is required.

Because the right pyriform fossa has been removed, it is first necessary to repair the pharyngeal defect up to the level of the left arytenoid (Fig. 20–9). Then the augmentation flap can be cut from high in the right hypopharynx and folded down to lie alongside the residual larynx. By sewing the flap to the residual larynx along its interarytenoid and posterior midline borders, the surgeon can increase the total amount of epithelium available for tubing, particularly at the narrowest (glottic) level (Fig. 20–10).

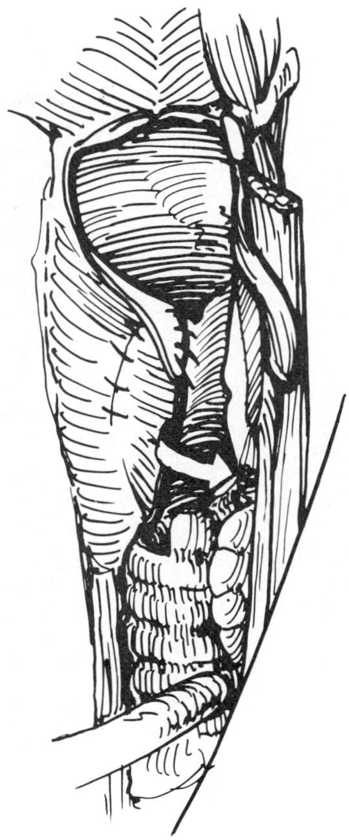

Figure 20–10. The myomucosal laryngeal remnant is tubed on itself. Note the flap from the pharynx, which is necessary to augment the tube when laryngeal mucosa is insufficient.

To prevent aspiration, we must avoid making the pharyngeal flap too wide. Only the laryngeal component of the shunt will be dynamic, and this is what we rely upon to prevent aspiration. It is also important to avoid making the base of the flap too low. The lip of the shunt is expected to lie at the level of the arytenoid, another factor in rendering the shunt resistant to saliva.

Several factors should be stressed to gain consistency in preventing aspiration. In the course of the resection, the left superior laryngeal nerve has not been destroyed, so the residual arytenoid retains sensory innervation and the cricothyroid muscle remains active. The left thyroid lobe has not been mobilized and the left recurrent laryngeal nerve remains undisturbed. Despite the loss of half the left vocal cord, most of the muscle bulk innervated by the left recurrent nerve has been preserved

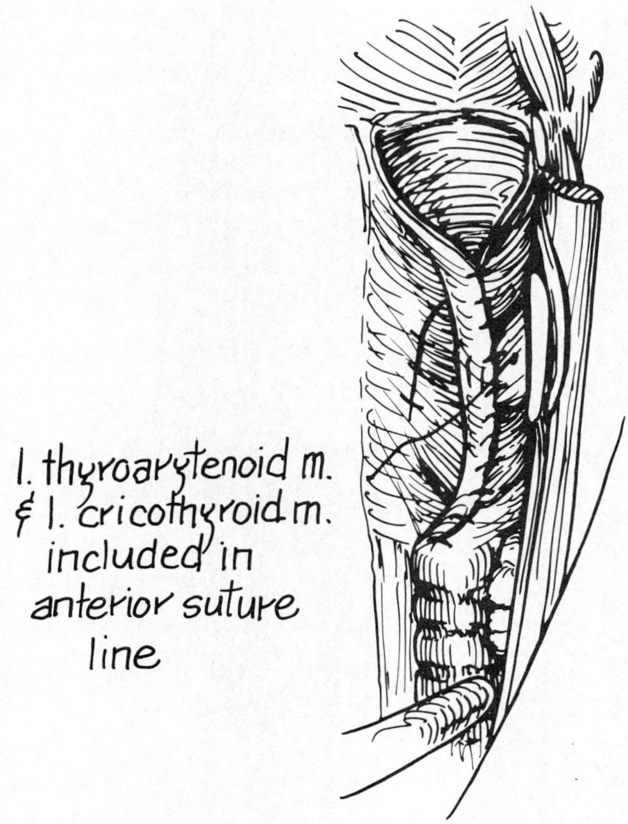

Figure 20–11. The laryngeal remnant has been tubed to make a dynamic tracheopharyngeal shunt.

(and not cauterized). Only the anterior fibers of the vocalis and thyroarytenoid muscles went with the specimen. The left lateral cricoarytenoid, posterior cricoarytenoid, and significant portions of the interarytenoid and thyroarytenoid muscles remain. By tailoring the resection to the tumor, the surgeon insured that no subglottic or upper tracheal mucosa was discarded unnecessarily. Thus the tube is dome-shaped below. Finally, the strap muscles on the left retain their innervation and their integrity. When they are sewn later to the suprahyoid musculature, they will help telescope the shunt upwards during deglutition.

Starting at the trachea, the shunt mucosa is tubed (Fig. 20–11). The seam of the tube is completed up to the level of the pharynx with 2–0 chromic catgut. To measure the diameter of the tube, the surgeon passes a No. 14 French catheter from the tracheostoma up into the pharynx. This is never left in place because the tube's epithelial continuity is enough to assure a patent shunt. A stent might cause epithelial necrosis if it were left in place; this would precipitate the very stenosis it was employed to avoid.

The pharyngotomy is closed transversely, or in a T, just as it would be in a total laryngec-

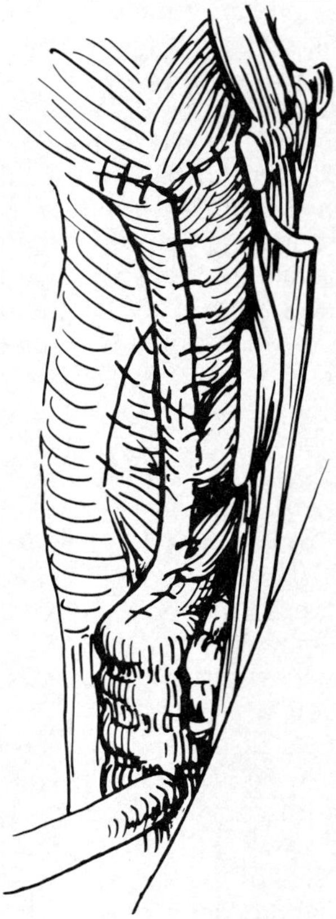

Figure 20–12. The pharyngotomy is closed in the usual fashion.

tomy (Fig. 20–12). The left strap muscles, which were reflected from the hyoid earlier, are now drawn across the upper closure and approximated to the suprahyoid muscles (Fig. 20–13). This reinforces the upper pharyngeal mucosal closure, but it may also be important to swallowing. The thyrohyoid muscle is still innervated and connected to the residual left thyroid ala. This ought to assure some elevation of the remaining pyriform fossa and a telescopic foreshortening of the shunt during deglutition.

Breathing after near-total laryngectomy will depend upon a permanent tracheostomy. This is an anterior tracheal wall stoma, not the end-on stoma of a total laryngectomy. Special attention should be paid to the creation of the stoma to minimize the prospect of contraction. The opening in the skin should be approximated to the opening in the anterior tracheal wall with 0 nylon sutures. These are simple sutures with respect to the tracheal wall and catch an entire tracheal ring. They are vertical mattress sutures with respect to the skin. Thus they gather skin over the edges of the tracheal opening so that no bare cartilage remains exposed.

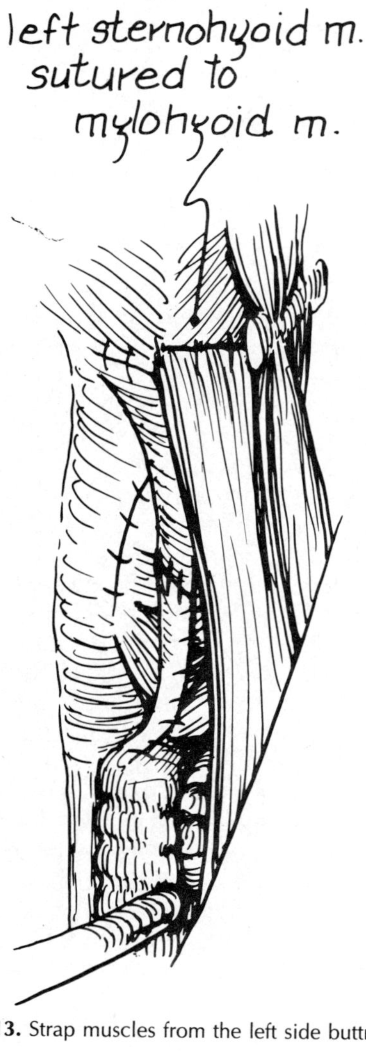

Figure 20–13. Strap muscles from the left side buttress the closure.

The neck wound is thoroughly irrigated, closed in layers, and drained (Fig. 20–14).

The early postoperative management is similar to that of a total laryngectomy. The speaking shunt is not a factor during the first week or two. It is closed by the swelling and its use is not encouraged or expected. Until the swelling decreases, tracheotomy self-care is well established, and the stoma is adequately healed, the shunt rests unused. In the early weeks, premature valving of the stoma by the patient attempting to speak simply inflames the healing of the stoma itself and complicates the overall rehabilitation. Our practice is to defer valving and speech until the first postoperative visit, at which time a comprehensive program of support is resumed.

DISCUSSION

Near-total laryngectomy fills a gap in our surgical approach to cancer of the larynx. In the range of previous surgical treatments, we have employed two general categories of operation—those that preserve voice and nasal breathing, and those that eliminate vocal function and require a tracheotomy. The former category includes laryngoscopic cordectomy, thyrotomy and cordectomy, vertical hemilaryngectomy, and supraglottic laryngectomy. The latter group consists of total laryngectomy and laryngopharyngectomy.

Near-total laryngectomy is perhaps the missing link between these two categories. Like the former group, it preserves the voice; like the latter, it sacrifices nasal respiration. No longer are we tempted to stretch the indications for hemilaryngectomy, risking recurrence to save the voice. The same may be said for cases in which we stretched the indications for supraglottic laryngectomy and risked aspiration to save the voice. Radical radiation and surgical salvage saved a few voices but at a greater overall cost with respect to life.[5] Near-total laryngectomy extricates us from the dilemma of surgical and radiotherapeutic brinkmanship in an effort to spare voice. At the time, we avoid the major drawback of total laryngectomy, loss of the voice. The price is a permanent tracheotomy. Therefore, this operation in no way competes for cases in which a conven-

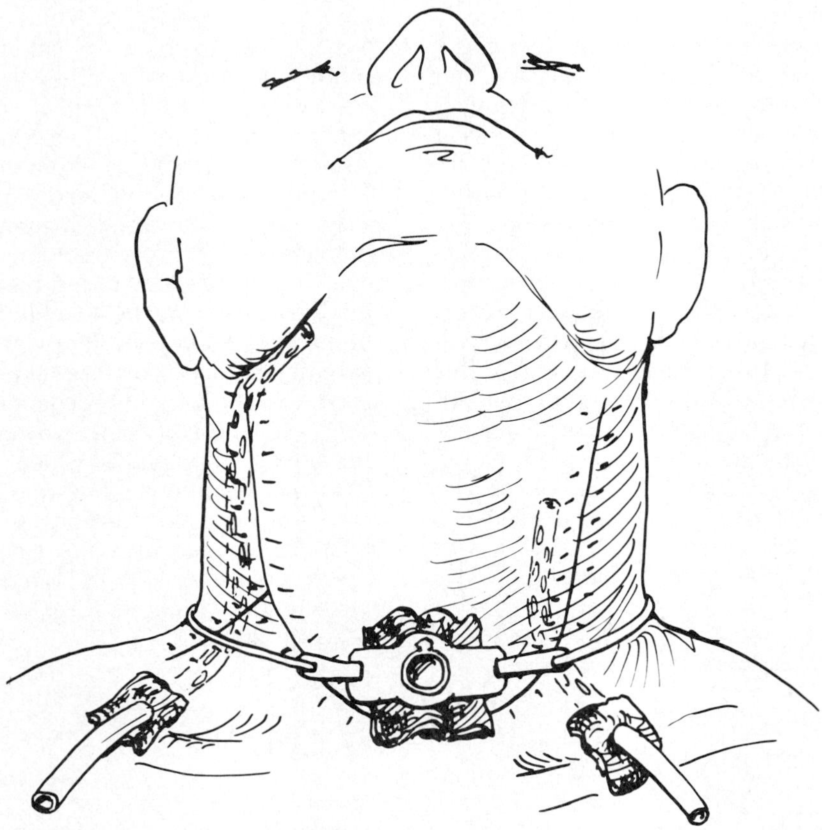

Figure 20–14. This closure is typical of the case in which a right neck dissection has also been performed.

tional partial laryngectomy is properly indicated. The indication for near-total laryngectomy is simply vocal cord fixation by cancer.

We have recently used the principle of near-total laryngectomy in cases in which the lateral and posterior extent of the tumor required pharyngeal reconstruction with a myocutaneous flap. Near-total laryngectomy and a shunt are eminently suitable as long as at least the pyriform fossa, into which the shunt connects, can be preserved.

The contraindication to near-total laryngectomy is interarytenoid involvement by cancer, such as might be seen in a postcricoid lesion or in pyriform carcinoma spreading to the interarytenoid region.

If vocal preservation is the object, we may well ask if the patient suitable for a near-total laryngectomy wouldn't be just as well off with a total laryngectomy, followed by a tracheoesophageal puncture and prosthetic valve.[6] A puncture and prosthesis is probably the best strategy after an oncologically necessary total laryngectomy; however, there are drawbacks. Puncture speech requires a second operation. The shunts popularized by Singer and Blom, Pange, and others enter the esophagus, so the voice must be generated by the pharyngoesophageal segment. The pharyngoesophageal segment is sometimes unsuited to this purpose, occasionally requiring a tertiary operation (myotomy). The principal deficiency is the dependence on a prosthesis. Not all patients are able to maintain a device. Inevitably, some do not possess the attitudes or the dexterity required for reinsertion and cleaning. The fistula is sometimes difficult to maintain, thus being abandoned or lost. Over the long haul, the prosthesis itself must be prescribed, fitted, and replaced with regularity as it ages. In the final analysis, dependence on a prosthesis requires the patient to assimilate its complexities. The near-total laryngectomy places the burden for managing complexities on the doctor. The biologic bridge between the airway and the foodway (the strip of mucosa we save) should not be discarded because a prosthetic replacement is feasible. It should only be sacrificed if oncologically necessary.

Although some patients will develop speech

after near-total laryngectomy without special instruction, none should fail to receive the services of a qualified speech pathologist. Patients learn what to expect at a preoperative interview, which provides important reassurance in the postoperative period. Later they learn how to initiate air flow. When speech does begin, many patients magnify their preoperative articulation errors and have a tendency to speak too rapidly. The speech therapist helps them to improve their articulation and valving. He or she can train them to slow their rate. Phonation is frequently improved by relaxation, proper phrasing, and attention to the elimination of stomal noise.

In the early months, valving is achieved with a finger to the stoma. Some patients must be taught which is the best finger to use and how to release for breathing. Ultimately, some patients can be fitted with the tracheostomal valve designed by Singer and Blom[7] to obviate the use of the hand.

So far, near-total laryngectomy has been described in the context of the unirradiated patient. Patients who fail radiation given for primary T3 laryngeal cancer probably are not candidates for near-total laryngectomy. Patients who began with T1 lesions, subsequently failing radiation and presenting with cord fixation (progression to T3), are different. For them, near-total laryngectomy may offer a surgical option that preserves the voice. Whenever confronted with radiation failure, surgeons must bear in mind the unpredictability of spread of the recurrent tumor. Near-total laryngectomy was designed for cancers behaving in their usual manner, the manner that has been demonstrated so well by numerous studies on whole organ serial sections of the larynx after total laryngectomy.[8]

RESULTS

The type of result to be expected from near-total laryngectomy may be appreciated from our first 33 cases (Table 20–1). With a mean follow-up of 22 months, we saw no local recurrences of cancer. Four patients died, one of pulmonary metastases without local recurrence and three of unrelated problems (two myocardial infarctions without evidence of disease and one pleural mesothelioma without evidence of disease). In three patients, cancer has recurred in the contralateral neck at six months, one year, and three years. Over two-thirds of the patients reported have had neck

Table 20–1. EXPERIENCE WITH NEAR-TOTAL LARYNGECTOMY

	Number of Patients
Total patients	33
Surviving patients	30
Using shunt for voice	30
Local recurrence of cancer*	0
Causes of death	
Myocardial infarct, NED.	1
Pleural mesothelioma, NED.	1
Multiple pulmonary metastases	1
Lesions	
T3 Glottic and transglottic	14
T3 Supraglottic	7
T3 Subglottic	2
Pyriform, aryepiglottic fold	10
Additional treatment	
Neck dissection	23
Preop. radiation	5
Postop. radiation	4
Aspiration	
None	23
Asymptomatic bubble	6
Caused cough†	2
Caused lung complication	0
Complications	
Pharyngocutaneous fistula	3
Stomal complications	2
Shunt complications	4
Cervical wound infection	1
Cerebrovascular accident	1

*Follow-up: mean, 22 months; longest, 88 months
†Successfully revised by endoscopy

dissections. Five patients had failed previous radiation and four received radiation postoperatively (for pyriform carcinomas with multiple postive neck nodes).

Our complications have been similar to those found for other patients with total laryngectomies and neck dissections. Three patients developed pharyngocutaneous fistulas, which eventually healed. Shunt complications arose in four patients; miscellaneous neck and stoma complications developed in four more. We assessed aspiration at six months postoperatively in all patients, finding none at all in 23. Significant aspiration occurred in two and minor degrees of aspiration were demonstrated in the remaining eight patients.

The two patients with significant aspiration deserve special mention. One suffered a complete wound disruption postoperatively and the other had a partial disruption. Both have undergone revision operations to arrest their aspiration. We have preserved the shunt and produced voice with satisfactory swallow. In both cases, the pathology was interesting. A breakdown had occurred between the seam of the speaking shunt and the opposing vertical closure seam in the lower hypopharynx. Thus, a side wall shunt-to-pharynx cleft had resulted. Meticulous attention to pharyngeal closure is recommended to avoid this complication, which appears to be a particular risk in irradiated patients with extensive resections for pyriform fossa cancer.

CONCLUSION

Near-total laryngectomy provides the surest and simplest way for vocal rehabilitation after surgery for lesions that fix the vocal cord. This procedure does not replace total laryngectomy, but it significantly reduces the indications for this and for extended conventional subtotal operations. Although it produces a speaking fistula, near-total laryngectomy is primarily a method of excision. The reconstruction is an obvious consequence of the desire to produce a predictable, dynamic, nonaspirating, tracheopharyngeal shunt in the simplest and most expeditious manner.

References

1. Pearson BW: Subtotal laryngectomy. Laryngoscope 91:1904–1911, 1981.
2. Woods RD, Pearson BW: Alaryngeal speech and the development of an internal tracheopharyngeal fistula. Otolaryngol Head Neck Surg 88:64–73, 1980.
3. Pearson BW: Laryngeal microcirculation and pathways of cancer spread. Laryngoscope 85:700–713, 1975.
4. Pearson BW et al.: Extended hemilaryngectomy for T_3 glottic carcinoma with preservation of speech and swallowing. Laryngoscope 90:1950–1961, 1980.
5. DeSanto LW, Pearson BW: Initial treatment of laryngeal cancer: Principles of selection. Minn Med 64:691–698, 1981.
6. Singer MI, Blom ED: An endoscopic technique for restoration of voice after laryngectomy. Ann Otol Rhinol Laryngol 89:529–533, 1980.
7. Blom ED et al.: Tracheostoma valve for postlaryngectomy voice rehabilitation. Ann Otol Rhinol Laryngol 91:576–578, 1982.
8. Van Nostrand AWP, Brodarec I: Laryngeal carcinoma—Modifications in surgical technique based on our understanding of tumor growth characteristics. J Otolaryngol 11:186–190, 1982.

21

Procedures for Voice Production After Laryngectomy

Thomas C. Calcaterra, M.D.

Since the first total laryngectomy by Theodor Billroth 100 years ago, surgeons have been concerned with the reconstruction of a vocal mechanism. It was known as early as 1874 that intelligible speech could be restored, provided that an air communication could be established between the trachea and pharynx.[1] Many different methods of constructing a partial or complete union of the upper airway and the alimentary tract have been described. These methods are based almost exclusively on the principle that air shunted from the pulmonary system to the pharynx or esophagus will produce vibration of the local tissues and that a tone sufficient for audible speech can thereby be generated.

The voice produced is similar in quality to esophageal speech but is much better controlled and provides more words per phrase. This is because the vibrating air stream is produced by pulmonary exhalation, as in normal speech, rather than by the air-gulping method of esophageal speech. In addition, the new voice technique can be learned almost immediately. It does not require the prolonged training with a speech therapist that is usually necessary for most candidates learning esophageal speech.

Although in the normal larynx the airway and the alimentary tract are conjoined at the level of the hypopharynx, aspiration is prevented during deglutition by a series of neuromuscular reflexes. These include a three-tiered sphincteric mechanism within the larynx and anterior laryngeal ascent effected by the hyoid musculature.[2] Obviously, these protective mechanisms are lost after total laryngectomy, and aspiration becomes a formidable problem when an attempt is made to reunite the airway with the alimentary tract for speech rehabilitation.

UNLINED FISTULA WITH AN INTERNAL PROSTHESIS

The earliest attempt to restore speech after total laryngectomy was described by Gussenbauer, who was a student of Billroth.[1] He constructed an unlined tunnel to the pharynx and inserted a modified Y-shaped tracheostomy tube with the upper tube extending into the pharynx (Fig. 21–1). During swallowing, an obturator was placed into the pharyngeal extension to prevent aspiration. The sound source was a reed located at the stomal end of the tracheostomy tube. As with most exposed pros-

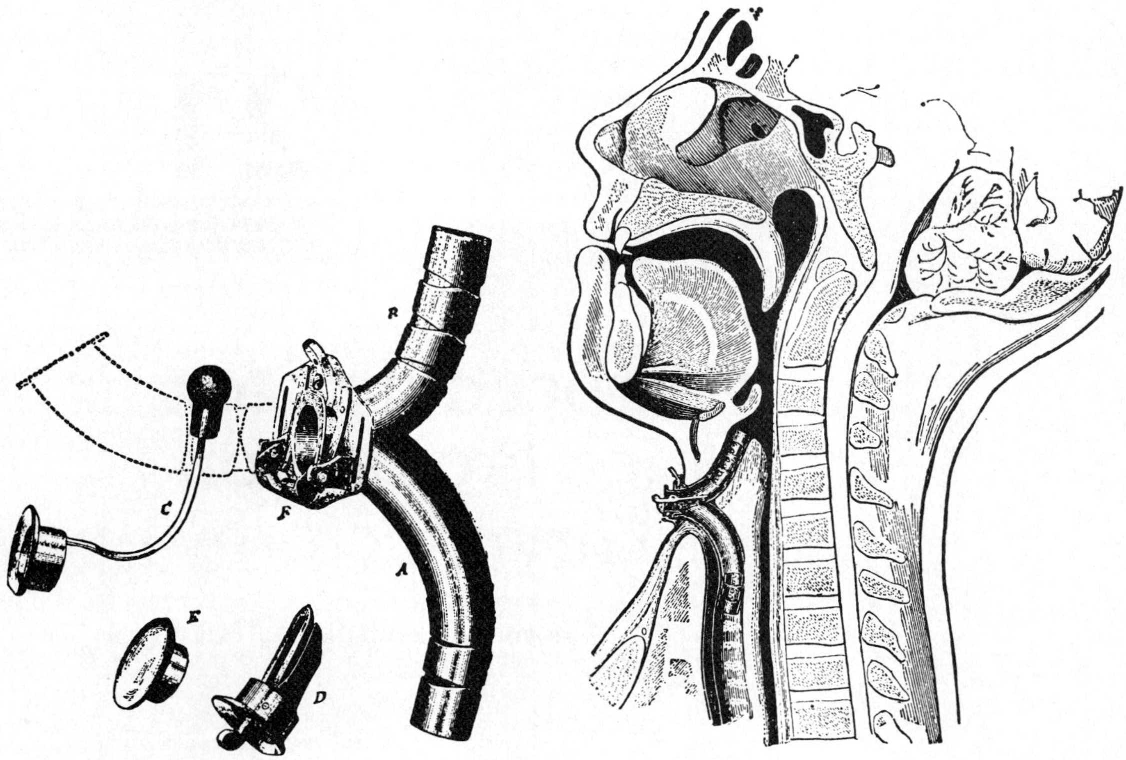

GUSSENBAUER'S ARTIFICIAL LARYNX. ARTIFICIAL LARYNX IN POSITION.

Figure 21–1. Metallic prosthesis with the upper tube inserted into the pharynx through an unlined fistula. (From Barton RT: Proc VIII Int Congr Oto-Rhino-Laryngol. 1965. Amsterdam, Excerpta Medica Foundation, 1966, p 731.)

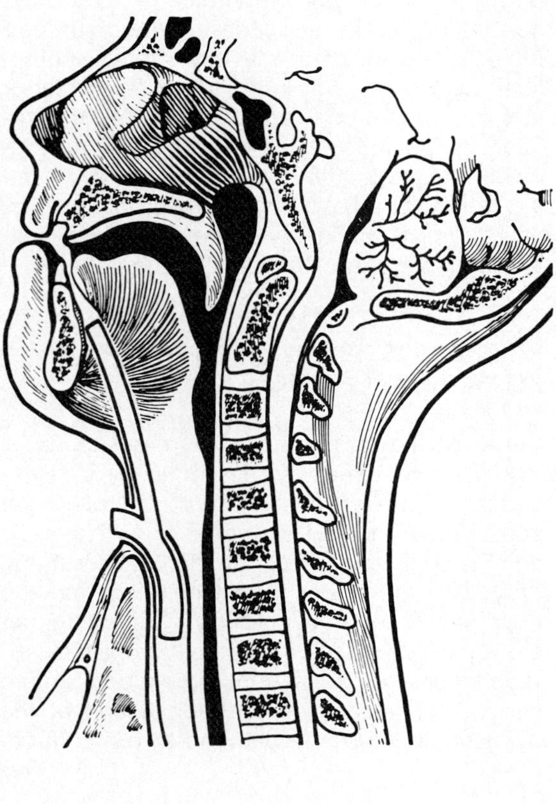

Figure 21–2. Silicone prosthesis with the upper extension opening into the floor of the mouth. (From Barton RT: Proc VIII Int Congr Oto-Rhino-Laryngol. 1965. Amsterdam, Excerpta Medica Foundation, 1966, p 734.)

thetic implants, the problems of poor tissue tolerance, leakage around the prosthesis, and stenosis upon removal were never overcome.

In 1965, Barton[3] described two innovative internal prostheses inserted through an unlined fistula. The first utilized an indwelling esophageal tube attached to a tracheostomy tube with a speaking valve. Expired air passed into the cervical esophageal tube and out through the mouth and nose. Aspiration was minimized by the upward angle of the connecting channel from the esophageal tube to the tracheostomy tube. This device required frequent cleaning by a physician.

The second prosthesis employed a silicone T-tube implanted under the skin and leading from the tracheostoma to an opening under the tongue (Fig. 21–2). Aspiration was prevented by having the patient cover the opening with his tongue while swallowing. No long-term follow-up was reported.

CERVICAL SKIN TUBE WITH AN EXTERNAL PROSTHESIS

Construction of a phonatory tunnel with local tissue was first described in 1952 by Briani,[4] who tubed and anastomosed to an anterior pharyngotomy (Fig. 21–3) a flap of anterior cervical skin pedicled superiorly. This fistulous tract was fitted with a device to shunt air from the tracheostoma to the hypopharynx for voice production.

MUCOUS MEMBRANE OR VEIN TUNNEL WITH A PROSTHESIS

In 1958, Conley[5] devised a tunnel of esophageal mucosa that excluded the muscular layer and opened either just above the tracheostoma or in the posterior wall of the trachea (Figs. 21–4 and 21–5). This tunnel received a special air outlet device attached to the tracheostomy tube. Conley believed that aspiration would be prevented by the air inlet being higher than the esophageal opening; this gravitational advantage was augmented by a sling of omohyoid muscle used to suspend the superior portion of the tunnel. Further, the shunt could collapse during swallowing. He later modified this operation and implanted an autogenous vein graft to connect the skin of the neck just above the tracheostoma with the lower portion of the cervical esophagus.[6] The vein graft was inserted by a specially adapted trocar and could be placed either at the time of laryngectomy or at a secondary procedure.

The sound source with this technique is the vibrating cervical esophagus; thus, the speech resembles conventional esophageal speech in quality. Comprehensive speech analysis indicated that approximately 98 per cent of the sentences spoken by the patients could be understood, a level of speech intelligibility that can be achieved by only a small percentage of esophageal speakers using the conventional gulping techniques.

Although aspiration was minimal, the most

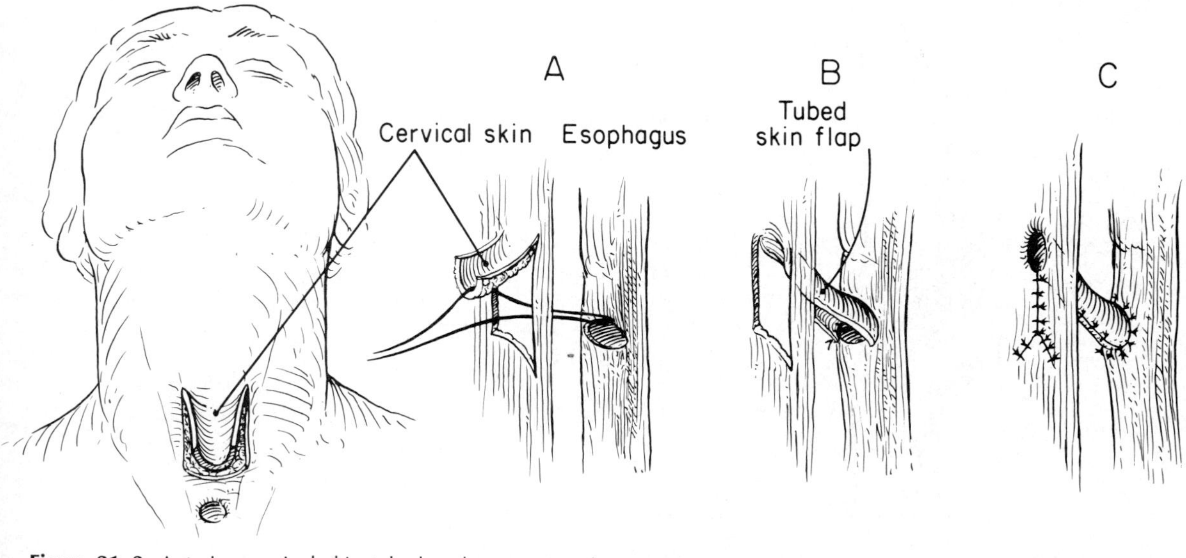

Figure 21–3. Anterior cervical skin tubed and anastomosed to an opening in the esophagus. (Adapted from Conley JJ: Trans Am Acad Ophthalmol Otolaryngol 73:288, 1969.)

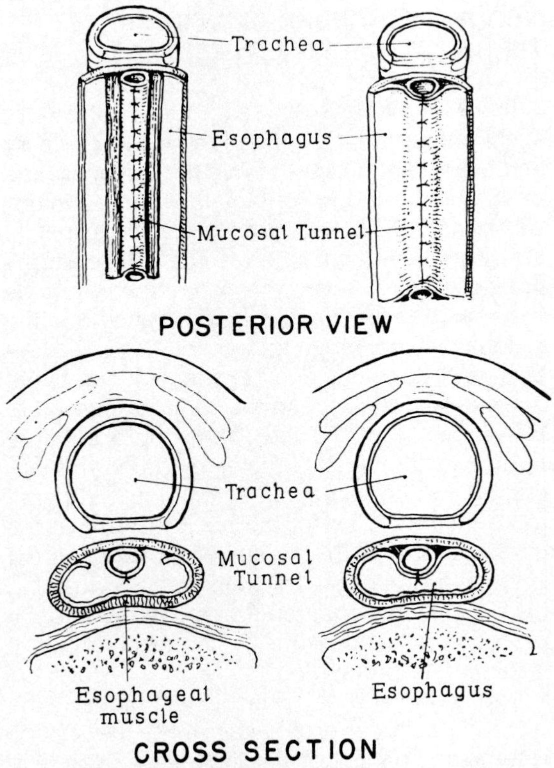

Figure 21–4. A mucous membrane tunnel fashioned from the esophagus. (From Conley JJ et al.: Ann Otol Rhinol Laryngol 67:655, 1958.)

distressing complication of this operation was the continual predisposition toward stenosis; it was necessary to maintain a small plastic catheter to maintain patency. If the patient allowed the catheter to dislodge, it was generally impossible to recannulate the tunnel.

CERVICAL SKIN TUBE WITHOUT A PROSTHESIS

Problems with indwelling prostheses and stenosis of the various fistulous tracts stimulated the search for other methods of channeling expired air to the pharynx. In 1960, Asai[7] described a method of vocal rehabilitation after laryngectomy that employed a buried cervical skin tube to connect the tracheostoma with a small pharyngostoma. This was originally described as a three-stage operation and was popularized in this country by Miller[8] (Fig. 21–6).

The first stage is ordinarily initiated at the end of a total laryngectomy. The upper end of the trachea serves as the opening for the air tunnel, which is sutured to the anterior cervical skin about 2 cm above the permanent trach-

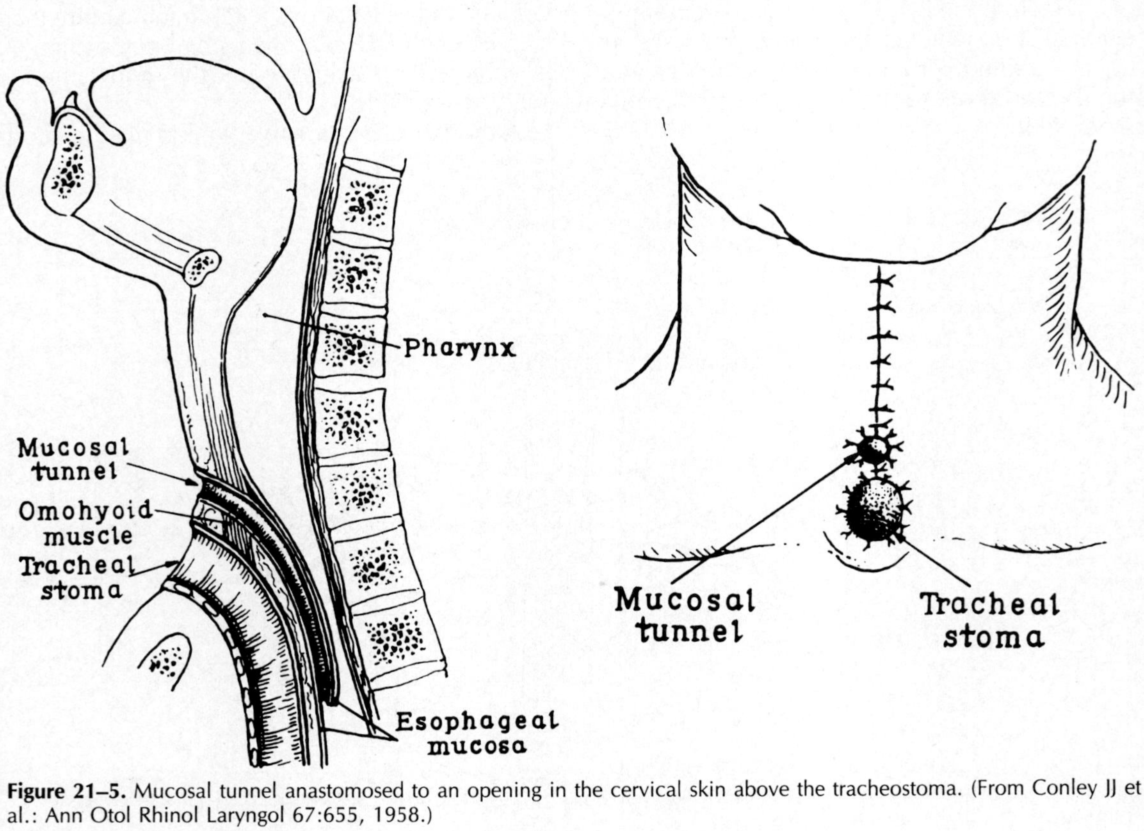

Figure 21–5. Mucosal tunnel anastomosed to an opening in the cervical skin above the tracheostoma. (From Conley JJ et al.: Ann Otol Rhinol Laryngol 67:655, 1958.)

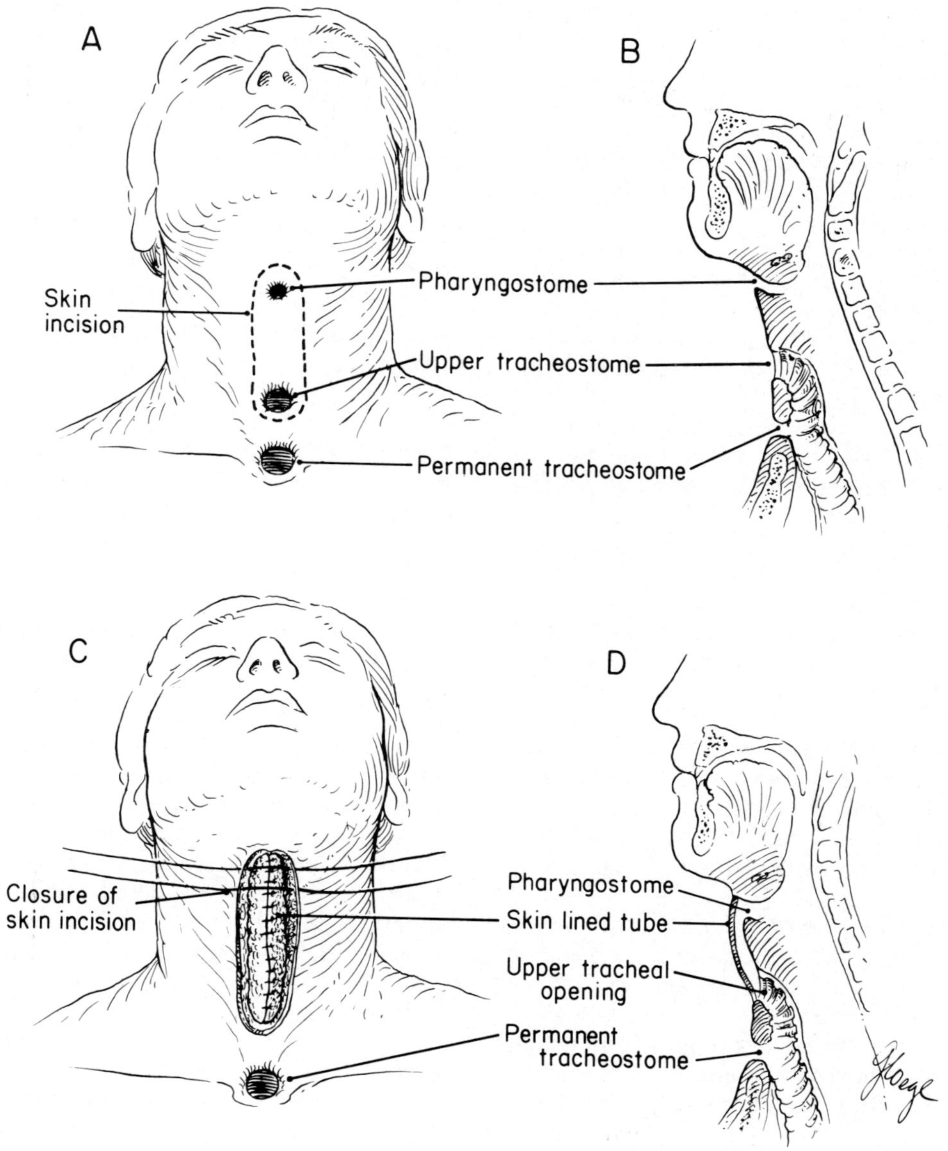

Figure 21–6. Three-stage operation employing a buried skin tube. *A* and *B*, Completion of both the first stage (upper tracheostoma) and the second stage (pharyngostoma). *C* and *D*, Completion of the third stage with skin tube buried. (Modified from Asai R: Arch Otolaryngol 95:114, 1972.)

eostoma constructed through the fourth or fifth tracheal ring.

The second stage is the creation of a small cervical fistula into the pharynx just under the base of the tongue. The surgeon attempts to incline this fistula inferiorly from the cutaneous opening to reduce salivary leakage and performs a skin-to-mucous-membrane anastomosis to prevent stenosis.

The third stage is the construction of a cervical skin tube that connects the pharyngostoma with the upper tracheal opening. The tube is formed by means of vertical incisions on each side of the midline of the neck, sized to allow an inside diameter of 2.5 cm. These incisions are joined above the pharyngeal stoma and below the tracheal stoma. The cut edges of this skin island are approximated with fine sutures, and the remaining cut edges are undermined and closed vertically in the midline, burying the skin tube.

The patient speaks by placing his finger over the permanent tracheostoma and exhaling. Expired air passes through the skin tube to the hypopharynx. Although the cervical esophagus has been documented as the sound source for conventional esophageal speech, both Asai[9] and Miller[10] deny that this anatomic area is the sound-producing focus for this operation. Asai believes the vibrating sound source to be the pharyngostoma. He has demonstrated support for this belief both by cineradiography and indirect mirror examination. He notes the voice to be louder and lower pitched with a wider pharyngostoma and softer and higher pitched with a smaller pharyngostoma. Miller states that the midportion of the skin tube is the site of maximum vibration.

Both authors found the speech to be highly intelligible. Although the potential pitch range is narrow, most patients are able to change pitch by varying expiratory air pressure and by altering tension of the tongue and pharynx musculature.

The results of three large series of patients are generally favorable. Miller reviewed 30 patients, Asai 72 patients, and Minnigerode 24 patients; all reported good voices in at least two-thirds of patients. None of the authors provided information regarding the long-term success of this speaking method.

Because the larynx is usually amputated just below the cricoid, the operation is considered to be contraindicated in the presence of substantial extension of subglottic cancer. When cervical skin has received high doses of irradiation, the skin tube often heals poorly. The bridge of skin between the two tracheal stomas may be easily jeopardized by previous irradiation, diabetes, or tissue handling that is not delicate.

The major late complication is aspiration, which can be sufficiently severe as to cause aspiration pneumonia. Most patients must compress the buried skin tube while swallowing, either manually or with an elastic bandage around the neck. Miller stated that aspiration can be reduced by placing the pharyngostoma beneath a ledge of the tongue. Schulthess[11] created this ledge or pseudoepiglottis with a pedicled cervical skin flap inverted into the pharynx above the pharyngostoma.

Another shortcoming of this operation is the frequent requirement of a permanent tracheostomy tube as a consequence of the stenotic tendency of the lower tracheostoma. In this event, a fenestra is placed in the upper arch of the tube to allow expired air to pass into the skin tube. Late stenosis of the skin tube, usually at the upper end, has also been a chronic problem. Operative revision may correct this stenosis. Kitamura et al.[12] retain the cricoid whenever possible for the upper tracheal stoma to serve as a natural stent to maintain patency of the skin tube. They also stress the importance of placing the pharyngostoma under the base of the tongue to reduce aspiration. Hair growth within the skin tube has been a nuisance in some male patients, but hair usually can be avulsed from below or destroyed by electrolysis preoperatively.

Although the entire technique can be accomplished in less than three stages, Miller currently completes the total laryngectomy with a high stoma. If the patient fails to acquire satisfactory esophageal speech, then the operation can be completed in two subsequent stages.

DISTANT SKIN TUBE WITHOUT A PROSTHESIS

Because the Asai operation usually cannot be employed in patients who have received high-dose irradiation and because multiple hospitalizations are required, McGrail and Oldfield[13] devised a one-stage operation for vocal rehabilitation with use of a medially based deltopectoral skin flap similar in principle to the technique for esophageal reconstruction by Bakamjian.[14] The procedure is performed at the completion of laryngectomy with or without radical neck dissection (Fig. 21–7).

A 2 cm pharyngostoma is left in the upper end of the pharyngeal closure. Should tracheal length be insufficient, partial or complete removal of the manubrium sterni is accomplished. A permanent tracheostoma is fashioned from an inferiorly based tracheal hinge flap about 2 cm below the cut end of the trachea. A deltopectoral skin flap based on the perforating branches of the internal mammary artery is raised to the shoulder tip. The sides of the flap are sutured to form a skin tube, and the distal end is sutured to the pharyngostoma. A second opening along the side of the tube is sutured to the distal end of the trachea. To prevent escape of expired air at the base of the tube, an epithelial shave and suture approximation is performed. The chest tube is buried beneath the cervical skin flaps, and split-thickness grafts are used to cover the donor site. Speech is accomplished by occlusion of the tracheostoma, shunting expired air into the hypopharynx via the chest tube.

This technique was employed in fifteen patients,[13] six of whom had the operation as a secondary procedure after laryngectomy. As with the Asai operation, aspiration was the major problem, although a modified epiglottis fashioned from the tip of the tube did help to control aspiration. No long-term results were reported, although in two patients stenosis developed at the upper end of the tube; this was treated by retrograde dilatation.

Bryce[15] reported a modification of the delto-

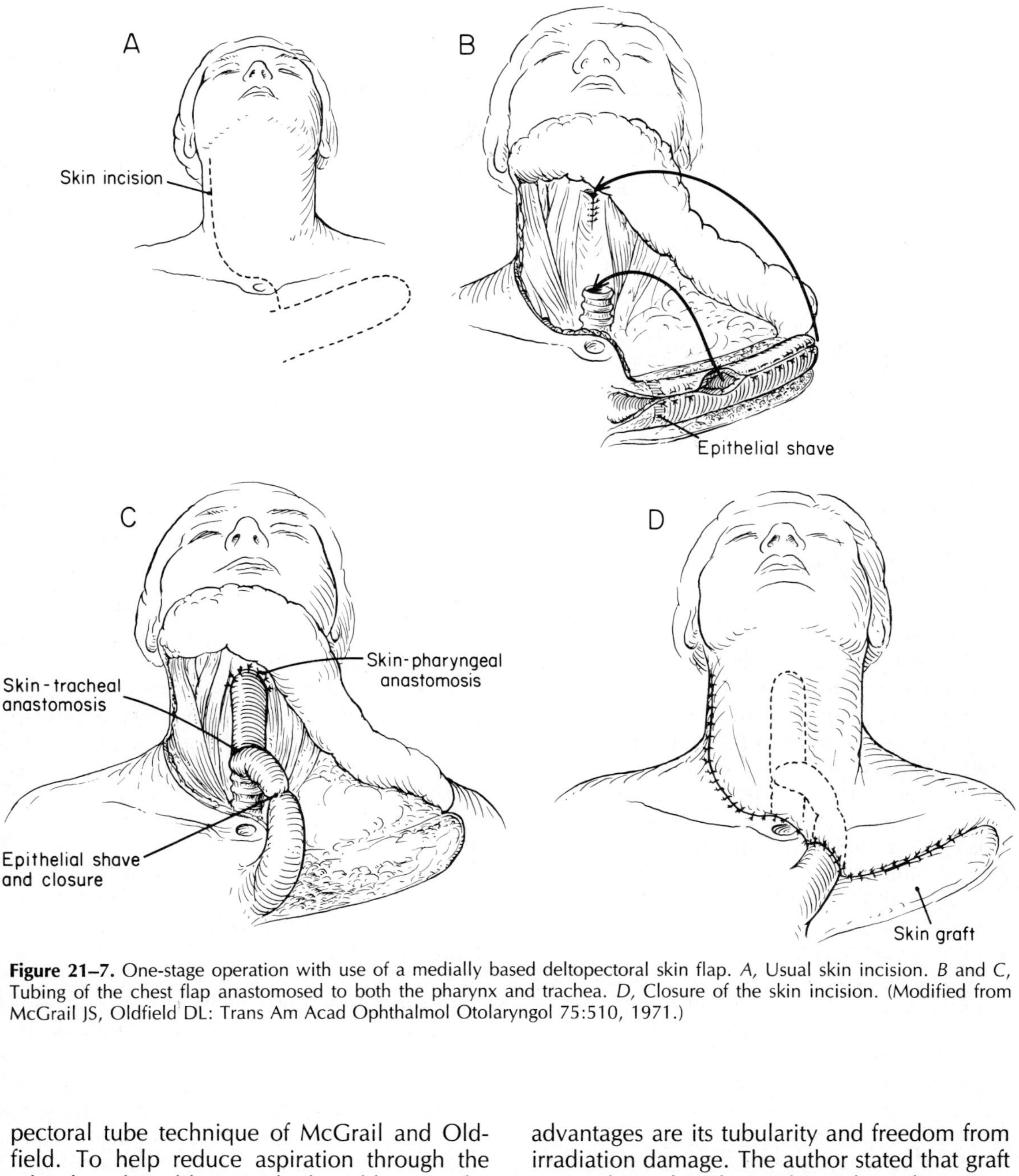

Figure 21–7. One-stage operation with use of a medially based deltopectoral skin flap. *A,* Usual skin incision. *B* and *C,* Tubing of the chest flap anastomosed to both the pharynx and trachea. *D,* Closure of the skin incision. (Modified from McGrail JS, Oldfield DL: Trans Am Acad Ophthalmol Otolaryngol 75:510, 1971.)

pectoral tube technique of McGrail and Oldfield. To help reduce aspiration through the tube, he advised leaving the hyoid bone at the time of laryngectomy and, when possible, retaining the tip of the epiglottis. The pectoral tube is then angled over the hyoid bone before approximation to the pharyngostoma (Fig. 21–8). Salivary leakage was controlled in the four patients reported; however, greater expiratory air pressure was necessary for phonation. The other limitation when the hyoid is retained is incomplete extirpation of the preepiglottic space.

Abu-Jaudeh[16] described the use of a penile skin graft as a phonatory tunnel. Its inherent advantages are its tubularity and freedom from irradiation damage. The author stated that graft material can be obtained simply without cosmetic or functional impairment of the donor organ.

SKIN OR MUCOUS MEMBRANE TUNNEL WITH AN INTERNAL PROSTHESIS

In 1968, Montgomery[17] described a dermal tunnel technique, similar to that originally described by Asai, for use in patients who had already undergone a laryngectomy (Fig. 21–9).

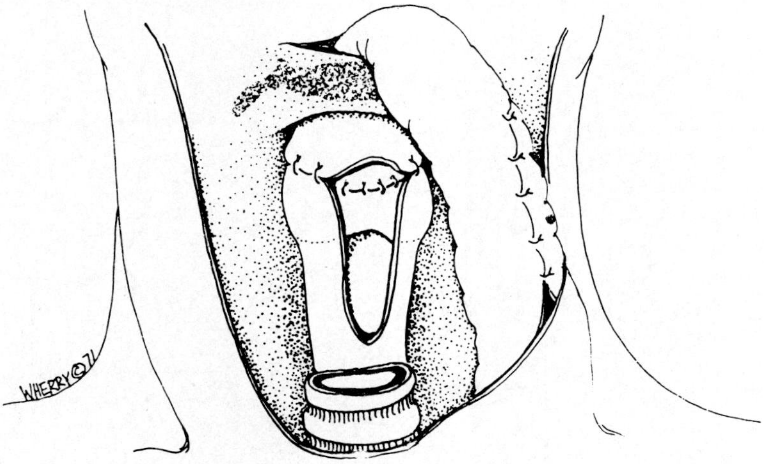

Figure 21–8. Tubed chest flap draped over the retained hyoid bone before anastomosis to the pharynx. (From Bryce DP: J Laryngol Otol 87:669, 1972.)

In the first stage, he constructed a pharyngostoma with two small apposing cervical skin flaps inverted into the pharynx. The original tracheostoma usually was enlarged by resection of a portion of the anterior wall of the trachea and suturing of the skin to the tracheal mucosa. In the second stage, a narrow, inverted-U incision encompassed the pharyngostoma and extended to the upper half of the tracheostoma. The margins were approximated to form a skin-lined tube, and the overlying anterior cervical defect was resurfaced with a nondelayed rotational cervical thoracic skin flap or a simple closure of the elevated anterior cervical skin. Because the interior outlet of the skin tube is flaccid, a silicone T-tube was inserted into the tracheostoma with the upper extension stenting the lower part of the skin tube.

Four years later, Montgomery[18] reported a modification of his earlier operation. Rather than constructing a simple skin-lined pharyngostoma after laryngectomy, he forms a rather elaborate mucous membrane tunnel concurrent with laryngectomy. As much hypopharyngeal mucous membrane as possible is conserved when the larynx is excised from the postcricoid region. A 2.5 cm flap of anterior hypopharyngeal mucous membrane is tubed, preserving the muscular layer for the pharyngeal closure (Fig. 21–10). The mucous membrane tube assumes a superior incline from its opening in the hypopharynx. Opposite the upper end of the tube, a circular incision is made in the anterior cervical skin with a trephine, and this opening is approximated with fine sutures to the upper end of the tube (Fig. 21–11).

If the patient acquires good esophageal speech, the pharyngostoma orifice can be excised and closed by a simple office procedure. If satisfactory esophageal speech is not learned, however, the second stage is carried out with a skin tube similar to that used in Montgomery's earlier operation. The silicone T-tube is also required as a permanent indwelling prosthesis.

The mucosal tube was constructed in 31 patients. Completion of the mucous membrane and skin phonatory tunnel was accomplished in 16 patients. In 10 of these patients, speech function resulted that was much superior to esophageal speech. No specific documentation regarding aspiration or late stenosis was reported.

ESOPHAGEAL TUBE WITHOUT A PROSTHESIS

An esophageal tube technique in dogs was investigated in 1969 by Calcaterra and Jafek.[19] Its purpose was to prevent the problems of aspiration and stenosis and to utilize tissues outside the usual portals of cervical irradiation. Stenosis was avoided with use of a full-thickness cervical esophageal flap that was tubed (Fig. 21–12) and sutured end-to-side to a fenestra excised in the membranous trachea (Fig. 21–13). A two-layer mucosa-to-mucosa anastomosis was accomplished with fine sutures. Aspiration was prevented by insertion of the tube upward about 4 cm from the esophageal opening and construction of a narrow lumen tube that would remain collapsed and perhaps would close with the esophageal contraction during peristalsis. The animals were followed for as long as a year. No evidence of aspiration was viewed by cine-esophagography or micro-

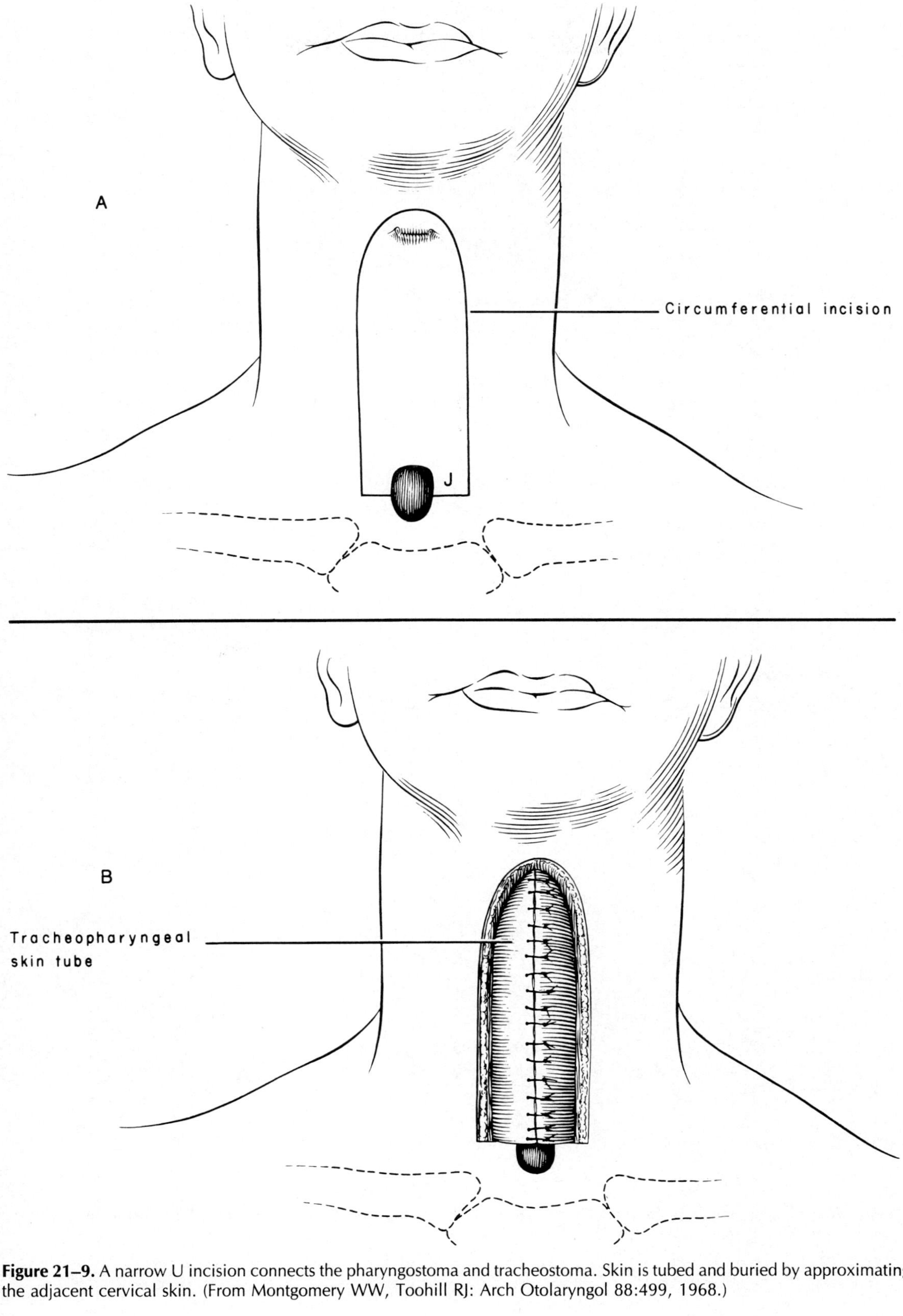

Figure 21–9. A narrow U incision connects the pharyngostoma and tracheostoma. Skin is tubed and buried by approximating the adjacent cervical skin. (From Montgomery WW, Toohill RJ: Arch Otolaryngol 88:499, 1968.)

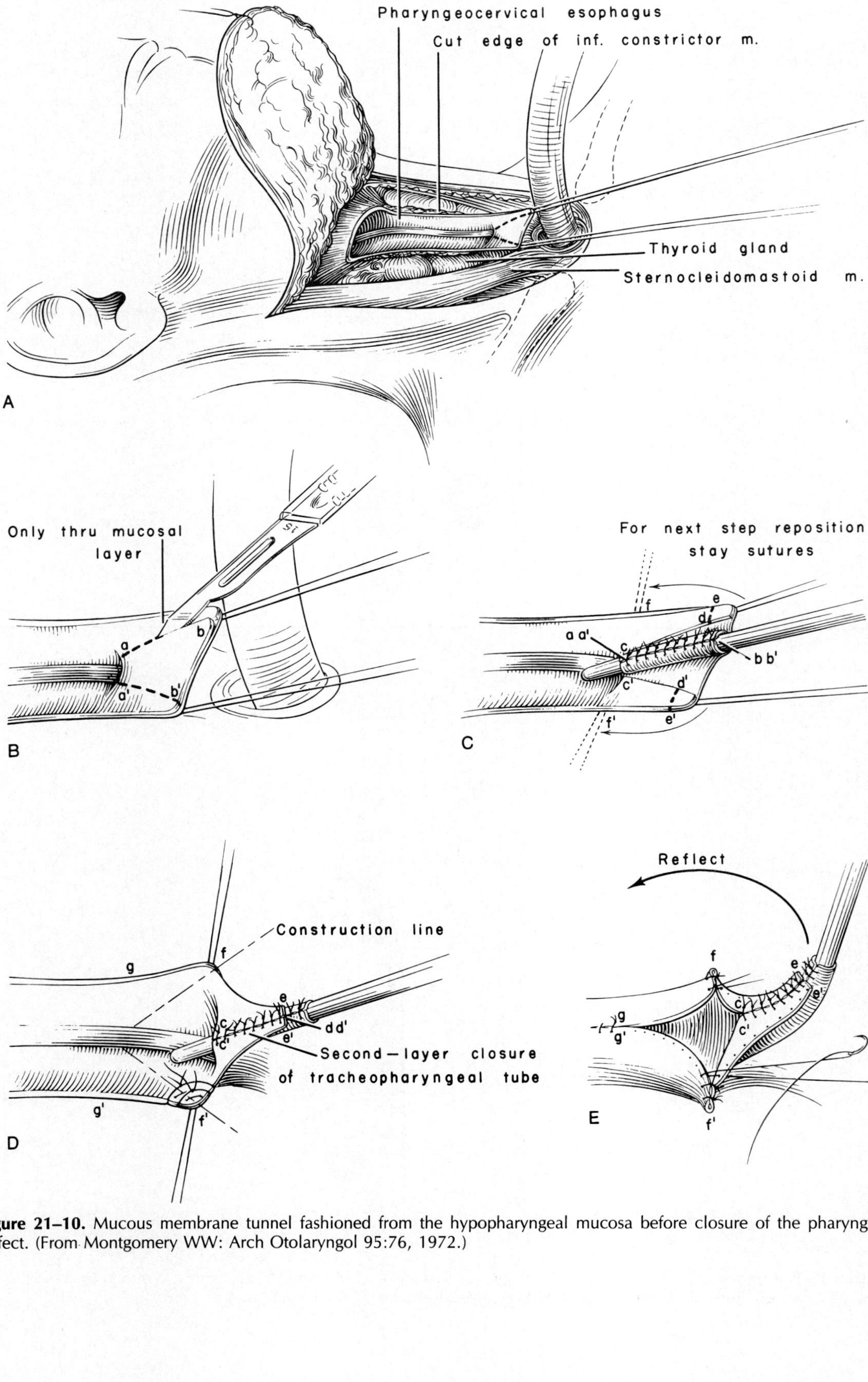

Figure 21–10. Mucous membrane tunnel fashioned from the hypopharyngeal mucosa before closure of the pharyngeal defect. (From Montgomery WW: Arch Otolaryngol 95:76, 1972.)

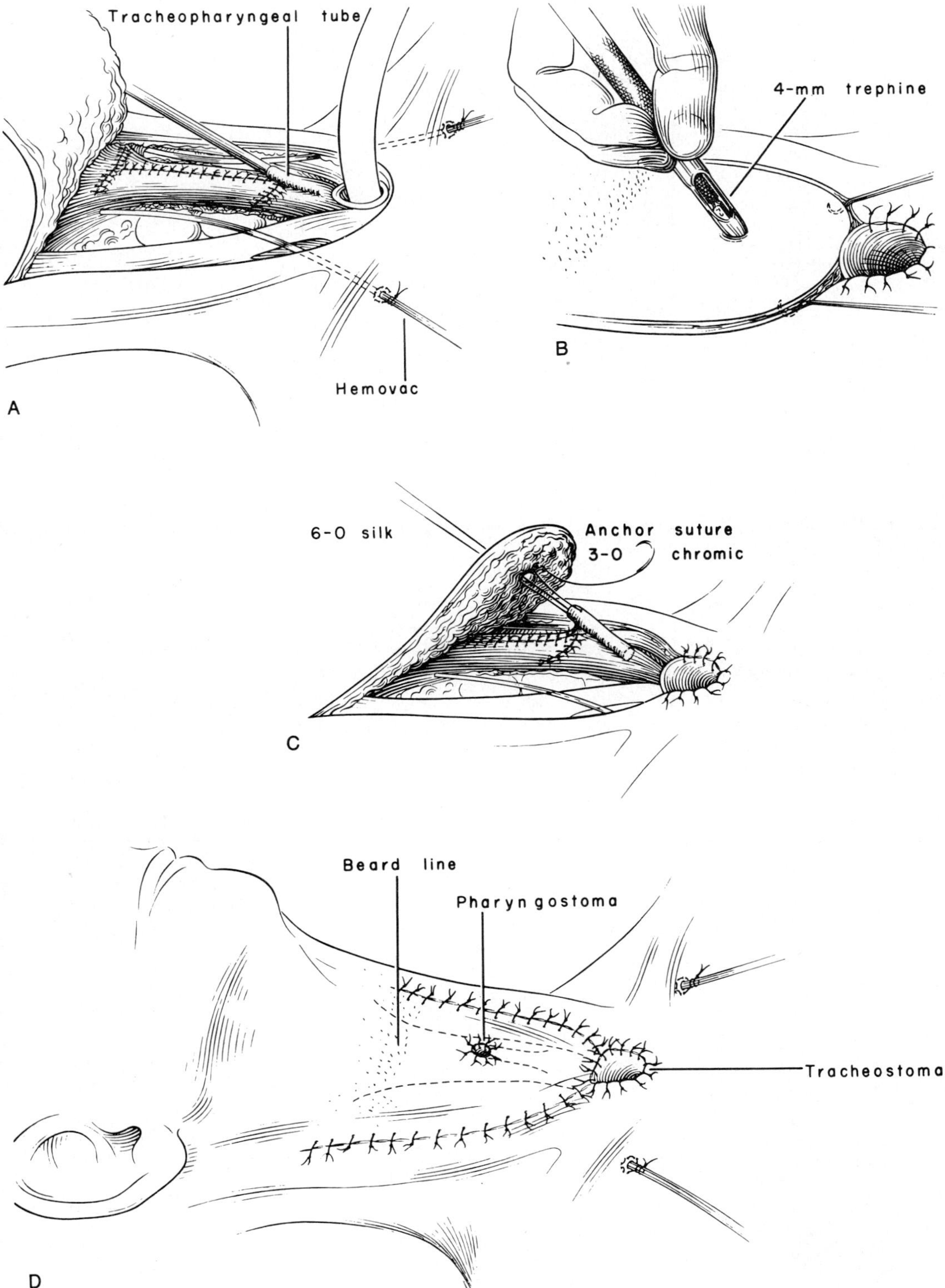

Figure 21–11. Mucous membrane tunnel anastomosed to a trephine opening in the anterior cervical skin. (From Montgomery WW: Arch Otolaryngol 95:76, 1972.)

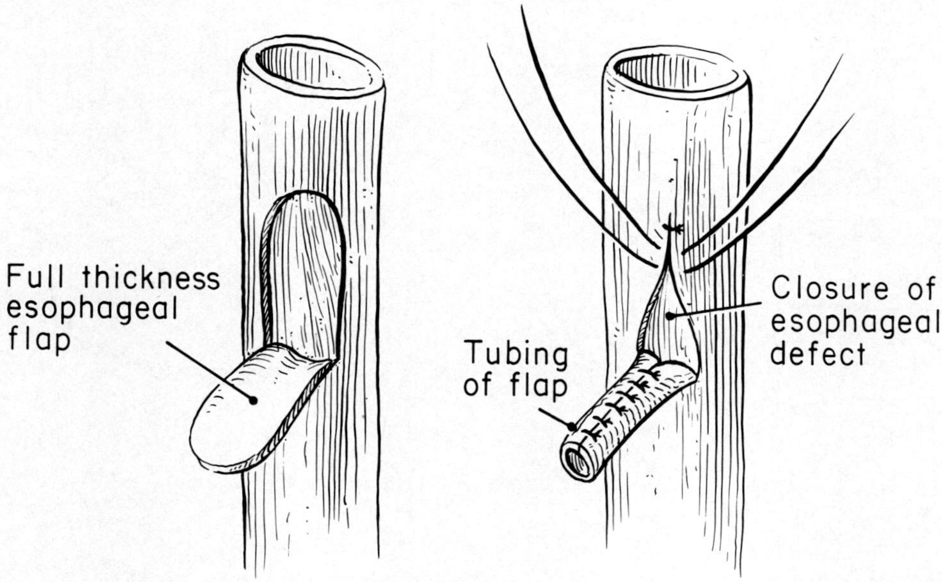

Figure 21–12. A full-thickness esophageal flap is tubed and esophageal defect closed primarily. (From Montgomery WW: Arch Otolaryngol 95:76, 1972.)

scopic examination of the lungs. Live endoscopic and postmorten examinations of the esophageal tubes revealed no stenosis. Serial sections of the tubes showed healthy mucous membrane linings and no evidence of tissue necrosis or scarring.

In an attempt to improve the vibratory or reed characteristics of the shunt, a bivalving

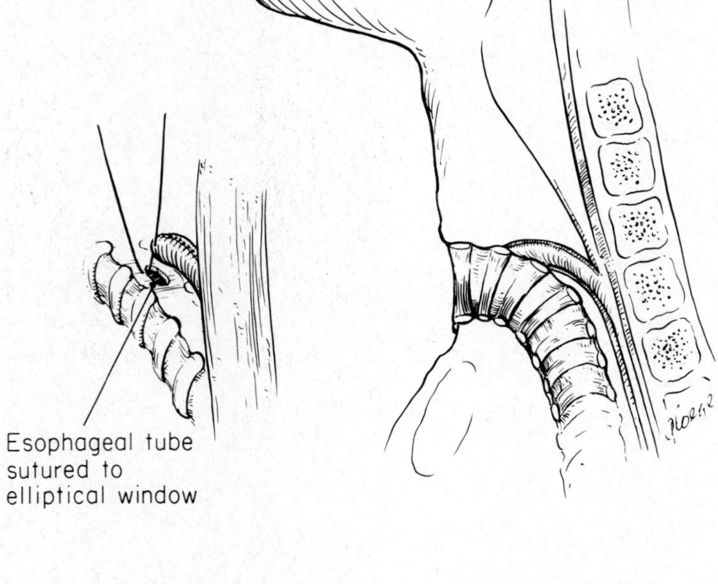

Figure 21–13. Anastomosis of esophageal tube to opening in the membranous trachea. (From Calcaterra TC, Jafek BW: Arch Otolaryngol 94:124, 1971.)

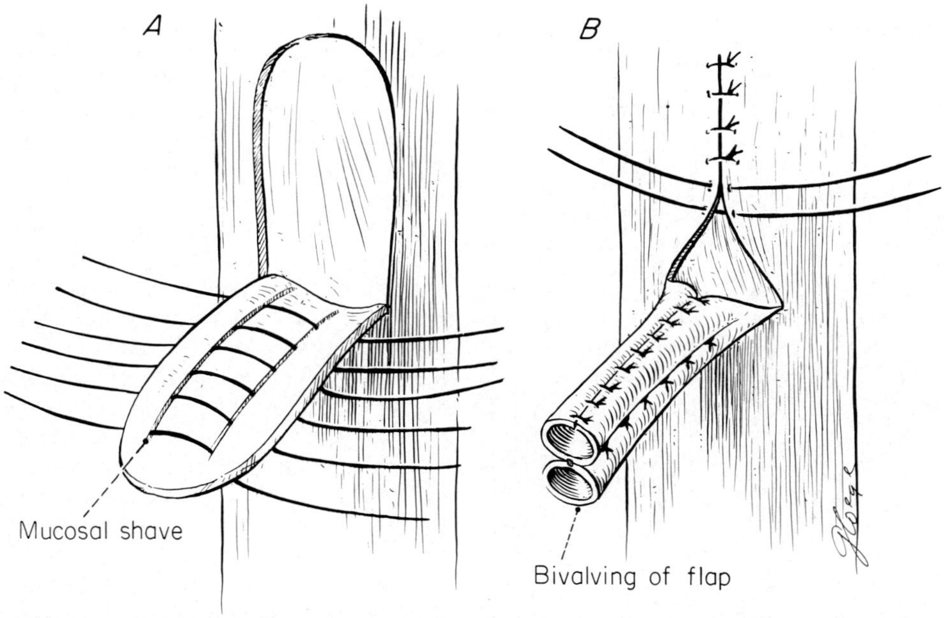

Figure 21–14. Creation of a valved tube by a mucosal shave. (From Calcaterra TC, Jafek BW: Arch Otolaryngol 94:124, 1971.)

technique was used. Before the esophageal flap was tubed, two narrow strips of mucosa were shaved longitudinally along the flap. These were approximated with fine sutures and the shunt completed in the usual manner (Fig. 21–14). On postmortem examination, the double lumen shunt was found to be patent.

The first clinical series of nine patients was reported by Komorn et al.[20] Three patients experienced aspiration, but revision of the shunt improved the reflux in two. Preexisting hiatal hernia appeared to be a factor predisposing the patient to aspiration.

Zwitman and Calcaterra[21] studied speech production with the tracheoesophageal shunt. Cinefluorographic analysis revealed that the esophagus remained constantly inflated during phonation, while the cricopharyngeal inlet remained contracted with only a narrow opening. Similar studies of conventional esophageal speakers have revealed the same anatomic configuration. Analysis of pitch revealed a pitch frequency of 60 to 70 Hz, which is within the range for esophageal speakers; however, the intensity as measured with a sound level meter was slightly higher. The authors concluded that the sound source is the cricopharyngeal sphincter, as it is for esophageal speakers.

The tracheoesophageal shunt speaker has a distinct advantage over the esophageal speaker with regard to the number of words produced per air charge. Like the normal laryngeal speaker, he is able to say 10 to 12 words per exhalation. He can hold "ah" for 20 seconds and can count up to 30 per exhalation. Esophageal speakers have a mean range of 3 to 6 words per air discharge. The gulping sounds and stoma noise heard with many esophageal speakers are absent in patients who have the tracheoesophageal shunt; however, the latter must manually occlude their tracheostomas whenever they wish to speak.

In 1974, Calcaterra reported long-term clinical results with the tracheoesophageal shunt in seven patients, all followed longer than one year.[22] Only two patients maintained patency of the shunt. Late stenosis developed at the tracheoesophageal anastomosis in four patients and, in one patient, complete necrosis of the shunt occurred after partial dehiscence of the laryngectomy closure.

The operation presently is restricted to postlaryngectomy patients who have failed to acquire satisfactory esophageal speech after at least a six-month trial. Delay of the shunt operation until after laryngectomy avoids the performance of a delicate reconstructive procedure after three to four hours of a radical extirpative operation. It also eliminates jeopardy of the shunt by complications such as pharyngeal fistula or infection. Early inferior recession of the trachea, which follows all laryngectomy operations, tends to reduce the ascending angle of the shunt. If shunt construction is delayed for six months, the position of the trachea is stabilized and the shunt angle will remain constant.

An omega incision is made over the tracheal

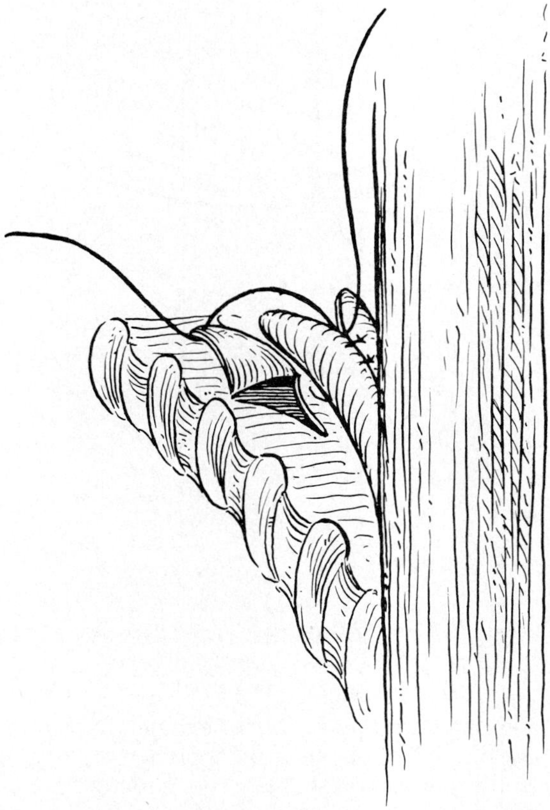

Figure 21–15. V-plasty closure of the esophageal-tracheal anastomosis to reduce tendency to stenosis. (From Calcaterra TC: Can J Otolaryngol 4:569, 1975.)

stoma and carried over the medial aspect of each clavicle. After adequate exposure has been achieved in the plane between the trachea and esophagus, an esophageal flap is tubed except for the distal centimeter. A V-shaped flap is fashioned in the membranous wall of the trachea and sutured into the distal unclosed portion of the esophageal tube (Fig. 21–15). This technique more than doubles the sutured length of the anastomosis and should reduce the tendency toward late stenosis. To prevent early stenosis, a silicone rubber (Silastic) tube is maintained for eight weeks. Long-term results with this modification are not available, but preliminary results are encouraging.

LATERAL CERVICAL ESOPHAGOSTOMY WITH AN EXTERNAL PROSTHESIS

In 1962, Lockhart[23] reported both animal experimentation and a clinical series with cervical esophagostomy as the method of vocal rehabilitation. A rubber nipple attached to a short cervical feeding tube placed at the time of laryngectomy is inserted momentarily into the tracheostoma. On exhalation, air passes up through the cricopharyngeus to produce an audible sound suitable for speech. Lockhart believed that this technique would accelerate the learning of esophageal speech.

Seeking a permanent method of diverting air from the trachea to the esophagus with an external appliance, Taub and Spiro[24] described a bivalved conduit worn at the base of the neck. The details of this air bypass mechanism will be discussed in Chapter 22 of this volume, Vocal Rehabilitation with Prosthetic Devices.

The cervical esophagostomy is placed through an incision along the anterior border of the sternocleidomastoid muscle. Dissection is carried anterior to the carotid sheath and the esophagus is opened laterally.

The sternal head of the sternocleidomastoid muscle is severed and rotated over the carotid vessels for their protection. A superior-based skin flap is raised from the posterior part of the incision, and the end is sutured to the circumference of the esophageal opening (Fig. 21–16). To reduce salivary leakage, the skin opening of the fistula is positioned higher than the esophageal opening. A soft rubber or Silastic stent is left in place.

This device can be fitted in about two weeks. The silicone tube inserted into the cervical esophagostomy has a one-way valve to prevent salivary leakage into the apparatus. The tracheostomy tube is fitted with an air bypass mechanism that permits patients to respire through the tube under normal air pressures and to vent air into the esophagus by increasing their expiratory air pressure.

The major limitations of this method of vocal rehabilitation are the inconvenience of an external appliance and salivary leakage from the cervical esophagostomy. Each patient must be carefully fitted to achieve airtight and watertight connections of the appliance to the trachea and esophagus. Salivary leakage is increased when the internal opening of the esophagostomy is above the cricopharyngeus, where pooling of saliva normally occurs; however, if the opening is placed too low in the esophagus, air distention of the stomach will occur.

Definite increased risk exists when the neck tissues have received previous irradiation, as there is a greater tendency for necrosis of the cervical skin flap used in the construction of

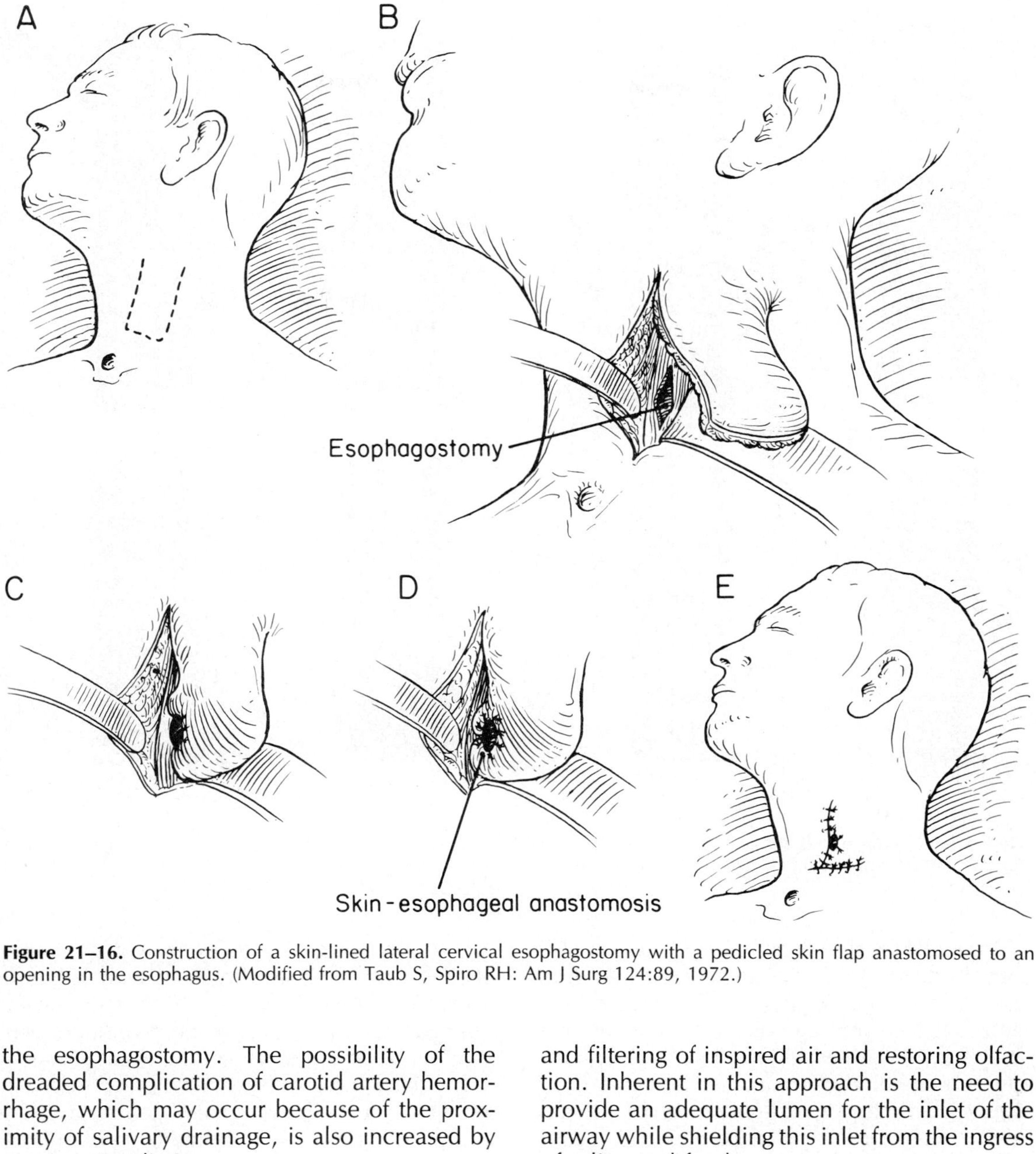

Figure 21–16. Construction of a skin-lined lateral cervical esophagostomy with a pedicled skin flap anastomosed to an opening in the esophagus. (Modified from Taub S, Spiro RH: Am J Surg 124:89, 1972.)

the esophagostomy. The possibility of the dreaded complication of carotid artery hemorrhage, which may occur because of the proximity of salivary drainage, is also increased by previous irradiation.

TRACHEOPHARYNGEAL ANASTOMOSIS

Clearly a most challenging goal in vocal rehabilitation after laryngectomy is the direct union of the trachea and pharynx without diverting the trachea to the outside of the neck. This would not only restore phonation but would also allow normal respiration through the nose and mouth, providing humidification and filtering of inspired air and restoring olfaction. Inherent in this approach is the need to provide an adequate lumen for the inlet of the airway while shielding this inlet from the ingress of saliva and food.

After clinical experience with tracheal replacements using alloplastic protheses, McCall and Whitaker,[25] working with dogs, reported an experimental study utilizing tubes of polyethylene, polyurethane, silicone rubber, and polytetrafluoroethylene (Teflon) for laryngeal replacement. The silicone rubber prosthesis produced the most favorable result, although the longest survival was only 16 days. Failure resulted in breakdown of the pharyngeal prosthetic anastomosis, malnutrition, and aspiration pneumonia.

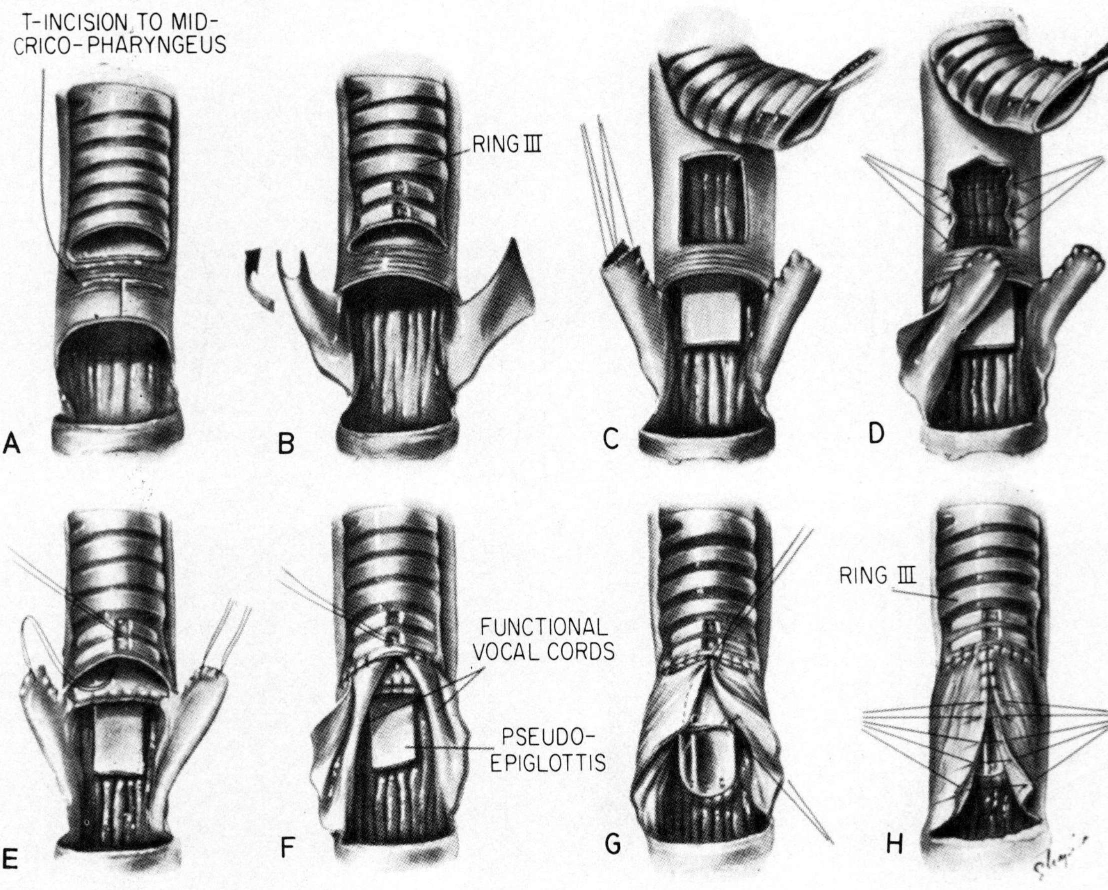

Figure 21–17. First two tracheal rings narrowed by wedge resection of cartilage. Pseudoepiglottis and vocal folds constructed from pharyngeal mucosa. (From Lapidot A et al.: Arch Otolaryngol 82:33, 1965.)

A comprehensive experimental study of laryngeal substitution in 87 laryngectomized dogs was carried out by Ogura, Shumrich, and Lapidot.[26] The senior author of this study had clearly demonstrated in his clinical experience that substantial portions of the larynx can be removed for cancer extirpation while the patient, after a period of adaptation and reeducation, can still retain the basic functions of respiration and phonation without significant aspiration. These investigators believed that some type of simplified, surgically constructed laryngeal substitute seemed feasible.

Four different methods of laryngeal substitution were investigated in dogs. The first group underwent laryngeal replacement by a plastic prosthesis, either of Teflon, nylon, polyester (Dacron), or polyolefin (Marlex). Regardless of the material used, every prosthesis was rejected in two and one-half months or less. Aspiration and late stenosis of the anastomosis were almost always present.

The second group of dogs had a simple tracheopharyngeal anastomosis with a stent, with no attempt to narrow the tracheal inlet. Although aspiration was prohibitive, there was little evidence of stenosis of the anastomosis.

The third group of dogs was studied to determine the effectiveness of simulated fixed cords in preventing aspiration by reducing the diameter of the inlet of the airway. This was accomplished by various methods of buckling the upper tracheal ring inward. When the tracheal diameter was narrowed to less than 50 per cent, decannulation of the tracheostomy tube was impossible. Less aspiration was observed than with the simple tracheopharyngeal anastomosis.

The most promising group of dogs underwent construction of a functioning sphincter or valve at the inlet of the trachea by transposition of the cricopharyngeal muscle. Cinefluoroscopic examination revealed minimal aspiration, and direct examination under light anesthesia showed that the sphincter closed partially during the act of swallowing. Follow-up extended to four and one-half months with apparent success. Upon permanent decannulation of the tracheostomy tube, the airway was adequate and the bark recognizable.

In 1965, Lapidot et al.[27] reported the first reconstruction of the larynx after total laryngectomy in a human being. His laryngeal reconstruction was designed to prevent aspiration by three techniques: (1) the upper two tracheal rings were partially collapsed by removal of a small anterior wedge, (2) a pseudoepiglottis was constructed with a superior-based flap of anterior cervical esophagus, and (3) bilateral mucosal flaps of pharyngeal mucosa were tubed and sutured anteriorly to form "vocal folds" (Fig. 21–17). This was performed in one stage and an acrylic mold conforming to the dimensions of the neolarynx was used as a stent. Postoperatively, the tracheal inlet was compromised by edema of the pseudoepiglottis. Although this was excised, a permanent pharyngeal airway was never established.

Lapidot et al.[28] followed in 1971 with an experimental study in dogs to create a pseudoepiglottis by means of a tongue pedicle flap designed to prevent aspiration after reconstruction of the larynx. Through a lateral pharyngotomy without laryngectomy, a large posteriorly based tongue flap was everted into the pharynx and sutured to an anterior esophageal flap (Fig. 21–18). In six of sixteen animals, a bridge of viable tissue could be maintained over the laryngeal inlet. The authors suggested that a similar flap could be used to shield a pharyngeal airway inlet after laryngectomy.

After a series of experiments in dogs and monkeys by Serafini,[29] Arslan reported his results in 35 patients who had undergone laryngeal reconstruction after a modified laryngectomy.[30] The operation was limited to patients who had an intrinsic lesion without evidence either of extension to the epiglottis or of cervical metastasis.

The operative technique used is the same as that used in the animal studies. A midline vertical incision is employed and the strap muscles are preserved. The perichondrium is dissected from the thyroid and cricoid cartilages and preserved after a tracheostomy at the fifth tracheal ring. The larynx is severed inferiorly between the cricoid and first tracheal ring and superiorly below the hyoid bone with preservation of the body of the epiglottis (Fig. 21–19A). The trachea is elevated about 4 cm, and the upper end is anastomosed to the pharyngeal defect (Fig. 21–19B). The first tracheal ring is firmly sutured to the hyoid bone for stabilization, and the tracheopharyngeal anastomosis is further supported by the midline approximation of the external perichondrium and strap muscles (Fig. 21–19C).

Spontaneous phonation was observed in all patients. Ninety per cent of the patients were able to swallow without a feeding tube, although some aspiration continued. About 30 per cent could ultimately have the tracheostomy removed. Electroacoustic and spectrographic analyses of the voices produced dem-

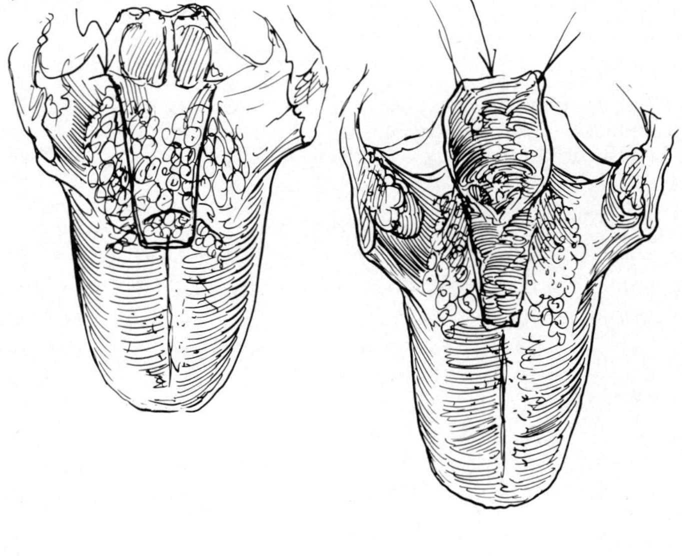

Figure 21–18. Eversion of a posterior-based tongue flap designed to cover the airway inlet. (From Lapidot A et al.: Arch Otolaryngol 94:197, 1971.)

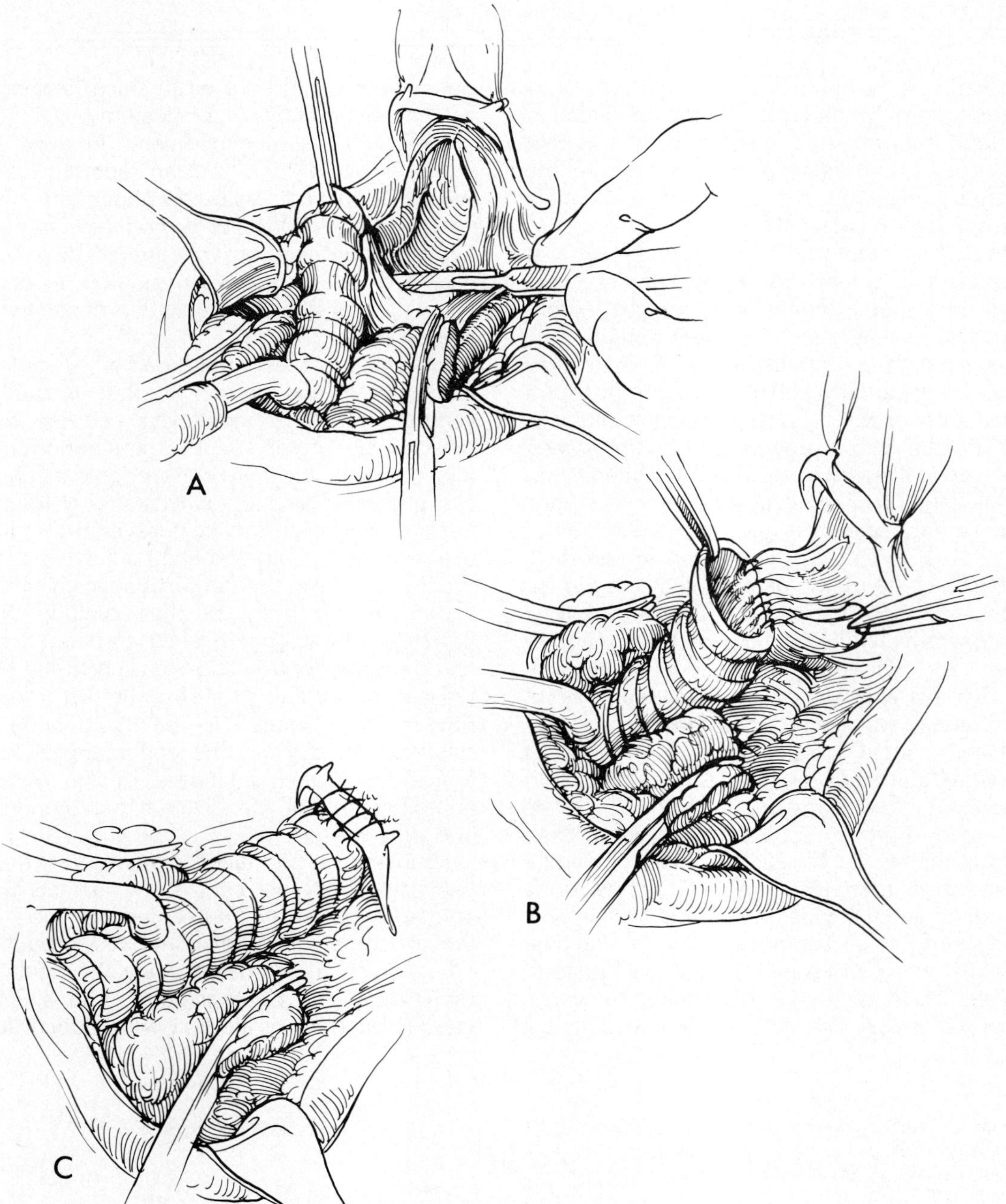

Figure 21–19. Laryngeal reconstruction. *A,* Completion of the laryngectomy with preservation of the hyoid bone, epiglottis, and the laryngeal perichondrium. *B,* Direct anastomosis of the upper trachea to the pharyngeal defect. *C,* Stabilization of the first tracheal ring to the hyoid bone. (Modified from Arslan M: Ann Otol Rhinol Laryngol 81:479, 1972.)

onstrated higher fundamental frequency and greater pitch range than with conventional esophageal speech.[31]

SUMMARY

The ultimate answer in total rehabilitation of the laryngectomized patient would be larynx transplantation. Because the problems of donor organ rejection and neural regeneration have not been overcome, this approach remains an experimental method.

A completely satisfactory method of vocal rehabilitation after total laryngectomy has not been achieved. All methods suffer to some degree from two common problems: (1) contamination of the airway by alimentary contents and (2) stenosis of the surgically reconstructed phonatory channel. The goal of reconstructive surgery should be directed primarily toward rehabilitation of speech, the patient's major handicap. Restoration of nasal and oral respiration without a tracheal cannula is of secondary importance, although it appears to be more challenging.

Most laryngologists today feel that since good esophageal speech effectively competes with most surgical methods of vocal rehabilitation, a trial period of training with a competent speech therapist should precede major surgical reconstruction. Worldwide interest in this problem is increasing and more innovative techniques will surely be forthcoming. It is hoped that a method can be devised to replace the larynx, not with a simple fistulous tract or prosthesis, but rather with a dynamic structure capable of the rudimentary, yet most important, laryngeal functions of phonation and sphincteric protection of the lower airway.

References

1. Gussenbauer C: Über die erste durch Th. Billroth am Menschen ausgeführte Kehlkopf—Exstirpation, und die Anwendung eines kunstlichen Kehlkopfes. Verh Dtsch Ges Chir, p 250, 1874.
2. Calcaterra TC: Laryngeal suspension after supraglottic laryngectomy. Arch Otolaryngol 94:306, 1971.
3. Barton RT: A review of attempted physiological restoration of voice following total laryngectomy. Proc VIII Int Congr Oto-Rhino-Laryngol, Tokyo, Oct 24–30, 1965. Amsterdam, Excerpta Medica Foundation, 1966, pp 731–734.
4. Briani AA: Riabilitazione fonetica di laringectomizzati a mezza dela corrente aerea esperatoria polmonare. Arch Ital Otolaryngol 63:469, 1952.
5. Conley JJ et al.: A new surgical technique for the vocal rehabilitation of the laryngectomized patient. Ann Otol 67:655, 1958.
6. Conley JJ: Vocal rehabilitation by autogenous vein graft. Ann Otol 68:990, 1959.
7. Asai R: Laryngoplasty. J Jap Broncho-Esophalog Soc 12:1, 1960.
8. Miller AH: First experiences with the Asai technique for vocal rehabilitation after total laryngectomy. Ann Otol Rhinol Laryngol 76:829, 1967.
9. Asai R: Laryngoplasty after total laryngectomy. Arch Otolaryngol 95:114, 1972.
10. Miller AH: Four years experience with the Asai technique for vocal rehabilitation for the laryngectomized patient. Ann Otol Rhinol Laryngol 85:567, 1971.
11. Schulthess GV: Pseudoepiglottis and pseudoglottis from pedicle skin flap: A modification of Asai's technique. Acta Otolaryngol [Stockh] 72:225, 1971.
12. Kitamura T et al.: Supracricoid laryngectomy. Laryngoscope 79:1027, 1970.
13. McGrail JS, Oldfield DL: One-stage operation for vocal rehabilitation at laryngectomy. Trans Am Acad Ophthalmol Otolaryngol 75:510, 1971.
14. Bakamjian VY: Total reconstruction of pharynx with medially based deltopectoral skin flap. NY State J Med 68:2771, 1968.
15. Bryce DP: The role of surgery in the management of carcinoma of the larynx. J Laryngol Otol 87:669, 1972.
16. Abu-Jaudeh CN: Modified Asai technique in one stage laryngectomy. J Laryngol Otol 86:263, 1972.
17. Montgomery WW, Toohill RJ: Voice rehabilitation after laryngectomy. Arch Otolaryngol 88:499, 1968.
18. Montgomery WW: Postlaryngectomy vocal rehabilitation. Arch Otolaryngol 95:76, 1972.
19. Calcaterra TC, Jafek BW: Tracheoesophageal shunt for speech rehabilitation after total laryngectomy. Arch Otolaryngol 94:124, 1971.
20. Komorn RM et al.: Vocal rehabilitation with a tracheoesophageal shunt. Arch Otolaryngol 97:303, 1973.
21. Zwitman DH, Calcaterra TC: Phonation using the tracheoesophageal shunt after total laryngectomy. J Speech Hear Disord 38:370, 1973.
22. Calcaterra TC: Tracheo-esophageal shunt for speech rehabilitation after total laryngectomy. Can J Otolaryngol 4:568, 1975.
23. Lockhart HB: The surgical rehabilitation of the laryngectomized patient. Laryngoscope 72:1585, 1962.
24. Taub S, Spiro RH: Vocal rehabilitation of laryngectomees. Am J Surg 124:87, 1972.
25. McCall JW, Whitaker CW: The use of prosthesis in the larynx and trachea: A preliminary report. Ann Otol Rhinol Laryngol 71:397, 1962.
26. Ogura JH et al.: Some observations on experimental laryngeal substitution in laryngectomized dogs. Ann Otol Rhinol Laryngol 71:532, 1962.
27. Lapidot A et al.: Reconstruction of the larynx following total laryngectomy. Arch Otolaryngol 82:33, 1965.
28. Lapidot A et al.: Dorsum of the tongue pedicle flap replacing the epiglottis. Arch Otolaryngol 94:197, 1971.
29. Serafini J: Restoration of laryngeal function after laryngectomy. Experimental research in animals. *In* Ruedi L (ed): Advances in Oto-Rhino-Laryngology. Basel/New York, S. Karger, 1969, pp 95–122.
30. Arslan M: Reconstructive laryngectomy: Report on the first 35 cases. Ann Otol Rhinol Laryngol 81:479, 1972.
31. Arslan M, Rossi M: Electroacoustical and spectrographical analysis of the voice of the human neolarynx. Acta Otolaryngol 73:230, 1972.

22

Vocal Rehabilitation with Prosthetic Devices

Mark I. Singer, M.D. and Eric D. Blom, Ph.D.

Advanced laryngeal carcinoma and its treatment have devastating effects on speech, swallowing, and respiration and pose numerous challenges for the clinician. The impact of loss of speech on the quality of life has few equals among medical handicaps. Speech provides an individual's presentation to society as well as his or her self-perception. Aphonia not only disrupts commerce with others but also changes relationships and dependencies, which may produce serious psychological stress and behavioral alteration. Failure to accommodate frequently results in permanent disability and withdrawal from society, sometimes leading to suicide.

The magnitude of this alteration in the quality of life may displace long-term considerations for survival. In a survey of normal individuals presented with a number of problems, including laryngectomy, nearly 20 per cent chose radiation therapy or conservative treatment with voice preservation instead of laryngectomy with its higher probability of survival.[1] The subjects easily substituted quality of life for improved quantity of life when confronting the dilemma of laryngeal carcinoma.

Voice preservation has been a concern inseparable from the effective therapy of laryngeal cancer, as seen in the evolution of treatment over nearly 100 years. Total laryngectomy is usually reserved for patients who are not likely to be cured by radiation therapy or by conservation surgical procedures. Rehabilitation of voice may consist of an artificial larynx, acquisition of esophageal voice, or a second operative procedure to restore continuity of the airway and alimentary tract. In addition, surgeons have developed neoglottic reconstructive procedures for total or near-total laryngectomy to diminish delays in secondary voice rehabilitation.[2, 3, 4, 5]

HISTORY OF VOCAL REHABILITATION

The intial reports of total laryngectomy were published by Watson (Edinburgh, 1866) and Billroth (Vienna, 1873). Watson treated a 36-year-old man who had syphilitic laryngeal stenosis by total laryngectomy. The patient reportedly died of pneumonia after three weeks. Billroth's reported total laryngectomy was for carcinoma of the larynx and followed an initial therapeutic failure with thyrotomy.[6] He used a diverting pharyngostomy to decrease the potentially fatal hazards of pulmonary infection from aspiration. The patient is reported to have sur-

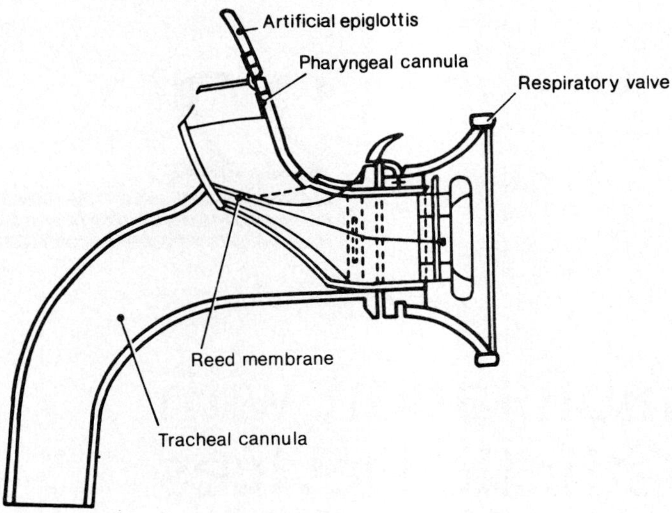

Figure 22–1. Gussenbauer's artificial larynx device. (From Singer MI: Laryngoscope 93:1454, 1983.)

vived the morbidity of the procedure, only to succumb to uncontrolled cancer several months later.

Gussenbauer, Billroth's assistant, reported the first laryngectomy in 1874 and also described a patient capable of speech three weeks after surgery with an artificial larynx or prosthesis that Gussenbauer had designed.[6] An earlier prototype "vocal cannula" had been developed by Vincenz Czerny (Heidelberg, 1870); it was effectively used in laryngectomized dogs. The cannula was merely a tube that connected the tracheostoma with the pharyngostoma for sound production.

Gussenbauer's prosthesis also consisted of a tracheal tube and a "laryngeal" (pharyngeal) tube that introduced expired air into the pharynx (Fig. 22–1). The pharyngeal extremity was covered by a lid or "epiglottis" that closed for swallowing and opened for speech. An important addition was a vibrating metal reed membrane or "tongue" that was inserted in the airstream for sound production.

Gussenbauer's report described a patient able to speak with an intelligible voice loud enough to be heard in the large hospital ward. Compared with the normal voice, the voice produced was a monotone. It had a different timbre and the patient was noted to fatigue easily after using the device. This landmark accomplishment recognized the need for a sound source and a reflux valve ("epiglottis") for laryngeal prostheses. A number of prosthetic instruments developed in Europe were generally of the design pioneered by Czerny and Gussenbauer. The operative technique continued to evolve in the late 19th century. By 1890, primary pharyngeal reconstruction replaced the external fistulas with subsequent improved deglutition.[7] New types of prostheses introduced sound into the buccal cavity or pharyngoesophagus by placement of a tube through the nose. The air supply was provided either by an external bellows or, more conveniently, by an exhalatory limb on a modified tracheotomy tube (Fig. 22–2). These methods were effective for ala-

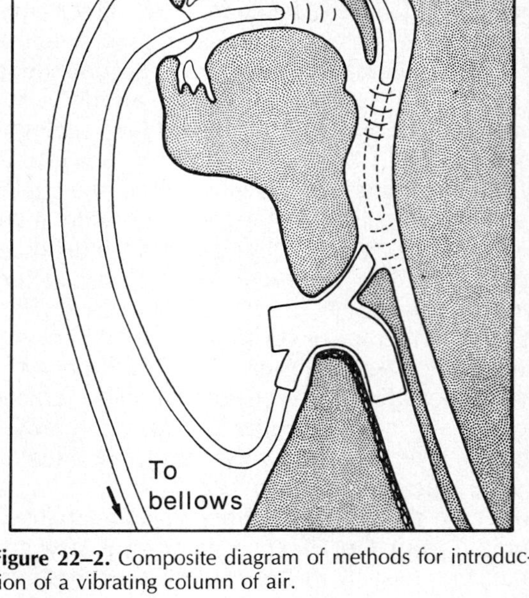

Figure 22–2. Composite diagram of methods for introduction of a vibrating column of air.

ryngeal voice production; however, with the closed pharyngoesophagus, esophageal speech became possible.

One of the earliest descriptions of esophageal voice was made by Seeman (Prague, 1919) in alaryngeal patients.[8] He noted that the source of sound was a specific region of the pharyngoesophagus. He called it the "pseudoglottis" or "pharyngoesophageal segment." This led to the first important physiologic measurements of this region by esophageal insufflation. The pharyngoesophageal segment represents the residuum following laryngectomy and has been extensively investigated by radiographic imaging, manometry, and electromyography.[9, 10]

Esophageal voice is the most widely used method of alaryngeal speech. The literature often states that this method is learned by 65 per cent to 80 per cent of laryngectomees. Reasons cited for failure have been lack of motivation, effects of irradiation, swallowing disorders, anatomic changes in the pharyngoesophagus, and inadequate speech therapy.[11] The complicated behavior of repeated esophageal inflation (injection or inhalation) and controlled release under varied intrathoracic pressures is a skill acquired by a smaller percentage of patients than previously reported. In a prospective study on laryngectomy rehabilitation, Gates and co-workers report that no more than 33 per cent of the patients acquire usable esophageal speech.[12]

If excellent esophageal speech were obtained by large numbers of laryngectomees with relative ease, the thought of aphonia after laryngectomy would produce far less anguish. Also, the need for voice-preserving surgical procedures would be reduced with less risk of recurrent disease or chronic pulmonary aspiration. The results of Gates et al. are supported by generally held clinical impressions of esophageal speech success. Educational or personal failure as primary arguments overlook the physiology of the region after laryngectomy. A realistic view must concede that it is the rare patient who lacks the interest to learn to speak again and that better methods must be developed.

The modern era of surgical and prosthetic rehabilitation of laryngectomized patients was introduced by the work of Briani in Italy in 1952.[13] The method involved the controlled development of a pharyngocutaneous fistula located superior to the level of the cricopharyngeus muscle. The fistula was linked to the tracheostoma by various prostheses of acrylic and polyethylene. Although this appears to be regression to the techniques of Billroth, the fistula was small and the prostheses did not require a vibratory membrane or reed. It was recognized that the pharyngeal mucosa could be activated by airflow to produce sound without introduction of an external or foreign sound source. An intrinsic sound source produced a less monotonous sound than the previous artificial larynges.

The following period of 25 years was marked by three directions of investigation. The main effort was characterized by secondary rehabilitative methods that used an internal shunt without a prosthesis or indwelling cannula. Internal shunt techniques were also undertaken as primary methods for vocal preservation after laryngectomy. Some clinicians insisted on the use of valved prostheses and external shunt techniques as a counter theme to these methods.

Conley proposed a new method using a mucosal tube from the esophagus, anastomosed

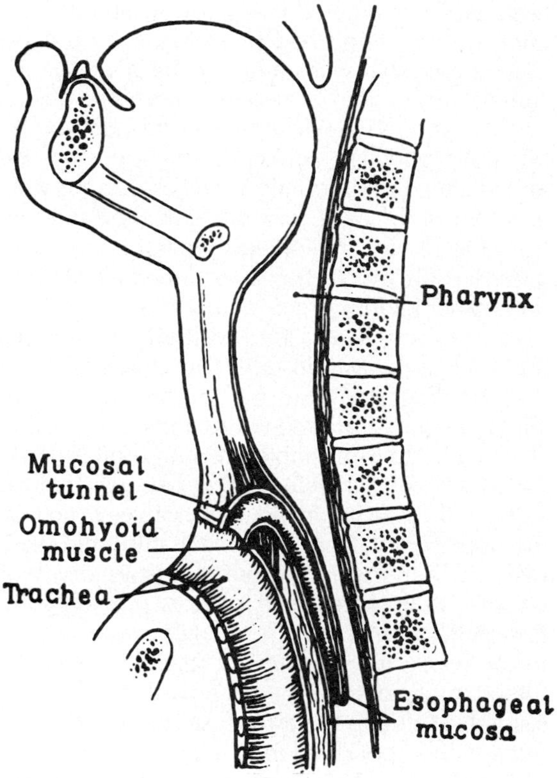

Figure 22–3. Esophageal mucosal tube looped over the omohyoid muscle and entering the membranous trachea. (From Conley JJ: Ann Otol Rhinol Laryngol 67:658, 1958.)

to the membranous trachea. This was later modified by the application of a vein graft[14, 15] (Fig. 22–3). Airflows for voice production required patent tracheoesophageal shunts and stenosis was a frequent problem. Aspiration of esophageal contents into the shunt and trachea presented another considerable problem, worsened with greater patency. Conley and coinvestigators developed an acrylic and rubber prosthesis, similar to the Briani device, to maintain shunt patency and to prevent free esophageal reflux. Continual maintenance problems of these customized prostheses prevented their enthusiastic acceptance.

Summarizing the problem, Conley wrote, "The technical problem to overcome consisted of creating a passageway that would permit the free flow of air from the trachea into the esophagus without the passage of food or saliva from the gullet into the trachea. The great inconvenience caused by an inadvertent small pharyngeal or esophageal fistula would unquestionably condemn any such uncontrolled communication."[14]

The best known of the external shunts utilizing a prosthesis was developed by Taub and reported in 1972.[16] A secondary esophagostoma was constructed in the lower lateral neck after an evaluation had been made by preoperative esophageal insufflation (Taub's test). Insufflation provided a means of assessing voice quality, and the cervical level corresponding to the most effective sound production was selected after air introduction. The esophagus was anastomosed to a 4 to 5 cm skin tube formed from the cervical region and separated from the great vessels by rotation of the medial head of the sternocleidomastoid muscle.

After three weeks, the prosthesis (known as the VoiceBak) was inserted by attaching it at the esophagostoma, using a trumpet-shaped silicone connector, and tightening it against the skin with an adjustable tension collar (Fig. 22–4). Tubing traveled to a one-way saliva valve and then to a regulator valve worn on the upper chest. The valve mechanism allowed two-way airflows for normal respiratory exchange. With increased expiratory pressure, the flow system was converted to a one-way system to the fistula for speech. The circuit was completed by another tube that passed from the regulator valve to the tracheostoma, which was fitted with a special adapter tube. The VoiceBak prosthesis was the first commercially available laryngeal prosthesis for a surgical-prosthetic restorative procedure.

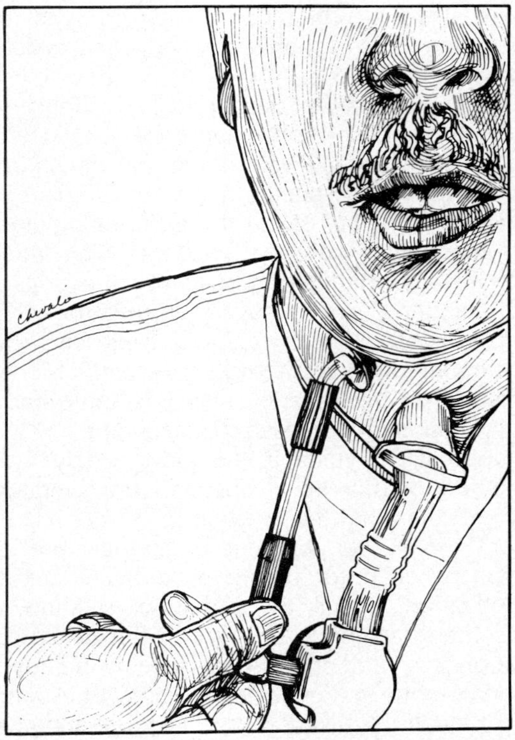

Figure 22–4. VoiceBak artificial larynx (after Taub). (From Singer MI: Laryngoscope 93:1458, 1983.)

Sisson and McConnell reported a method of voice restoration that capitalized on the controlled pharyngostoma used in patients who had received unplanned radiation therapy.[17] A custom valve system was fitted into the tracheostoma, and an extension was inserted into the pharyngostoma with a seal placed on the skin to prevent salivary leakage. The fistula limb contained an antireflux valve designed by McConnell. The air was readily directed to the hypopharynx for speech. This method permitted rapid voice acquisition after laryngectomy without requiring secondary closure of the control fistula.

The authors reported that eight of fifteen patients were satisfactory speakers with this method. Long-term use of the method deteriorated because of the need for time-consuming maintenance of the custom devices and eventual lack of patient compliance. The resultant speech was of higher fundamental frequency than conventional esophageal speech and intelligibility was reported to be comparable. These findings were unexpected because earlier concepts of alaryngeal speech production indicated that the sound source was situated lower in the pharyngoesophagus than the controlled pharyngocutaneous fistulas. Fluoroscopic studies clearly identified the location of sound production in some individuals as at the level of the base of the tongue, or within the fistula itself.[18] This finding supported the view that apposition of mucosal surfaces, often in multiple locations, was independent of the cricopharyngeus muscle or pharyngoesophageal segment and was an effective source of alaryngeal sound.

The experience with the prosthetic valved shunts can be contrasted with progress in internal shunt techniques in the period from 1968 to 1980. As experience was gained with conservation laryngeal procedures, European and Japanese investigators proposed subtotal laryngectomy or so-called reconstructive neoglottic surgery.[2–5, 19–21] A primary near-total resection of the larynx was feasible with reconstruction of the pharynx and trachea to permit not only a phonatory shunt but also reconstruction of the oronasal respiratory tract.

The remarkable function of the larynx may be preserved by conservation procedures and may sometimes be simulated by neoglottic reconstructive techniques. When the tumor invades the boundary of the laryngeal ventricle, crossing a number of lymphatic regions, voice-preserving procedures are limited by the need for eradicating the disease. Extended procedures are further complicated by crippling aspiration as the laryngeal sphincter mechanism is dismantled, although local function is preserved. It is not surprising that a reconstruction using irradiated tissues, constantly bathed in contaminated secretions and partially devitalized by the tumor resection, does not achieve a true simulation of glottic and supraglottic function.

A vocal rehabilitative method must be measured by its capacity to answer a number of critical problems. Rehabilitation must not limit adequate cancer treatment in terms of the extent of surgical resection or tolerance to conventional-dose radiation therapy. Resulting deglutition should be normal and rapidly reacquired postoperatively. Patients should be free of dependence on complicated valves, tubes, and external devices; frequent endoscopy, dilatations, and revisions should not be required.

To solve many of these problems, the authors of this chapter have proposed a surgical technique of endoscopic tracheoesophageal puncture. Speech is restored by use of a prosthesis incorporating a silicone valve.[22] This method of phonation is presented here.

PATIENT SELECTION FOR TRACHEOESOPHAGEAL PHONATION WITH A SILICONE VALVE

Past experience has affected the current approach to voice restoration described here. The successes and failures were carefully considered against the background of a cancer patient in need of rehabilitation. A simple, reproducible technique was needed if large numbers of laryngectomees were to benefit. Considerations of safety, conventional cancer treatment standards, and rapid uncomplicated return to near-normal life without excessive cost are foremost in the development of the voice restoration method.

In 1979, we proposed an uncomplicated surgical technique and simple silicone valve apparatus. These answer many of the historical problems that we have reviewed and open new areas for research.[22] Initially, patients who are dissatisfied with their alaryngeal communication skills are selected. This patient population includes the artificial larynx user and the partly successful esophageal speaker, as well as the individual confined to writing notes. Evaluation measures used include: (1) general health status, (2) interest in a further rehabilitative method, (3) anatomic factors, (4) oncology treatment plan, and (5) esophageal distention test.

Laryngeal cancer patients tend to be in the upper decades of life, so that overall health status is important. Multiple disabilities or concurrent illnesses assume greater significance. A further surgical procedure and mechanical valve system may only further incapacitate them. Chronic obstructive pulmonary disease is commonly associated with this population and, although not a serious limitation, is complicated by copious tracheal secretions, cough, dyspnea, and limited pulmonary reserves.

Although alcoholism is seen frequently in this patient population, it does not contraindicate rehabilitation; it often affects general reliability and compliance, however. Diabetes and atherosclerosis are common problems, but they do not increase the failure rate to any extent. Osteoarthritis may affect manual dexterity and does affect mastery of the stoma and its prostheses. Concurrent neurologic disorders that affect speech production or deglutition and that cause tremor are limiting factors for tracheoesophageal phonation.

Patients accustomed to the ease of an artificial larynx or the independence of esophageal speech must realize that the mechanical devices (silicone tracheal valves) require regular maintenance. Reclusive individuals or severely depressed patients may be incapacitated and unable to maintain acceptable personal hygiene, an important prerequisite for tracheoesophageal valve use.

The laryngectomized neck must be examined from the standpoint of healthy skin and an acceptable tracheostoma. The effects of multiple neck procedures, including fistula closures, radical dissections, and revisions may promote cutaneous breakdown or hypersensitivities. The tracheostoma should have at least a single greatest diameter of 1 cm and be located 1 cm or more above the jugular notch of the manubrium. The heavily irradiated stoma (to a dose of 6,000 rads) is acceptable; however, crusting and secretions will be initial problems that the patient must be able to manage. Tracheal wall breakdown may occur in heavily irradiated patients, who will require an indwelling tracheal cannula.

Patients who do not maintain their stomas or who refuse to tolerate cannulation when necessary are not likely to succeed. Irregularly shaped tracheostomies require stomaplasty and patients who have indwelling tubes require conversion to silicone tubes after dilation for convenient use of the silicone voice prosthesis. Prominent sternal heads of the sternocleidomastoid muscles are not a problem for valve placement and use. Irradiated patients have a satisfactory prognosis for voice acquisition. Adjunctive chemotherapy creates no additional problems. Pharyngeal replacement procedures using cutaneous flaps, myocutaneous flaps, or visceral interpositions have no intrinsic reason for failure, although vocal quality through a reconstructed pharynx may not be as acceptable as with the conventional pharyngoesophageal reconstruction.

Poor tumor prognosis should not prevent vocal rehabilitation by tracheoesophageal puncture. Cervical recurrences are not incompatible with this method. Regional pharyngeal or tracheal recurrences are absolute contraindications. Second primary tumors, partial glossectomies, or maxillectomies present individual considerations but are not strict contraindications.

The response of the pharyngoesophagus to air flow is important for adequate voice after a tracheoesophageal fistula is established. Esophageal distention may result in hypertonicity of the pharyngoesophageal region, as has been estimated to occur in 12 per cent of cases.[23] A simple test may be done by esophageal insufflation with direct observation of patient response relative to voice production, fluency, and gastric filling. A repeatable technique, uncomplicated and brief, should be used. The nasal airway is topically anesthetized and a soft catheter (French 14) is inserted through the nose to the level of the upper thoracic esophagus. The patient is comfortably positioned and asked to release any regurgitated air at the mouth. The catheter is insufflated at pressure ranging from 10 to 30 cm H_2O for 5 s, and the resultant airflows will either audibly escape the oral cavity or distend the stomach. This maneuver is repeated two to three times and the catheter is pulled retrograde 2 to 3 cm and repeatedly inflated until the tip is located at the upper hypopharynx, which is signaled by sound released that resembles a whisper.

The sound emanating from a freely vibrating hypopharynx is relatively low in frequency, resembling esophageal voice. It may then be articulated by the patient as speech in a short spoken task such as counting. With gradual increases in insufflation pressures and airflows, the speech should continue fluently, occasionally breaking or stopping for short intervals but resuming spontaneously.

Gastric filling without voice production may occur if the catheter tip is below the midthoracic esophagus. It should be withdrawn to a point that corresponds with the tracheostoma. At this level, labored monosyllabic speech with frequent breaks and prolonged pauses indicates pharyngoesophageal hypertonicity, a condition that prevents fluent tracheopharyngeal phonation. Pharyngeal constrictor myotomy is proposed to resolve this problem.[23]

If the resultant speech is a whisper, the catheter tip should be checked to be sure it is not in the oropharynx or upper hypopharynx. Although fluency will be noted in this circumstance, the pharyngoesophagus is bypassed and an assessment of tracheoesophageal airflows is not made. The catheter should be advanced 2 to 3 cm and the test repeated, invariably resulting in different sound quality that resembles voice rather than whisper.

The esophageal distention test does not always predict vocal quality. It provides a preoperative assessment of pharyngoesophageal response to airflows, an occurrence that is not unique to this region. We cannot state at this time the accuracy with which the insufflation maneuver will predict acquisition of satisfactory tracheoesophageal phonation, but we can safely say that successful speakers result from preoperative findings of free flows with few breaks in fluency. Individuals who have tightness with insufflation frequently fail to achieve fluent speech, but they may do so in some cases. In this setting, the distention test may be helpful in planning for a delay in voice acquisition.

THE ENDOSCOPIC PUNCTURE TECHNIQUE FOR VOICE RESTORATION

The endoscopic method is the preferred way to establish a tracheoesophageal fistula safely without the risk of cervical or mediastinal infection.[24] The endoscope compresses the esophageal mucosa against the posterior tracheal wall, permitting an easier field for establishment of the tracheoesophageal fistula. In addition, it is advantageous to endoscope the postlaryngectomy patient for a second look, because the incidence of recurrence or second primary is high. A rigid esophagoscope is preferred as a working instrument and a general anesthetic is recommended. An esophagoscope no larger than 7 mm is selected because the hypopharyngeal inlet at the base of the tongue is commonly narrow postlaryngectomy. A suitable instrument length is 30 cm and an aperture is placed at the introduction end to facilitate the puncture technique.

The esophagoscope is inserted to the midesophagus and then withdrawn to a point where the aperture is adjacent to the membranous tracheal wall and immediately inferior to the mucocutaneous junction of the skin and trachea. The instrument and window are palpable through the stoma at the membranous trachea. A 14-gauge intravenous needle is then fashioned into a gentle "C" to clear the superior edge of the manubrium sterni. The puncture should be placed 5 mm from the mucocutaneous junction of the tracheostoma (Fig. 22–5).

As the endoscopist views the field through the esophagoscope, the needle will press the tracheal wall and distort the esophageal mucosa. The mucosa protrudes into the stabilized endoscope aperture, providing a single perforation while the needle advances in the esophagoscope, safely shielded in the lumen. A polyethylene catheter from the intravenous set or a monofilament suture is introduced into the needle from the tracheal side and is recovered in the esophagoscope by the endoscopist. The needle is removed and the polyethylene catheter is threaded through the tip of a urethral

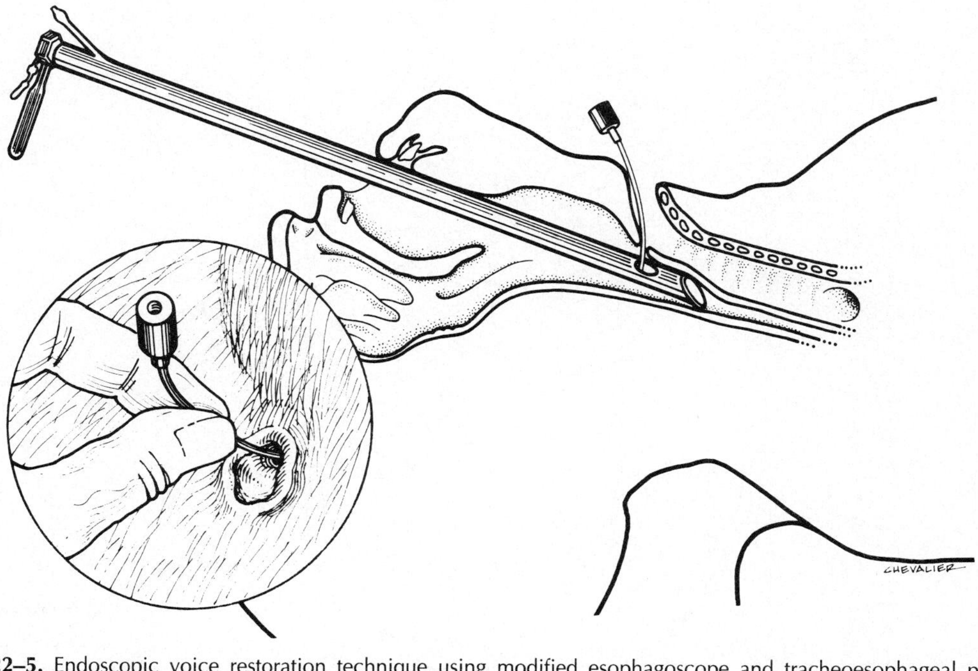

Figure 22–5. Endoscopic voice restoration technique using modified esophagoscope and tracheoesophageal puncture. (From Singer MI, Blom ED: Ann Otol Rhinol Laryngol 89:530, 1980.)

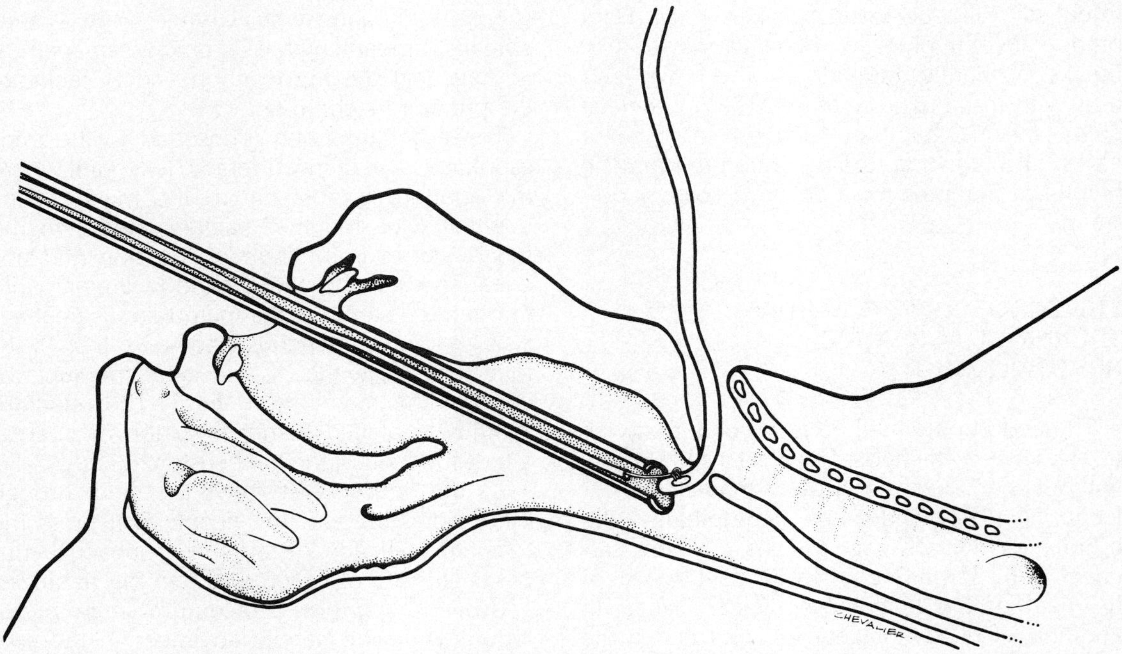

Figure 22–6. Retrograde advancement of catheter through the tracheoesophageal puncture. (From Singer MI, Blom ED: Ann Otol Rhinol Laryngol 89:531, 1980.)

catheter (French 14). The puncture site is dilated at the tracheal wall with the endoscope in place, and the polyethylene catheter is used to guide the urethral catheter retrograde into the pharynx after it crosses the tracheoesophageal walls (Fig. 22–6).

The tracheoesophageal stent is fixed by bringing the polyethylene catheter through the nose

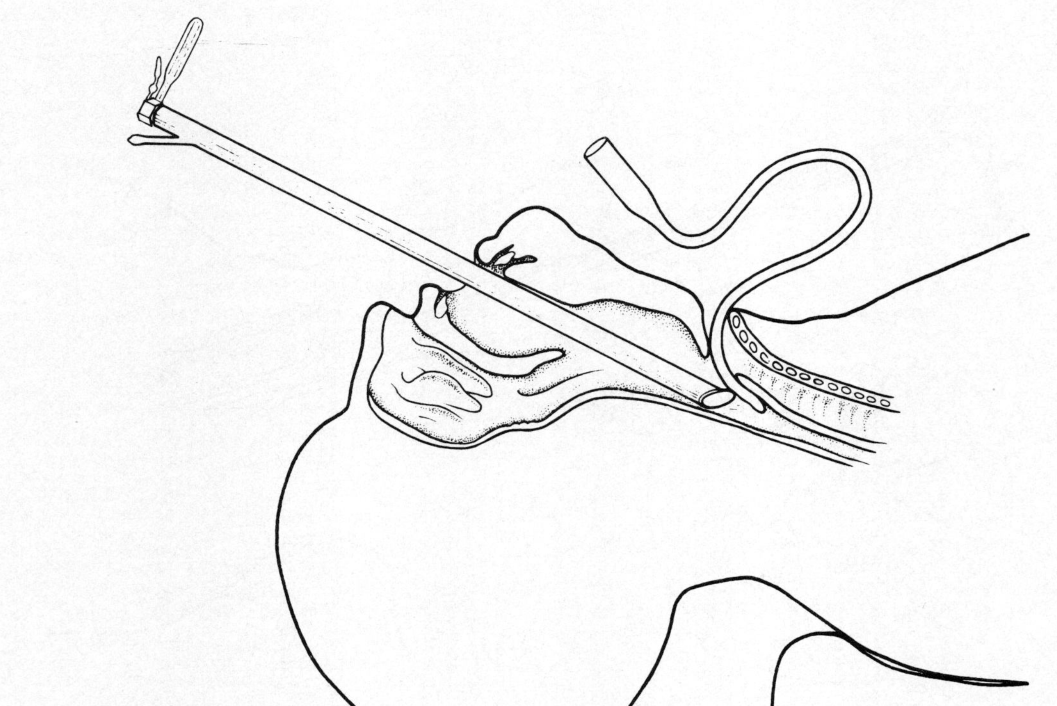

Figure 22–7. Catheter stent of tracheoesophageal puncture directed into distal esophagus.

from the nasopharynx for a later pull-out. Alternatively, it may be removed from the stent catheter, which is then directed into the esophagus by a dilator or by reintroduction of the esophagoscope (Fig. 22–7).

The tracheoesophageal fistula will mature sufficiently after 48 hours with the stent catheter in place. The patient may eat normally during this period but is monitored for tracheal reaction, evidenced by increased tracheobronchial secretions. Esophageal speech or artificial laryngeal communication is unaffected by this procedure and is encouraged in the postoperative period.

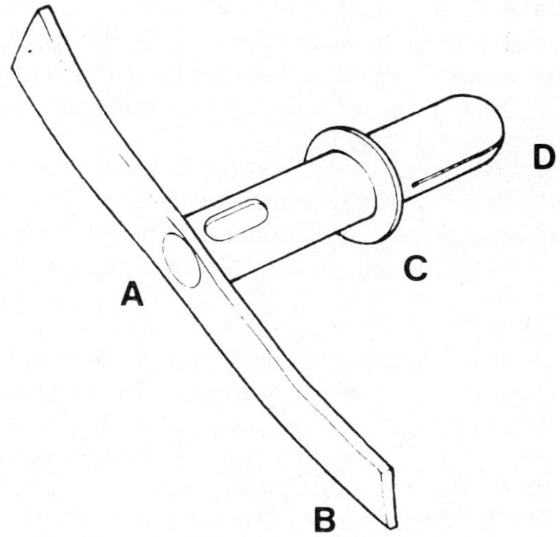

Figure 22–8. Blom-Singer silicone voice prosthesis (duckbill), showing airflow port (A), retention flanges (B), retention collar (C), and slit valve (D).

THE LARYNGEAL (VOICE) PROSTHESIS

The laryngeal prosthesis need only restore the sphincter aspect of the larynx because the sound source can be substituted for by the pharyngoesophageal mucosa. A one-way valve of silicone was developed from using a slit design that closes by natural recoil of the material. The initial Blom-Singer voice prosthesis consisted of a silicone tube of 5.4 mm diameter and lengths varying from 2.2 to 4.3 cm (Fig. 22–8). A single slit valve at the pharyngeal end of the prosthesis opens under positive pressure, permitting airflows of 100 ml per s at pressures of 40 to 60 cm H_2O. The valve closes tightly when airflow stops, after speaking ceases. This type of valve has been descriptively termed a *duckbill.* A port (5 by 3 mm) at the tracheal extremity faces the exhaled tracheal air stream; two flanges or straps are present both for fixation to the peritracheal skin and for prevention of tracheal aspiration. The end is open for insertion and ease of cleaning secretions.

This valve prosthesis occupies the tracheoesophageal puncture and usually is horizontal or has a slight antegrade inclination. It remains

Figure 22–9. Trapdoor voice prosthesis (low pressure valve).

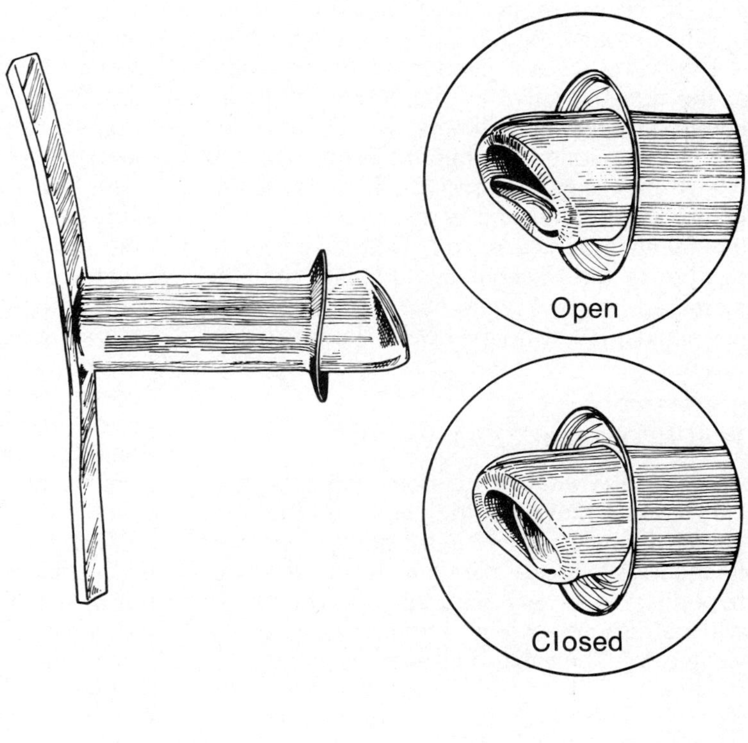

closed during swallowing and maintains a competent barrier to swallowed liquids or foods. The leaves of the slit valve open more efficiently with increasing airflows, permitting relatively effortless alaryngeal speech.

The silicone valve is comfortable and convenient to maintain. After two to three days, it can be removed for cleaning and then returned. The environment of the pharynx affects the silicone minimally; replacement is required after two to three months of continuous use.

A second voice prosthesis was developed to reduce the resistance to airflow. The opening pressure of the duckbill valve is two to three times greater than that of the normal vocal folds. Effective speech production was possible with the initial valve, but with the use of a stoma-closing valve to eliminate manual occlusion, some individuals did not tolerate well the higher airflow resistances. The duckbill slit valve concept gave way to a simple trap valve.

The lumen was enlarged to 6.3 mm diameter with a recessed, hinged trapdoor of silicone sheeting at the intraesophageal end (Fig. 22–9). As with the other valve, the elastic recoil of the silicone closes the valve after airflow has stopped, while it opens with a resistance of 30 cm H_2O/liters per second (LPS), which approximates that of the normal human larynx during phonation. The addition of a collar prevented extrusion of the prosthesis from the esophagus and permitted minimal entry into the lumen. Also, the flexible collar improved the seal around the voice prosthesis at the intraesophageal orifice, decreasing the possibility of reflux of saliva around the tube and into the trachea.

The trap valve was fitted in a manner similar to the duckbill valve by measuring the tracheoesophageal wall thickness. The collar of the valve is positioned just into the esophagus and opens upon entering the lumen. It also resists inappropriate extrusion of the prosthesis from the tracheoesophageal wall. This valve is comparable to the duckbill in durability, but the increased airflows with decreased resistance permit adaptability to the stoma-closing device.

INSERTION OF THE TRACHEOESOPHAGEAL VALVE

After the two-day maturation period, the stent catheter is removed in the clinic and the horizontal distance is measured from the posterior tracheal wall at the puncture to the posterior hypopharyngeal wall (Fig. 22–10). This length will correspond, within 3 mm, to one of the valve sizes. The valve is inserted, is felt to enter

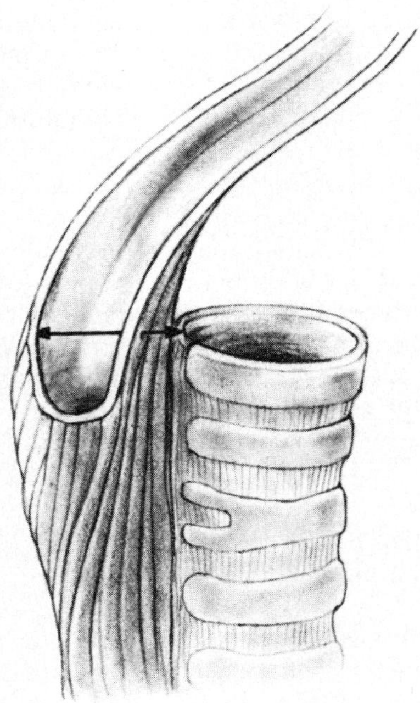

Figure 22–10. Distance across tracheoesophageal common wall for correct voice prosthesis sizing.

the esophagus, and is fixed to the skin by tape. The patient is given instruction on beginning tracheoesophageal speech.

The initial training program consists mainly of teaching the patient to exhale air under increased pressures so as to open the valve and thereby produce pharyngoesophageal sound. Also, the patient must appreciate the critical importance of precise valve placement, orientation, and fixation. Instruction on stoma care and valve maintenance and replacement are crucial to effective compliance with the tracheoesophageal prosthetic valve method.

Exhalation must be accompanied by effective manual occlusion of the stoma to efficiently divert air across the valve. Stoma coverage must eliminate air escape, which is distracting, but must not be so firm as to distort the pharyngoesophagus and prevent valve opening or effective airflows. This aspect of the rehabilitative program requires empiric trials and practice for the most effective seal and valve function. Speech re-education is not difficult because the postlaryngectomy vocal tract remains functional for articulation as intelligible speech in spite of the requisite change in the source of sound.

Most patients will experience little difficulty except for accommodation to pharyngeal airflows. When the intratracheal pressures needed for voice production are uncomfortably elevated, the status of the pharyngoesophagus must be assessed or the valve checked for optimum function. The simplest method is to remove the valve and observe the tracheoesophageal puncture for patency. The stoma is covered and, without the valve, air is directed through the open tracheoesophageal tunnel. The flow will usually travel superiorly producing effortless sound and voice, but the air may be directed to the stomach producing a characteristic gastric rumble and feeling of distention.

With satisfactory voice production, the tracheoesophageal measurement is rechecked, valve length selected, and orientation for effective airflow noted. The airflow port on the valve should not be buried in the tracheoesophageal puncture; this can be avoided by angling the retention flanges superiorly or using a tracheostoma valve housing (see below). If the valve is too short, the duckbill slit may be partially contained within the tracheoesophageal puncture and opening will be restricted. This problem is corrected by using a silicone valve of increased length or a collar that stabilizes the prosthesis against the esophageal wall anteriorly. If the valve is too long, either the tip will embed in the posterior pharyngeal wall, which impedes opening, or it will be distorted, increasing the elastic recoil of the duckbill and demanding increasingly higher opening pressures. The former problem is managed by using a tube 3 to 5 mm shorter, if the esophageal anteroposterior diameter will accommodate it, or by increasing the length by 0.3 to 1.0 cm to direct airflows down and away from the posterior wall. The latter problem may be corrected by rotating the valve 45 to 90 degrees to permit the duckbill to open laterally rather than vertically, eliminating the higher recoil effect.

If speech failure results from gastric overfilling secondary to pharyngoesophageal hypertonicity, the problem is related to the status of the pharyngeal constrictor muscles. This difficulty appears in 12 per cent of patients but may exist in varying degrees in up to 40 per cent of patients and often explains esophageal speech failure as well.[25] In a later section, we review the problem of disordered pharyngoesophageal sphincter behavior and present therapeutic recommendations.

SELF-CLOSING TRACHEOSTOMA VALVE

As our experience with the various methods for postlaryngectomy voice rehabilitation increases, intermittent tracheostoma occlusion assumes growing importance. Manual stoma occlusion is undesirable from a hygienic standpoint and draws attention to the alaryngeal condition. A valve system is required that will close the trachea for phonation but remain open for normal breathing. Also, the desired system should accommodate increased rates of flow with exertion and the sudden increased pressures generated by coughing.

Blom, Singer, and Hamaker described a tracheostoma valve that meets these important physiologic criteria.[26] The initial concept of this valve was to avoid intubation of the sensitive postlaryngectomy tracheostoma and consequently to decrease the incidence of tracheitis, bleeding, and increased mucorrhea. Experience with medical grade adhesives in the peritracheal skin confirmed the feasibility of an adhesive bond between skin and valve that would be tolerated by irradiated patients.

A flexible valve housing has been developed to conform to various stoma sizes and shapes (Fig. 22–11). The housing is bonded to the parastomal skin with a disk of hypoallergenic adhesive and a liquid skin cement applied directly to the skin. The housing accepts and engages the valve assembly firmly enough to prevent dislocation with increased tracheal pressures during speech or cough. A curved diaphragm of latex, which is airflow sensitive and responds to variations in expiratory exchange, is attached to the center of the valve assembly.

The normal respiratory position of the valve is fully open for comfortable inspiratory and expiratory airflows. As the airflow increases for speech production, the diaphragm unfurls and seats against the inner rim of the valve assembly, sealing the tracheostoma. When airflows decrease, the diaphragm returns to the open position. When the wearer must cough, the thin diaphragm will partially evert through the assembly to release air pressure; it then easily repositions itself with the following inspiration. Individual respiratory needs during exertion are accommodated by substituting diaphragms of different thickness with corresponding changes in valve compliance.

The principal problem that prevents effective use of the tracheostoma valve is increased intratracheal pressures when the airway is closed. This is related to vocal tract resistance and stems from two sources: (1) voice prosthesis resistance and (2) excessive pharyngeal constrictor tone. The tonicity of the pharynx following esophageal distention has been mentioned

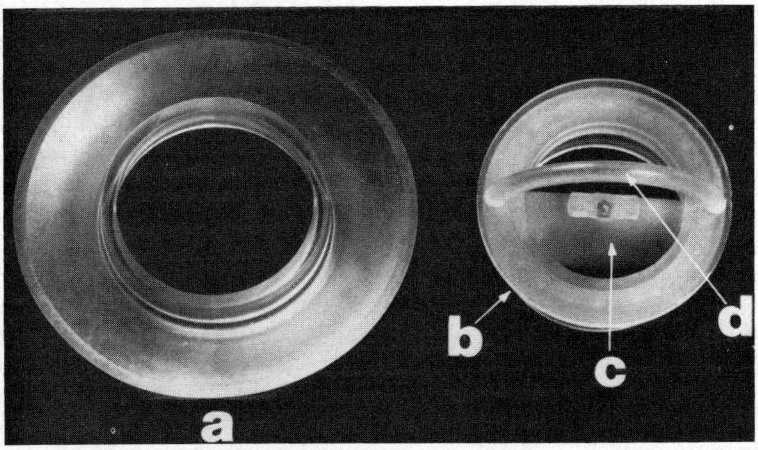

Figure 22–11. Self-closing tracheostoma valve showing housing (a), valve casing (b), diaphragm (c), and clothing bar (d). (From Blom ED et al.: Ann Otol Rhinol Laryngol 91:576, 1982.)

earlier and will be reviewed further. The problem of resistance of the voice prosthesis has been solved by the trapdoor valve modification in many cases.

In vitro measurements of the airway resistance offered by the Blom-Singer voice prosthesis with the duckbill valve and the Panje voice button consistently demonstrated values considerably higher than the normal laryngeal pressures,[27] which range from 30 to 43 cm H_2O/LPS. The opposition to airflow through the Blom-Singer prosthesis ranged from 45 to 120 cm H_2O/LPS, while resistance through the Panje voice button ranged higher, from 285 to 430 cm H_2O/LPS. This higher resistance stimulated the design of the trapdoor voice prosthesis, which reduced airway resistance to levels comparable to those cited for the normal human larynx during phonation.

RESULTS OF THE ENDOSCOPIC PROSTHESIS METHOD OF VOICE RESTORATION

In 1981, we reported our accumulated experience with 129 patients as well as that of other investigators.[25, 28–30] Successful acquisition of voice after total laryngectomy was noted in 113 patients or 88 per cent of the series. The criteria for success were fluency and intelligibility of the speakers. Acoustic, aerodynamic, and intelligibility studies of tracheoesophageal speakers were analyzed in a number of other publications.[31–33] In general, the parameters studied showed values that were equal to or better than those in excellent esophageal speakers.

Nine patients failed to maintain the voice prosthesis, although speech was initially acquired. These failures resulted from inability to manage the tracheostoma and voice prosthesis. A customized vocal prosthesis might have solved the mechanical problem for some of these patients, but the risk of aspiration of saliva or of the prosthesis itself would have been increased.[34]

Although 20 per cent of the patients experienced occasional extrusion of the voice prosthesis, it was replaced after dilatation of the tracheoesophageal puncture. Additional supervision of stoma care regimen was then provided. The addition of a prosthesis collar in 1981 reduced the extrusion rate to less than 10 per cent.

Postoperative problems have not been significant. Some patients initially experience inflammation of the stoma and narrowing of the lumen. This narrowing is managed by insertion of a soft tracheal cannula. Transient tracheitis may occur, requiring increased local hygiene measures and, occasionally, antibiotics. No cases of cervical or mediastinal abscess formation, uncontrolled fistulization, or dysphagia have been observed.

The most important problem is tracheal reflux and aspiration. Although salivary contamination of the trachea occurs, no patients have experienced aspiration pneumonia. Two patients developed intractable aspiration with a functioning valve in place and required a second procedure to close the fistula. Three patients reported intermittent aspiration from three months to one year postoperatively. They were treated by repeated electrocauterization of the tracheoesophageal fistula to increase stenosis and provide tight valve fitting. Nine patients experienced minimal aspiration that responded to a single electrocautery treatment. Tracheoesophageal puncture leakage has been negligible with the collar model of the voice prosthesis.

Although the tracheoesophageal puncture was patent and the voice prosthesis was properly fitted and functional, 16 patients failed to develop satisfactory speech. These esophageal speech failures were unable to support airflows across the pharyngoesophagus for fluent speech production. The pharyngoesophageal transition zone failed to relax for airflow or became hypertonic, as had been suggested earlier by the esophageal distention test.

HYPERTONIC TRACHEOESOPHAGEAL SPEECH FAILURE

The tracheoesophageal puncture phonation system depends on airflow introduced into the esophagus inferior to the cricopharyngeal and pharyngeal constrictor muscles. Such airflow with esophageal distention is readily pinched off by the upper esophageal sphincter. Procedures that bypass this region, such as the VoiceBak prosthesis or the methods of Conley and Asai, do not confront this problem.[35] On the other hand, bypass of the tonic pharyngoesophageal region diminishes the quality of resultant speech toward a less intelligible whisper. This has sometimes been overcome by inserting an artificial vibrator or reed in the system.[36]

Surgeons often insist that the pharynx after laryngectomy is a passive or even a flail structure, devoid of cricopharyngeal muscle and only partially buttressed by remnants of the inferior pharyngeal constrictor muscle. Pharyngeal closure techniques to decrease the likelihood of the most serious early complication of laryngectomy (dehiscence of the pharyngeal closure with subsequent uncontrolled fistulization) are frequently debated. Many clinicians advocate a T-shaped mucosal closure to decrease suture line stress, while others support the concept of a straight line vertical or horizontal closure.[37] Most apply a multiple layer reconstruction and fastidiously buttress the closure with pharyngeal constrictor remnants, strap muscles, or even the thyroid gland (Fig. 22–12).

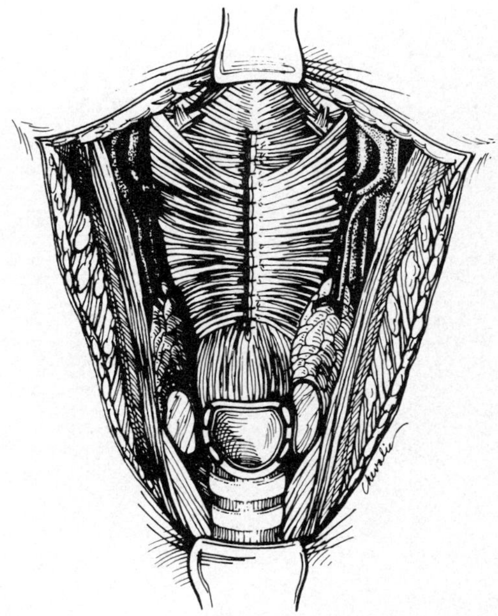

Figure 22–12. Diagrammatic representation of three-layer pharyngeal closure with pharyngeal constrictor muscle reconstitution.

The reconstituted pharyngeal musculature is partially denervated anterolaterally, but the pharyngeal plexus innervation remains intact. Gates demonstrated that manometric measurements of the pharyngoesophageal high pressure zone in a resting state did not differ statistically in successful versus failed esophageal speakers.[38]. The pressure profile examined by a computerized force-summing probe was distinctly different from normal subjects but demonstrated the presence of definite resting tones of 70 ± 18 mm Hg and variability of relaxation among patients. It is not unreasonable to assume that the pharyngeal muscle remnants have enough tone to function as an effective sphincter in the alaryngeal state.

In the group of patients that had failed tracheoesophageal speech, videofluoroscopy consistently identified a retropharyngeal mass corresponding radiographically with the inferior pharyngeal constrictor muscles. The axial length ranged from 1 to 4 cm and became increasingly prominent with greater esophageal distention (Fig. 22–13). The effect of this mass can close the pharyngeal lumen and prevent the airflow needed for satisfactory voice production.

A parapharyngeal nerve block was developed to assess constrictor relaxation and subsequent vocalization. Lidocaine (Xylocaine, 2 per cent) was injected into the retropharyngeal space at locations corresponding to C2 and C4, lateral to the pharynx (Fig. 22–14). After a few minutes, a reduction in the muscle mass was seen radiographically and voicing was possible through the tracheoesophageal puncture. In the

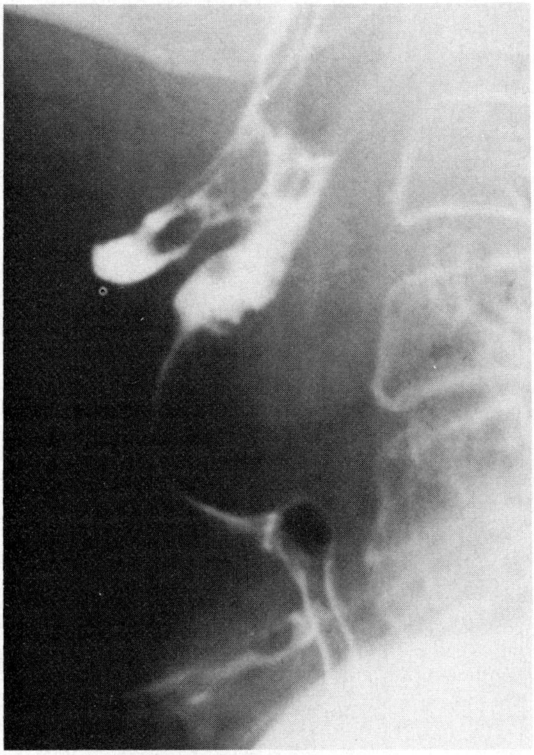

Figure 22–13. Radiographic appearance of pharyngeal constrictor closure of upper esophagus during insufflation (retropharyngeal "bar"). (From Singer MI, Blom ED: Arch Otolaryngol 107:671, 1981.)

few cases where the block had no effect, it was repeated on the contralateral side, with certainty of the retropharyngeal plane gauged by palpating the cervical spine with the injecting needle. A positive block and subsequent voice production are indications for a pharyngeal constrictor myotomy.

TECHNIQUE OF PHARYNGEAL CONSTRICTOR MYOTOMY

The surgical technique of pharyngeal constrictor myotomy is similar to that described for cricopharyngeal myotomy for dysphagia. A mercury-filled dilator is placed as a stent in the pharyngoesophagus, and an incision is placed in the scar from the flap used at the initial laryngectomy.[23] The flap is elevated to the level of the base of the tongue and within 1 cm of the tracheostoma. The dilator is readily palpated as a guide to the pharynx in the laryngectomized state.

A variable thickness of scar tissue resembling a pseudocapsule around the neopharynx is encountered; this tissue is dissected to separate the pharynx from the carotid artery, which is often adjacent to the pharynx after laryngectomy. The carotid artery is retracted laterally and the pharynx is rotated over the dilator medially. It is advisable to dissect posteriorly to the prevertebral space to enter the retropharyngeal plane, subsequently opening the field for a fastidious myotomy.

The pharyngeal constrictor muscles are 3 to 5 mm thick, located adjacent to the submucosa, deep to a layer of fibroadipose tissue, and investing fascia, which must be divided. The constrictor muscles are identified by their oblique fiber disposition and axial length of 3 to 5 cm. The entire constrictor muscle group is divided from the tongue base (identified by the flare into the hypopharynx at its widest part) to the level of the esophageal inlet (identified by a characteristic narrowing at the lip of the cervical esophagus) (Fig. 22–15). The incision is made completely through the fibers at the posterolateral aspect of the pharynx and avoids disrupting the submucosal venous plexus. The muscle is not resected or sutured and the wound is drained with a suction catheter for 24 hours.

A diet is resumed after 48 hours and voicing may begin on the third day. The resultant voice is fluent, effortless, immediate, and usually characterized by low fundamental frequency. All in a present series of 75 patients who underwent the secondary procedure achieved satisfactory tracheoesophageal phonation and have maintained it without deterioration.

Observations of the myotomized patients have yielded some important information. Independent of the method of pharyngeal closure at the laryngectomy, the constrictor muscles will form a pseudoinsertion on the anterior mucosal closure resembling a raphe. This has been observed in patients in whom the muscles were not purposely closed as a third layer and occasionally interfered with successful voice acquisition.

Of the patients submitted to pharyngeal constrictor myotomy, five were subsequently able to develop conventional esophageal voice following the procedure and others improved their fluency, a finding recently noted by others as well.[39] The implication of this contradicts the widely held theories that esophageal speech depends on an intact cricopharyngeal muscle and that failure has no anatomic or physiologic basis.[9] It is reasonable to assume that esophageal speech acquisition is highly dependent on the tolerance of the pharyngoesophagus to distention and that elevation of the pharyngoeso-

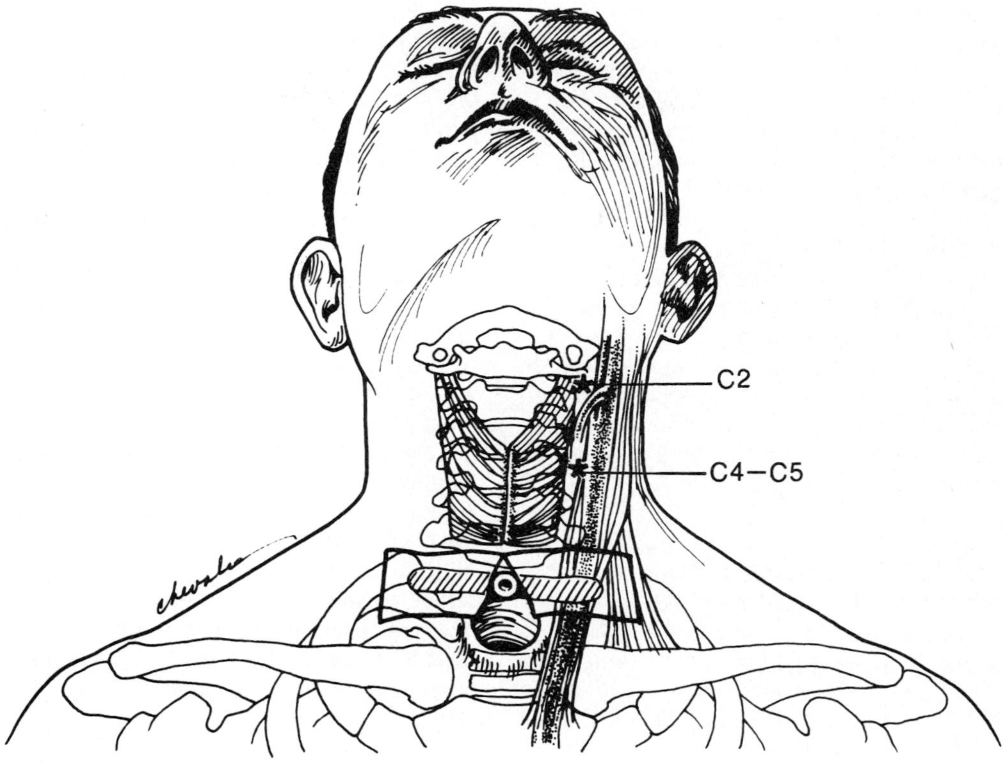

Figure 22–14. Pharyngeal nerve plexus block. Sites marked by stars (C2, C4-C5). Note voice prosthesis in place at tracheoesophageal puncture. (Adapted from Singer MI, Blom ED: Arch Otolaryngol 107:672, 1981.)

phageal resting tone may hinder voice production in a reflexive manner wholly independent of training or motivation. The hypertonicity problem is usually not associated with volunteered complaints of dysphagia or repeated need for esophageal dilatations. When carefully interviewed, however, many patients will report occasional nasal regurgitation, delays of swallowing two to three times normal, or the sensation of having to swallow over an obstruction. The postmyotomy patient is usually relieved of these problems of motility of the laryngectomized pharynx after muscle relaxation.

When the muscular sphincter ring is broken more posteriorly (distal to its natural anatomic insertion), maximum hypotonicity may be achieved and voices approaching a whisper may result as the pharynx is rendered increasingly flaccid. On the other hand, if the myotomy is more anterior, residual tonicity may prevent satisfactory voice acquisition and a contralateral approach may be required.

Based on these observations, pharyngeal

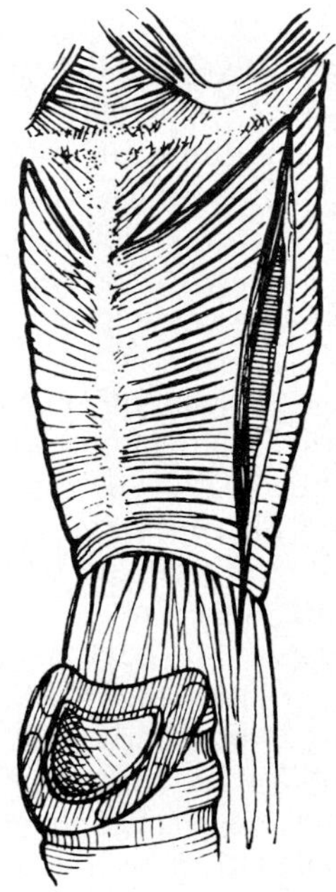

Figure 22–15. Posterolateral pharyngeal constrictor myotomy extending from the cervical esophagus to the superior hypopharynx.

constrictor myotomy is added to the initial laryngectomy procedure to enhance the achievement of either conventional esophageal voice or secondary development of tracheo-esophageal phonation. The surgical field for laryngectomy provides an opportunity for a thorough, safe, and technically easy myotomy when the pharynx is open. The mucosa can be protected by stretching it over the operator's finger as a guide. The incision is placed in the posterior midline, which is advantageous for preservation of the vascularity of the musculature and subsequently underlying mucosa. If the pharyngeal constrictor musculature is devitalized by an anterolateral myotomy, the likelihood of subsequent mucosal breakdown and fistulization may be increased.[40]

A PROSTHETIC APPROACH FOR PRIMARY SPEECH PRESERVATION

The near-total laryngectomies or neoglottic reconstructions were designed to avoid prosthetic devices and permit rapid speech acquisition. Unfortunately, problems of uncontrolled aspiration and pharyngeal secretions demanded custom tracheal devices or fistula valves. Success rates are further diminished by frequent revision procedures, conversion to conventional total laryngectomy, deteriorating speech results, ineffectiveness in an irradiated milieu, and higher local recurrence rates. Application of the silicone valve prosthesis to a primary tracheoesophageal puncture at laryngectomy may hold some promise for rapid speech rehabilitation. This approach does not compromise the classic wide-field laryngectomy, has no prolonged period of postoperative aspiration, and causes no delay in receiving radiation therapy.

Thirty unselected patients underwent this approach; nineteen (63 per cent) were considered successful. They achieved voice rapidly and maintained the silicone valve without dislodgment. Five patients received unplanned radiation therapy and seven received postoperative radiation therapy. Six patients (20 per cent) were considered partially successful. Of this group, three patients had satisfactory speech but lost the valve after two weeks with resultant closure of the tracheoesophageal puncture. One individual had delayed speech development at six weeks, one lost the prosthesis at six weeks with closure of the tracheoesophageal puncture, and one developed regional and distant metastases.

Five patients were considered absolute failures because of inability to establish speech postoperatively with the valve prosthesis. This problem was characterized by mechanical difficulty with the new stoma and inability to master stoma and valve hygiene in the initial postoperative state.

From this experience, some general comments can be offered. The method will result in satisfactorily fluent speech by trachoesophageal phonation; however, continued use is limited by the inability of newly laryngectomized patients to manage a stoma and a prosthesis simultaneously. There were no problems related to uncontrolled aspiration and no major delays in adjunctive radiation therapy. Four fistulas (13 per cent) occurred.

When the tracheoesophageal valve method for phonation should be applied as a primary method cannot be ascertained from the experience to date. Although the success rates are not as satisfactory as with the secondary application of the method, they are actually equivalent to some of the primary methods previously reported.

SUMMARY

The unique sound-generating capacity of the larynx must always be considered secondary to its vital function of protecting the airways during swallowing. Only after airway protection was achieved did total laryngectomy become a reasonably safe treatment method. The evolution of laryngeal cancer treatment has been associated with numerous techniques to preserve the ability to speak.

Alaryngeal patients may develop voice from the pharyngoesophageal mucous membranes or pseudoglottis, but efficient activation of this requires skilled air trapping or a tracheal shunt. The valve prosthesis serves its purpose well by providing reliable airway protection and voice production by the vibrating effect of expired pulmonary air on the pharyngoesophageal membranes.

The pharynx and esophagus are reported to require driving pressures ranging from 15 to 120 cm H_2O for voice production. When the esophagus is coupled by the tracheoesophageal puncture to the pulmonary system, the patient's lung volume is again available as a reliable generator of voice. In addition, the control of exhalatory forces and airflows optimizes the quality of the subsequent alaryngeal speech. Through complex motor function, the pharyngoesophagus is capable of variable adjustments of tone with varying airflows resulting in a more natural voice quality.

The laryngeal cancer patient faces the dilemma of an uncertain future with life-threatening disease as well as voicelessness. Life as he has known it is forever altered. Laryngectomy represents a loss not only of body integrity but also of an innate human trait. The restoration of voice is a goal pursued as vigorously as more effective treatments for laryngeal cancer. The planned fistulas, shunts, cannulas, valves, and artificial larynges, along with diligent efforts of speech clinicians, vividly reflect the need to improve the status of these indivduals. A historical review illustrates the repeated refinements of previous ideas and the improved understanding of the mechanisms of voice production.

The surgical residua of total laryngectomy can be used for effective rehabilitation. The combination of modern technology, a simple tracheoesophageal shunt, and skilled patient instruction will permit rehabilitation, with a voice that is intelligible and natural for most laryngectomees. Future trends will undoubtedly advance current methods. Emphasis on improved laryngectomy techniques must continue in order to provide suitable therapy for the cancer while maintaining the continuity of the airway and digestive tract for sound production.

References

1. McNeil BJ et al.: Speech and survival: Tradeoffs between quality and quantity of life in laryngeal cancer. N Engl J Med 305:982–987, 1981.
2. Staffieri M, Serafini I: La riabilitazione chirurgica della voce e della respirazione dopo laringectomia totale. XXIX Cong Nazionale. Bologna, Associazione Otologi Ospedalieri Italian, 1976, pp 57–111.
3. Arslan M, Serafini I: Restoration of laryngeal functions after total laryngectomy. Report on the first 25 cases. Laryngoscope 82:1349, 1972.
4. Mozolewski ES et al.: Arytenoid vocal shunt in laryngectomized patients. Laryngoscope 85:853, 1975.
5. Amatsu M.: A one stage surgical technique for post laryngectomy voice rehabilitation. Laryngoscope 90: 1378–1386, 1980.
6. Gussenbauer C: Über die erste durch Th. Billroth am Menschen ausgeführte Kehlkopf—Extirpation und die Anwendung eines kunstlichen Kehlkopfes. Arch Klin Chir 17:343–356, 1874.
7. Gluck T.: Der gangewaertige Stand der Chirugie des Kehlkopfes Pharynx—Oesophagus und der Traachea. Monatsschr Ohrenh 38:89, 1904.
8. Seeman M.: Speech and voice without larynx. Cas Lek Cesk 41:369–372, 1922.
9. Diedrich WM, Youngstrom KA: Alaryngeal Speech. Springfield IL, Charles C Thomas, 1966, pp 129–148.
10. Robe EY et al.: A study of certain factors in the development of speech after laryngectomy. Laryngoscope 66:173–186, 1956.
11. Snidecor JC: Some scientific foundations for voice restoration. Laryngoscope 85:640–647, 1975.
12. Gates GA et al.: Current status of laryngectomee rehabilitation: I. Results of therapy. Am J Otolaryngol 3:1–14, 1982.
13. Briani AA: Riabilitazione fonetica di laringectomizzati a mezzo della corrente aerea espiratioria polmonare. Arch Ital Otol 63:469, 1952.
14. Conley JJ et al.: A new surgical technique for vocal rehabilitation of the laryngectomized patient. Ann Otol Rhinol Laryngol 67:655–664, 1958.
15. Conley JJ: Vocal rehabilitation by autogenous vein graft. Ann Otol Rhinol Laryngol 68:990–995, 1959.
16. Taub S, Spiro RH: Vocal rehabilitation of laryngectomees: Preliminary report of a new technique. Am J Surg 124:87–90, 1972.
17. Sisson GA et al.: Voice rehabilitation after laryngectomy. Arch Otolaryngol 101:178–181, 1975.
18. McConnel FMS et al.: Three years experience with a hypopharyngeal pseudoglottis for vocal rehabilitation after laryngectomy. Trans Amer Acad Ophthalmol Otol 84:63–67, 1977.
19. Iwai H, Koike Y: Primary laryngoplasty. Laryngoscope 85:929, 1975.
20. Labayle J: Restorative total laryngectomy. *In* Shedd, DP, Weinberg B (eds): Surgical Prosthetic Approaches to Speech Rehabilitation. Boston, GK Hall Medical Publishers, 1980, pp 55–66.
21. Piguet JJ: Functional laryngectomy, *In* Shedd DP, Weinberg B (eds): Surgical Prosthetic Approaches to Speech Rehabilitation. Boston, GK Hall Medical Publishers, 1980, pp 41–53.
22. Singer MI, Blom ED: Tracheoesophageal puncture: A surgical prosthetic method for post laryngectomy speech restoration. Third International Symposium on Plastic and Reconstructive Surgery of the Head and Neck, New Orleans, 1979.
23. Singer MI, Blom ED: Selective myotomy for voice restoration after total laryngectomy. Arch Otolaryngol 107:670–673, 1981.
24. Singer MI, Blom ED: An endoscopic technique for restoration of voice after laryngectomy. Ann Otol Rhinol Laryngol 89:529–533, 1980.
25. Singer MI et al.: Further experience of the voice restoration after total laryngectomy. Ann Otol Rhinol Laryngol 90:498–502, 1981.
26. Blom ED et al.: Tracheostoma valve for post laryngectomy voice rehabilitation. Ann Otol Rhinol Laryngol 91:576–578, 1982.
27. Weinberg B.: Airway resistance of the voice button. Arch Otolaryngol 108:498–500, 1982.
28. Wood BG et al.: Tracheoesophageal puncture for alaryngeal voice restoration. Ann Otol Rhinol Laryngol 90:492–494, 1981.
29. Wetmore SJ et al.: The Singer-Blom voice restoration procedure. Arch Otolaryngol 107:674–678, 1981.
30. Johns ME, Cantrell RW: Voice restoration of the total laryngectomy patient: The Singer-Blom technique. Otolaryngol Head Neck Surg 89:82–86, 1981.
31. Dudley BL et al.: An intelligibility study of tracheoesophageal puncture speakers and esophageal speakers. Annual Convention, American Speech-Language-Hearing Association, Detroit, 1980.
32. Robbins J et al.: An acoustic study of voice after tracheoesophageal puncture. Annual Convention, American Speech-Language-Hearing Association, Detroit, 1980.

33. Weinberg B et al.: Airway resistance during esophageal phonation. J Speech Hear Disord 47:194–199, 1982.
34. Shapiro MJ, Ramanathan VR: Tracheostoma vent voice prosthesis. Laryngoscope 92:1126, 1982.
35. Asai, R.: Asai's new voice production method: A substitution for human speech. Eighth International Congress of Otorhinolaryngology, Tokyo, 1965.
36. Shedd DP et al.: Reed fistula method of speech rehabilitation after laryngectomy. Am. J. Surg 124: 510–514, 1972.
37. Applebaum EL, Levin HL: Pharyngeal reconstruction after laryngectomy. Laryngoscope 87:1884–1890, 1977.
38. Welch RW et al.: Manometry of the normal upper esophageal sphincter and its alterations in laryngectomy. J Clin Invest 63:1036–1041, 1979.
39. Chodosh PL: Pharyngeal myotomy for vocal rehabilitation post-laryngectomy. Laryngoscope, 94:52–57, 1984.
40. Singer MI et al: Muscle flap reconstruction of the pharynx after total laryngectomy. American Society for Head and Neck Surgery, May, 1982.

23

Experience with the Panje Voice Prosthesis

William R. Panje, M.D. and D. R. VanDemark, Ph.D.

The Panje Voice Prosthesis, used in conjunction with appropriate speech therapy, provides an effective primary means of voice rehabilitation for the total laryngectomy patient. The Panje prosthesis, called a voice button, is a miniature, biflanged, one-way silicone valve that was developed and first used by one of the authors (WRP) in 1979. It makes possible tracheoesophageal speech by the laryngectomee while successfully preventing excessive aspiration of food and liquid into the trachea.

The voice button not only provides good results in voice rehabilitation, but it does so without certain disadvantages associated with other techniques of verbal communication utilized by laryngectomees. For example, unamplified esophageal speech has been considered the most appropriate method of communication for the laryngectomee, but a lack of voice volume restricts this means of communication to close proximity interactions in quiet surroundings. In addition, approximately 50 per cent of laryngectomees are unable to acquire useful and acceptable esophageal speech[1] while most of the patients who do may require six to nine months of training to attain a stable level of speech proficiency.[2] The Panje prosthesis enables the laryngectomee to acquire adequate voice production, with more volume, in less time than required for unamplified esophageal speech. Artificial laryngeal devices provide another way of communicating postlaryngectomy but produce a mechanical, robotlike sound, low in volume, and difficult to understand. A hand-held electromechanical device that needs frequent battery replacement is required. The voice button eliminates electromechanical devices, provides a more normal range of voice tone, inflection, and expressiveness, and allows speech at a higher volume that is easier to understand.

The Panje Voice Prosthesis also improves on certain devices that enable the laryngectomee to utilize tracheoesophageal fistula speech. Tracheoesophageal fistula speech is essentially esophageal speech created by driving tracheal air through a fistula created between the trachea and esophagus. The fistula eliminates the need for gulping and rebelching air to produce the pharyngoesophageal vibrations that create new speech sound. A number of devices have been developed for use in conjunction with a permanent tracheoesophageal fistula to produce tracheoesophageal fistula speech.[3] Many of these devices are expensive, bulky, and difficult to clean. With some of these, aspiration and stenosis have been serious problems. The voice button procedures and device enable the laryngectomee to achieve tracheoesophageal fistula speech with the following advantages:

1. The fistula is created by an outpatient procedure that can be done in 15 to 30 min and requires no special instrumentation.

2. The fistula can be created at the time of laryngectomy, avoiding a nasogastric feeding tube and allowing early speech rehabilitation.

3. The prosthesis is self-contained within the tracheostoma.

4. Usually, there is no specific size requirement for the prosthesis.

5. If it becomes necessary to discontinue use of the prosthesis for any reason, the fistula site will, in nearly all cases, heal spontaneously.

For successful results with the voice button, the otolaryngologist and speech pathologist must work as a team. This will optimize the chances for complete vocal rehabilitation of the laryngectomy patient. In the attempt to regain speech with the Panje prosthesis, it is very important for the patient to obtain some measure of successful voice production as soon as possible after creation of the fistula. By helping the patient to believe that he or she can return to a productive life as an individual who can successfully communicate, this will provide motivation to continue the rehabilitation process. In our studies, we have found that patients who have had the guidance and counsel of the speech pathologist during the initial tracheoesophageal fistula speech production are more successful in their early speech efforts and are less likely to become discouraged with the process of voice rehabilitation.

Table 23–1. INDICATIONS FOR PANJE SURGICAL TECHNIQUE AND PROSTHESIS

1.	Total laryngectomy
2.	No evidence of locally persistent or recurrent cancer
3.	Tracheostoma area greater than 1.5 sq cm
4.	Good manual dexterity
5.	Adequate pulmonary function
6.	No irradiation for prior three to six months
7.	No concurrent chemotherapy
8.	Positive nitrogen balance
9.	Good communication lacking
10.	Good attitude and personal hygiene

PATIENT SELECTION

Patients to be considered for the Panje Voice Prosthesis should be evaluated in terms of the following requirements (Table 23–1). The patient selected should:

1. Have total laryngectomy.

2. Have no evidence of locally persistent or recurrent cancer (metastatic cancer is not a contraindication of the procedure).

3. Have a tracheostoma area of 1.5 sq cm (for example, 1.5 by 1 cm or 3 by 0.5 cm). The stoma must be of adequate size for insertion of the voice button, yet be small enough for occlusion of the stoma by the patient.

4. Have good manual dexterity in occluding the tracheostoma with a finger or thumb (this would exclude patients with severe arthritis or tremorous conditions).

5. Have good pulmonary status (this excludes patients with severe chronic pulmonary disease, asthma, and recurrent pneumonia).

6. Have not had radiation therapy for the prior three to six months and will not be undergoing radiation or chemotherapy at the time of tracheoesophageal fistula formation. A patient in negative nitrogen balance should also be excluded from fistula formation because of increased chance of wound infection and widening of tracheoesophageal puncture site.

7. Have communication skills that are not satisfactory to the patient (the patient is not doing well with esophageal speech, or desires better speech with which to communicate more readily). Be cautious of performing tracheoesophageal fistula in long-term esophageal speakers who will need extensive retraining for voice button speech. We usually employ a communication rating chart for the laryngectomee (Table 23–2). Unless the patient falls into classifications 1-A, 1-B, or 2-B of Table 23–2, we feel that the tracheoesophageal fistula procedure should at least be attempted.

In addition, excessively tense patients or patients with psychological problems should be considered with caution.

Each patient who has had a laryngectomy and who is considered as a potential candidate for the Panje prosthesis should be evaluated by both the speech pathologist and the otolaryngology–head and neck surgeon. The speech pathologist assesses the patient in terms of adequacy of current speech, ability to close the stoma, air supply, general tension, and hygiene. The surgeon evaluates the patient with regard to stoma size, evidence of further disease, and appropriateness of surgical site.

The criteria presented herein can assist in the selection of patients most suitable to receive the Panje Voice Prosthesis; however, predicting which of selected patients will achieve good tracheoesophageal fistula speech with the voice button appears to be just as difficult as attempt-

Table 23–2. COMMUNICATION RATING CHART*

Mechanical Speech (Electrolarynx)	Esophageal Speech	Tracheoesophageal Fistula Speech (TEF)
1-A. Does well, desires no additional form of communication	1-B. Learns esophageal speech easily, communicates effectively, meets needs	1-C. Learns TEF easily, communicates effectively, meets needs
2-A. Does well, desires different mode of communication	2-B. Learns esophageal speech with some difficulty, limited intelligibility, meets needs	2-C. Learns TEF easily, communicates effectively, learns esophageal speech for auxillary communication needs (short responses)
3-A. Does moderately well, doesn't like electrolarynx	3-B. Learns esophageal speech well, limited intelligibility, does not meet needs	3-C. Learns TEF, but communicates only moderately well; needs additional therapy proportionate to communication needs
4-A. Does poorly, limited intelligibility	4-B. Has difficulty learning esophageal speech	4-C. Learns TEF poorly with therapy; consider introduction of esophageal speech if vibrating source is adequate
5-A. Refuses to use electrolarynx	5-B. Limited or no speech therapy available	5-C. Cannot achieve sound with TEF (a) determine source of problem (refer back to otolaryngologist) (b) if irreversible, consider best alternative method of communication
	6-B. Does not desire to learn esophageal speech (some patients find esophageal speech offensive)	

*Unless the patient falls into classification 1-A, 1-B, or 2-B, we feel the TE fistula procedure should be attempted.

ing to predict which patients will succeed with esophageal speech. The factors that influence the development of esophageal speech will also influence the development of tracheoesophageal fistula speech. These factors include patient age, stage of disease, extent of radical neck dissection, extent of radiation therapy, upper esophageal sphincter function, hearing capacity, patient motivation, degree of personal stress, and quality of training.[4]

PATIENT PREPARATION

After the laryngectomee has been selected for the Panje prosthesis, he or she should be given a written description of the voice button and the surgical procedure required to insert the prosthesis. Then, in a meeting with the otolaryngology–head and neck surgeon and the speech pathologist, the daily use of the prosthesis is thoroughly discussed, and the patient is instructed in the care of the prosthesis and of the fistula. We have found it helpful to show the patient a short video tape that further explains the procedure and that demonstrates the use of the voice button by patients. (This video tape and other materials for patient education are available through the authors.) Also at this meeting, the patient is instructed to eat only a small breakfast on the day of surgery.

SURGICAL PROCEDURE FOR THE ESTABLISHED LARYNGECTOMEE

The procedure that creates the tracheoesophageal fistula, making possible the placement of the voice button, is a simple outpatient tracheoesophageal stab operative technique.[5, 6] Surgical instrumentation includes a headlight, air suction equipment, soft tissue surgical instruments, and the supplies and instruments listed in Table 23–3.

Thirty minutes before the procedure is begun, the patient is given by mouth 30 mg of codeine to decrease the cough reflex and 5 mg of diazepam (Valium) to reduce anxiety. The upper aerodigestive system is anesthetized by having the patient swallow 15 ml of 2 per cent viscous lidocaine with 0.5 per cent dyclonine hydrochloride (Dyclone) gargle. The trachea, oral cavity, and pharynx are sprayed copiously with 5 per cent cocaine solution.

Once the patient is under local anesthesia, he or she swallows an appropriately sized Hurst or Maloney dilator that has been previously

Table 23–3. SUPPLIES, EQUIPMENT, AND INSTRUMENTS FOR VOICE BUTTON FISTULA

Supplies, medications, and solutions
Codeine 30 mg orally one-half hour before procedure to suppress cough reflex
Cocaine solution 5 per cent in atomizer
Lidocaine 1 per cent with epinephrine 1:100,000
Viscous lidocaine 2 per cent, 15 ml
Dyclonine hydrochloride 0.5 per cent, 30 ml
Normal saline solution
Tap water
Equipment
Hurst esophageal dilators (mercury emptied), sizes 34, 38, 40, 42, 44, and 46 French
Catheter coudé, size as requested by surgeon, usually 14 Fr, or Foley catheter 14 Fr with 5 ml balloon
Fishing line, 30-lb test or 24-lb test, or silk suture size 4 (not 4-0)
Chromic suture size 4-0 on micropoint double-armed needle × 4
Headlight
Surgeon's gloves
Shaving mirror
Drinking cup
Cautery
22-gauge spinal needle
Panje Voice Prosthesis and inserter if requested
Sterile voice button fistula instrument tray
Irrigation basin
Mayo drape, sterile
Table cover, sterile
Suction tubing
Instruments
One Bard-Parker knife handle No. 3
One single tooth conjunctival forceps
One bayonet forceps
One curved Stevens scissors
One straight Mayo (suture) scissors
One Webster needle holder
One ruler
Four small Tyrell iris single-prong skin hooks
Four curved mosquito hemostats
One Frazier suction tip, 10 Fr
One 3 ml Luer-Lok syringe
Bard-Parker knife blades No. 15 or No. 11
Cotton-tipped applicators, 6 inch
4 × 4 gauze sponges
Three glass medicine cups
Disposable 18-gauge needle
Disposable 22-gauge spinal needle, 3 inch
Disposable 25-gauge × 1.25 inch needle
Disposable 27-gauge needle
Pynchon suction (tonsil)
One curved Kelly hemostat

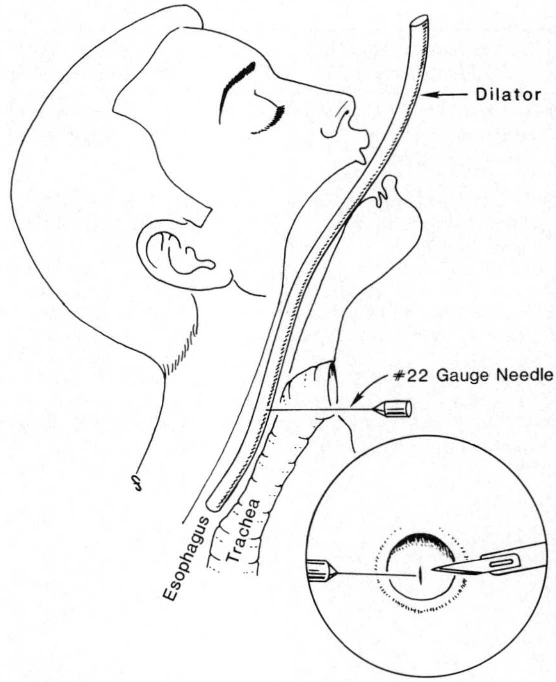

Figure 23–1. Insertion of spinal needle through tracheoesophageal wall into dilator. *Inset,* vertical incision along needle.

emptied of mercury (Fig. 23–1). The size of the dilator can range from 34 French for a small person to 46 French for a large individual. If the patient cannot swallow a 34 French dilator, the surgeon should consider trying to actively dilate the patient up to a 34 French dilator before attempting the fistula operation. Thus, the patient may have to wait until the esophagus has been dilated to an appropriate size before the operation is performed. With the patient in the supine position, the face should be pointed straight ahead, not to one side. Wearing a headlight and looking into the tracheostoma, the surgeon will note that as the esophageal tube passes the tracheostoma, a bulge will develop at the posterosuperior verge of the stoma and will proceed inferiorly as the dilator is advanced. It is crucial to determine the point of maximum bulge of the posterior tracheal wall because this will represent the anterior midpoint (maximum lumen diameter) of the esophagus.

The midpoint of the esophagus is injected through the membranous tracheal wall with 0.5 ml of 1 per cent lidocaine with epinephrine. A 22-gauge spinal needle is then inserted through the intended fistula site into the rubber esophageal tube. It is critical that the dilator not contain mercury when the spinal needle is inserted. The spinal needle should be inserted into the rubber dilator approximately 1.5 to 2 cm below the superior verge of the tracheostoma. The fistula is usually then located just above the level of the lower verge of the stoma. With a No. 15 Bard-Parker blade, a midpoint incision is made vertically along the spinal needle down to the esophageal dilator. The incision is approximately 7 to 10 mm in length.

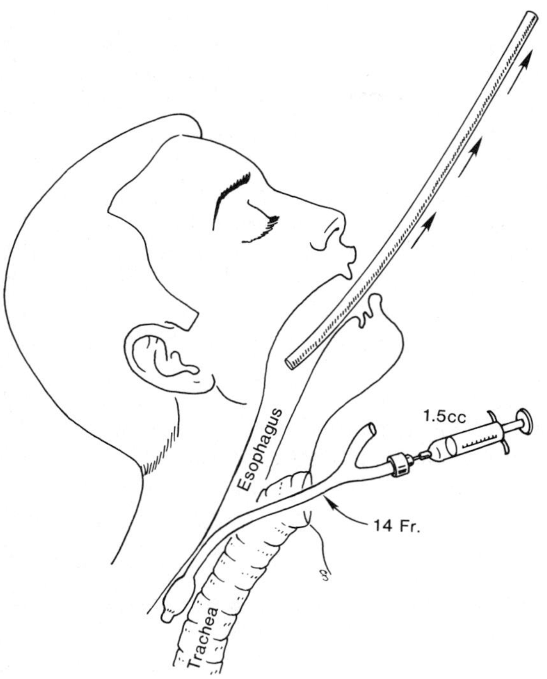

Figure 23–2. Removal of dilator and insertion of 14 French Foley catheter through fistula; 1.5 cc of solution is used to fill catheter bag.

When the fistula has been established, a 14 French Foley catheter is passed through the fistula site and inserted 6 to 8 cm toward the stomach (Fig. 23–2). Simultaneously, the esophageal dilator is removed. The balloon of the catheter is filled with 1.5 ml of fluid, preventing inadvertent extrusion of the catheter during the healing period.

The catheter is tied to the patient's neck in the same manner as a tracheostomy tube would be. It is important to occlude the catheter by tying the string (size 4 silk) tightly to avoid regurgitation of fluids and to prevent the escape of water from the balloon through the catheter. The upper part of the Foley catheter is then cut away.

The cut edges of the fistula do not need to be sutured together unless there is excessive bleeding. The tracheal and esophageal mucosa will heal together over the catheter in 10 to 14 days.

POSTOPERATIVE CARE AND PATIENT TEACHING

At the completion of the procedure, the patient is given a few sips of water. If the fistula leaks excessively when the patient swallows, then the 14 French Foley catheter should be replaced by a larger one. The patient is instructed to return in two or three days. During that visit, the catheter is removed and the surgical site is cleaned. The next smaller size of catheter is inserted (e.g., 18 French to 16 French, or 16 French to 14 French). This reduction in the size of the catheter should be made every three days until a 14 French Foley catheter can be inserted. The patient is advised not to attempt speech during this period. Since the upper aerodigestive tract has been surgically violated, the patient is placed on a five-to-seven-day course of prophylactic antibiotics.

The patient is instructed not to remove the catheter and is told that if the catheter does inadvertently become dislodged, it should be immediately reinserted. The catheter should not come out unless the balloon bursts or the catheter is intentionally cut. The patient is warned that during the first twenty-four postoperative hours there may be some leakage of liquids around the catheter upon drinking. This leakage can be reduced by eating solid food at the same time liquids are taken. Therefore, during the first two or three days after the procedure, fluids should be taken only with meals. It is emphasized that food should be well chewed while the patient is wearing the partially filled Foley catheter.

Approximately 10 to 14 days after formation of the fistula, the patient returns and the final catheter is removed. At that time, if the fistula is healed, the patient can be introduced to tracheoesophageal speech.

SURGICAL PROCEDURE AT TIME OF LARYNGECTOMY

Tracheoesophageal speech results that are excellent to good have been achieved in the established laryngectomee. Recently, initial reports have suggested that even better success can be achieved when the tracheoesophageal fistula is performed at the time of laryngectomy. We have also found this to be true in properly prepared patients (Fig. 23–3).

One of the authors (WRP) essentially performs a tracheoesophagostomy in nearly all patients at the time of laryngectomy. A simple instrument made by modifying a ring forceps allows the surgeon to make the tracheoesophagostomy (Fig. 23–4) 1.5 to 2 cm inferior to the superior cut edge of the trachea (Fig. 23–5).[7]

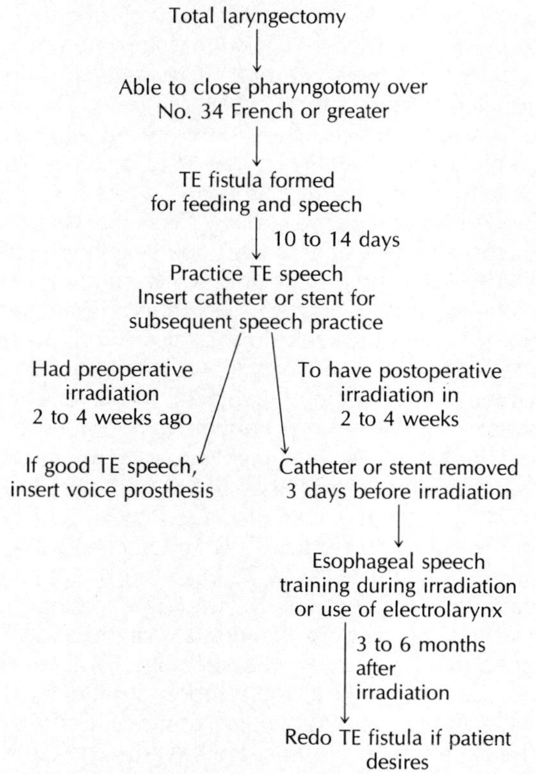

Figure 23–3. Patient selection for tracheoesophageal (TE) fistula at time of laryngectomy.

The cup part of the forceps is introduced into the esophagus through the resultant pharyngotomy following removal of the larynx; the other arm of the forceps (the U-shaped part of the clamp) is inserted into the trachea and with gentle approximation of the clamp the tracheoesophageal tissues become aligned for creation of the fistula. A No. 15 or No. 11 knife blade is used to make a 1 cm vertical incision in the midpart of the U-shaped clamp. The cup arm of the forceps prevents inadvertent cutting of the posterior esophageal wall and also allows for proper insertion of a 14 to 16 French feeding tube into the stomach. The feeding tube is sutured or tied to the neck with string in such a manner as not to cross over the tracheostoma. If the feeding tube traverses the stoma, an inordinate amount of crusting can develop in the postoperative period. At seven to ten days postoperatively, the feeding catheter is removed and a 14 to 16 French catheter coudé or a Panje fistula stent (Xomed, Inc.) is then inserted through the fistula. Tracheoesophageal fistula speech can usually be introduced at this time if the wound has healed well. The catheter or stent is removed from the fistula only during those times the patient is practicing tracheoesophageal fistula speech, as outlined in the following section on initial voice production. Again, we are not anxious to place the voice prosthesis until the patient has achieved good tracheoesophageal fistula speech and can comfortably manage obturating the fistula with the catheter.

We have been able to establish fistulae in 23 patients at the time of laryngectomy. Of the 23, if the pharynx and cervical esophagus could be closed over a 34 to 36 Hurst dilator (16 patients), the patient has been able to achieve tracheoesophageal fistula speech. Although too early to prove, our belief is that this selected population of laryngectomees (immediate tracheoesophageal fistula and closure over a 34 Hurst dilator) will have better long-term success with the voice prosthesis as well as with subsequent or concomitant development of esophageal speech.

INITIAL VOICE PRODUCTION

At this point, the speech pathologist plays an important role in helping the patient achieve initial tracheoesophageal fistula speech. The

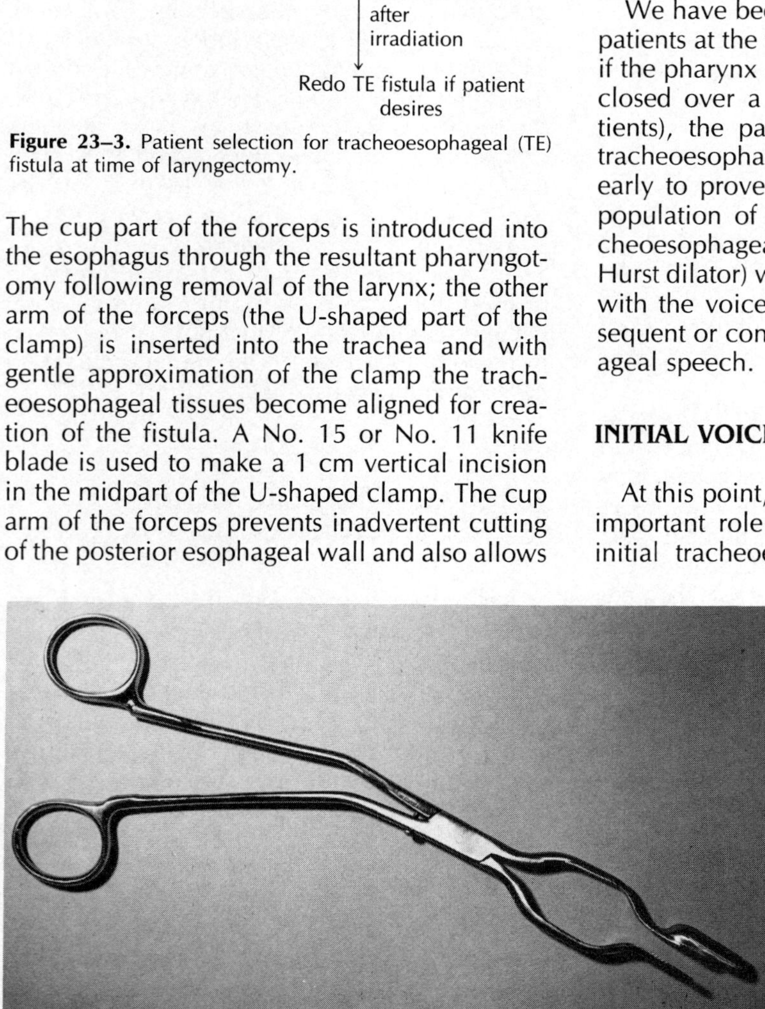

Figure 23–4. Panje-Shagets tracheoesophageal fistula clamp, modified from ring forceps, used at time of laryngectomy for doing a tracheoesophagotomy.

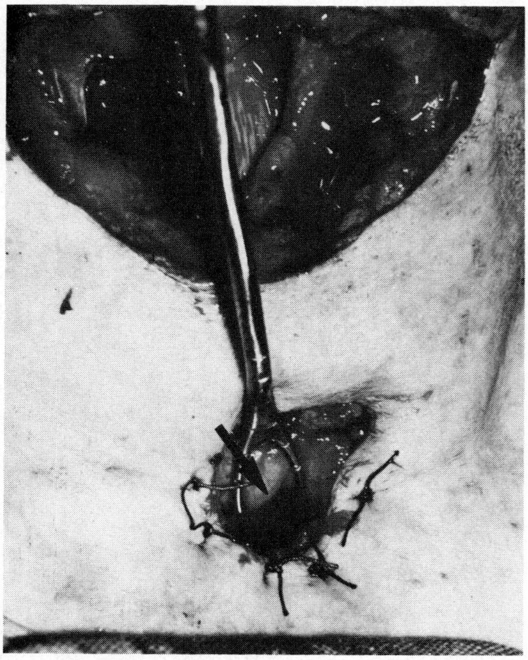

Figure 23–5. Using tracheoesophageal fistula clamp at time of laryngectomy, cup part of forcep is in esophageal lumen. Vertical incision will be made through the center *(arrow)* of the modified part of the ring clamp placed in the trachea.

method used by the speech pathologist to first introduce the patient to tracheoesophageal fistula speech will be an important factor in the overall success of the voice rehabilitation process. We have found the following method to be effective (Table 23–4).

After the catheter has been removed, the initial voice production session begins. It is preferable for the speech pathologist to work with the patient alone, since the presence of the patient's spouse or family member can create an unnecessary anxiety to be successful, thereby causing tension in the patient.

First, the patient is advised that a relaxed approach will bring better results. Then, the patient is told to inhale and the speech pathologist occludes the tracheostoma. The patient then exhales while attempting to say "ahh." Once the "ahh" sound has been successfully achieved, the speech therapist shows the patient how to occlude the stoma.

The patient is advised to use the nondominant hand, closing the stoma with either the thumb or index finger. It is explained that airtight coverage of the stoma is necessary, without pressing too hard. If the patient presses too forcefully on the stoma during exhalation, production of sound may be significantly reduced because the esophagus cannot effectively expand to produce adequate vibrations. The patient is reminded that relaxation is important for success.

After receiving these instructions, the patient is asked to cover his or her stoma and to again produce the "ahh" sound. There should be success in four or five trials. If not, the patient is instructed to relax and, if necessary, to lie down for a short period. Then a new attempt is made. If necessary, the catheter can be reinserted to make sure the fistula is open.

If the patient continues to be unsuccessful after a series of trials and relaxation periods, then the speech pathologist can attach a catheter to a Politzer's bag and insert the catheter back into the stoma through the tracheoesophageal fistula. By manually squeezing the Politzer's bag, the speech pathologist can force air into the tracheoesophageal area. Usually sound is attained. This success can help the patient to release tension and relax. After utilization of this maneuver, sound can usually be produced by digital closing of the stoma during expiration. If necessary, a tube can be passed from the mouth to the fistula site while delivering air through the catheter. Usually an area of adequate sound can be elicited if the patient is to become a successful tracheoesophageal speaker.

After success has been attained in producing the "ahh" sound while occluding the tracheostoma during exhalation through the naked fistula, the patient practices saying this sound against the clock, attempting to draw it out as long as possible. Then, the patient is asked to produce the vowels a, e, i, and o, and to practice repeating them. Next, short verses of a well-known song are sung (e.g., *Twinkle, Twinkle Little Star, Jingle Bells*). Finally, the patient is asked to produce short sentences.

If the patient is successful in all of these voice productions, then the voice button is inserted

Table 23–4. INITIATION OF TRACHEOESOPHAGEAL SPEECH

1. Catheter or stent is removed.
2. Patient takes small breath.
3. Speech pathologist or surgeon occludes tracheostoma with minimal digital pressure.
4. Patient attempts to say "ahh."
5. Patient instructed in stomal occlusion.
6. Patient attempts to say "ahh," then "a, e, i, o," and attempts to sing short songs.
7. Short sentences are produced.
8. Patient practices speech four to six times per day for 15 to 30 min each time at home or at work.
9. Catheter or stent replaced after practice session.

immediately. If the patient is not able to successfully accomplish all of the above verbal tasks during this initial voice production session, then insertion of the voice button is delayed for two to three weeks. Instead of inserting the prosthesis, a 14 French catheter coudé or a silicone tracheoesophageal fistula stent (Xomed, Inc.) is placed through the fistula. The patient is taught how to remove the catheter and how to replace it. The patient is sent home with the following instructions:

1. At least four to six times per day, remove the catheter and practice the phonatory exercises that were attempted during the initial voice production session. Each practice session should be no longer than 30 min. The catheter should not be left out for more than 30 min.

2. Do not eat or drink anything while the catheter is out.

The patient returns for reevaluation in two to three weeks. If the edges of the fistula site are well healed and the patient is speaking comfortably (counting to 15 or 20, holding "ahh" for at least 9 s, speaking in short sentences), then the voice button is inserted.

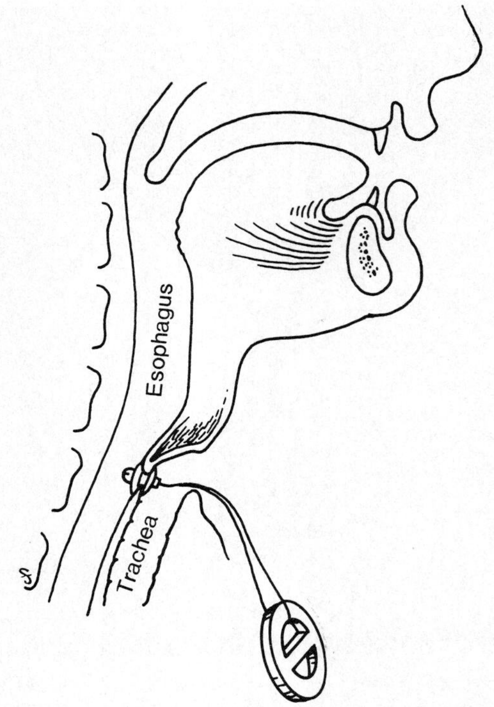

Figure 23–6. Position of voice button within tracheoesophageal fistula.

INSERTING THE PROSTHESIS

First, a prosthesis of the appropriate length is chosen. The Panje Voice Prosthesis is made in three lengths based on interflange distance (short, 7 mm; medium, 9 mm; long, 12 mm). Most patients require a medium or a long prosthesis. If the patient is not retaining the prosthesis, then the next longer one should be tried.

When the catheter has been removed, the voice button is inserted in the fistula (Fig. 23–6). The patient is instructed in the insertion of the prosthesis. The string attached to the prosthesis should be taped to the patient's body so that it does not become entangled during dressing, sleeping, or talking.

The most common difficulty encountered in inserting the prosthesis is failure to insert it far enough into the fistula. In some cases, difficulty with insertion can be caused by less than optimal placement of the fistula site. Another problem with prosthesis insertion can be caused by the use of an older rubber catheter that enlarges with age (this is usually not a problem with the silicone stent), causing the fistula site to become too large. Usually if the fistula is left open (by removal of catheter) for a short period of time, the size of the opening will decrease and the prosthesis will fit. In some cases, the fistula site may become slightly edematous, especially if the patient has attempted to insert the prosthesis several times. Thus, the fistula becomes slightly smaller and the patient is unsuccessful with insertion. In such a case, the catheter or stent should be reinserted for a short period. The patient should carry a catheter or stent to insert in the fistula in case the prosthesis cannot be retained.

After insertion of the voice button, most patients find that voice production requires a bit more effort than it does with the naked fistula. For this reason, the patient should feel confident in voice production before the prosthesis is inserted.

Once the Panje Voice Prosthesis is inserted into the tracheoesophageal fistula, the patient may experience the need for an inordinate amount of pulmonary force to achieve sound. In fact, some patients may not be able to make any sound after insertion of the voice button, whereas without the prosthesis they have had acceptable speech. Some investigators feel that the reason for failure to achieve tracheoesophageal fistula speech by patients wearing the voice button is that the prosthesis produces excessive resistance to pulmonary air flow into the esophagus.[8] We, as well as other investigators, have

Table 23–5. REASONS FOR EXCESSIVE PULMONARY FORCE FOR PHONATION

1. TE* fistula speech not properly introduced
2. Excessive digital-stomal force on phonation
3. Improper placement of voice prosthesis
   a. TE fistula made too near the superior tracheostomal verge
   b. Fistula not dilated with catheter or stent before placement of voice prosthesis
   c. Voice prosthesis not seated properly within fistula
   d. Inappropriate voice prosthesis size
   e. Redundant esophageal mucosa
4. Defective voice prosthesis
   a. Valve slits not completed back to esophageal flange
   b. Accumulation of debris within lumen
   c. Calcification of valve tip
5. Pharyngoesophageal spasm, scar, or tumor

*TE = tracheoesophageal

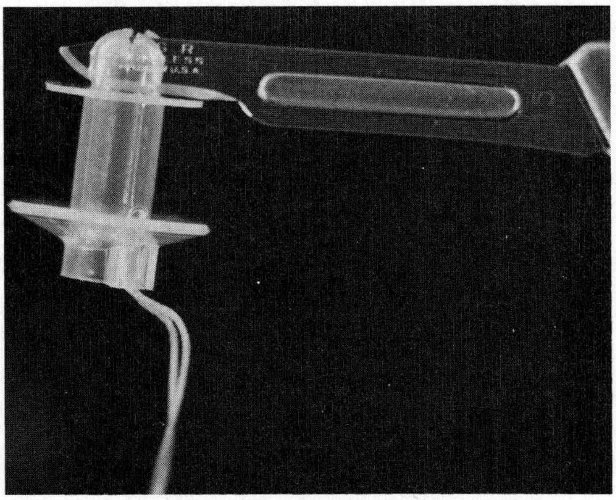

Figure 23–7. Using No. 15 knife blade to complete the valve slit cuts to the level of the esophageal flange of voice button.

not found this to be a major reason for failure to achieve speech with the voice prosthesis. In fact, the opening pressure of the Panje Voice Prosthesis is quite similar to that of the Blom-Singer prosthesis.[9] Our patient results, as well as comparative studies between the voice prosthesis and the Blom-Singer duckbill prosthesis, have demonstrated essentially no difference in the ability to achieve or sustain speech as well as intelligibility.[10, 11] We conclude that if the surgeon or speech pathologist encounters a tracheoesophageal fistula patient with inordinate difficulty in achieving speech after voice prosthesis placement, reasons other than prosthesis airway resistance should be explored.

Table 23–5 lists, in descending order of rate of occurrence, most of the reasons for failure of phonation after placement of the Panje Voice Prosthesis. Note that a defective voice prosthesis, which can occur with any manufactured appliance, is encountered in a minority of cases. In these cases, we have found that the valve splits are not extended back to the esophageal flange. Simple finger manipulation of the rounded end of the valve will, in the majority of cases, cause the valve slits to separate back to the esophageal flange. If the valve slits do not open all the way, then the surgeon or speech pathologist should cut the slits back to the esophageal flange using a razor blade or surgical knife (Fig. 23–7).

In some cases, especially in those patients wearing the voice button continuously for three to six months without removing it, esophageal mucosa may build up over the valve tip or stiffening and encrusting may occur. This is noted by the patient's slowly progressive need for increased pulmonary force for sustained phonation. Removal of the prosthesis will show whether the valve has become calcified. Also, if the patient still has difficulty in phonating after removal of the prosthesis, having once had good tracheoesophageal fistula speech, then tissue redundancy at the fistula site should be expected. Simple surgical excision of this redundant material will, in most cases, allow for proper reinsertion of a new voice button and return of speech. Sudden onset of voice loss is usually more compatible with food blockage of the prosthetic lumen, partial dislodgement of the prosthesis, or improper seating of the prosthesis. The patient may not be properly cleaning the prosthesis or may need a longer prosthesis.

A video fluoroscopy of the pharynx and esophagus can be helpful in assessing those laryngectomees who have previously had a tracheoesophageal fistula but have not achieved sound production with or without the prosthesis in place. If the esophagram demonstrates no air reservoir development at the tracheoesophageal fistula upon attempting voicing, then the surgeon should suspect pharyngeal spasm, scar, or possibly recurrent tumor (Fig. 23–8).

To determine if aphonia following tracheoesophageal fistula is due to spasm, the following procedure can be utilized. The pharyngoesophageal segment between the tracheostoma and the base of the tongue is anesthetized with 1 percent lidocaine (Xylocaine). Approximately 6 to 10 ml of the local anesthetic should be distributed along one side of the pharyngoesophageal segment so as to avoid any cardiovascular side effects from bilateral carotid bulb anesthesia. The surgeon should wait approxi-

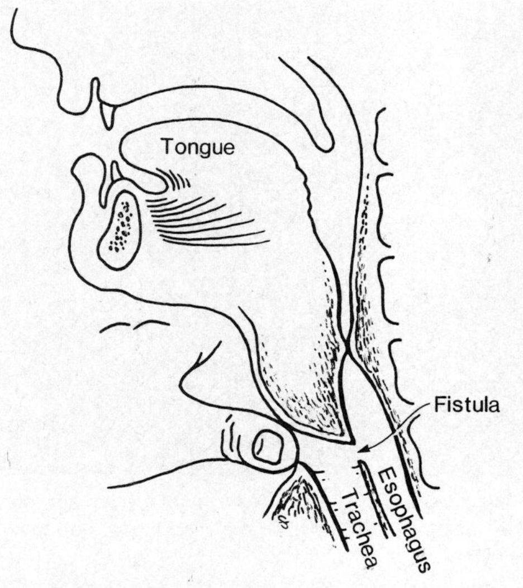

Figure 23–8. Esophagram in tracheoesophageal fistula, patient attempting phonation without success. Note lack of air reservoir and valving at level of fistula.

mately 5 min and then have the patient attempt to vocalize. If the patient is able to produce sound, then an air reservoir will usually be seen at the level of the tracheoesophageal fistula, with the development of a constriction just immediately above the pharyngoesophageal dilation (Fig. 23–9). In these cases, a pharyngeal myectomy will usually allow for development of tracheoesophageal fistula speech.[12] If no sound is produced following pharyngoesophageal anesthesia, then the clinician should suspect scar or tumor as the cause of aphonia, rather than spasm.

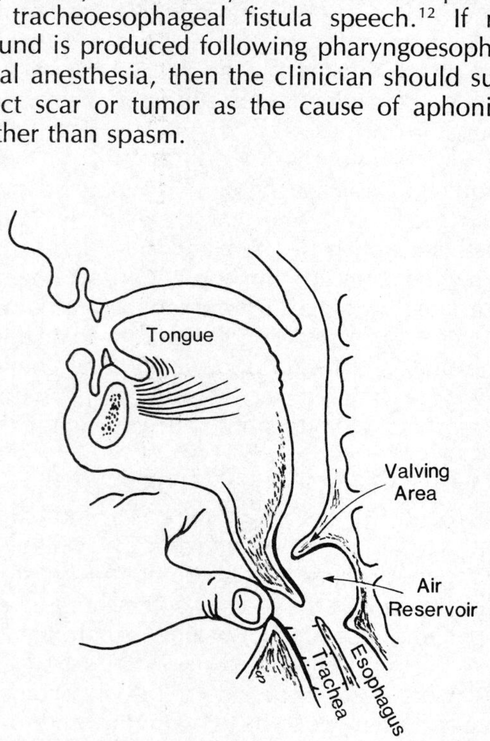

Figure 23–9. Esophagram of good tracheoesophageal speaker.

If no tumor is present, esophageal dilations offer some help in establishing tracheoesophageal fistula speech with the scarred pharyngoesophageal segment. Speech developed following dilation is usually of poor quality, however, and basic phonatory skills, consisting of duration of phonation, consistency of production, and number of syllables per breath expulsion, are also usually quite reduced.

If the patient with a tracheoesophageal scarred segment appears to be a good operative candidate, has good motivation, and appears to be best served by tracheoesophageal fistula speech, then we have found that, in a limited number of patients, excision of the pharyngoesophageal scar may be beneficial for sound production. If the patient's cervical esophagus is severely narrowed, as is frequently seen in the patient who has had extralaryngeal cancer in which a large part of the pharynx has been removed, then the patient may be a candidate for skin flap replacement to increase the lumen diameter of the esophagus.

CARE OF THE PROSTHESIS

Because the Panje Voice Prosthesis is made of silicone, it does not need to be changed daily.[13] The patient is instructed to wear the prosthesis at all times and is taught how to clear it in situ. If a daily cleaning regime is followed, then the prosthesis can remain in place for one month between removals. When leakage begins to occur through the prosthesis, it must be replaced by a new one.

To clean the prosthesis in situ, a small eyebrow tweezer is used to remove crusts from the tracheal side of the prosthesis. This should be done once per day. To prevent inadvertent aspiration of the tweezer, a large coat button is attached to the tweezer with a string.

The most effective way to clean the voice button while it is in the fistula is to use a pipe cleaner. This also should be done once per day. Before the pipe cleaner is inserted into the prosthesis, the end of the pipe cleaner must be checked to make certain that it does not have a sharp point.

The patient is advised not to remove the voice button from the fistula unless there is difficulty in attaining speech. Frequent removal and reinsertion (once advocated, now condemned) will cause irritation at the fistula and will result in thickening of the tracheoesophageal tissue.

The green or clear plastic disc and the string attached to the voice prosthesis should be taped to the chest. This prevents entangling of the string during vocalization, which can dislodge the prosthesis.

RESULTS AND DISCUSSION

The Panje Voice Prosthesis procedure provides a highly successful, reproducible, reversible, and inexpensive method of voice rehabilitation for the laryngectomee. Our success rate for establishing the fistula in 120 cases has been 100 per cent (Table 23–6). A success rate of 85 per cent can be expected for initial sound production (having the patient phonate against the occluded tracheostoma without the voice button in place). Of the patients who achieve success with initial sound production, only 5 per cent to 10 per cent will be unable to wear the voice button because of a thick tracheoesophageal wall, inability to insert the prosthesis, or incorrect stoma size. The success rate for short-term use of the voice button (using effective tracheoesophageal fistula speech for less than six months) approaches 78 per cent. The rate for long-term success with the prosthesis (using effective tracheoesophageal speech for more than six months) is 52 per cent. Reasons for failure with the voice button include inability to retain the prosthesis, poor phonatory qualities, inability to attain good stomal occlusion, and the patient's decision not to use the voice button. In the last case, the patients may have been more comfortable with the original method of communication (electrolarynx, esophageal speech), may not have liked volume or pitch of speech, or may have found salivary soiling of the occluding digit repulsive, even though they successfully attained effective speech with the prosthesis.

Because the voice button is a prosthesis, it does require care and cleaning, as do other prostheses such as dentures and contact lenses. The voice button will eventually wear out and need replacement. Another limitation of the voice button is that the patient must cover the stoma with a thumb or finger in order to produce speech. These limitations, however, are considered by the laryngectomee to be minor, in light of the fact that the voice button makes it possible to regain effective verbal communication.

The voice quality produced by the patient using the Panje prosthesis is comparable to that of esophageal speech but, in contrast to esophageal speech, the voice button patient can use normal phrasing. Thus, general intelligibility is much higher with the voice button than with esophageal speech or the electrolarynx. Also, the volume of speech with the voice button is, in some patients, comparable to that of a person with a larynx and is louder than esophageal or electrolarynx speech. The pitch of speech produced by the voice button will vary with patient pharyngoesophageal tension and with head position. The range of pitch is limited in comparison with normal phonation.

We believe that greater success with the Panje Voice Prosthesis can be attained by a coordinated effort of the speech pathologist, or knowledgeable nurse, and the otolaryngology–head and neck surgeon. Such an approach can help the laryngectomee to maintain the confidence and motivation necessary to achieve voice rehabilitation at the highest level of success and in the shortest possible length of time.

Table 23–6. RESULTS OF PANJE VOICE PROSTHESIS PROCEDURE

Number of Patients*	Result
97/97	Established TE† fistula as an outpatient
23/23	Established TE fistula at time of laryngectomy
102/120	Produced TE sound
8/120	Unable to wear Panje Voice Prosthesis
94/120	Intelligible TE-prosthesis speech
62/120	Intelligible TE-prosthesis speech six months or longer

*Values given as number of patients/total patients
†TE = tracheoesophageal

References

1. Smith JK et al.: Speech recovery in laryngectomized patients. Laryngoscope 76:1540–1546, 1966.
2. Diedrick WM, Youngstrom KA: Alaryngeal Speech. Springfield IL, CC Thomas, 1968.
3. Dworkin JP, Sparker A: Surgical vocal rehabilitation following laryngectomy: A state-of-the-art report. Clin Otolaryngol 5:339–350, 1980.
4. Gates, GA et al.: Current status of laryngectomee rehabilitation: Causes of failure. Am J Otolaryngol 3:8–14, 1982.
5. Panje WR: Prosthetic vocal rehabilitation following laryngectomy: The voice button. Ann Otol Rhinol Laryngol 90:116–120, 1981.
6. Knapp BA, Panje WR: A voice button for laryngectomees. AORN J 36:183–192, 1982.
7. Panje WR, Shagets, F: Tracheoesophagostomy after laryngectomy for feeding and speech. Otolaryngol Head Neck Surg, 1984 (in press).
8. Weinberg B: Airway resistance of the voice button. Arch Otolaryngol 108:498–500, 1982.
9. Herrmann I: Glottoplasty. Presented at International Conference Surgical Speech Rehabilitation, Charing Cross, Cromwell Hospital, London, November 1982.

10. Maves MD, Lingeman, RE: Primary vocal rehabilitation using the Blom-Singer and Panje Voice Prosthesis. Ann Otol Rhinol Laryngol 91:458–460, 1982.
11. Kotsamis C et al.: A comparison between the Blom-Singer and Panje tracheoesophageal prostheses. (Abstract.) Otolaryngol Head Neck Surg 90:207, 1982.
12. Singer MI, Blom ED: Selective myotomy for voice restoration procedure. Arch Otolaryngol 107:674–676, 1981.
13. Panje WR: Surgical-prosthetic restoration of voice following laryngectomy. New Horizons Otolaryngol Head Neck Surg 1(2):1–9, January 1983.

PART IV

RELATED TOPICS AND SPECIAL PROBLEMS

24

Surgery for Aspiration

Richard L. Goode, M.D. and Paul A. Levine, M.D.

The human larynx performs three important functions: (1) airway protection, (2) respiration, and (3) phonation. When the protective mechanisms of the larynx are functionally impaired, the patient may experience aspiration, the taking of foreign matter into the lungs with the respiratory current. The degree of aspiration dictates the necessity for and type of therapy, since aspiration may vary from inconsequential to life-threatening.

Before considering those techniques that may be helpful in averting or controlling the aspiration process, it is most helpful to briefly consider what anatomic and neurologic functions may be altered for aspiration to exist. First, from a phylogenetic point of view, it is important to note that the low position of the larynx in the adult human neck, as compared to its position in mammalian species, makes it inherently less efficient in separating deglutition from respiration. During the act of swallowing, the larynx must be elevated under the posteriorly displaced base of tongue; this provides the first line of laryngeal protection. As the bolus reaches the hypopharynx, the broad, flat epiglottis directs the food laterally, away from the glottis and toward the pyriform sinuses. Important in this process is the role of the arytenoids and the aryepiglottic folds, which when adducted provide a gutter between themselves and the lateral pharyngeal wall. In the intrinsic larynx itself, the most important glottic ingress protection is provided by true cord adduction, with a less potent blockade provided by false cord apposition. These processes, in association with normal laryngeal and pharyngeal sensation and normal motor function of the superior, middle, and inferior constrictors, the cricopharyngeus muscle, and the esophageal musculature, provide for normal deglutition without aspiration. Any variation from the norm may result in minimal-to-catastrophic aspiration.

Etiology of Aspiration. The etiology of aspiration falls into four basic categories: (1) neurologic disorders, (2) laryngeal or pharyngeal tumors, (3) anatomic losses secondary to surgery (usually head and neck tumor surgery), and (4) trauma.

Any neurologic disease involving the vagus nerve from the nucleus ambiguus to its peripheral endings may cause some degree of aspiration. This picture can be complicated by paralysis of cranial nerves IX, XI, and XII. The most common disease entities include cerebrovascular accidents, amyotrophic lateral sclerosis, multiple sclerosis, cerebral palsy, muscular dystrophy, pseudobulbar palsy, and poliomyelitis. In these conditions, aspiration usually occurs, caused by both pharyngeal and laryngeal motor impairment. Hypopharyngeal pooling with an incompetent glottis provides a perfect milieu for aspiration. Aspiration can rarely occur from a purely sensory deficit, such as a unilateral superior laryngeal nerve paralysis. This most commonly produces a relatively minor transitory swallowing dysfunction.

Disruption of the function of the recurrent laryngeal nerve is not limited only to natural disease, since the trauma of surgery is an all too frequent cause of recurrent laryngeal nerve paralysis. Thyroid surgery is the foremost cause of both unilateral and bilateral recurrent laryngeal nerve paralysis; surgery of the left chest is also a common etiology. Aspiration often will occur during the early phase of laryngeal nerve paralysis when the vocal cord is in the intermediate position.

Any significant hypopharyngeal or laryngeal tumor will cause some degree of aspiration by impairment of glottic mobility, interruption of passage of the bolus to the cricopharyngeus, loss of hypopharyngeal sensation, and pooling of saliva and food debris in vulnerable hypopharyngeal areas. In the same way, any tumor involving the cricopharyngeal region or the cervical esophagus can cause pooling and aspiration secondary to laryngeal overflow.

In conjunction with the above considerations, major head and neck cancer resections produce significant anatomic deficiencies that may lead to aspiration. Supraglottic laryngectomy, vertical hemilaryngectomy and its variations, and base of tongue and pharyngeal resections with atonic, insensitive flap reconstruction all impair the normal process of deglutition by the physical removal of important defenses against aspiration.

Less commonly, direct trauma to the larynx and pharynx may provide a setting for aspiration. This can occur by a resulting incompetent larynx or by an immobile larynx and pharynx. The most difficult of these injuries to rehabilitate are those associated with severe acid and lye ingestion, in which the motor function and sensation of the larynx and pharynx are altered by the resulting burns and subsequent dense fibrosis.

Indications for and Timing of Surgery. While the indications for surgical intervention are similar in aspiration secondary to all etiologic factors, the timing of the surgical procedure is, indeed, different. A patient suffering from aspiration secondary to a neurologic disorder requires surgical intervention only when unable to protect the airway satisfactorily enough to prevent life-threatening aspiration pneumonia or when oral alimentation is insufficient to maintain body weight at an acceptable level. Such intervention should be considered only when the clinical picture is not expected to improve in a relatively short period of time. For example, a patient suffering from a recent cerebrovascular accident may be able to compensate for his dysphagia and aspiration in a relatively short period of time with minor treatment modalities. In contrast, a patient with multiple sclerosis cannot be expected to show improvement of these functions.

On the other hand, the timing of aspiration surgery in relation to a major head and neck resection should not be ex post facto but should be planned before the primary resection and carried out before the aspiration process begins. The astute cancer surgeon will anticipate his needs preoperatively and will include aspiration-prevention techniques in his primary procedure. On occasion, in spite of excellent preoperative planning, significant aspiration cannot be prevented. It is then fruitless to attempt laryngeal suspension, for example, after primary healing and radiation therapy. Therefore, the first chance is the best chance and, sometimes, the only chance to compensate for major anatomic deficiencies.

Evaluation. An evaluation can only be considered complete after a head and neck examination with complete cranial nerve and laryngeal assessment. This examination need not always include direct laryngoscopy, because often the best evaluation of laryngeal function is obtained indirectly. If an indirect mirror examination is not satisfactory, fiberoptic laryngoscopy performed in the office under local anesthesia will probably provide more information than will direct laryngoscopy under a general anesthetic.

Radiologic evaluation may consist of a cineesophagram employing either thin barium sulfate or propyliodone suspension (oily Dionosil). If the patient is severely aspirating, to the point of being critically ill, a dye study will do no more than confirm the clinical assessment and will probably further jeopardize the patient's already compromised pulmonary status. Conversely, with mild-to-moderate aspiration, a dye contrast study can be valuable in assessing the motor function or dysfunction of the constrictors, cricopharyngeus muscle, and esophageal musculature, along with the delineation of the hypopharynx and esophagus to rule out neoplasm, stricture, diverticulum, or cricopharyngeal spasm contributing to the aspiration. A laryngogram probably offers little value unless an adequate physical examination cannot be performed.

MEDICAL TREATMENT OF ASPIRATION

The keystone of treatment for significant aspiration is prevention. By eliminating eating by mouth and minimizing regurgitation of stomach contents into the upper esophagus and pharynx, aspiration pneumonia, the major complication, can essentially be eliminated. Obviously, adequate nutritional intake must be maintained; thus, soft, small feeding tubes are an essential part of the medical treatment of aspiration.

Feeding Tubes. We have found silicone rubber tubes extremely satisfactory for nasogastric feeding. The silicone rubber is a soft, well-tolerated material. The tubes selected should be small in diameter (about 14 French); however, larger sizes also are available. A disadvantage of these tubes is that they are difficult to insert because of their softness; however, a stylet is available to aid in insertion. If we expect aspiration to last a month or less, we consider a feeding tube satisfactory treatment.

An alternate solution consists of a cut-off 14 or 16 French Robinson catheter attached to a 50-ml syringe (Fig. 24–1). After lubricating the tube, the patient inserts the tube slowly through the mouth so that it lies in the upper esophagus just below the level of the cricopharyngeus muscle. Practice is required for the patient to suppress the gag reflex so that the tube may be passed; this may be facilitated by the use of 4 per cent lidocaine (Xylocaine) spray prior to insertion. Initially, 5 ml of sterile saline should be injected through the tube to make sure it is not in the larynx. Coughing by the patient suggests the tube is in the larynx rather than the upper esophagus; if so, the tube must be removed and reinserted. In addition, the patient should attempt to speak after the tube is inserted; hoarseness following tube insertion indicates that the tube is between the vocal cords rather than in the upper esophagus. In damaged larynges, where vocalization is already abnormal, this may be difficult to assess and the use of a saline injection through the tube prior to initiating feeding is essential. Once the patient is sure the tube is in the right place, he fills the syringe with the feeding solution and slowly injects it through the tube. The syringe is refilled as many times as necessary to complete the feeding; some patients prefer attaching the tube to a gravity flow feeding container. This method does not require that a nasogastric tube be constantly in place—the patient feeds himself as often as necessary to achieve and maintain an adequate weight. Another advantage of this type of short feeding tube is that it diminishes the likelihood of gastric regurgitation because no tube passes through the gastroesophageal junction. If the patient is not able to learn this technique and a nasogastric tube must be used, it is important for the patient to sit or lie at a 45 degree or greater angle during feedings and for several hours afterward. We recommend a 45 degree elevation of the head of the bed at all times for patients receiving nasogastric tube feedings. Gastric emptying times may be prolonged in these patients; therefore, regurgitation can occur hours after feeding. Feedings should be given slowly enough so that gastric distention or regurgitation does not occur. This may require that feedings be given eight to twelve times a day, or as a continuous drip in some patients. A variety of nasogastric feeding solutions exist and some may be better tolerated than others by any given patient in regard to bloating, diarrhea, and regurgitation; consultation with a dietitian may be helpful in difficult cases. The use of cimetidine with or without antacids to diminish gastric acidity will minimize the effects of aspiration; the lower the pH of aspirated gastric contents, the worse the irritation to the lungs.

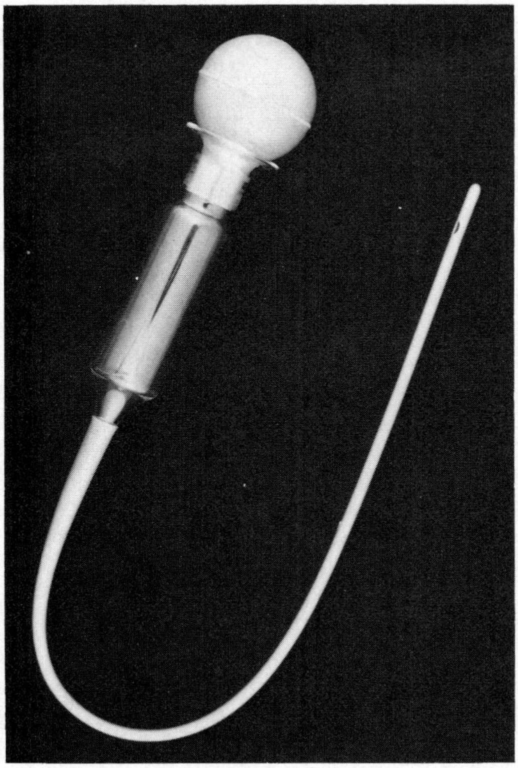

Figure 24–1. Feeding apparatus made by using a 50-cc syringe and a Robinson catheter.

Experimenting with the location of the nasogastric tube may minimize regurgitation. In some cases, insertion of the feeding tube into the duodenum improves the situation; however, a dumping syndrome may be produced, particularly if concentrated solutions are given too rapidly. Injecting a small amount of barium compound into the nasogastric tube followed by an x-ray of the abdomen and lower chest will show the exact location of the tube; on occasion, tubes are found coiled up in the lower esophagus, predisposing to reflux.

Aspiration of saliva can be minimized by the use of anticholinergics. We find that 15 mg of probantheline bromide (Pro-Banthine) given by tube 30 min before meals helps decrease saliva. A dental saliva sucker connected to a suction pump may be handy at mealtime to suction out excess saliva; most patients will realize the importance of spitting out excess saliva to minimize aspiration and coughing. Irradiation to the submaxillary and parotid glands will decrease saliva to a variable extent; 1500 rads over a five-day period is a common dose.

Initiation of Eating by Mouth. Periodically, the ability of a patient suffering aspiration to take food by mouth must be assessed. The ease with which the patient swallows saliva will provide information on when to initiate oral feedings; if the saliva is not being swallowed, food will probably not be taken well.

A few important rules that apply to the patient who is beginning to eat again are as follows:

1. Start with foods that are easy to swallow and that produce minimal pulmonary irritation if aspirated. Usually these are fluids such as carbonated clear beverages (7-Up, ginger ale) or semisolids such as raw or poached eggs. Water and milk seem to be more easily aspirated than other fluids. Egg nog, pudding, ice cream, apple sauce, gelatin, and consommé are all good choices. A certain amount of trial and error is inevitable.

2. Proper positioning is important. The patient should be sitting up with the head slightly flexed at the neck—for some reason, swallowing is easier in this position.

3. Prior to placing the food in the mouth, the patient must clear out any excess secretions using suction and cough, then take several deep breaths and hold his breath.

4. A small portion of the selected food is placed on the back of the tongue, toward the undamaged side if there is one, using a long-handled spoon or the syringe with short tube.

5. The patient forcibly attempts to swallow the food with at least three swallows and then coughs to clear his airway of any aspirated food.

6. The process is repeated until success is achieved or until it is obvious that eating by mouth is not possible at that time.

The physician should be present at these initial swallowing sessions to make sure the patient follows these rules. Results are better when the physician, who understands the problem best, takes an active role in the swallowing rehabilitation process. Later, a family member or nurse can supervise the swallowing sessions if necessary.

When attempts at eating by mouth are initiated, it may be helpful to temporarily remove the nasogastric tube, if present, to make eating easier. If a tracheotomy tube is present, it should be removed and the stoma sealed with a pressure dressing unless contraindicated; plugging the tracheotomy tube opening during swallowing attempts is less effective.

SURGICAL TREATMENT OF ASPIRATION

If conservative, noninvasive therapy has failed or is inappropriate for a patient's needs, multiple surgical procedures are available that can correct, compensate for, or bypass the route of aspiration. These techniques include: (1) vocal cord injection, (2) insertion of a cuffed tracheotomy tube, (3) hypopharyngostomy or esophagostomy, (4) cricopharyngeal myotomy, (5) desalivation procedures, (6) laryngeal suspension, (7) glottic closure, (8) arytenoid-epiglottic flap procedure, (9) laryngeal diversion, and (10) laryngectomy.

Vocal Cord Injection. The advent of paraffin injection into the vocal cord region provided a simple, yet effective, means of treating aspiration caused by the intermediately positioned vocal cord; this technique was devised by Brunings in 1911.[1] He established the concept of injection of a nonresorbable, relatively nonreactive foreign body into the lateral region of the vocal cord. This augmented its size and pushed the cord medially, providing a midline cord for apposition with the normal vocal cord. This technique was employed initially only for chronic vocal cord paralysis. In 1962, Arnold[2] generated new interest in this technique by employing a mixture of glycerin and polytetrafluoroethylene (Teflon) to attain the same goal.

Since most otolaryngologists have been, and still are, loathe to inject a permanent material into vocal cords that might regain mobility, especially in cases of so-called idiopathic vocal cord paralysis, Lewy and Mathews in 1965[3] described immediate and temporary restoration of glottic function by the use of glycerin as the bulk medium. This technique provided for a rapid reinstitution of an effective cough and reduction of aspiration, but it was limited in that the duration of effectiveness was measured in days. The technique, therefore, had to be repeated quite frequently before the decision was made to employ the permanent Teflon injection. More recently, in the latter half of 1978, Schramm et al.[4] introduced the injection of a paste of absorbable gelatin sponge (Gelfoam) that provides for temporary glottic closure over a period of six to ten weeks. This provided the otolaryngologist with a longer temporary technique for restoring the protective and phonatory functions of the glottis.

The permanent injection that has evolved to date is Teflon paste via the Arnold-Brunings syringe. This provides a method to improve glottic competency for the permanently paralyzed vocal cord, to improve function after vertical hemilaryngectomy, and to augment a surgically reconstructed vocal cord that does not quite provide glottic competence. A more comprehensive discussion of this technique will be found in Chapter 7 of this volume.

Tracheotomy and Insertion of a Cuffed Tube. The insertion of a tracheotomy tube with a low pressure balloon cuff is indicated when severe aspiration persists despite medical treatment (Fig. 24–2). The low pressure cuff is left inflated around the clock if necessary.

The tracheotomy performs two functions. First, it allows for suctioning, mist, and positive pressure ventilation; all may be important in treating recurrent aspiration penumonia. Second, the inflated balloon cuff decreases the amount of liquids or solids that can pass into the tracheobronchial tree. Some aspiration usually does occur because a continuously perfect seal with the balloon is difficult to achieve.

The use of a cuffed tracheotomy tube does not make eating by mouth easier, although it may minimize the complications of aspiration. Usually, eating by mouth is easiest after the tracheotomy tube has been removed and the stoma closed. A low pressure balloon cuff on the tube is essential to prevent tracheal stenosis; it should be inflated with just enough air to get an adequate seal within the trachea.

Hypopharyngostomy and Esophagostomy. After one month of nasogastric tube use, if progress in eating by mouth is poor and the patient is not able to pass the short tube, cervical esophagostomy may be indicated. Long-term use of a nasogastric tube has several disadvantages; it is obvious in appearance and irritating to the nose and hypopharyngeal structures.

Gastrostomy has been classically used to eliminate the need for a nasogastric tube. Although particularly useful in cases of esophageal obstruction due to tumor or stricture, gastrostomies have certain disadvantages. A tube or obturator must be continuously in place and leakage of the stomach's acid contents around the tube can cause excoriation of the abdominal skin. The location of the tube under the clothes is not particularly convenient for feedings and, since the peritoneal cavity must be entered for placement, peritonitis becomes a possible postoperative complication.

Cervical esophagostomy is recommended to eliminate the nasogastric tube and the disadvantages of gastrostomy. The procedure can be subdivided into two types; (1) pyriform sinus hypopharyngostomy, and (2) cervical esophagostomy. In each, the basic procedure is the same—a fistula is created between the hypopharynx or esophagus and the lateral neck so that a tube can be inserted for feeding. Technically, the two procedures are different and each has certain advantages in use.

In both types of procedure, the problem of leakage is minimal and the secretions are not irritating. They can be performed in all cases where gastrostomy is considered, except for cases of esophageal cancer or marked stenosis of the esophagus or hypopharynx. The presence of irradiated neck tissue is not a contraindication, although healing is slower. Early and late complications have been rare in our experience and in the literature and consist of local cellulitis or hematoma. One case of bleeding from a branch of the internal jugular vein has been reported.[5]

Pyriform Sinus Hypopharyngostomy. The pyriform sinus hypopharyngostomy is considered in cases where it is planned that a tube will be in place for weeks or months but will ultimately be removed. After premedicating the patient and spraying the hypopharynx with a topical anesthetic, the surgeon places a curved Yankaeur tonsil suction down into the pyriform sinus on one side and rotates it laterally so it can be palpated in the neck. A good location is at the posterior edge of the thyroid cartilage, just below the superior border of the thyroid cartilage. The bulge of the suction tip is felt under the skin and infiltration of 1 per cent lidocaine with 1:100,000 epinephrine is done in this area. A stab wound is made through skin and platysma, just in front of the sternocleidomastoid muscle. Using blunt dissection with a clamp, the surgeon separates the fascial and muscle planes over the suction tip down to the hypopharyngeal mucosa. The dissection passes between the carotid sheath and the thyroid cartilage. The pharynx is grasped with a Babcock clamp and a small incision is made into the hypopharynx. A silicone rubber feeding tube is inserted and passed into the stomach. It is important to place the external skin incision higher than the hypopharyngeal incision, providing a downward course to the tract, which helps in replacing the tube.

In two weeks, the tract becomes lined so that the tube can be removed between feedings if desired. Removal is not recommended because the tube often ends up in the mouth rather than the stomach. If it is left out too long, the tract will contract so that passage of the tube becomes difficult. The silicone rubber feeding tube can stay in place for months without irritation; however, we recommend changing it at two month intervals. Using a large syringe or gravity feeder, the patient may feed himself or be fed by a nurse or family member. The tube can be left in place indefinitely.

This procedure offers the advantages that it can be done under local anesthesia within 20

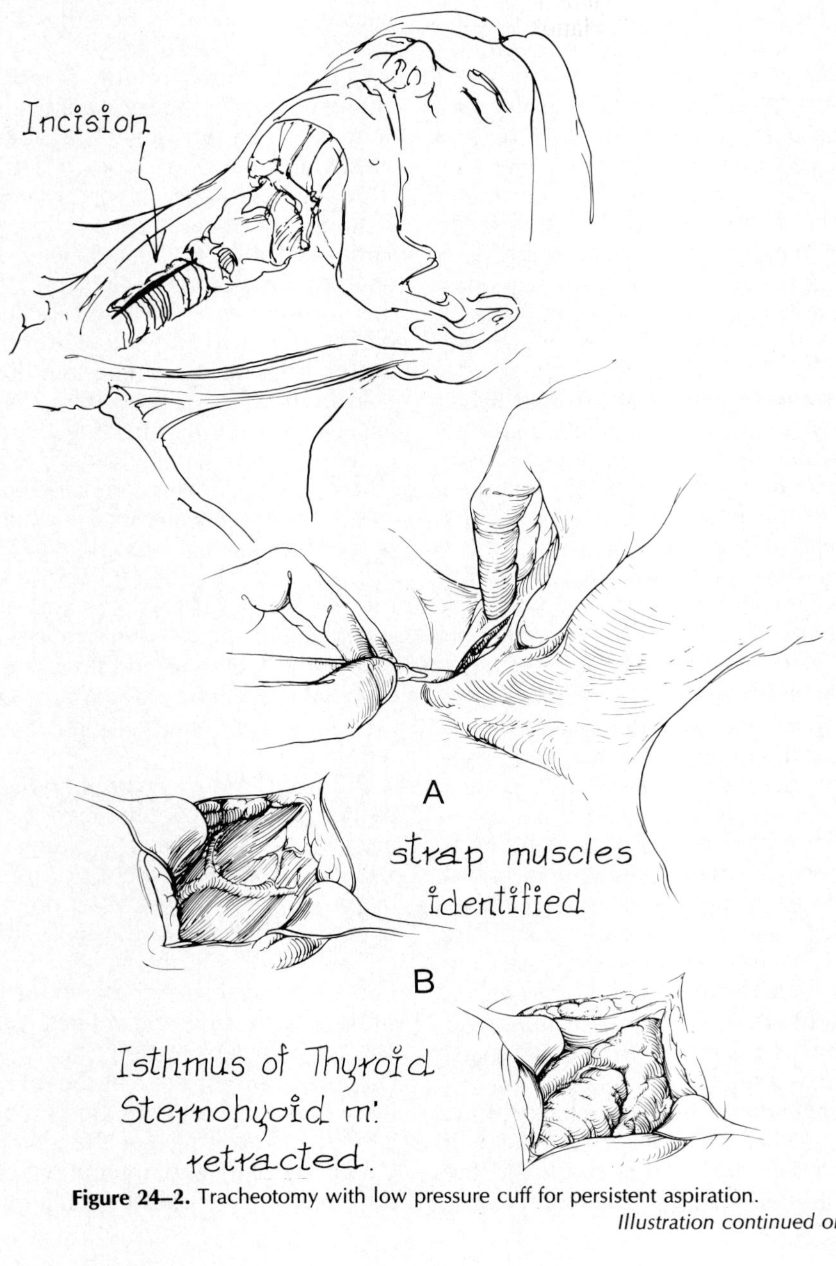

Figure 24–2. Tracheotomy with low pressure cuff for persistent aspiration.

Illustration continued on opposite page

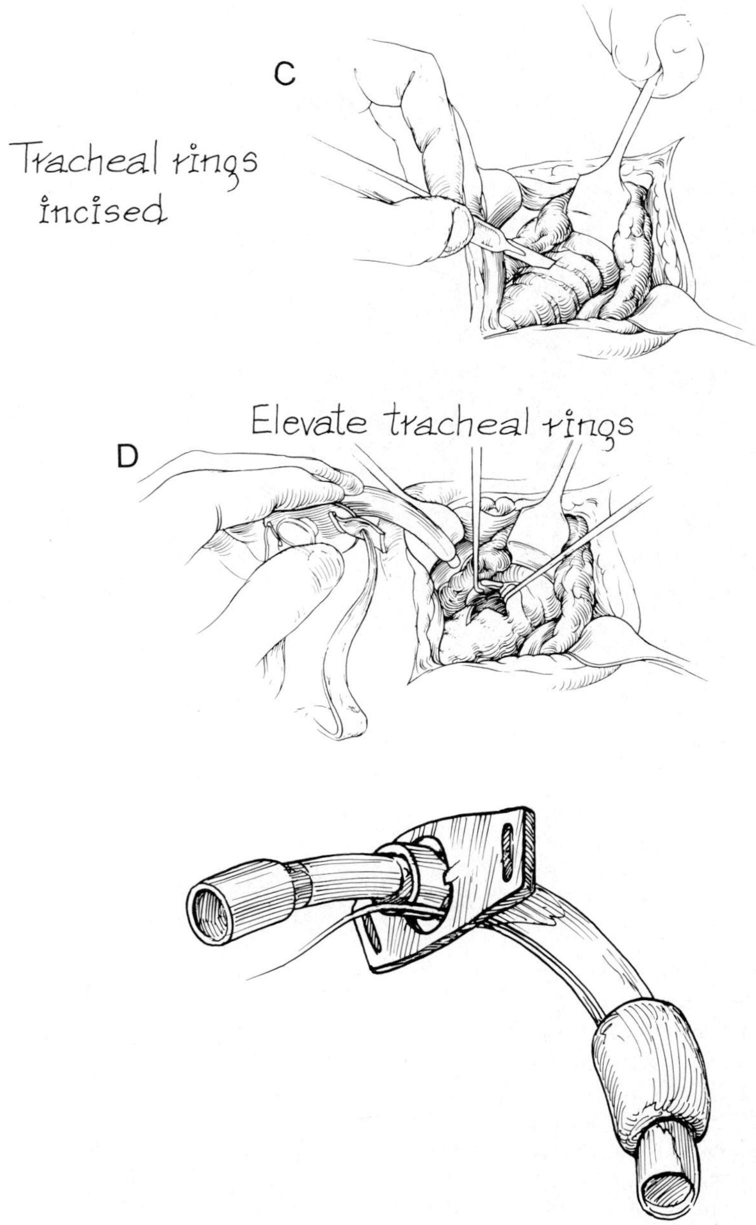

Figure 24–2 *Continued*

minutes and may be conveniently added to any operation around the head and neck, particularly in cases where long-term postoperative tube feedings are likely. In major head and neck surgery cases where postoperative swallowing is likely to be a problem, placement of a prophylactic feeding pharyngostomy or esophagostomy should be considered. The tube is easily accessible for feedings since it is close to the head and is not covered by clothing. When the tube is pulled, the fistulous tract closes so that no further operations are required.

Cervical Esophagostomy. The cervical esophagostomy is made into the esophagus just below the level of the cricopharyngeus muscle.[6] Under general anesthesia, a horizontal incision is made in the lateral neck at about the level of the cricoid cartilage. The deep dissection proceeds anterior to the carotid sheath down to the posterolateral esophagus. The posterior aspect of the esophagus is sought so that the

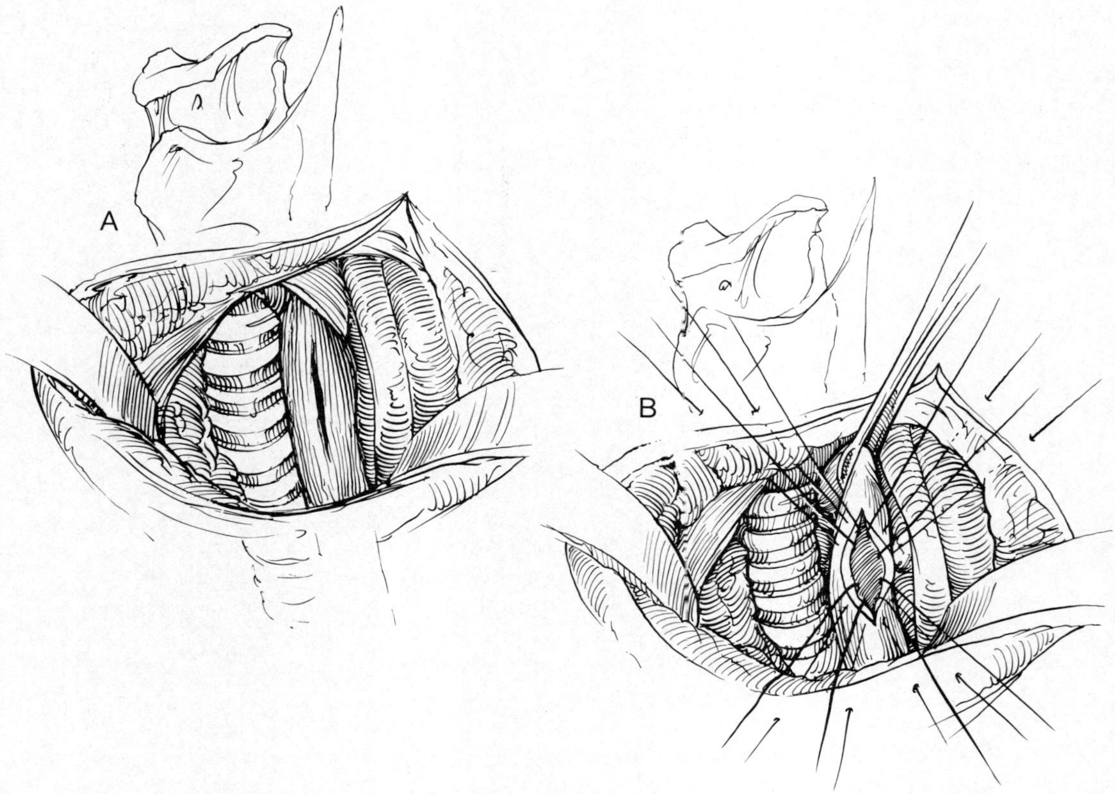

Figure 24–3. Cervical esophagostomy technique to create a permanent tract for the feeding tube.

recurrent laryngeal nerve in the tracheoesophageal sulcus is avoided. Babcock clamps are placed on the esophagus wall and the esophagus is opened between them (Fig. 24–3). This is usually simplified by having a large nasogastric tube in place prior to the procedure. The skin is undermined around the external skin incision and the edges of the skin sewn to the esophageal wall to create a fistula lined with skin and mucosa. Rotation skin flaps may be used to line the tract.[7] The anterior aspect of the sternocleidomastoid muscle should be rotated over the carotid sheath adjacent to the tract for additional protection; a silicone rubber feeding tube is inserted. This produces a low fistula in which the likelihood of stenosis is much smaller than with pyriform sinus hypopharyngostomy. This fistula is better cosmetically because of its low-lying location, and there is less irritation because the tract is lined. The procedure requires about an hour to perform. This procedure is designed for patients who will need a tube indefinitely, usually for neurologic problems (cerebrovascular acci-

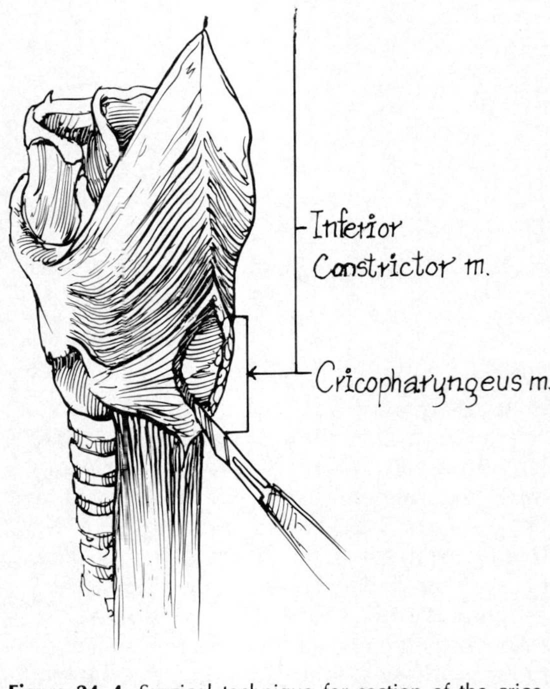

Figure 24–4. Surgical technique for section of the cricopharyngeus muscle.

dents, amyotrophic lateral sclerosis, multiple sclerosis, cerebral palsy, etc). In most cases, section of the cricopharyngeus muscle (Fig. 24–4) is done at the time to help improve residual swallowing.

Cricopharyngeal Myotomy. Section of the cricopharyngeus muscle is helpful in cases of aspiration where cricopharyngeal spasm exists, usually due to vagus nerve dysfunction. It may also help in preventing postoperative aspiration following supraglottic laryngectomy or base of tongue and pharynx resection, and it is commonly performed as part of these procedures.

Diagnosis of cricopharyngeal spasm requires a contrast esophagram, preferably a cine-esophagram. Oily Dionosil should be used because it is less irritating than barium compound when aspirated. The radiologic evaluation must continue long enough for the radiologist to evaluate whether the cricopharyngeus muscle opens normally at the right time. Too often, the examination is stopped at the first sign of aspiration and the status of the cricopharyngeus muscle remains unknown. Since it is known prior to the radiologic examination that the patient aspirates, the radiologist must be informed of this and the reason for the examination.

The best candidates for cricopharyngeal myotomy are patients in whom the muscle does not open or opens only partially despite several swallows of contrast material: hypertrophy of the muscle may be seen.

The approach is the same as for cervical esophagostomy, and the two procedures are often combined. The muscle is sectioned posteriorly to avoid trauma to the recurrent nerve (if it is still functional). All muscle fibers are cut down to the mucosa for a distance of 1 cm above and below the muscle (Fig. 24–4). To minimize reattachment of the cut muscle, the cut ends should be dissected free from the mucosa for 5 to 10 mm, folded back onto themselves, and sutured in this position. Placement of a large dilator prior to surgery makes the procedure easier.[8]

A postoperative cine-esophagram is required in unsuccessful cases to see whether the cricopharyngeus muscle has been adequately sectioned. Failure may follow an inadequate muscle section; if so, the operation may be repeated on the opposite side.

Desalivation Procedures. A variety of surgical techniques that decrease salivary secretions have been described. Several, by virtue of their simplicity and low morbidity, are useful in treating the patient suffering aspiration.

Salivary Gland Excision. Excision of the submaxillary gland is technically not difficult and can be performed under local anesthesia. Removal of one or both glands will decrease total salivary secretions but is likely to be ineffective because of the persistence of parotid secretions. Parotidectomy is more difficult than submaxillary excision, requires a general anesthetic, and carries the risk of facial nerve injury. This therapy is too radical for patients afflicted by other serious disease.

Ductal Ligation. Ligation of the parotid duct has been used for years in the treatment of salivary fistulas and chronic parotitis. Laage-Hellman[9] initially described its use in controlling secretions following cancer surgery. Wallenborn et al.[10] and Baron[11] showed histologic evidence of acinar atrophy secondary to the ligation, explaining the effectiveness of the procedure in producing parotid atrophy. Similar histologic findings are seen in the submaxillary gland following ductal ligation.[12] Patients with actively secreting glands may experience pain after ductal ligation. This pain is associated with feeding and disappears after several weeks. Diamant[13] advocated the use of irradiation followed by ductal ligation to prevent postligation pain. The use of anticholinergics just before meals and at bedtime, beginning before surgery and continuing for three weeks afterward, may be equally effective.

Nerve Sectioning. Nerve sectioning techniques may be used to interrupt the efferent parasympathetic nerve supply to the glands. Section of these nerves causes a prompt decrease in salivary secretion with later glandular atrophy.

The efferent parasympathetic nerve supply to the submaxillary and sublingual glands originates in the superior salivatory nucleus of the pons and travels via the facial nerve to the chorda tympani and then to the lingual nerve. From here, the axons pass to the submaxillary ganglion, synapse, and are distributed to the submaxillary and sublingual glands.

Chorda tympani section in the middle ear appears to be the site of choice for submaxillary gland denervation.[14] It is easily reached and sectioned in 15 min under local anesthesia using routine otologic techniques. No special techniques or new operations need be learned. Operative morbidity is minimal, and interruption of the parasympathetic pathway to the ipsilateral parotid gland, by section of the tympanic nerve in the middle ear, can be conveniently done at the same time.

The loss of taste that occurs with chorda

tympani section is not significant when unilateral. In head and neck cancer cases, a unilateral radical neck dissection is often present; therefore, chorda tympani section on that side is not required, since the gland is absent. Bilateral chorda tympani section does produce a decrease in taste sensation and thus has limited usefulness.

The parasympathetic nerve supply to the parotid arises in the salivatory nucleus in the medulla, passes out via the glossopharyngeal nerve to the petrosal ganglion, where it leaves with the tympanic nerve and passes through the tympanic plexus and lesser superficial petrosal nerve to reach the otic ganglion. From here, it goes with the auriculotemporal nerve to supply the parotid gland. An alternate parasympathetic route to the parotid via the chorda tympani appears to be present.

Section of the tympanic nerve in the middle ear, as used in the treatment of Frey's syndrome, appears to be the method of choice to denervate the parotid gland for the same reasons as chorda tympani section.[14] No undesirable side effects occur with tympanic nerve section, and Wallenborn's careful histologic studies confirm that tympanic nerve section produces significant parotid atrophy.

Laryngeal Suspension. Laryngeal suspension as a technique to improve function following surgical resection of the anterior floor of the mouth was first described by Edgerton and Duncan[15] and DesPrez and Kiehn[16] in 1959. Jabaley and Hoopes[17] simplified the procedure and reported two successful cases in 1969. Calcaterra[18] described the use of laryngeal suspension to minimize postoperative aspiration in four cases of supraglottic laryngectomy. Two wire sutures were placed through each thyroid lamina and tied to a single hole placed in the mentum of the mandible. A cricopharyngeal myotomy was also performed.

Laryngeal suspension is intended to help compensate for the loss of the laryngeal elevator muscles, upper larynx, or base of tongue following radical cancer surgery. Removal of these structures produces a decrease in sensation and produces a relative ptosis of the larynx during swallowing that contributes to aspiration.

By pulling the larynx upward and forward under the base of the tongue, postoperative aspiration is minimized and swallowing improved.[19] Obviously, the procedure must be used at the time of the resection since postoperative scarring minimizes its value later.

Technique of Laryngeal Suspension. A Tevdek suture, 0 or 2-0, is placed through each thyroid cartilage lamina and then through two holes drilled in the lower aspect of the mandible, just anterior to the mental foramen on each side (Fig. 24–5). The sutures are placed through the thyroid cartilage and both perichondrial

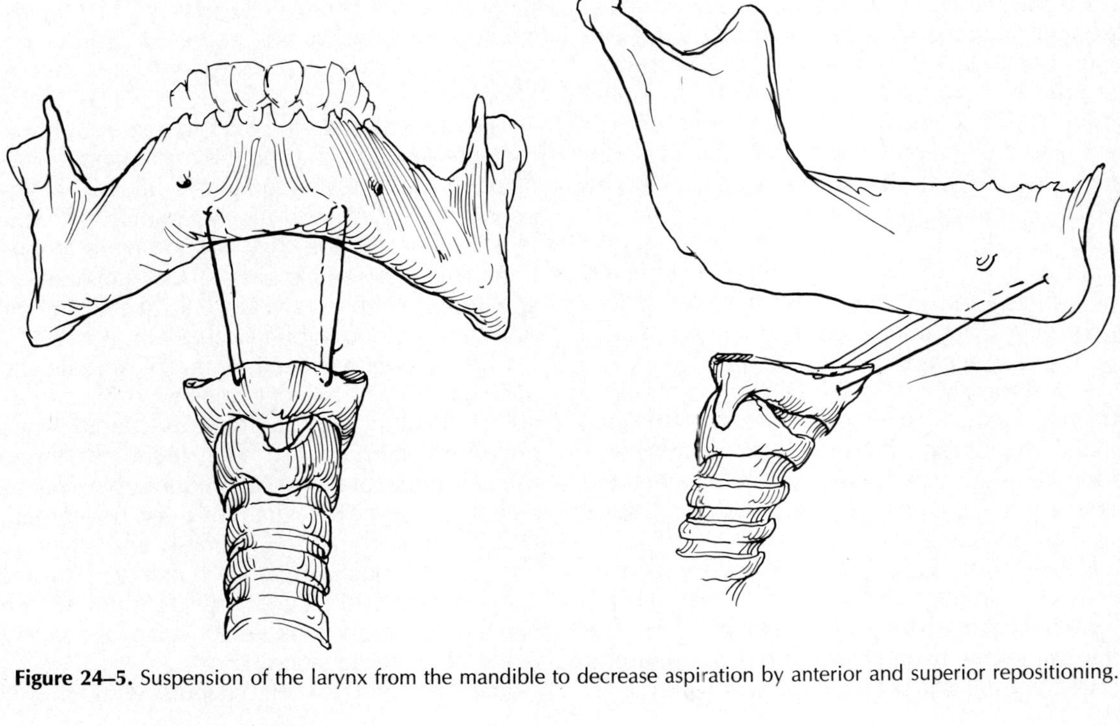

Figure 24–5. Suspension of the larynx from the mandible to decrease aspiration by anterior and superior repositioning.

layers under the intrinsic laryngeal structures using a large noncutting curved needle; care must be taken not to tether the vocal cord or arytenoid. The sutures are placed in the posterior third of the thyroid cartilage to maximize anterior displacement and tilt the larynx forward; this opens the inferior constrictor and cricopharyngeal muscles. In each suture, 8 to 10 mm of cartilage are included to minimize later pulling through. A cricopharyngeal myotomy is also performed.

The sutures are tightened to moderate tension, using a surgeon's knot followed by at least four square knots. The procedure usually elevates the larynx 1.5 to 3 cm. The suspension sutures are placed prior to closure of the primary defect but are not tightened. After the internal closure is completed, the suspension sutures are tightened, taking tension off the internal suture line. In theory, laryngeal obstruction could develop if the larynx were pulled too high under the tongue, but this has not occurred in our experience; some postoperative dropping of the larynx does occur. Unilateral suspension may be performed in cases where reaching the other side is technically difficult. In these cases, two sutures are placed on the one side.

Whenever suspension is performed, a tracheotomy is also done. Care is taken to elevate the larynx with a tracheotomy hook to the desired position prior to performing the procedure so that the tracheotomy will support the larynx in the elevated position during the postoperative period. The laryngeal depressor muscles are arbitrarily sectioned to minimize later dropping.

Other Surgical Techniques. In patients with chronic, life-endangering aspiration, for whom the techniques described above are ineffective, more drastic techniques should be considered prior to performing a total laryngectomy, the ultimate surgical technique to permanently prevent aspiration. Since surgical extirpation of a noncancerous larynx is most distasteful to the laryngologist, even under the most extreme circumstances, techniques to be considered before total laryngectomy include: (1) Montgomery's technique of glottic closure[20] including the modification by Sasaki et al.,[2] (2) Habal and Murray's[22, 23] epiglottic flap to the arytenoids, and (3) Lindeman's[24, 25] laryngeal diversion.

Glottic Closure. In 1975, Montgomery[20] described a technique to prevent aspiration and to reestablish swallowing function in the patient who is seriously aspirating. The technique requires formation of a permanent tracheotomy using multiple flaps and the standard thyrotomy approach to the glottis. Another method of performing a permanent tracheotomy with skin and mucosal flaps has recently been introduced by Fee and Ward[26] and can be used with this procedure. The approach is via a horizontal cervical skin incision at midlevel of the thyroid cartilage. After the strap muscles have been retracted laterally from the midline, the thyroid cartilage and cricothyroid membrane are exposed. If the thyroid cartilage has not undergone complete ossification, it is incised in the vertical midline with a No. 10 surgical blade or, more commonly, with an electric oscillating saw. The airway is then entered by a small horizontal incision in the cricothyroid membrane, and the thyrotomy incision is made in the anterior midline under direct vocal cord visualization. An oral endotracheal tube is recommended by Montgomery for glottic support prior to the membranous laryngeal incision, but we have not found this necessary; the membranous incision may be made via laryngotomy scissors or Pott's angled scissors. The exact midline is assured with an upward pull of the open scissors blade in the anterior commissure cleft prior to blade closure.

The thyroid laminae are then retracted using a self-retaining retractor. Next, an incision is made, either with a No. 15 surgical blade or cutting electrocautery, along the medial convexities of the true and false cords, continuing across the posterior commissure. The glottis is then denuded of a circumferential strip of epithelium between these two parallel incisions (Fig. 24–6). It is important to make sure there is complete removal of the mucosa from both ventricles and saccules.

The key step in this technique is the suture placement for the glottic closure. A 3-0 nylon suture is passed through the anterior aspect of one thyroid lamina and the true vocal cord of the same side. It is then inserted into the anterior portion of the opposite cord and passed through both the vocalis muscle and the vocal process posteriorly. The needle is then brought posteriorly through the initially sutured vocal cord and thyroid lamina, anterior to the vocal process. The same stitch is placed in the contralateral thyroid lamina (Fig. 24–7). The sutures are then tied on the lateral thyroid cartilage lamina.

The mucosal margins of the false cord incisions may be reapproximated with 3-0 chromic catgut sutures. The rest of the closure is standard technique. It should be noted that this technique has limited value in nonossified thy-

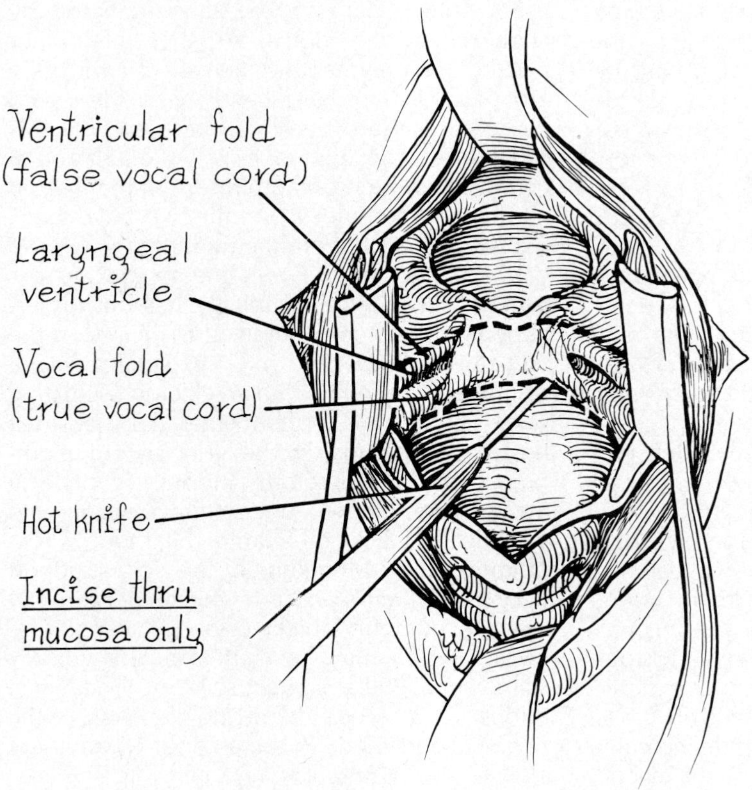

Figure 24–6. Technique to prepare the glottis for temporary or permanent closure.

roid cartilage, as is seen in children. Since this problem is uncommon in children and significant ossification usually occurs in adulthood, these limitations provide little drawback.

If this procedure fails, it is usually due to the persistence of a glottic space in the posterior commissure. For this reason, Sasaki et al.[21] have developed a modification of this technique that may provide better glottic closure posteriorly.

In this procedure, after removing the mucous membranes circumferentially from false to true cords, the glottis is closed with an interrupted

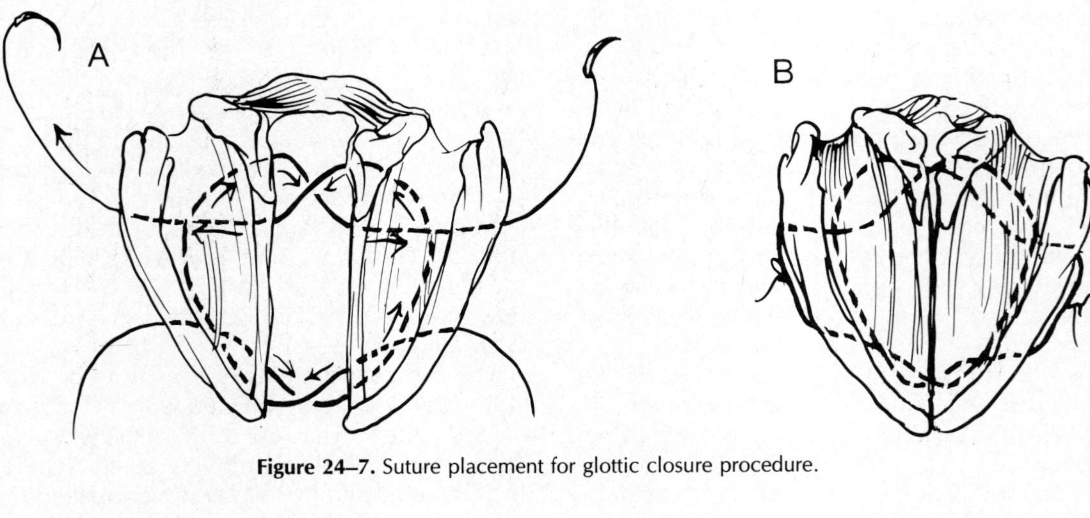

Figure 24–7. Suture placement for glottic closure procedure.

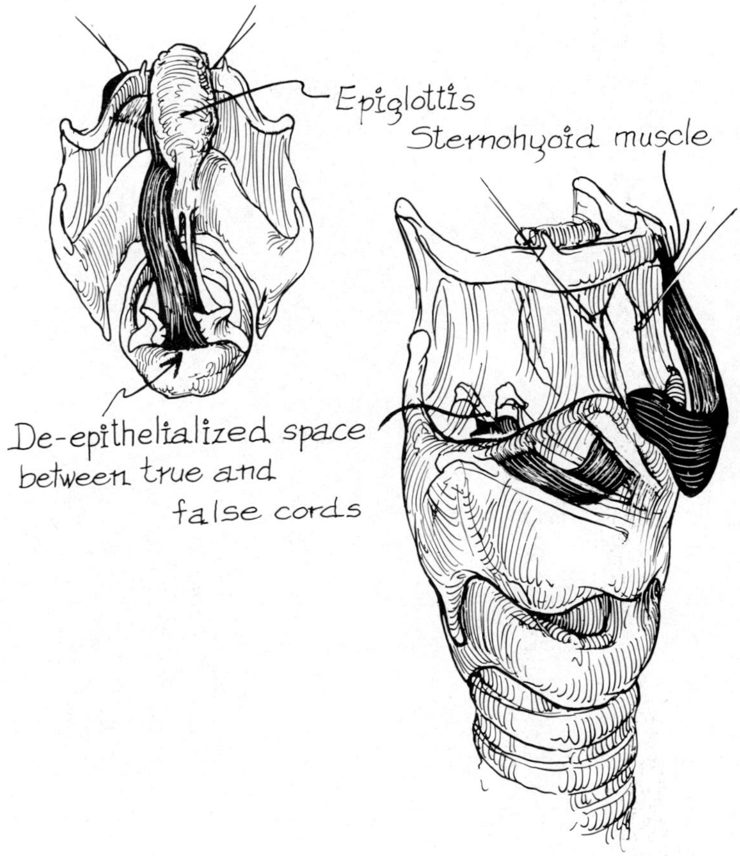

Figure 24–8. Superiorly based sternohyoid muscle flap for glottic closure.

4-0 polyglycolic acid (Dexon) suture line, approximating the cut mucosal edges at the false cord level. A superiorly based sternohyoid muscle flap is then developed and placed through the thyroid notch; this step may be facilitated by resecting a margin of thyroid cartilage for easier insertion of the muscle flap. The edge of the muscle flap is then sutured to the denuded interarytenoid muscle in the midline of the posterior commissure, prior to suturing the cut edges of the true vocal cord with 4-0 Dexon vertical mattress sutures (Fig. 24–8).

The advantages of this modification, according to the authors, are that it provides a three-layer rather than a two-layer closure, fills in the ventricular cavity dead space, and obviates the need for the through-and-through traction sutures of Montgomery that may pull through the thyroid cartilage. This modification also helps prevent postoperative patency of the posterior commissure by the introduction of the viable sternohyoid muscle flap.

Although both of these procedures are theoretically reversible, those patients who have required them rarely recover from the underlying disease that necessitated the glottic closure. Therefore, reversal of this procedure has yet to be carried out.

Arytenoid-Epiglottic Flap Procedure. Three years before Montgomery published his glottic technique, Habal and Murray presented a case report of their arytenoid-epiglottic flap procedure.[22] This initial report was followed three years later by a report describing six additional patients and offering some insight into the problems and limitations of the procedure.[23]

The surgical technique is a relatively straightforward one. Through a suprahyoid skin incision, the sternohyoid muscle is divided and the hyoid is pulled cephalad. Next, the hypopharynx is entered via the thyrohyoid membrane, i.e., by an anterior pharyngotomy approach. The edges of the epiglottis, aryepiglottic folds, and the arytenoids are then de-epithelialized and the cut mucosal surface of the epiglottis is sutured to the arytenoid-aryepiglottic fold complex with absorbable suture. A second layer closure is obtained by rotating pyriform sinus mucosal flaps, and the wound is closed in the standard manner (Fig. 24–9).

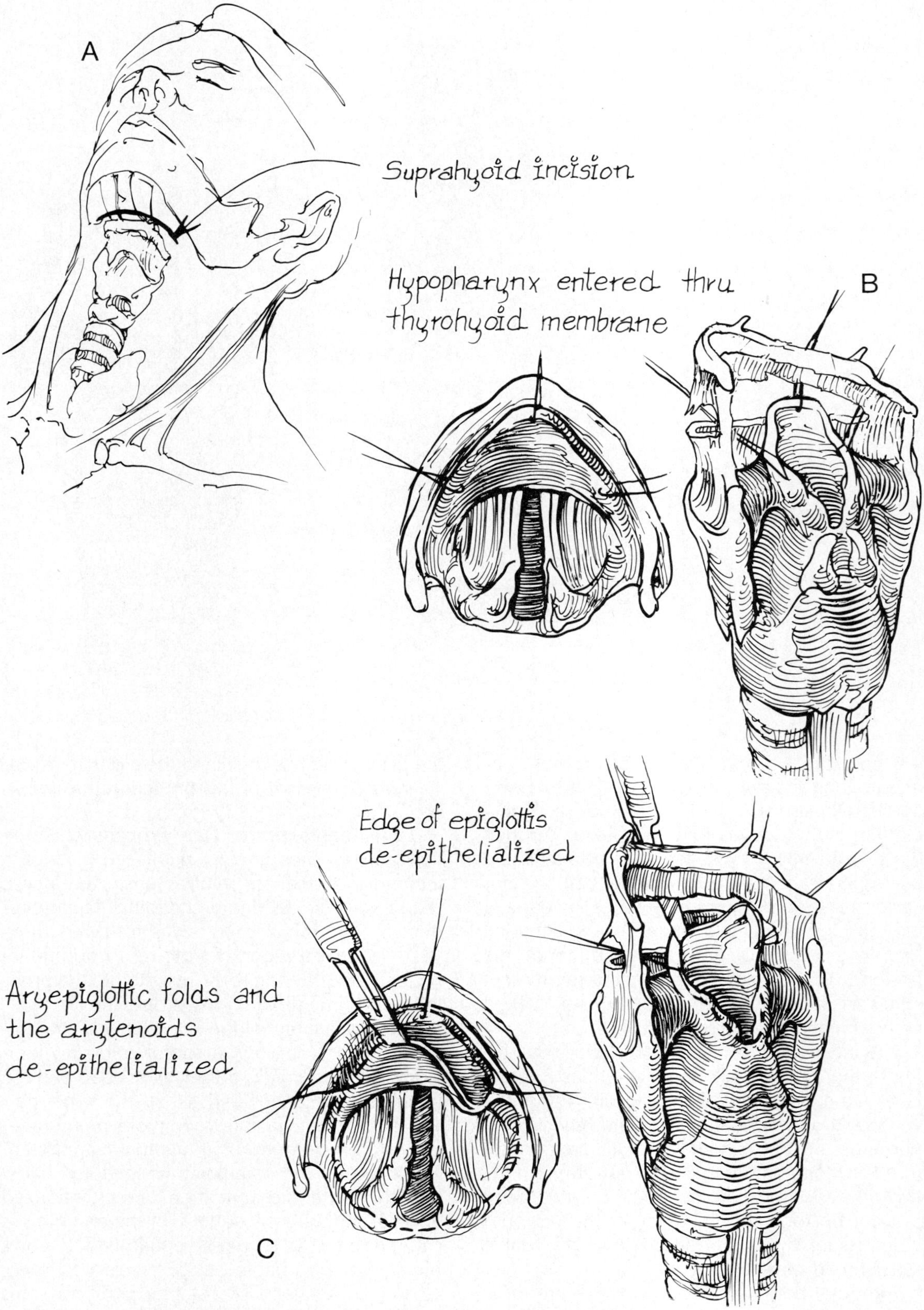

Figure 24–9. Arytenoid epiglottic flap procedure. *A,* Suprahyoid skin incision. *B,* Entry through the vallecula. *C,* De-epithelialization of the epiglottis.

Illustration continued on opposite page

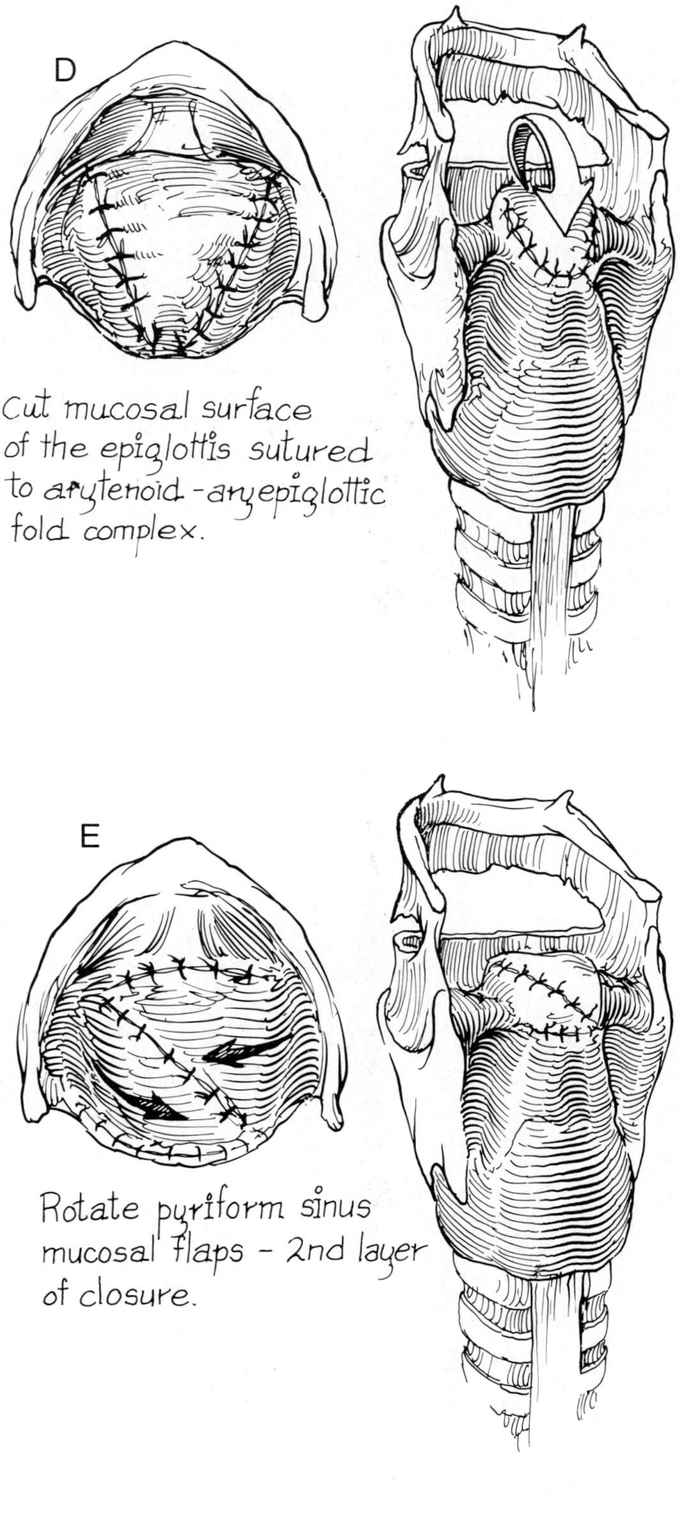

Figure 24–9 *Continued. D,* Closure of epiglottic mucosa to arytenoid-aryepiglottic fold complex. *E,* Second layer of closure with pyriform sinus mucosal flaps.

Habal and Murray were able to detach the arytenoid-epiglottic flap in one case and reestablish a normal airway after a few dilations of the laryngeal introitus. They reported a failure rate of one in three in obtaining complete laryngeal closure. This procedure provides another option for blocking the larynx from aspiration, with proven reversibility.

Laryngeal Diversion. In 1975[24] and again in 1976,[25] Lindeman reported a technique of laryngeal diversion. This procedure theoretically has better potential for reversibility because the intrinsic larynx is not surgically altered.

The procedure involves tracheal exposure via a midline skin incision from just below the cricoid to just above the suprasternal notch. The trachea is exposed and freed circumferentially for a 4 cm length, with careful preservation of both recurrent laryngeal nerves. These nerves are carefully retracted laterally. The trachea is separated between the third and fourth tracheal rings; the endotracheal tube is removed and an anode tube placed in the lower tracheal segment for ventilation. At this point or earlier, an esophageal dilator, No. 32 or No. 34, is passed to aid in access to the anterior esophageal wall. A vertical incision, slightly larger than the diameter of the trachea, is then created in the anterior esophagus at a location that will easily be reached by the upper transected trachea. An end-to-side tracheoesophageal anastomosis is then performed, the author's preference being 3-0 nylon one-layer closure, with all ties outside the lumen. The strap muscles are then reapproximated over the anastomosis site, and the distal trachea is pulled up just below the anastomosis site and sutured to the strap muscles for temporary support. A permanent tracheotomy is then performed by immobilizing the lower trachea segment to the skin edges and creating a permanent tracheostoma (Fig. 24–10).

Lindeman's procedure is reversed by sacrificing the lower tracheal ring of the upper segment (the one directly involved with the tracheoesophageal anastomosis) and the superior ring of the permanent tracheotomy. The esophagus is then closed in the standard fashion with a strap muscle placed between the closure and the trachea. The trachea is reconstructed by an end-to-end anastomosis, without requiring laryngeal release. A tracheotomy at a lower level is not performed.

A modification of this procedure in patients who have had a high tracheotomy performed prior to the diversion procedure has also been

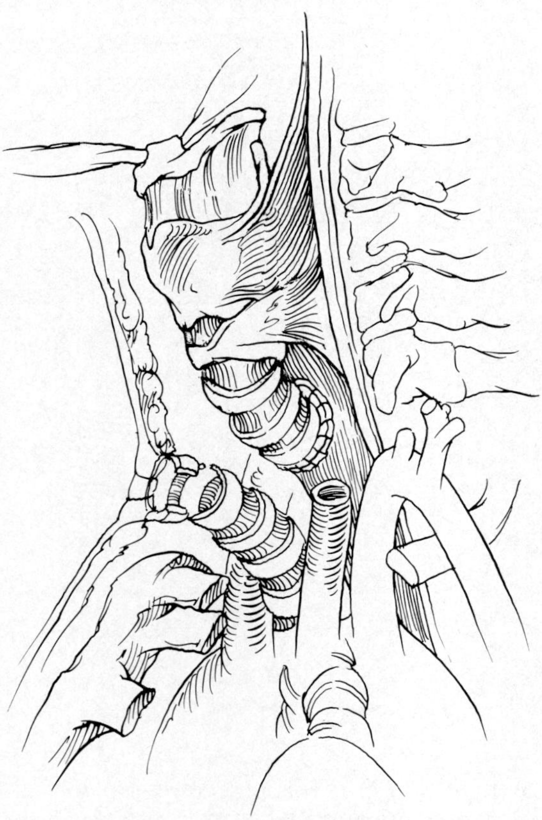

Figure 24–10. Lindeman procedure for laryngeal diversion by tracheoesophageal anastomosis and permanent tracheostoma.

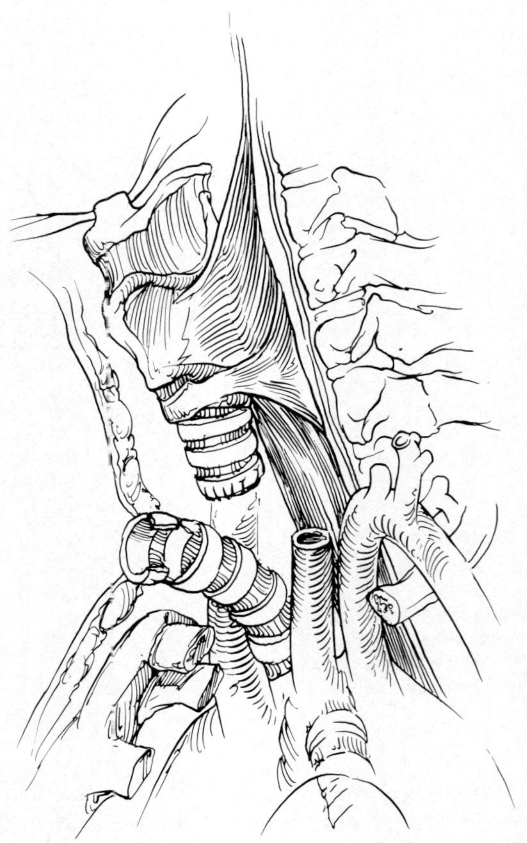

Figure 24–11. Technique for reversal of Lindeman's procedure by creating a blind pouch of the proximal trachea.

developed. In these cases, since an insufficient length of upper trachea is available, a blind pouch of the proximal trachea is created. This has worked equally well (Fig. 24–11).

The advantage of this procedure is that it is definitely reversible; Lindeman et al. reconstructed two cases with excellent results. The intrinsic laryngeal structure is not modified, as with the Montgomery and Habal procedures, theoretically simplifying reversibility. Most importantly, the otolaryngologist can follow the return of function of the larynx, hypopharynx, and cricopharyngeus muscle by direct vision and contrast studies. None of the important structures are covered or surgically modified.

This procedure is not without its risks. Danger of permanent damage to the recurrent laryngeal nerves exists, both initially while the anastomosis is being performed and again during the reconstruction. Bilateral recurrent laryngeal nerve paralysis would negate all the above-mentioned advantages for potential reversibility.

Ideally, this procedure should be performed in an aspirating patient who has not yet had a tracheotomy; if a tracheotomy is performed in a patient who may later be a candidate for the tracheoesophageal anastomosis, avoidance of a high tracheotomy should be considered to allow enough length of trachea superiorly to perform the anastomosis.

Laryngectomy. Of all the procedures discussed, a laryngectomy provides the greatest guarantee of aspiration prevention. Not only does the total removal of a partially disabled or nondisabled larynx run contrary to the thoughts of most laryngologists, but unlike the other procedures discussed, a total laryngectomy is not reversible. To sentence a patient to esophageal speech or an electric larynx for the rest of his life as treatment for nonmalignant disease seems unkind and insensitive. If a total laryngectomy is deemed the treatment of choice, every effort should be made to provide aggressive vocal rehabilitation (see recent advances in voice prostheses discussed elsewhere in this book).

CONCLUSION

Clinically significant aspiration is a taxing situation for both physician and patient. While the obvious surgical therapy, after a trial of conservative medical therapy, would logically seem to be a cuffed tracheotomy, this therapeutic regimen is often unsuccessful in patients with severe aspiration. Although a laryngectomy would guarantee no further aspiration of saliva and food, most physicians avoid removing a larynx that is free of neoplastic disease.

The surgical techniques presented in this chapter have all been used successfully to treat severe aspiration; however, each technique poses potential risks. Each surgeon is limited in his experience by the paucity of patients who require these procedures for life-threatening aspiration. More time and further experience will test the value of these procedures and possibly other clinicians will develop simpler techniques for this complex problem.

References

1. Brunings W: Ueber eine neue behandlungsmethode der Recurrenslahmung. Verh Dtsch Laryng 18: 151(583), 1911.
2. Arnold G: Vocal rehabilitation of paralytic dysphonia. Arch Otolaryngol 73:290–294, 1961.
3. Lewy RB, Mathews R: Immediate temporary restoration of glottic valve function. Laryngoscope 75:1348–1351, 1965.
4. Schramm VL et al.: Gelfoam paste injection for vocal cord paralysis: Temporary rehabilitation of glottic incompetence. Laryngoscope 88:1268–1273, 1978.
5. Pevoin FM: Complications of cervical esophagostomy. Arch Otolaryngol 90:79, 1969.
6. Acquarelli MJ et al.: Cervical esophagostomy. Arch Otolaryngol 96:453–456, 1972.
7. Dobie RA et al.: Skin flap esophagostomy. Arch Otolaryngol 105:200–202, 1979.
8. Thawley SE, Ogura JH: Cricopharyngeal myotomy. Laryngoscope 88:872–874, 1978.
9. Laage-Hellman JE: Ligatur au ductus Stenoni som terpeutisk atgard. Svenska lak-tidning 52:3150, 1955.
10. Wallenborn WM et al.: Experimental production of parotid gland atrophy by ligation of Stensen's duct and by irradiation. Laryngoscope 74:644–655, 1964.
11. Baron HC, Ober WB: Parotid gland atrophy. Arch Surg 85:1042–1044, 1962.
12. Tamarin A: Secretory cell alterations associated with submaxillary gland duct ligation. *In* Schneyer LH, Schneyer CA (eds): Secretory Mechanisms of Salivary Glands. New York, London, Academic Press, 1967.
13. Diamant H: Ligation of the parotid duct in recurrent parotitis. Acta Otolaryngol (Stockh) 49:375–380, 1958.
14. Goode RL, Smith RA: The surgical management of sialorrhea. Laryngoscope 80:1078–1089, 1970.
15. Edgerton MT, Duncan MM: Reconstruction with loss of the hyomandibular complex in excision of large cancers. Arch Surg 78:425–436, 1959.
16. DesPrez JD, Kiehn CL: Methods of reconstruction following resection of anterior oral cavity and mandible for malignancy. Plast Reconstr Surg 24:238, 1959.
17. Jabaley ME, Hoopes JE: A simple technique for laryngeal suspension after partial or complete resection of the hyomandibular complex. Am J Surg 118:685, 1969.
18. Calcaterra T: Laryngeal suspension after supraglottic laryngectomy. Arch Otolaryngol 94:306, 1971.

19. Goode RL: Laryngeal suspension in head and neck surgery. Laryngoscope 86:349–355, 1976.
20. Montgomery WW: Surgery to prevent aspiration. Arch Otolaryngol 101:679–682, 1975.
21. Sasaki CT et al.: Surgical closure of the larynx for intractable aspiration. Arch Otolaryngol 106:422–423, 1980.
22. Habal MB, Murray JE: Surgical treatment of life-endangering chronic aspiration pneumonia: Use of an epiglottic flap to the arytenoids. Plast Reconstr Surg 49:305–311, 1972.
23. Vecchione TR et al.: Further experiences with the arytenoid-epiglottic flap for chronic aspiration pneumonia. Plast Reconstr Surg 55:318–323, 1975.
24. Lindeman RC: Diverting the paralyzed larynx: A reversible procedure for intractable aspiration. Laryngoscope 85:157–180, 1975.
25. Lindeman RC et al.: Clinical experience with the tracheoesophageal anastomosis for intractable aspiration. Ann Otol Rhinol Laryngol 85:609–612, 1976.
26. Fee W, Ward PH: Permanent tracheostomy: A new surgical technique. Ann Otol Rhinol Laryngol 86:635–638, 1977.

25

Radiation Therapy for Carcinoma of the Larynx

Carlos A. Perez, M.D. and James E. Marks, M.D.

Irradiation is widely used in the treatment of head and neck cancer, particularly laryngeal carcinoma, either alone in the early stages of disease or combined with surgery in more advanced tumors.

Ionizing radiations transfer energy to the cells through fast particles that excite and ionize atoms in the absorber, depending on the energy of the incident radiation and the electrons activated (34 eV necessary to form an ion pair in air). Effects of irradiation can occur directly on the cell or be mediated by radical formation in water. When ionization occurs, a variety of ions in solution are formed with the appearance of free radicals (H^+, OH^-, NH to O^+, H_2O_2).

The critical target in cell death is the nucleus, where molecular damage to the DNA and the RNA results. This biochemical injury produces biologic effects in the cell that, depending on the dose of radiation given, will induce nuclear changes that may result in mitotic delay, cell cycle changes, mutations or chromosome destruction, or (to a lesser extent) changes that may affect membrane permeability and enzyme and protein synthesis. If the damage to the DNA is beyond repair, the cell is killed (lethal damage). If the injury is subsequently repaired, however, after a period of delay the cell will return to a normal proliferative cycle (sublethal damage). On occasion, the cell may be severely affected by irradiation, and any modification in its environment will cause it to die (potentially lethal damage).

Biologically speaking, cell kill by irradiation is defined as the loss of unlimited proliferative capacity. In mathematical expression, this loss of cell viability follows an exponential function, so that a specified dose of radiation will kill a constant fraction of cells (Fig. 25–1). This means that the fraction of cells killed may be independent of the number of cells that are irradiated; by the same token, the absolute number of cells killed by a given dose of radiation will be greater when the initial number of cells is larger. A cell survival curve may be straight (single hit will result in death of the cell) or it may have an initial shoulder, indicating that one target must be hit more than once by the ionizing event or that several targets need to be destroyed before the cell is inactivated. The shoulder observed in the initial portion of the cell curve may indicate (1) repair of sublethal damage, (2) progression of some cells through the cell cycle, or (3) repopulation from surviving cells. The major factor is the repair of sublethal damage.

Various conditions will influence the effects of irradiation on cells: (1) the oxygen enhancement effect, (2) the position of the cell in the proliferative cycle, (3) the dose fractionation

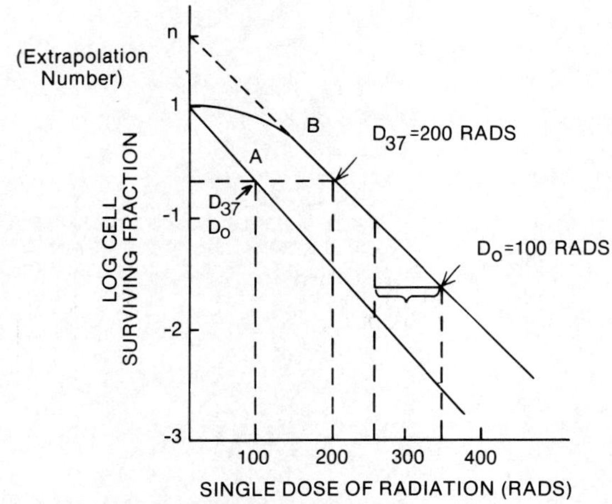

Figure 25–1. Theoretical cell survival curve depicting a single hit (*line A*) or multihit (*line B*) type of survival.

and dose-time relationship, (4) the linear energy transfer (LET) of particles, and (5) the presence of radiation sensitizers or protectors. Standard radiobiology textbooks are suggested for additional reading.[1]

Cells that are closer to capillaries are better oxygenated and will be more sensitive to radiation. Cells in the center of the tumor tend to be hypoxic and doses of radiation about three times as high as those required for well-oxygenated cells are necessary to produce the same lethal effect (Fig. 25–2). During fractionated radiotherapy or with split course schedules, tumor regression and revascularization result in reoxygenation of some of the hypoxic tumor cells.

High LET particles, such as neutrons and pi-mesons, have a larger mass than x-rays (photons) or electrons and a greater ionizing capacity per unit track. Because of this property, heavier particles produce a greater cell kill. In addition, the oxygen enhancement effect is minimal for these particles, hypoxic cells being nearly as sensitive as well-oxygenated cells. Since the damage induced is nearly always lethal, there is no significant repair between fractions (Fig. 25–3).

The potential application of chemotherapeutic agents that may be effective against epithelial tumors of the head and neck is under investigation.[2, 3] In Chapters 26 and 27 of this volume, Panettiere discusses this work.

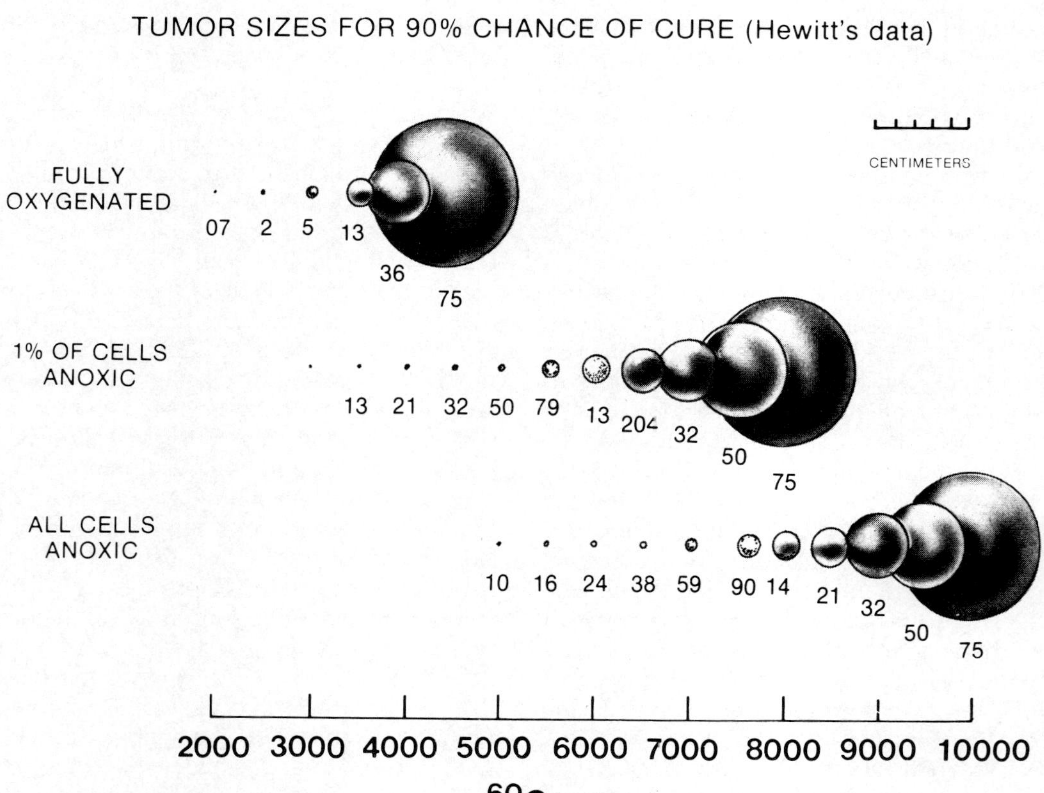

Figure 25–2. The dose of irradiation necessary to eradicate a tumor, depending on the size and proportion of anoxic or hypoxic cells. Even a small fraction of hypoxic cells will significantly increase resistance of the tumor to irradiation. (From Fowler J et al.: Br J Radiol 36:79, 1963.)

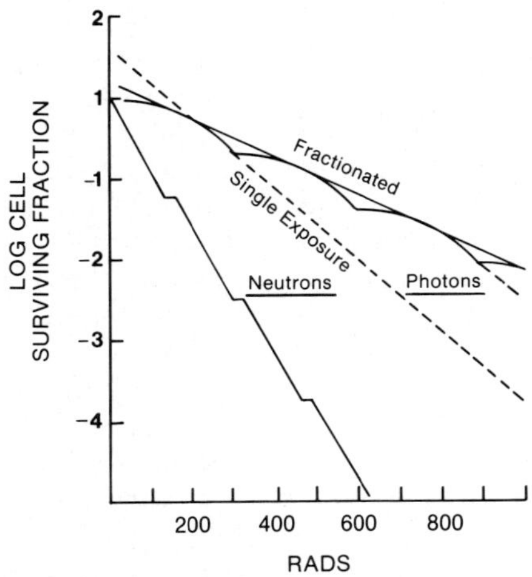

Figure 25–3. Example of cell survival with single or fractionated irradiation with photons or neutrons. Cell lethality is the same with single or fractionated doses because neutrons are associated with minimal repair of sublethal damage between fractions.

COMBINED SURGERY AND RADIOTHERAPY

Biologic Basis of Preoperative and Postoperative Irradiation. In a simple model, a malignant tumor in man is composed of a central hypoxic area and a better oxygenated periphery, with microextension into the adjacent tissues. Some tumors have a propensity for spread along the lymphatics or through the blood vessels.

The surgeon may not accomplish a complete removal of all extensions of the tumor in a surgical resection. Furthermore, surgery raises the possibility that viable tumor cells may be mechanically disseminated in the operative field or into the lymphatics or the general circulation through manipulation of the tumor.

The radiotherapist, on the other hand, may effectively control small tumors and peripheral extensions of larger lesions. Large tumors, because of their fraction of hypoxic cells, will require extremely high doses of irradiation, which may damage surrounding normal tissues. Such tumors may not be eradicated by conventional radiotherapy. The combination of moderate doses of radiation with an operation has been advocated to treat a variety of malignant tumors, on the bases that the fraction of well-oxygenated cells may be reduced by a factor of 10^6 to 10^7 and that the surgeon will remove the central hypoxic tumor. This should result in improved local and regional tumor control with less anatomic and functional deficit. Furthermore, if malignant cells have not disseminated before the patient is treated, these cells will be rendered nonviable and mechanical spread at the time of the surgical procedure should not result in distant metastasis.[4, 5] Postoperative irradiation may accomplish local and regional tumor kill, thereby reducing the recurrence rate, but has no effect on the incidence of distant metastasis.

Indications for Combined Therapy. It is important to identify the patient subpopulations that, from either biologic or clinical considerations, may benefit from combined irradiation and surgery. These include patients in whom local or regional recurrrence will develop, either because of tumor cell dissemination in the operative area or because microextensions of the tumor that are clinically unrecognized will not be removed by the surgical procedure. Also, large tumors that initially cannot be removed because of involvement of vital adjacent structures may occasionally be rendered resectable after relatively high doses of irradiation.

Patients with a high propensity toward development of distant metastasis early in the evolution of the tumor, as in carcinoma of the breast or lung, may not greatly benefit from preoperative radiation. This situation does not exist in head and neck cancer and specifically not in cancer of the larynx, where the tumors tend to invade adjacent structures and the regional lymphatics before distant dissemination takes place. Strong et al.[6] reported a 22 per cent frequency of recurrence in the necks of 111 patients treated with 2000 rads in five fractions prior to surgery, compared with a 33 per cent neck failure rate in a control group of 164 patients treated with surgery alone.

Adjuvant preoperative or postoperative radiation should be given to patients with large tumors or palpable lymph node metastases because the possibility of cure is lower in these patients.[7] Tables 25–1 and 25–2 summarize the advantages and disadvantages of preoperative and postoperative irradiation.

Table 25–1. PREOPERATIVE IRRADIATION

Advantages
Inactivation of viable cells that may be disseminated at surgery
Better tissue vascularization and oxygenation
Disadvantages
Regression of tumor may result in inadequate resection
Interference with wound healing

Table 25–2. POSTOPERATIVE IRRADIATION

Advantages	
	No distortion of operative field
	Full extent of tumor can be determined at surgery
	No interference with wound healing
Disadvantage	
	Cellular oxygenation may be compromised because of fibrosis and decreased vascularity after surgery

The use of ionizing radiation in combination with surgery raises several technical considerations:

1. Location and size of primary tumor. Small laryngeal carcinomas that are controlled in over 90 per cent of patients by either irradiation or surgery should not receive combined therapy.

2. Probability of regional lymph node metastasis. Only patients with a significant probability of having lymphatic metastases will show decreased regional recurrence with combined therapy. It is critical to be familiar with the pathways of dissemination so that they are included in the irradiated volume.

3. Optimal dose and fractionation of irradiation. A relatively high dose (tumor dose of 4500 to 5000 rads) must be delivered in order to achieve tumor eradication. The dose delivered should not be so excessive that it hinders the surgical procedure or wound healing. Also, the combined therapy should result in minimal anatomic and physiologic deficit. In general, daily fractionation should be in the range of 200 rads ± 10 per cent.

4. Timing of surgical procedure. The surgical procedure should be timed to allow subsidence of the acute effects of irradiation, which can interfere with the patient's general condition or nutritional status or with the healing of the surgical incision. On the other hand, surgery should not be delayed to the time when tumor repopulation and regrowth will occur. In general, an interval of four to six weeks after doses of 4500 to 5000 rads will be adequate.

EFFECTS OF IRRADIATION ON THE NORMAL TISSUES OF THE NECK AND LARYNX

Reactions in the oropharyngeal and laryngeal mucosa are related to damage to the germinal cell layers of the epithelium and to vascular changes. The acute phase of the radiation reaction manifests increased vascular permeability and interstitial edema with associated inflammatory changes. During the first three to four weeks, erythema of the mucosa is followed by studded mucositis. At this point, the patient begins to complain of a sore throat. After 4000 rads, a patchy fibrinous exudate may be seen, becoming more confluent with doses of over 5000 rads. Late effects of irradiation are secondary to nonreversible damage to the microvasculature and to proliferation of connective tissue. Atrophy of the mucosa, telangiectasis, and ulceration may be observed with relatively large doses of radiation (over 6000 rads). Hyperkeratosis of the vocal cords may be observed. With higher doses, there is some edema of the vocal cords and arytenoids. In general, the larynx tolerates relatively high doses of irradiation (6500 to 7000 rads) if the volume treated is small (less than 40 cm^2).[8] Higher doses of irradiation may result in severe laryngeal edema or, occasionally, chondritis or cartilage necrosis.

Skin reactions range from erythema and dry desquamation to moist desquamation and ulceration with necrosis, depending on the type of radiation and energy used, the area treated, and the doses and fractionation used. When orthovoltage (below 300 kVp) or electron energies are used, erythema will appear with doses of about 3000 rads in three weeks, dry desquamation with slightly higher doses, and moist desquamation with 4500 to 5000 rads. With cobalt-60, high energy x-rays (above 4 Mev), neutrons, and electrons, subcutaneous fibrosis is frequently observed with doses over 5000 rads.

Severe ulceration and necrosis of skin should never be seen after therapeutic exposures. Sometimes, however, they have been observed after high doses of irradiation.

Moderate doses of irradiation (3000 to 4000 rads) cause transient epilation, which usually repairs in three to four months. The other skin appendages, as well as the fingernails, follow the same recovery pattern. With larger doses of irradiation (over 5000 rads), total epilation as well as depopulation of sebaceous and sweat glands may be observed.

Erythema and dry desquamation will heal in three to four weeks. Moist desquamation may take longer to disappear, depending on the area involved; however, most patients will show complete recovery in six to eight weeks.

Chronic and late effects of irradiation are characterized by atrophy and depigmentation of the dermis or epidermis, telangiectasias, and, sometimes, hyperkeratosis. This is frequently associated with the loss of hair follicles, sebaceous glands, and sweat glands. On occasion, there are necrosis and ulceration of the skin that will not heal because of the high dose of irradiation. A resection of the area may be required and a skin graft with a vascular pedicle must be done to insure healing.

HISTORICAL REVIEW

Radiotherapy began during the years between 1895 and 1898 with the discovery of radioactivity by Becquerel, x-rays by Roentgen, and radium by the Curies. Early in the present century, attempts were made to treat cancers of the larynx by external irradiation using x-ray tubes designed specifically for this purpose.[9, 10] Despite these early attempts, it was not until 1922 that Regaud and Coutard[11, 12] recorded the first series of 32 patients treated by irradiation. They treated these original patients with multiple small daily increments of dose, which resulted in preservation of the normal tissues of the larynx and destruction of the tumor in the 22 patients whose tumors were cured. By 1926, the group at the Curie Foundation in Paris had treated a total of 77 patients; the 22 who survived four or more years had important historical significance.[11] This experience in carcinoma of the larynx formed the groundwork for fractionated radiation in the treatment of malignant tumors. In the decades following this initial experience, other authors in Scandinavia, England, and the United States carried on the original work of Coutard with different types of kilovoltage equipment.[13, 14] The same fractionated courses of radiation continued with the advent of megavoltage radiation from cobalt-60 and linear accelerators. Today there is considerable standardization of technique for radiotherapy of carcinoma of the larynx. Because of its simplicity and demonstrated success, fractionated external irradiation remains the treatment of choice for early cancers of the larynx.

Another experience not to be overlooked in treating cancers of the larynx is the use of radium. Interstitial implantation of radium needles into the larynx was shown, on occasion, to be successful in the treatment of laryngeal cancer. In 1928, Finzi and Harmer[15] demonstrated that radium could be used to treat early cancers of the larynx. They created a fenestration in the thyroid cartilage for implantation of the tubes in immediate proximity to the cancer. This technique was used extensively at Manchester, England, to treat a group of cases, but it never gained the degree of popularity achieved by external irradiation because of the necessity for operative intervention.

TREATMENT

Carcinoma in situ. Stutsman and McGavran[16] reported satisfactory results with conservative management of eleven selected patients with in situ or superficially invasive carcinoma of the true vocal cord. In a review of 354 laryngeal specimens by serial longitudinal step blocks, Bauer[17] demonstrated carcinoma in situ in 76 per cent of the patients with nonkeratinizing carcinoma of the larynx and in 26 per cent of those with keratinizing carcinoma. He concluded that carcinoma in situ is a common route of intramucosal spread, particularly of the nonkeratinizing lesions, and that a biopsy finding of in situ carcinoma usually indicates the presence of an invasive tumor elsewhere in the laryngeal mucosa. Further, if the patient is not extremely reliable, if very close follow-up cannot be assured, or if there is concern regarding invasion or the aggressiveness of the tumor, either irradiation or a limited surgical procedure will always be a better approach. In this type of patient, the lesion will be treated as T1 invasive carcinoma, with small portals (5×5 cm) to a dose of 6000 rads tumor dose in six weeks. Pene and Fletcher[18] reported survival and tumor control in 86 patients treated for carcinoma in situ with radiation alone compared with those described for stage T1 and T2 invasive carcinoma of the vocal cords. Only one patient died of cancer. The failure rate was 11 per cent for 63 T1 lesions and 26 per cent for 23 T2 tumors. All of the patients but one (who refused treatment) with recurrent tumor were salvaged by surgical procedures (eight laryngectomies, two cordectomies, and one hemilaryngectomy).

Glottic Carcinoma. Because of the paucity of lymphatics in the region of the true vocal cord, lymphatic metastasis in early glottic carcinoma is unusual. Therefore, tumor size (or volume) and fixation, instead of lymphatic metastasis, primarily affect prognosis and radiocurability for glottic carcinoma[9, 19–21] (Table 25–3). The two-dimensional extent of the tumor can easily be determined by indirect and direct laryngoscopy; the third dimension, or penetrability, of the tumor can be estimated by determining the degree of vocal cord fixation, which occurs when there is extensive infiltration of the muscle.[22, 23] It has been reported that treatment by irradiation controls the primary tumor

Table 25–3. RESULTS OF RADIATION THERAPY FOR GLOTTIC CARCINOMA*

Vocal Cord Status	Three-Year NED† Number of Patients	Three-Year NED† Per Cent	Five-Year NED† Number of Patients	Five-Year NED† Per Cent
Anterior two-thirds vocal cord involved	240/255	94	191/208	92
Anterior two-thirds cord and/or anterior commissure involved	46/56	82	34/42	81
Entire cord or posterior third vocal cord involved	70/93	75	57/75	76
Totals	356/404	88	282/325	87

*From Wang CC: Am J Roentgenol 120:158, 1974.
†NED = No evidence of disease.

Table 25–4. GLOTTIC CARCINOMA—CONTROL, SALVAGE, VOICE, AND SURVIVAL

Investigators	T and N Control Range	T and N Control Total	Salvage Range	Salvage Total	Voice Preserved Range	Voice Preserved Total	Five-Year Survival Range	Five-Year Survival Mean
Radiation alone for mobile cord								
Wang, Marks, Goffinet, Horiot, Shaw	77%–91%	706/810 (87%)	83%–89%	87/104 (84%)	83%–91%	511/581 (88%)	80%–90%	85%
Radiation alone for impaired cord mobility								
Wang, Horiot, Goffinet	64%–75%	162/226 (72%)	65%–75%	34/50 (68%)	64%–75%	162/226 (72%)	—	64%
Radiation alone for fixed cord								
Wang	—	12/45 (27%)	—	12/27 (44%)	—	27%	—	27%
Hemilaryngectomy for fixed cord								
Lesinski, Kirchner	60%–72%	26/40 (65%)	33%–60%	6/14 (43%)	—	65%	60%–66%	63%

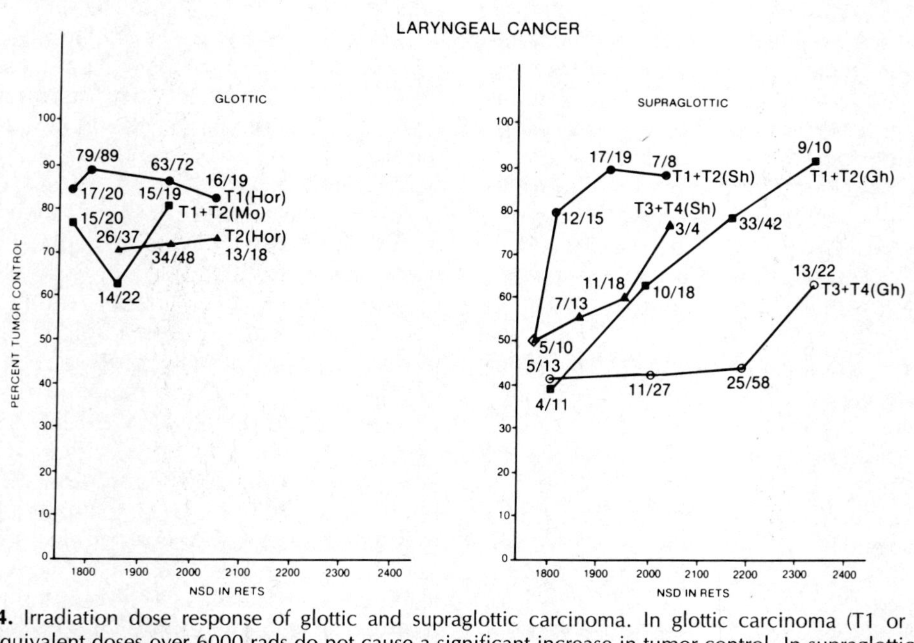

Figure 25–4. Irradiation dose response of glottic and supraglottic carcinoma. In glottic carcinoma (T1 or T2 tumors), biological equivalent doses over 6000 rads do not cause a significant increase in tumor control. In supraglottic carcinoma, tumor control is increased with higher doses of irradiation.

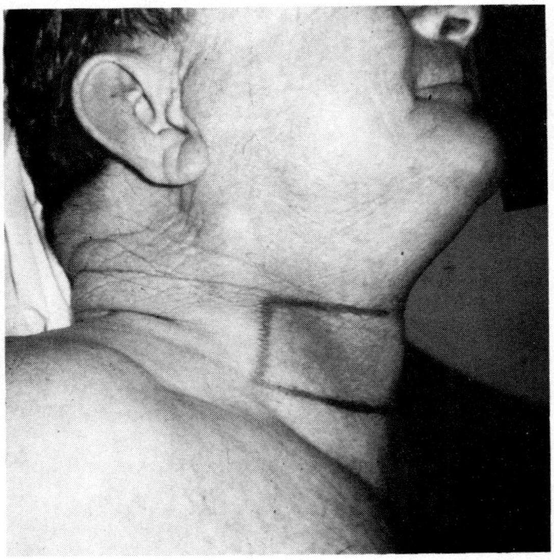

Figure 25–5. Portal used for treatment of localized glottic carcinoma.

and preserves voice in up to 90 per cent of tumors that are localized to one true vocal cord without infiltration of the vocalis muscle, in 80 per cent of tumors extending to the anterior commissure, in 60 per cent of tumors causing decreased mobility of the cord, and in 30 per cent of tumors with fixation of the vocal cord (Table 25–4).[19–21, 24–26] Partial fixation of the true vocal cord is a relative contraindication to treatment with irradiation alone, because hemilaryngectomy with preservation of voice probably achieves local control superior to that achieved by irradiation alone.[23, 26]

The low incidence of lymphatic metastasis with early glottic cancer makes it unnecessary to treat neck lymphatics in those patients without palpable lymph nodes. The larynx alone is irradiated to doses between 6000 and 7000 rads in six to seven weeks. Dosages within this range do not change local control of the primary tumor by stage, indicating a significant lack of dose response for early glottic cancer[20, 27] (Fig. 25–4).

The field size is approximately 5 × 5 cm and includes the intrinsic larynx. The portals extend from the thyroid notch to the inferior margin of the cricoid, posteriorly to the horn of the thyroid cartilage including the arytenoids, and anteriorly with falloff on the skin (Fig. 25–5). If there is involvement of the anterior commissure or exophytic subglottic extension, the lower margin is extended at least 1 cm below the cricoid ring.

With a small T1 lesion, a single unilateral port can be employed (Fig. 25–6A); with anterior commissure involvement, bilateral ports should always be used (Fig. 25–6B). Open fields will result in higher doses in the anterior commissure (about 20 per cent) because of the sloping contour of the neck; this can be corrected by the use of wedges (usually 15 to 30 degrees) (Fig. 25–6C).

In patients with extremely short necks, the customary lateral port arrangement may not be adequate, and anterior oblique fields with wedges may yield a better dose distribution. Also, electrons may be employed, although the radiotherapist and physicist must be acutely aware of the perturbations in dose distribution that may take place with this modality.

Irradiation with cobalt-60 or 4 to 6 Mev photons will be adequate in most instances. Epp et al.[28] recently reported on the perturbation that the glottic air gap may have in the dose distribution of 8 to 10 Mev photons with the loss of electronic equilibrium and a reduction of 10 per cent to 15 per cent in the dose to the opposite vocal cord. This may explain some of the infield recurrences seen after seemingly adequate doses of irradiation for small glottic lesions.

Hemilaryngectomy may salvage 70 per cent to 75 per cent of patients with T1 and T2 glottic carcinoma who develop a local recurrence after irradiation, preserving their voices.[29] The remaining patients require total laryngectomy.[25]

Mittal et al.[30] reported the results at the Mallinckrodt Institute of Radiology in 177 patients with invasive epidermoid carcinoma of the true vocal cords with normal mobility treated with irradiation alone. Patients were treated with lateral ports, 5 × 5 cm, to doses in the range of 6000 to 6600 rads in six to six and one-half weeks. A series of 119 patients with tumor limited to one vocal cord had an initial tumor control rate of 85 per cent; 28 patients with involvement of the anterior commissure had a rate of 82 per cent; 30 patients with involvement of both true vocal cords had 77 per cent tumor control. Of the 30 patients who failed, 23 (77 per cent) were salvaged, in most instances by a hemilaryngectomy. Thus, the overall tumor control was 96 per cent and voice preservation 90 per cent. The results are summarized in Table 25–5 and Fig. 25–7. Recurrences were seen more frequently in men (18 per cent in 163) than in women (7 per cent in 14). The survival rate was 20 per cent higher in women than in men. Of 61 patients treated with 250 kV x-rays, 23 per cent failed, in contrast to 13 per cent of 54 patients treated

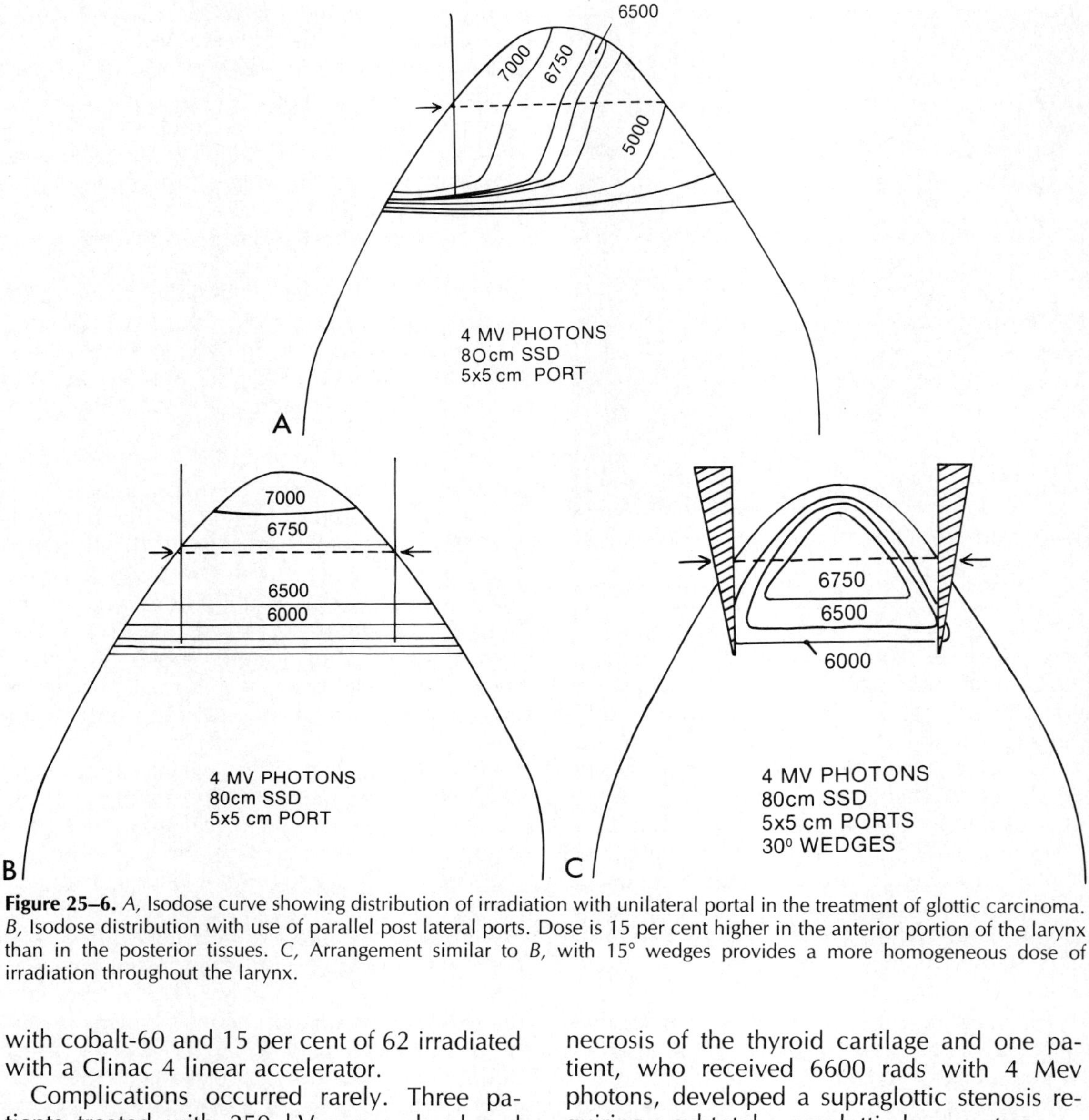

Figure 25–6. *A,* Isodose curve showing distribution of irradiation with unilateral portal in the treatment of glottic carcinoma. *B,* Isodose distribution with use of parallel post lateral ports. Dose is 15 per cent higher in the anterior portion of the larynx than in the posterior tissues. *C,* Arrangement similar to *B,* with 15° wedges provides a more homogeneous dose of irradiation throughout the larynx.

with cobalt-60 and 15 per cent of 62 irradiated with a Clinac 4 linear accelerator.

Complications occurred rarely. Three patients treated with 250 kV x-rays developed necrosis of the thyroid cartilage and one patient, who received 6600 rads with 4 Mev photons, developed a supraglottic stenosis requiring a subtotal supraglottic laryngectomy.

Table 25–5. EARLY CARCINOMA OF TRUE VOCAL CORDS

Mucosal Extent of Disease	Control with Initial Radiation	Initial Failure	Recurring Patients Salvaged	Ultimate Tumor Control	Voice Preservation
One cord only $n = 119$*	101 (85%)	18 (15%)	16 (89%)	117 (98%)	111 (93%)
One cord + A.C.† $n = 28$	23 (82%)	5 (18%)	3 (60%)	26 (93%)	26 (93%)
Both cords $n = 30$	23 (77%)	7 (23%)	4 (57%)	27 (90%)	23 (77%)
Totals $n = 177$	147 (83%)	30 (17%)	23 (77%)	170 (96%)	160 (90%)

*n = Number of patients.
†A.C. = Anterior commissure.
From Mittal B et al.: Int J Radiat Oncol Biol Phys 9:998–1002, 1983.

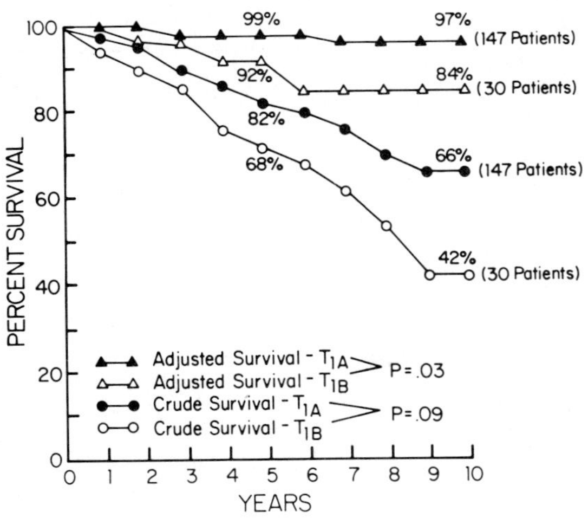

Figure 25–7. Survival by T-stage. (From Mittal B et al.: Int J Radiat Oncol Biol Phys 9:1000, 1983.)

Of 121 patients evaluated for voice quality, 77 per cent had good voice and 22 per cent fair voice (minimal or moderate hoarseness). Only one patient was known to have persistent severe hoarseness. Of seven patients who had salvage hemilaryngectomies, six had fair voices and one had a voice of poor quality.

Of the 177 patients, 32 (18 per cent) developed second primary malignant tumors, only 2 in the head and neck (trachea and pharyngeal wall). Most common second primaries were in the lung, prostate, and colorectal area, and there were five patients with leukemia.

Thus, radiotherapy appears to effectively control limited carcinoma of the true vocal cord. Following therapy, these patients must be followed closely, for 75 per cent of the failures can be salvaged with a hemilaryngectomy.

Transglottic Carcinoma. In general, lesions with fixation of the vocal cord and transglottic extension, even if small, are more successfully treated with surgery. Hemilaryngectomy for small transglottic laryngocarcinomas[26] and total laryngectomy for large transglottic laryngocarcinomas are the prime methods used to control the primary tumor; irradiation, therefore, is adjuvant.[31–33]

If, however, laryngectomy is contraindicated, either because of medical reasons or patient refusal, radiotherapy is utilized in the management of these tumors. A total dose of 7000 rads in approximately eight weeks will be necessary to achieve moderate to high local tumor control. The portals for the treatment of the primary tumor, with an adequate margin, will be demonstrated by the extent of the lesion. The neck lymphatics should be included in the irradiated field, to a dose of at least 5000 rads if lymph nodes are not palpable. If nodes are palpable, they should be included in the high dose irradiation volume (6500 to 7000 rads). This must be done, keeping in mind that more complications and impairment of voice will be observed with higher doses and larger volume treated. The portals must include the entire neck because nodal metastasis may appear not only in the midjugular area but also in the subdigastric or low cervical regions. At Washington University, lower doses have been utilized with results that do not differ significantly from those obtained with laryngectomy alone (Table 25–4). Palpable lymph nodes are best treated by radical neck dissection; however, a neck dissection is probably not necessary for patients without palpable lymph nodes. Doses of 5000 rads in five weeks prevent the subsequent appearance of lymphatic metastases in 95 per cent of patients whose necks are electively irradiated.[34, 35] In patients treated surgically, irradiation may also be delivered preoperatively or postoperatively to prevent recurrence in the laryngeal remnant, pharynx, tracheostoma, and neck. Special attention should be given to elective irradiation of the neck in patients whose primary tumors indicate the potential for lymphatic metastases. This can be estimated by studying the pathologic characteristics of the primary tumor; the incidence of lymphatic metastases for transglottic carcinomas varies between 40 per cent and 50 per cent when the tumor has infiltrating margins, poor differentiation, nerve sheath invasion, or size greater than 2 cm.[36]

Mittal et al.[37] reported on 152 patients with transglottic carcinoma treated at the Mallinckrodt Institute of Radiology between 1968 and 1978. Of these patients, 98 were treated by total laryngectomy, usually combined with a radical neck dissection and in many instances with preoperative or postoperative irradiation; 30 patients were treated with voice conservation procedures and 21 with radiotherapy alone. Three patients died during treatment. The sites of failure are shown in Table 25–6.

In 29 patients treated with total laryngectomy and 24 with voice conservation procedures, no lymph node dissection was done. The failure rate in the ipsilateral neck was 13 per cent and in the contralateral neck, 6 per cent. In 69 patients treated with total laryngectomy and 6 treated with voice conservation procedures, the neck dissection was carried out. The incidence of neck failures was 4 per cent in the ipsilateral and 2 per cent in the contralateral neck. There

Table 25–6. TRANSGLOTTIC CARCINOMA—SALVAGE OF FAILURES ABOVE THE CLAVICLE*

Treatment	Number of Patients	Initial Failures		Ultimate Failures		Patients with Initial Failures	Patients Salvaged
		P/S†	*Neck*	*P/S*	*Neck*		
Total laryngectomy ± neck dissection ± irradiation	98	11 (11%)	10 (10%)	11 (11%)	9 (9%)	20	1 (5%)
Voice conservation surgery ± neck dissection ± irradiation	30	7 (23%)	3 (10%)	4 (13%)	2 (7%)	10	4 (40%)
Irradiation alone	21‡	8 (38%)	0 (0%)	3 (14%)	0 (0%)	8	5 (63%)

*From Mittal B et al. In press.
†P/S = Failure at primary site or stoma.
‡Three additional patients died during treatment.

were two patients (3 per cent) with bilateral neck failures. Of the 21 patients treated with radiotherapy alone, no neck dissections were carried out. No failures were observed in either the ipsilateral or the contralateral necks.

Of the patients who presented initially with stage N0 necks and who received radiotherapy, only 10 per cent developed ipsilateral or contralateral node metastases. Of 13 patients with T4 primary tumors, 4 did not receive radiotherapy and 2 developed ipsilateral neck node metastases.

The voice conservation procedure, along with radiotherapy, yielded a 60 per cent rate of preservation of voice in these patients (Table 25–7).

Figure 25–8, A and B, shows the survival rate according to the stage of the primary tumor or the cervical lymph node. Note that 39 patients requiring tracheostomy had a five-year survival of 33 per cent, in contrast to 52 per cent in 113 patients who did not require such a procedure.

Supraglottic Carcinoma. The ability of irradiation to cure a supraglottic cancer depends on the size and morphologic characteristics of the primary tumor. Control of the primary tumor and regional nodes, with voice preservation, is excellent for small exophytic tumors treated by irradiation, whereas both tumor control and voice quality decline significantly for ulcerating and larger infrahyoid tumors.[24, 38–41] Irradiation of supraglottic cancers followed by surgical salvage for irradiation failures has been advocated,[25, 38] but the rationale for this approach is weakened by the fact that surgical salvage of an irradiation failure is usually achieved by laryngectomy, with loss of voice, and is successful in only approximately half of the cases.[42, 43] The clinician's ability to recognize radioresponsive supraglottic lesions determines the degree of success that may be achieved

Table 25–7. TRANSGLOTTIC CARCINOMA—TREATMENT METHOD AND VOICE PRESERVATION*

Primary Treatment Method	Number of Patients	Cause of Voice Loss			Voice Preservation
		Primary Treatment	*Recurrence at Primary Site*	*Treatment Complication*	
Total laryngectomy ± neck dissection ± irradiation	98	98 (100%)	0	0	0
Voice conservation surgery ± neck dissection ± irradiation	30	0	7 (23%)	5† (17%)	18 (60%)
Irradiation alone	24	0	8 (33%)	0	16 (67%)

*From Mittal B et al. In press.
†Four patients required permanent tracheostomy, three because of laryngeal edema and one because of laryngeal stenosis. One patient required total laryngectomy because of recurrent aspiration due to laryngeal incompetence.

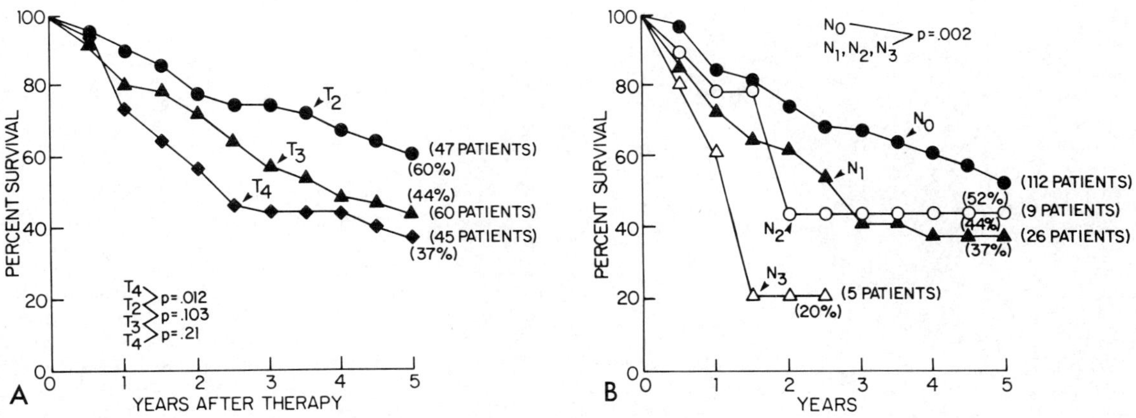

Figure 25–8. Observed survival. *A,* By T-stage. *B,* By N-stage.

using irradiation alone to treat supraglottic cancer.[38, 44] Radiotherapy can be effectively utilized in the following tumors: (1) small exophytic lesions with no palpable neck nodes; (2) nonfixed larger tumors originating in the suprahyoid epiglottis,[44] and (3) lesions of moderate size when there is question of deep infiltration. In the latter instance, the clinician may start radiotherapy and, in four to five weeks, reevaluate the patient to make sure the lesion is primarily exophytic and mobile. If this is the case, the patient can be treated with irradiation alone to doses of 6500–7000 rads with progressively reduced ports. The third dimension (penetrability) of an ulcerating tumor may be greater than that of an exophytic tumor, and the combination of increased volume and poor tumor response makes control with irradiation difficult in a significant number of these lesions. If infiltration or impairment of vocal cord mobility persists, irradiation should be considered a preoperative measure and a supraglottic or total laryngectomy should be performed. Frequent causes of failure to control supraglottic carcinoma with radiotherapy alone are (1) tumor extension into the vallecula, base of the tongue, or preepiglottic space; (2) large infiltrating tumors; (3) inadequate portals (geographic miss); and (4) low doses of irradiation.[44]

In some patients with marginal lesions involving the aryepiglottic fold, partial laryngopharyngectomy may be performed. Conservative surgery, more effective than irradiation alone for the control of ulcerating compartmentalized and noncompartmentalized tumors of the supraglottic larynx, results in local control and voice preservation in approximately three-quarters of the patients[45] (Table 25–8).

Table 25–8. SUPRAGLOTTIC CARCINOMA—CONTROL, SALVAGE, VOICE, AND SURVIVAL

	T and N Control		Salvage		Voice Preserved		Five-Year Survival	
Investigators	***Range***	***Total***	***Range***	***Total***	***Range***	***Total***	***Range***	***Total***
Radiation alone for T1 and T2 lesions								
Fu, Wang, Fletcher, Ghossein	66%–79%	230/312 (74%)	—	9/16 (56%)	66%–79%	74%	70%–74%	98/137 (72%)
Conservation surgery for T1 and T2 lesions								
Marks	—	62/84 (74%)	—	—	—	74%	—	62%
Radiation alone for T3 and T4 lesions								
Wang, Fletcher, Ghossein, Fu, Shukovsky	22%–68%	156/391 (40%)	16%–48%	25/112 (22%)	22%–68%	40%	22%–43%	83/251 (33%)
Conservation surgery for T3 and T4 lesions								
Marks	—	51/76 (67%)	—	—	—	67%	—	47%

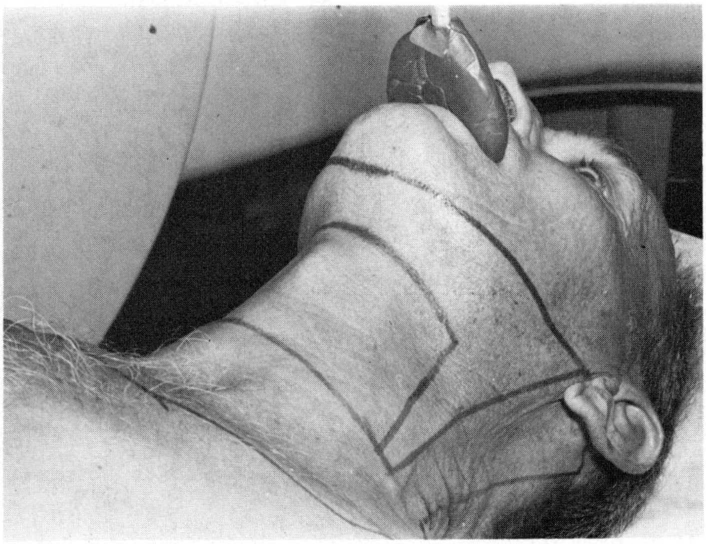

Figure 25–9. Example of portals used in treatment of supraglottic carcinoma. Large fields are used to irradiate the entire upper neck nodes and the primary tumor. After 4500 rads, the posterior margin is moved anteriorly to exclude spinal cord. Depending on the status of the lymph nodes (whether palpable or not), reduced fields are employed to deliver additional dose to complete 6500 to 7000 rads to the primary laryngeal tumor. Lower necks are treated with a separate AP portal that extends to slightly below clavicles. If no palpable nodes are present, a midline 2-cm wide block is used to shield spinal cord.

The supraglottic larynx has a rich lymphatic supply, and the incidence of palpable cervical lymph nodes in the ipsilateral neck is approximately 25 per cent for central supraglottic and 50 per cent for marginal supraglottic cancer.[45] Therefore, the ipsilateral neck must be treated routinely by surgery or irradiation. Neck dissection is preferred for patients with palpable cervical lymph nodes, while irradiation is acceptable for patients without palpable cervical nodes. Doses of 5000 rads in five weeks can prevent the subsequent appearance of tumor in the neck.[34, 35] Evidence of lymphatic metastasis is the most important prognostic factor in carcinoma of the supraglottic larynx because it predicts the development of primary or nodal recurrence and distant metastasis.[9, 45, 46]

The portals used for the supraglottic tumors will vary depending on the anatomic site of origin, tumor size, and presence or absence of neck nodes. The volume treated will extend from the base of the tongue, including the entire epiglottis, to the lower margin of the cricoid, so that the true vocal cords are included (Fig. 25–9). Opposing lateral fields provide good dose distribution, although, if the tumor is unilateral, unequal loading with a higher maximum dose can be used. Since even small lesions tend to permeate the regional lymphatics, the upper and midjugular lymph nodes should be covered in the irradiated volume, to a minimal tumor dose of 5000 rads. In selected patients treated with irradiation alone, the ports can be reduced and the additional boost delivered to the primary laryngeal tumor only. Tumor doses ranging from 6500 to 7000 rads in seven weeks, five weekly fractions, are necessary for high probability of local control (Fig. 25–10).[47, 48]

Fletcher et al.,[38] Fu et al.,[39] Ghossein et al.,[40] Shukovsky,[48] and Wang[49] have reported control rates and survivals of 85 per cent to 90 per cent for T1, 70 per cent for T2, and 50 per cent for

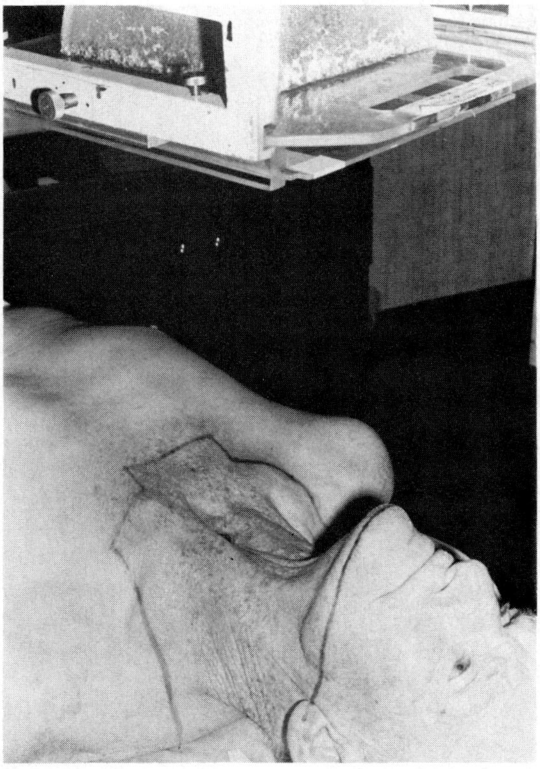

Figure 25–10. Example of portal used for treatment of stomal recurrence and neck nodes following total laryngectomy.

T3 lesions with irradiation alone (Table 25–10). At Washington University, similar results have been obtained with a combination of low-dose preoperative radiation (3000 rads in three weeks) and a supraglottic laryngectomy.[33, 45, 50]

When preoperative irradiation is used, all the anterior cervical lymph nodes should be treated with opposing lateral portals so that each neck receives a minimal dose of 4500 rads, which is adequate to control subclinical disease in the electively treated neck. The lower neck fields can be treated with an anteroposterior portal using a small midline block to shield the cervical spinal cord (Fig. 25–9).

If patients initially treated with surgery show evidence of tumor extension near the surgical margins or metastatic cervical lymph nodes, postoperative irradiation should be given to decrease local and regional recurrence. Doses ranging from 5000 to 6000 rads in five to six weeks will be necessary. The entire neck field should be treated in the manner described above. Irradiation should begin when treatment of the surgical wound is completed and the general condition of the patient is adequate to tolerate radiotherapy (usually three to six weeks after operation).

Subglottic Carcinoma. Small subglottic carcinomas (either primary or extension from a glottic tumor) not associated with vocal cord fixation can be successfully irradiated to control the tumor and preserve the voice. Once the vocal cord becomes fixed or the tumor becomes extensive or if metastatic cervical lymph nodes are present, laryngectomy and radical neck dissection are preferred to irradiation alone.[51]

If radiotherapy is indicated, the field should be extended inferiorly about 2 to 3 cm distal to the cricoid to include the tumor with an adequate margin. Careful evaluation with direct laryngoscopy and laryngograms or tomograms should be made to avoid geographic misses. The upper margin of the field will be the thyroid notch; posteriorly, the margin will be the border of the thyroid cartilage and arytenoid, covering the postcricoid space inferiorly. After 6000 rads, the posterior margin of the field should be moved anteriorly to exclude the arytenoids so as to reduce edema induced by irradiation.

Doses in the range of 7000 rads will be necessary to control the lesion. Opposing lateral fields will provide the best dose distribution. The midjugular nodes should be electively treated with a dose of 5000 rads tumor dose (TD) since subglottic lesions have been shown to metastasize in approximately 20 per cent of patients.[36] In patients with palpable neck nodes, the entire neck should be treated to minimal doses of 4500 rads (preoperative or postoperative irradiation) in combination with laryngectomy and radical neck dissection.

Irradiation After Hemilaryngectomy. Lee et al.[52] reported on the results of irradiation in 18 patients treated prophylactically because of positive margins[53] following a hemilaryngectomy. They also reported on 12 patients treated for a biopsy-proven gross recurrence of laryngeal carcinoma, which occurred five weeks to eight years after a hemilaryngectomy. The usual irradiation technique consisted of treating the larynx through 5 × 5 cm ports and, in a few instances, larger fields encompassing the intrinsic larynx and adjacent tissues. Doses ranging from 6000 to 7000 rads were delivered in six to seven weeks, at 200-rad daily increments, five fractions per week.

Of the patients treated electively for tumor at the margin following a laryngectomy, five (28 per cent) had recurrence after irradiation. Of the twelve patients treated for gross recurrence, five (42 per cent) failed (Table 25–9). Two of the patients irradiated for positive margins and one of the five failing with gross recurrent tumor were salvaged by a total laryngectomy. Thus, the ultimate tumor control was 83 per cent for the electively treated patients and 67 per cent for those irradiated for posthemilaryngectomy recurrence. Three of the patients with residual tumor at the margin had relatively extensive lesions, with involvement of the false cord.

Table 25–9. RESULTS OF IRRADIATION AFTER HEMILARYNGECTOMY*

Reason for Irradiation	Number of Patients	Recurrence After Irradiation	Salvaged by Total Laryngectomy	Ultimate Control of Cancer
Positive margin in hemilaryngectomy specimen	18	5/18 (28%)	2/5	15/18 (83%)
Gross recurrence after hemilaryngectomy	12	5/12 (42%)	1/5	8/12 (67%)

*From Lee F et al.: Laryngoscope 90:1536, 1980.

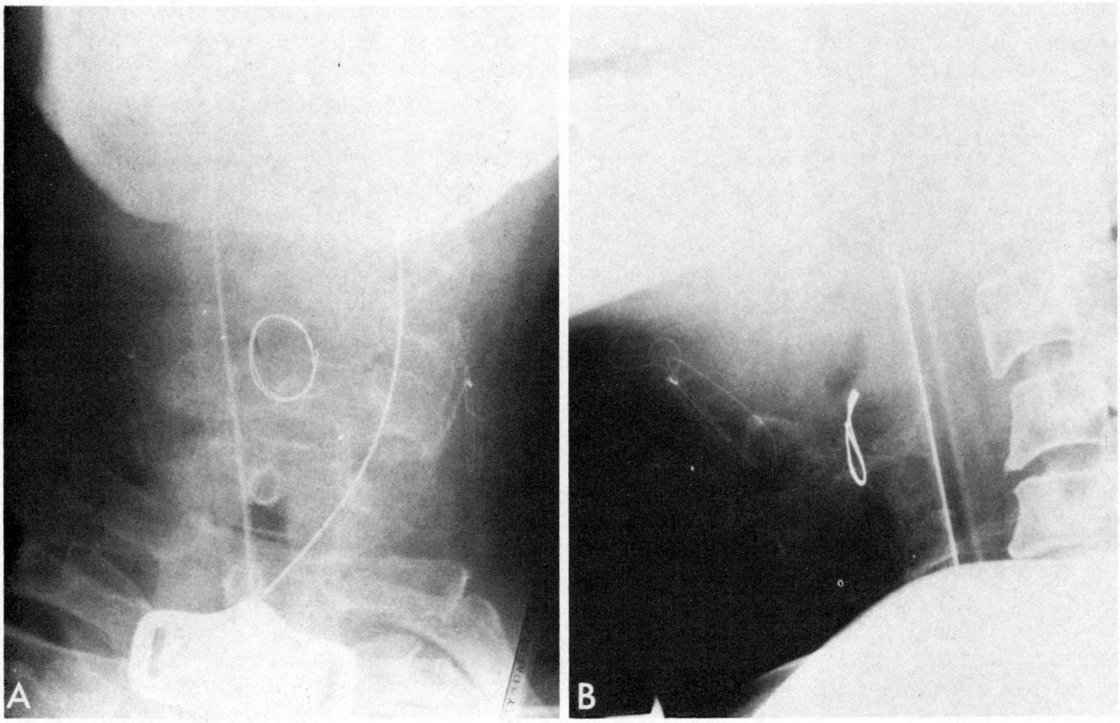

Figure 25–11. Radiographs of neck showing a coil of Iridium-192 implanted in larynx of patient with small recurrence in the arytenoid following supraglottic laryngectomy for epidermoid carcinoma. Dose of 6000 rads was delivered with this method.

Irradiation was well tolerated, with only one patient developing a severe complication—laryngeal edema and subglottic stenosis that required a tracheostomy. Five other patients developed less severe complications associated with scar tissue in the supraglottic or glottic area; one additional patient developed laryngeal edema requiring temporary tracheostomy.

Radiotherapy for Postsurgical Recurrence. Irradiation can effectively control small recurrences in the larynx (for instance, following a hemilaryngectomy, a partial horizontal laryngectomy, or in neck node recurrence). In cases of isolated small laryngeal recurrence, limited fields encompassing the tumor and an adequate margin encompassing the compartment under consideration will be adequate (Fig. 25–10). Doses ranging from 6500 to 7000 rads in seven to eight weeks will be necessary to control the tumor. In cases of lymph node recurrence, the entire neck should be irradiated to doses of 6000 rads followed by a boost of 1000 to 1500 rads, preferably with electrons (13 to 16 Mev energy), to the area of gross recurrence. If a patient has received high doses of external irradiation and additional nonsurgical treatment is required for a laryngeal or neck recurrence, innovative intracavitary techniques, with in situ implantation or radioactive sources, may be employed (Fig. 25–11, A and B).

COMPLICATIONS OF RADIOTHERAPY

Moderate doses of irradiation produce acute mucositis of the pharynx and larynx as well as minimal transient edema of the vocal cords and arytenoids. These side effects usually subside within four to six weeks after completion of radiotherapy.

More significant complications are edema of the larynx or arytenoids (about 5 per cent) and chondritis, which is noted in about 2 per cent of the patients. Necrosis of the thyroid cartilage occurs in 1 per cent to 2 per cent of the patients treated with definitive radiotherapy. Severe complications are seldom noted below biologic equivalent doses of 1900 rets[8, 24, 40, 48] and are uncommon with field sizes smaller than 50 cm^2.[8, 48] Radiation complications are more common with larger tumors that are infiltrating or ulcerated and that have produced some fixation of the vocal cord.

Most complications can be treated conservatively. Exceptions are chondritis and cartilage necrosis, which, may require a total laryngectomy to relieve pain and infection. Also, because of occasional glottic edema, some patients may require emergency tracheostomy to relieve acute airway obstruction.

Patients treated with a combination of irradiation and surgery may exhibit delayed wound healing and fistula formation, depending on the dose of irradiation and the timing of surgery. These complications are significantly more common in patients on whom pharyngeal surgery is performed.[54] Aspiration pneumonia and respiratory difficulties are seen in 10 per cent to 15 per cent of the patients treated with supraglottic laryngectomy; this operation is generally contraindicated in elderly patients with poor pulmonary function.

Preservation of voice in patients with laryngeal carcinoma is extremely important and should be included in the evaluation of treatment methods. Approximately 75 per cent to 80 per cent of the irradiated patients have good voice quality. Marks et al.[45] reported preservation of voice in 71 per cent of 160 patients treated by low-dose preoperative irradiation and a supraglottic laryngectomy.

ADJUVANT CHEMOTHERAPY

Interest is growing in the use of systemic chemotherapy to treat patients with advanced head and neck cancer. As treatment of local and cervical lymph node metastases becomes more effective, the patients survive longer and distant metastases appear clinically with greater frequency. About 15 per cent of the patients with supraglottic or transglottic carcinoma will develop distant metastases.

Several drugs, particularly methotrexate, bleomycin sulfate, cisplatin (*cis*-diamminedichloroplatinum), and vincristine sulfate, have been shown to induce partial responses in patients with advanced head and neck epithelial tumors.[2,3] Combinations of these drugs have been used in noncontrolled clinical trials; preliminary results suggest prolongation of disease-free survival and fewer distant metastases. Well-designed studies are needed to evaluate the potential benefit of multidrug chemotherapy in the management of head and neck malignancy.

NEW RADIOTHERAPEUTIC MODALITIES

Hyperbaric Oxygen. Hyperbaric oxygen has been used to increase the lethal effect of irradiation on hypoxic cells. Henk et al.[55] reported on a randomized study of patients with head and neck cancer treated by irradiation in air (151 patients) or in hyperbaric oxygen (143 patients). Twenty-eight of the patients treated in air and 21 of those treated with hyperbaric oxygen had a primary laryngeal carcinoma. Many radiotherapists consider the fractionation of irradiation (3500 rads in 10 fractions in three weeks) to be less than ideal for patients treated in air, since the time is not adequate to allow for reoxygenation. Survival was similar in both groups; however, the recurrence-free rate at five years was 64 per cent in patients with carcinoma of the larynx treated with hyperbaric oxygen, compared to 49 per cent in those treated in air. The overall results in the 294 patients showed comparable survival in both groups and a recurrence-free rate at five years of 53 per cent in the hyperbaric oxygen group and 30 per cent in the control patients treated with air. The patients with hyperbaric oxygen had more complications than those in the control group. In the hyperbaric oxygen group, eleven patients developed perichondritis and four patients had severe laryngeal edema, in contrast to one patient with perichondritis and three with severe laryngeal edema in the group treated in air.

Neutrons. A report by Catterall et al.[56] describes the preliminary results of a randomized study at Hammersmith comparing neutron versus conventional megavoltage radiation in the treatment of advanced head and neck tumors. Of the 70 patients treated with neutrons, 53 (76 per cent) have shown tumor control at two years in the irradiated volume in comparison with 12 of 63 patients (19 per cent) treated with megavoltage conventional radiation. Although the tumor control is very encouraging, the higher incidence of late complications in the patients treated with neutrons has caused concern. A total of ten major complications has been described in this group in contrast to only two in those patients treated with megavoltage radiation. Note, however, that the percentage of uncomplicated tumor control in the neutron patients is significantly higher. Further studies are required to evaluate this new therapeutic modality, both alone and in combination with high-energy electron or photon beams.

Hypoxic Sensitizers. Recently, several compounds with electron affinity that selectively sensitize hypoxic cells to the effects of irradiation have been synthesized. Two drugs have been used in some clinical trials in patients: metronidazole (Flagyl) and misonidazole (Roche Ro-07-0582). These compounds mimic oxygen, must be present at pharmacologic levels (50 to 75 μg/ml) at the time of irradiation, and have been shown to effectively sensitize hypoxic cells to radiation in in vitro and animal tumor experiments. Wasserman et al.[57] recently published preliminary observations on a phase I study of patients to determine toxicity, reporting that these drugs may induce a significant degree of peripheral neurotoxicity in patients treated with large doses. The maximum total dose of misonidazole reported to be acceptable in patients is 12 to 15g/m^2 body surface. Since the total individual dose is 1.5 to 2 g/m^2, it follows that no more than six to ten doses can be given. This schedule has demanded modifications in the customary daily radiotherapy fractionation regimens (for instance, administering misonidazole and 400 rads in one fraction followed by conventional fractionation the rest of the week, to total doses of 5500 rads). Because of this unconventional fractionation, further studies will be necessary before the hypoxic sensitizers can be used on a broader scale. Also, institutions presently participating in this study must have the capability of measuring by spectrophotometry or high pressure liquid chromatography the plasma levels of the drug prior to the irradiation.

Hyperthermia. Temperatures of 41°C or higher have been sporadically used against cancer since the turn of the century. Numerous experiments in cultured cells and in animal tumors demonstrate the potential of hyperthermia to destroy normal and tumor cells.[32] Also, temperatures higher than 42°C sensitize mammalian cells to x-rays. This sensitization is more selective for cells in relatively resistant late S phase and those with a low oxygen tension. Hyperthermia reduces or eliminates the repair of sublethal and potentially lethal damage induced by x-rays. In addition, hyperthermia can enhance greatly the cytotoxic effect of hypoxic sensitizers with electron affinity and a variety of chemotherapeutic agents.[58]

Preliminary studies at Washington University School of Medicine indicate that some recurrent epithelial tumors of the head and neck may be sensitive to combined treatment with irradiation and hyperthermia. In our phase I and II studies, we have delivered a total tumor dose of 3200 to 4000 rads divided into eight equal fractions of 400 rads, delivered every 72 h, and followed by exposure to 915 MHz microwave hyperthermia at 42.5°C for 60 min.[59]

Unfortunately, at present, several technical problems must be conquered before hyperthermia can be used more effectively to treat head and neck tumors. The available microwave applicators have limited tissue penetrability (1.5 cm for 2450 MHz, 3 cm for 915 MHz, and about 4 cm for 433 MHz). Radio frequency (RF) generators could offer a better dose distribution, but experience with this equipment is extremely limited. Ultrasound can also produce heat, but the distribution is greatly disturbed by the presence of bone or air cavities. In addition, clinical thermometry and the effect that blood flow has in the distribution of heat have not been adequately elucidated. Until further clinical experiences are accumulated, all four of these therapeutic modalities must be considered experimental and their use should be strictly investigational under controlled conditions.

References

1. Hall EJ: Radiobiology for the Radiologist, 2nd ed. Hagerstown MD, Harper and Row, 1978.
2. Taylor SG IV et al.: Methotrexate (M) with Leucovorin (L) as an adjuvant to surgery (S) and radiotherapy (R) in locally advanced squamous carcinoma of the head and neck. (Abstract). Proc Am Assoc Cancer Res Am Soc Clin Oncol 18:346, March 1977. Baltimore, Williams & Wilkins.
3. Wittes RE et al.: Combination chemotherapy with *cis*-diamminedichloroplatinum (II) and bleomycin in tumors of the head and neck. Oncology 32:202–207, 1975.
4. Perez CA: Preoperative irradiation in the treatment of cancer. *In* Vaeth JM (ed): Frontiers of Radiation Therapy and Oncology. Vol 5. Baltimore, University Park Press, 1970, pp 1–19.
5. Powers WE, Tolmach LJ: Preoperative radiation therapy: Biological basis and experimental investigations. Nature 201:272–273, 1964.
6. Strong EW et al.: Preoperative x-ray therapy as an adjuvant to radical neck dissection. Cancer 19:1509–1516, 1966.
7. Hendrickson FR: The results of low dose preoperative radiotherapy for advanced carcinoma of the larynx. *In* Vaeth JM (ed): Frontiers of Radiation Therapy and Oncology. Vol 5. Baltimore, University Park Press, 1970, pp 123–129.
8. Fletcher GH, Klein R: Dose-time-volume relationship in squamous-cell carcinoma of the larynx. Radiology 82:1032–1042, 1964.
9. Lederman M: Radiotherapy of cancer of the larynx. J Laryngol Otol 83:867–896, 1970.
10. Newton Company Catalogue, 1910–1911, p 58.
11. Coutard H: Roentgenotherapy of epitheliomas of the tonsillar region, hypopharynx and larynx from 1920 to 1926. Am J Roentgenol 28:313–331, 1932.
12. Regaud C et al.: Rapport sur la curietherapie et la roentgenotherapie dans le cancer du larynx. Ann Mal Orielle Larynx 41:967–969, 1922.
13. Lenz M: Radiotherapy of cancer of the larynx. Am J Surg 30:259–265, 1935.
14. Nielsen J, Strandberg O: Roentgen treatment of cancer of the larynx. Acta Radiol (Stockh) 23:189–208, 1942.
15. Finzi NH, Harmer D: Radium treatment of intrinsic carcinoma of the larynx. Br Med J 2:886–889, 1928.

16. Stutsman AC, McGavran MH: Ultraconservative management of superficially invasive epidermoid carcinoma of the true vocal cord. Ann Otol Rhinol Laryngol 80:507–512, 1971.
17. Bauer WC: Concomitant carcinoma *in situ* and invasive carcinoma of the larynx. Can J Otolaryngol 3:533–542, 1974.
18. Pene F, Fletcher GH: Results in irradiation of the *in situ* carcinomas of the vocal cords. Cancer 37:2586–2590, 1976.
19. Fletcher GH et al.: Reasons for irradiation failure in squamous cell carcinomas of the larynx. Laryngoscope 85:987–1003, 1975.
20. Horiot J-C et al.: Analysis of failures in early vocal cord cancer. Radiology 103:663–665, 1972.
21. Wang CC: Treatment of glottic carcinoma by megavoltage radiation therapy and results. Am J Roentgenol 120:157–168, 1974.
22. Kirchner JA: One hundred laryngeal cancers studied by serial section. Ann Otol Rhinol Laryngol 78:689–709, 1969.
23. Kirchner JA, Som ML: Clinical significance of fixed vocal cord. Laryngoscope 81:1029–1044, 1971.
24. Goffinet DR et al.: Carcinoma of the larynx: Results of radiation therapy in 213 patients. Am J Roentgenol 117:553–564, 1973.
25. Hendrickson RG et al.: Primary squamous cell carcinoma of the larynx. Laryngoscope 85:1650–1666, 1975.
26. Lesinski SG et al.: Hemilaryngectomy for T_3 (fixed cord) epidermoid carcinoma of the larynx. Laryngoscope 86:1563–1571, 1976.
27. Marks JE et al.: Glottic cancer: An analysis of recurrence as related to dose, time, and fractionation. Am J Roentgenol 117:540–547, 1973.
28. Epp ER et al.: Underdosing of lesions resulting from lack of electronic equilibrium in upper respiratory air cavities irradiated by 10 MV x-ray beams. Int J Radiat Oncol Biol Phys 2:613–619, 1977.
29. Biller HJ et al.: Hemilaryngectomy following radiation failure for carcinoma of the vocal cords. Laryngoscope 80:249–253, 1970.
30. Mittal B et al.: Role of radiation in the management of early vocal cord carcinoma. Int J Radiat Oncol Biol Phys 9:997–1002, 1983.
31. Goldman JL et al.: Combined therapy for cancer of the laryngopharynx. Arch Otolaryngol 92:221–225, 1970.
32. Leeper DB, Henle KJ: Hyperthermia: Effects of different temperatures on normal and tumor cells. Proc First Int Symp Cancer Therapy by Hyperthermia and Radiation. Philadelphia, American College of Radiology, 1975, pp 47–60.
33. Ogura JH, Biller HF: Preoperative irradiation for laryngeal and laryngopharyngeal cancers. Laryngoscope 80:802–810, 1970.
34. Barkley HT et al.: Management of cervical lymph node metastases in squamous cell carcinoma of the tonsillar fossa, base of tongue, supraglottic larynx, and hypopharynx. Am J Surg 124:462–467, 1972.
35. Fletcher GH: Elective irradiation of subclinical disease in cancers of the head and neck. Cancer 29: 1450–1454, 1972.
36. McGavran MH et al.: The incidence of cervical lymph node metastases from epidermoid carcinoma of the larynx and their relationship to certain characteristics of the primary tumor. Cancer 14:55–66, 1961.
37. Mittal B et al.: Transglottic carcinoma. Int J Radiat Oncol Biol Phys, in press.
38. Fletcher GH et al.: The place of radiotherapy in the management of squamous cell carcinoma of the supraglottic larynx. Am J Roentgenol 108:19–26, 1970.
39. Fu KK et al.: Results of integrated management of supraglottic carcinoma. Cancer 40:2874–2881, 1977.
40. Ghossein A et al.: Local control and site of failure in radically irradiated supraglottic laryngeal cancer. Radiology 112:187–192, 1974.
41. Niederer J et al.: Failure analysis of radical radiation therapy of supraglottic cancer. Int J Radiat Oncol Biol Phys 2:621–629, 1977.
42. DeSanto LW et al.: Surgical salvage after radiation for laryngeal cancer. Laryngoscope 86:649–657, 1976.
43. Skolnik EM et al.: Radiation failures in cancer of the larynx. Ann Otol Rhinol Laryngol 84:804–811, 1975.
44. Fletcher GH, Hamberger AD: Causes of failure in irradiation of squamous-cell carcinoma of the supraglottic larynx. Radiology 111:697–700, 1974.
45. Marks JE et al.: Carcinoma of the supraglottic larynx. Am J Roentgenol 132:255–260, 1979.
46. Marks JE, Sessions DG: Radiation therapy of carcinoma of the larynx. *In* Brady LW, Perez CA (eds): Basis and Clinical Practice of Radiation Oncology. In preparation.
47. Herring DF: The consequences of dose response curves for tumor control and normal tissue injury on the precision necessary in patient management. Laryngoscope 85:1112–1118, 1975.
48. Shukovsky LJ: Dose, time, volume relationship in squamous cell carcinoma of the supraglottic larynx. Am J Roentgenol 108:17–19, 1970.
49. Wang CC: Megavoltage radiation therapy for supraglottic carcinoma: Results of treatment. Radiology 109:183–186, 1973.
50. Biller HF, Ogura JH: Planned preoperative irradiation for laryngeal and laryngopharyngeal carcinoma. *In* Vaeth JM (ed): Frontiers of Radiation Therapy and Oncology. Vol 5. Baltimore, University Park Press, 1970, pp 100–105.
51. Sessions DG et al.: Carcinoma of the subglottic area. Laryngoscope 85:1417–1423, 1975.
52. Lee F et al.: Radiation of the larynx after hemilaryngectomy. Laryngoscope 90:1534–1539, 1980.
53. Bauer WC et al.: The significance of positive margins in hemilaryngectomy specimens. Laryngoscope 85:1–13, 1975.
54. Gall AM et al.: Complications following surgery for cancer of the larynx and hypopharynx. Cancer 39:624–631, 1977.
55. Henk JM et al.: Radiotherapy and hyperbaric oxygen in head and neck cancer: Final report of first controlled clinical trial. Lancet 2:101–103, 1977.
56. Catterall M et al.: Second report on results of a randomized clinical trial of fast neutrons compared with chi or gamma rays in treatment of advanced tumors of head and neck. Br Med J 1:1642–1645, 1977.
57. Wasserman TH et al.: Initial clinical and pharmacologic evaluation of misonidazole (Ro-07-0582), a hypoxic cell radiosensitizer. Int J Radiat Oncol Biol Phys 5:775–786, 1979.
58. Conner WG et al.: Prospects for hyperthermia in human cancer therapy: Part II. Implications of biological and physical data for applications of hyperthermia to man. Radiology 123:497–503, 1977.
59. Perez CA et al.: Clinical applications of irradiation combined with local hyperthermia. Cancer 52:1597–1603, 1983.

26

General Principles of Chemotherapy and Immunotherapy

Frank J. Panettiere, M.D.

Chemotherapy and (perhaps) immunotherapy are, to a large extent, complementary to surgery and radiotherapy. Where the latter are primarily aimed at local control, drug therapy has a more generalized effect. Surgery and radiation therapy are like rifle bullets; drug therapy is like buckshot. To optimally use these weapons, a physician needs to have a good working knowledge of the effects of each.

This chapter will present an overview of the effects of chemotherapy, emphasizing its limitations as total body therapy and its toxicity. It will also summarize current concepts of tumor cell kinetics. Because of the current interest in tumor cell immunology and immunotherapy, their basic principles will also be reviewed. This will help give a frame of reference as to their status today. Moreover, understanding this fundamental information should help the reader participate in future developments of these rapidly progressing fields.

GENERAL PRINCIPLES OF CHEMOTHERAPY

The large variety of chemotherapy drugs available today differ greatly in structure and, to some extent, in therapeutic and toxic effects. Generally, these drugs were developed as agents to take advantage of processes that tend to be more vulnerable to attack in malignant cells than in normal cells. There is no "magic bullet." Therefore, in varying degrees, normal cells share cytocidal effects with malignant cells.[1] Actually, it is drug toxicity against normal cells that limits us in how much drug we can apply to malignant cells.

This leads to one basic principle of chemotherapy: since normal cells share toxic effects with malignant cells, the clinician should use the highest dose tolerable by the patient and his normal cells. The hope is that this dose will cause irreparable toxicity to the patient's malignant cells. If the highest tolerable dose is ineffective in causing beneficial results for the patient, then this particular drug regimen should be discontinued immediately and something else should be tried. This basic principle makes chemotherapy quite different from the drug therapy of other illnesses. When the physician uses pain killers, tranquilizers, or antimicrobials, the appropriate therapeutic approach usually begins with a small but likely-to-be-effective dose that can be increased if necessary. Choosing the lowest effective dose is appropriate in treating most patients with high blood pressure or insomnia; it is totally wrong in treating malignancies. If drug therapy of a malignancy proves (through observation of tumor growth) ineffective because of an inadequate dose, then, every time an inadequate dose is given, the tumor is allowed to grow further. By using the highest dose the patient can tolerate, the physician saves the time involved in progressively increasing the dose, which might eventually have proved ineffective in any case. If such a maximal dose causes tumor shrinkage, then the clinician might rationally follow it with smaller and less toxic doses. If that initial high dose proves ineffective, however, no time need be wasted on a nonbeneficial regimen and another can be started without delay.

Another important principle that makes chemotherapy complementary to surgery and radiotherapy is that, generally, it is total body therapy. There are important exceptions to this, such as local perfusion chemotherapy. Another exception, which pertains to most anticancer drugs, is the effect of the so-called blood-brain barrier. Although chemotherapy drugs can cause tumor regression in primary sites and elsewhere, the concentration that penetrates the blood-brain barrier may be inadequate to prevent growth of brain metastases. Too often, excellent peripheral tumor regression is seen while progressive tumor in the central nervous system is attributed to alcoholism, anxiety, or a stroke.[2] Such brain metastases will often respond quite beneficially to steroids initially and, for several months, to radiotherapy. Drugs now known to be able to cross the blood-brain barrier in therapeutic levels are the nitrosoureas (BCNU, CCNU, and methyl CCNU), procarbazine hydrochloride (Matulane) and dacarbazine (DTIC-Dome). Unfortunately, these have not been found significantly useful in treating the various forms of epidermoid carcinoma of the head and neck.[3]

Another limitation to the effect of chemotherapy as possible total body therapy is a more common problem. For a chemotherapy drug to exert its effect, it must reach the tumor cell. Poorly perfused tumors are less likely to respond to chemotherapy drugs for two important reasons. First, the drug may not diffuse far enough to reach the tumor in concentrations sufficient to be effective. Second, the impaired blood supply to the tumor impairs the removal of toxic metabolites from the tumor cell. This may suppress the tumor cell's metabolic activities. Since chemotherapeutic drugs act against cell metabolic processes, such a relatively inert tumor cell would be less susceptible to drug effect. Thus, chemotherapy is likely to be most effective when used initially, before surgery or radiotherapy has caused impairment of the tumor's vascular supply.

The general and widespread effects of chemotherapy can be looked upon as an advantage, because even occult deposits of tumor might be susceptible to the drugs. Metastases that are not within a surgical or radiotherapy field are affected; however, these widespread effects also form the major factor limiting current-day chemotherapy. Unlike surgery and radiotherapy, the full weight of the chemotherapeutic attack is not limited to the tumor area itself. Much of it is wasted in peripheral sites that do not harbor malignant cells. In these areas, unwanted effects occur, which, of course, result in toxicity, the major limiting factor.[4]

GENERAL PRINCIPLES OF TOXICITY

Chemotherapeutic drugs are most effective against rapidly metabolizing cells, whether they are malignant or normal. It is for this reason that the patient's rapidly renewing cell populations, such as those in the bone marrow, the intestinal mucosa, and the hair follicles, tend to be most sensitive to the chemotherapy drugs. On the other hand, cells that do not undergo rapid replacement, such as cells in muscles and in the brain, tend to be resistant to the effects of chemotherapy agents.

Myelosuppression. The most important toxic effect of most of these drugs is myelosuppression. If chemotherapeutic drugs cause life-threatening or fatal toxicity, it is almost invariably caused either by drug-induced granulocytopenia (leading to fatal infections) or by thrombocytopenia (leading to hemorrhage). Chemotherapeutic drugs neither affect the mature granulocyte nor the latter stages of granulocyte development in the bone marrow; only the more immature granulocyte percursors are susceptible. The more mature cells can, therefore, live out a normal life span. For this reason, the fall of the circulating white blood count is delayed after the administration of chemotherapeutic drugs. For some drugs, the low point in the blood count may occur a week or two after the chemotherapy drug is administered. For other drugs, no fall in blood counts may be observed for a month or more. The review of Creaven and Mihich gives specific data as to the timing of these and other toxic effects of chemotherapy.[5]

Early recognition and treatment of granulocytopenia are very important; however, there is a basic problem in such recognition. Normally, the physician depends upon granulocytes to aid in the detection of infection. Examples abound: an elevated white blood count helps us diagnose appendicitis; white blood cells in the urine indicate that a patient has a urinary tract infection; râles, consolidation, and radiographic shadows in the lung (all of which result from a leukocyte exudation) help us to recognize pneumonia. Therefore, the physician giving chemotherapy to patients must be ever aware that, if a patient is markedly granulocytopenic, the usual clinical signs of infection cannot be entirely depended upon. The physician must obtain a white blood count whenever an infection is remotely suspected.

The seriousness of granulocytopenia and infection is further compounded by the setting in which such infections may occur. Chemotherapeutic drugs may often, as an additional toxic effect, cause disruption of the gastrointestinal mucosa, resulting in portals for the entrance of microorganisms. Moreover, patients with tumors of the head and neck often have chronic infections, which are kept under control by the host's normal resistance. The infections may rapidly become uncontrolled if granulocytopenia is induced.

A significant infectious process associated with marked granulocytopenia can be a medical emergency, and death can occur within 24 hours unless aggressive therapy is undertaken. Generally, combinations of maximal dose antibiotics are utilized. More recently, some centers have been testing utilization of leukocyte transfusions for this purpose. This requires the use of blood cell separators to obtain adequate numbers of granulocytes from blood donors. This technology is not yet widely available. Moreover, it is not yet proven that this offers any definite advantage over intensive antibiotic therapy alone.

It is generally recognized that platelet transfusions are the appropriate mode of therapy for drug-induced thrombocytopenia. Platelet transfusion therapy is not generally required for those who have platelet counts above 20,000. Today a controversy still remains as to the precise indications for platelet transfusion in those with drug-induced thrombocytopenia. Reasonable guidelines might be that platelet transfusion is indicated (1) when there is active bleeding associated with thrombocytopenia but with normal quantities of other clotting factors, (2) when the platelet count is falling very rapidly, although it has not yet reached dangerous levels, or (3) when the platelet count falls below 20,000.

Gastrointestinal Toxicity. Drug-induced gastrointestinal toxicity usually takes the form of nausea and vomiting. Although claims are made for various types of antiemetic therapy, there is no overwhelming evidence of superiority of any particular regimen, except perhaps for metoclopramide hydrochloride (Reglan) at repeated 2 mg/kg doses.[6] Otherwise, the antiemetic routinely used by a physician for other indications would be an appropriate alternative for chemotherapy-induced vomiting. There are two important clinical considerations worthy of emphasis. First, the patient who has a high likelihood of vomiting after a chemotherapy dose should be advised to eat or drink something before the chemotherapy drug is given. The patient should be advised that vomiting something is far more comfortable than the so-called "dry heaves." The second important consideration is the possibility of dehydration. If vomiting is severe, fluid loss may be significant. This can be a special problem in patients whose cancer of the head and neck, or its previous therapy, has already rendered the fluid intake marginal.

Nephrotoxicity. Dehydration can also increase the toxicity of nephrotoxic drugs, especially those that are primarily excreted by the kidneys. Decreased total body fluid decreases urine output and slows such drug excretion. This can result in prolongation of drug effect and add an unexpectedly increased risk of severe toxicity.

CELL CYCLE KINETICS

An appreciation of cell cycle kinetics is important in the understanding of the effects of chemotherapy drugs and is even more important in designing programs utilizing multiple drugs with proper timing. The subjct has been reviewed by Valeriote and Edelstein.[7]

Both normal cells and tumor cells may be either *clonogenic* or *nonclonogenic*. The clonogenic cell is able to divide and form daughter cells, while the nonclonogenic cell does not have this property. An example of a clonogenic cell is the myeloblast (normally found in the bone marrow), which has the characteristic

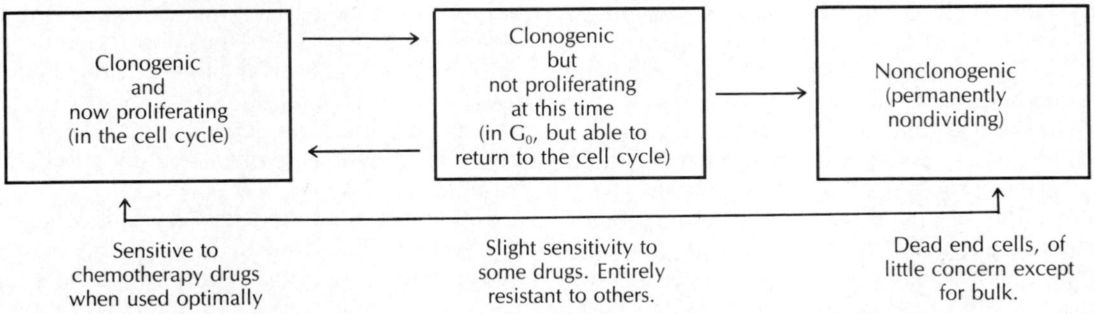

Figure 26–1. The three cell compartments in a tumor. A reasonable strategy is to kill cells in the clonogenic and now proliferating compartment and to recruit new cells into the vulnerable compartment from the previously nonproliferating clonogenic cells. A future therapeutic approach would be to drive tumor cells to mature in the dead end nonclonogenic compartment.

ability to reproduce itself as well as to produce families of more mature granulocytes. In the tumor, as in the normal cell, there are some cells that are clonogenic and others that are nonclonogenic or "dead-end cells." The clonogenic cells are cells that proliferate and replace themselves, causing enlargement of the tumor mass.

Clonogenic cells themselves can be reasonably separated into two categories: (1) those that are currently actively proliferating and (2) those that, although able to do so, are not proliferating at the particular time. The proliferating clonogenic cells are those primarily affected by chemotherapeutic drugs[8] (Fig. 26–1).

All proliferating cells, normal and neoplastic, go through a similar cycle. Classically, the cell cycle has four phases (Fig. 26–2). Just after a new cell is created by mitosis, it enters the G_1 (gap) phase. The G_1 phase of the cell cycle varies most in duration, lasting anywhere from hours to weeks. After the completion of G_1, a period of active DNA synthesis occurs to prepare for cell replication. This synthesis phase is known as the S phase. After the S phase is

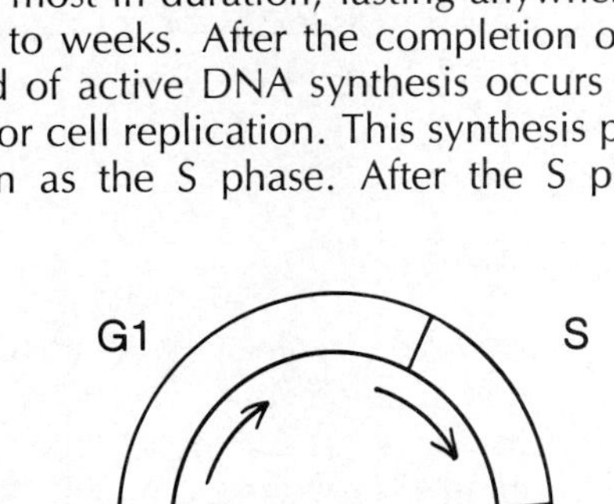

Figure 26–2. The cell cycle. Mitosis of the M phase produces two daughter cells, each of which should progress through its own cell cycle.

completed, there is another gap phase known as G_2. The G_2 phase terminates at mitosis (the M phase) when the cell, which had synthesized enough DNA for two cells during the preceding S phase, now divides into two separate daughter cells. The cell that is not currently active in its metabolic cycle is said to be in the G_0 (or G zero) phase. It is uncertain whether or not G_0 is indeed a very long G_1 phase.

An example of a normal situation would be shown by the cells in the normal undisturbed skin. Many of these cells are resting in G_0; however, if the skin is injured, the adjacent cells will soon leave the G_0 phase and enter the cell cycle, repeatedly dividing until the previously destroyed cells have been replaced. A new steady state is then achieved, with the majority of the cells again resting in G_0.

Understanding the cell cycle helps in understanding the actions of various classes of anticancer drugs. It also gives us the opportunity to utilize them in a rational fashion. Some anticancer drugs have been designated cycle *phase nonspecific*. That is, they are equally effective at any phase of the cell cycle. Such drugs include alkylating agents such as nitrogen mustard; they attack vital processes in the cell, whether or not it is metabolically active at the time. If the cell can repair the damage caused by a cycle phase nonspecific drug before the cell needs the particular metabolic function that has been damaged, the cell can recover from potentially lethal damage.

The second type of anticancer drugs have been designated cycle *phase specific*. These drugs are effective only during certain phases of the cell cycle.[9] One example, methotrexate, interferes with folic acid metabolism, which is vital during DNA synthesis. Therefore, methotrexate can lethally damage a cell if enough of the active drug gets into susceptible portions of the cell during its S phase. At other times in the cell cycle, methotrexate has no toxic effect at all. Another important example is vincristine sulfate (Oncovin), which attacks the mitotic spindle. If vincristine is present in the cell when mitosis is being attempted, its effect against the mitotic spindle prevents mitosis and the cell dies. Vincristine does not have any effect at any other time during the cell cycle. Normally, the M phase, when vincristine is active, lasts only one hour. This is often a very small proportion of the time for the total cell cycle, which may be many hours or days.

Phase specific drugs are often limited in effectiveness if given in single doses. Unless the drug persists for a long time in the patient, only a small proportion of the cells might be affected by its action. For this reason, frequent doses, or sometimes continuous infusions, may reasonably be employed. The problem is that normal cells go through the same cell cycle; therefore, maneuvers to prolong the exposure of malignant cells to such drugs can also prolong the exposure of normal cells to the same drugs and increase risk to the normal cells.

Not only do phase specific drugs affect cells in specific phases of the cell cycle, but they also tend to block cell progression through one or more portions of the cycle. Much of the information concerning this comes from the work of Barranco et al., who showed the potentially beneficial effects of blocking cells at a specific point in the cycle.[10] For this purpose, a drug is utilized to prevent cells from passing a certain single point in the cell cycle. As a result, cells are progressively accumulated before the block. An important example is a low dose of bleomycin sulfate (Blenoxane), which in vivo reversibly blocks cells at the S and G_2 boundary. If low doses of bleomycin are maintained in contact with cells, those cells located in other stages of the cell cycle are essentially unaffected; thus, they progress through the cell cycle until they reach the S and G_2 boundary, where they are blocked from further progression through the cell cycle. If this continues for a long enough period of time, then a high proportion of cells will be blocked at the S and G_2 boundary. As long as only low doses of bleomycin are utilized, the block is a reversible one. After the bleomycin is discontinued, the cells that had been blocked at the S and G_2 boundary continue around the cell cycle as a tight group or wave of cells relatively synchronized in phase. The potential advantage of this maneuver is that there will be a much higher proportion of cells at each specific phase of the cell cycle than would be the situation with the normal random distribution of cells passing through the cell cycle (Fig. 26–3).

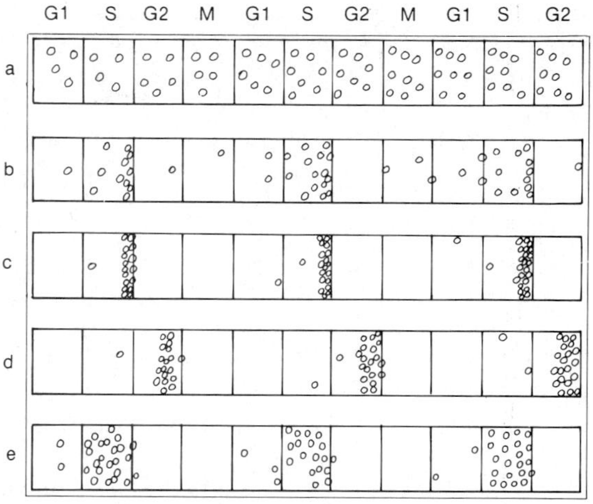

Figure 26–3. The effect of synchrony block. This cell cycle is displayed linearly instead of in a circle. *a,* The normal situation where cells randomly are in different phases of the cell cycle. *b,* The situation soon after a drug (such as bleomycin) has been introduced to prevent cells from progressing through the cycle, blocking them at the boundary between S and G_2. Note how cells before the block pile up at the boundary. This progressively depletes cells in the other phases of the cell cycle. *c,* After more time has passed, essentially all cells have progressed in the cycle until stopped at the boundary between S and G_2. *d,* The blocking agent has been discontinued. A partially synchronized wave of cells begins its progression through the cell cycle. *e,* The partially synchronized wave of cells has reached the S phase. If an S-phase drug, such as methrotrexate, is given at this time, a high proportion of cells would be susceptible to its toxic effects.

If the physician can estimate when this enriched population of cells will reach the S phase of the cell cycle, then a higher than usual proportion of cells would be susceptible to the toxic effects of an S phase specific drug administered at that time. Certainly, normal cells would also be migrating through their cell cycles after their release from the synchrony block. But if the kinetics of the normal cell and the tumor cell are significantly different, they will have different rates of progression through the cell cycle. In such a case, the wave of normal cells would not be in the susceptible phase of the cycle at the same time as the malignant cells are. Ideally, a cell cycle specific drug may be given at a time when tumor cells are much more affected than normal cells are.

In addition to knowing which drug is active at which phase of the cell cycle, of critical importance is knowledge of the cell cycle parameters. We need to know them both for normal cells and for the specific human malignancy under treatment. To determine such parameters of malignancies growing in humans requires repeated biopsies. Although many human tumor types are not often readily accessible to repeated biopsies, tumors of the head and neck region frequently are accessible. Data such as those of Straus and Moran, as well as those of Terz et al., have been quite useful in attempts to develop clinically useful protocols capitalizing upon these cell cycle kinetic principles.[11, 12]

Klein and Lennartz showed the usefulness of these theories in animals and in humans with malignancies.[13] Costanzi and his associates made use of these principles in the therapy of epidermoid carcinomas of the head and neck region.[14] Their regimen involved a continuous infusion of bleomycin to synchronize cells. Then, after a specific interval calculated according to available data on head and neck tumor progression, one of the S phase specific drugs (methotrexate or hydroxyurea) was given. Although the therapeutic effect of their regimen was not strikingly better than the effect when methotrexate is used without such a synchronizing procedure, there was a definite advantage to the patient in that there was less toxicity. It would appear that because the synchronized wave of normal cells was away from the S phase when the cycle specific drug was given, a relatively small proportion of normal cells was susceptible to the toxic effects of methotrexate or hydroxyurea. This would explain why the drugs were less toxic than they are when used against a random population of cells in all phases of the cycle.

Another important kinetic concept to understand is recruitment. As mentioned above, a clonogenic cell may be one of two varieties, proliferating or nonproliferating. Only the actively proliferating cells are susceptible to the metabolic attack of anticancer drugs that are cell cycle specific; however, if an initial dose of therapy kills a large fraction of proliferating cells, the death of such cells will result in the recruitment of nonproliferating cells into the proliferating cell cycle. When cells come into the cell cycle to replace the drug-killed cells, they too become susceptible to the attack of the cell cycle specific agent. If we learn how to exploit this phenomenon of recruitment appropriately, with the proper timing of drug therapy, we should be able to progressively destroy the cells of a tumor, even though only a very small fraction was initially susceptible to the chemotherapeutic attack.

A clinical problem is that as a disease progresses, proportionately more and more cells go into G_0 and leave the active cell cycle. The normal situation is that initially, when a tumor is microscopic, essentially all of the cells are in the cell cycle. Soon, however, the cells begin outgrowing their own blood supply. This results in an ever-increasing proportion of cells that are not actively proliferating because of impaired nutrition and buildup of toxic metabolites in their environment. As mentioned previously, when surgery or radiotherapy further impairs the blood supply to the tumor, an even higher proportion of cells leave the cell cycle. Therefore, the large tumor and the tumor that recurs following surgery or radiotherapy have a small proportion of cells in the cell cycle where they are sensitive to such drugs.

The problem is further aggravated by nutritional factors. Typically, the patient with an advanced head and neck cancer is one who, even prior to development of cancer, was in poor nutritional state resulting from an inadequate diet. This situation is then markedly aggravated by the location of the primary tumor around the entrance into the alimentary tract and also by the effects of previous surgery or radiotherapy. Although there are no data to prove this, it is expected that impaired nutrition would even further decrease the proportion of cells in the susceptible phases of the cell cycle. In addition, the poor nutritional state will serve to greatly increase the risk of toxicity, because impaired nutrition results in impaired resistance to the toxic effects of therapy. Performance status is a general assessment of the patient's overall physical capacity. It ranges from the patient whose tumor has caused no impairment

Table 26–1. PERFORMANCE STATUS*

Patient Status	Karnofsky Grade
Fully active. Able to do all predisease activities	90–100
Can do light sedentary work but restricted in strenuous physical activities	70–80
Ambulatory, out of bed more than 30% of waking hours. Cannot accomplish gainful employment	50–60
Requires bed and chair more than 50% of waking hours. Capable of limited self-care	30–40
Totally bed or chair confined. Incapable of any self-care	10–20
Dead	

*As originally devised by Karnofsky, Performance Status was divided into eleven catagories (0% to 100%). Today, most physicians feel this provides more categories than are clinically useful, and many use only three catagories: Karnofsky 70–100, Karnofsky 30–60, and Karnofsky less than 30. The above is a compromise frequently in use.

at all, to one who has mild or moderate impairment, to one who is moribund or dead (Table 26–1). In every chemotherapy program in which performance status was assessed, the patient's pretreatment performance status was one of the most important factors, if not the single most important factor, in predicting whether or not he would respond favorably to therapy.

IMMUNE FACTORS AND IMMUNOTHERAPY

There is no question today that immune factors have a significant impact on morbidity and mortality in cancer patients, and that immunotherapy is effective in managing some tumors in animals. Although there have been reports suggesting benefits from immunotherapy in human breast cancer and lung cancer, at this time there is no incontrovertible evidence that immunotherapy is definitely beneficial for any patient, including the patient with epidermoid tumors of the head and neck. Nevertheless, because immunotherapy may, in the future, prove to be a beneficial treatment modality, a brief discussion of the situation is warranted here.

There is a good theoretic basis for the difficulty in proving the effectiveness of immune stimulation in management of the typical cancer patient. Animal data clearly indicate that immune stimulation is effective only if the malignant cells are too few to be detected clinically. Thus, by the time a patient is seen with gross tumor, the tumor is unlikely to respond to immune stimulation. Therefore, immune factors seem to be most useful in treatment when a tumor is a subclinical size, either prior to its clinical appearance or after the therapeutic elimination of all grossly visible disease.

The relationship between immune factors and tumor growth is suggested by recipients of renal transplants. These patients, who are clinically immunosuppressed, show a very high rate of cancer development. Additionally, patients with gross cancer of various types have evidence of immune impairment as manifested by multiple tests.

As mentioned previously, immunotherapy is theoretically most effective against very small, early cancers. There is no clinical setting in which immune stimulation would be attempted for the patient who does not yet have any gross evidence of disease. One situation in which immunotherapy could reasonably be instituted is immediately after attempted definitive surgery for a tumor with a very high probability of recurrence. Whatever residual tumor might then be left behind should be of a small enough volume to be affected by immune stimulation. Therefore, a most rational use of immunotherapy would be a situation in which, even though all known disease has been resected, there is a high probability of recurrence without further therapy.

As indicated above, based on current knowledge, patients with gross advanced disease are not likely to be helped by immunotherapy. The observation of Suen et al.[15] that 100 patients with gross head and neck epidermoid tumors were not benefited by bacille Calmette-Guérin (BCG) immunotherapy is one example that confirms this expectation; however, if the nutritional status of patients with gross tumors can be improved, this alone may help them improve their own immunologic responsiveness. Such an improvement in immunologic reactivity may, or may not, be beneficial against the tumor itself. In any case, it should help to improve the patient's resistance against secondary infections.

Most of the immunotherapy agents that have been tried are nonspecific, broad spectrum stimulants of immune reactivity. These include BCG, the vaccine that is used to stimulate immunity against tuberculosis. BCG has been shown to have a broad spectrum effect and to stimulate immunity, not only against tuberculosis but also against a wide variety of other substances. Most commonly, BCG is given by means of skin scarification with the living organism. The technique of administering BCG immunization is described in Table 26–2.

BCG (administered in this manner) poses a potential problem because it contains living microorganisms that might cause infection. To try to prevent this problem, nonviable fractions of BCG have been developed that seem to retain immune-stimulating properties. Most commonly used has been the methanol extractible residue of BCG known as MER. MER, because it is not the whole microorganism, cannot cause infection; however, this agent is very toxic to the area into which it is injected and frequently causes multiple, painful skin ulcerations. *Corynebacterium parvum* is another bacterium used as an immune stimulant; its major toxic side effects are fever and chills. Like BCG, its place in human immunotherapy, if any, is not established. Another nonspecific

Table 26–2. BCG IMMUNIZATION BY SCARIFICATION

1. The site of scarification is rotated among the four limbs
2. The area is cleansed with soap and water or acetone and shaved if necessary
3. A 2 inch (5 cm) square is drawn
4. Utilizing the cutting edge of an 18-gauge needle at the bevel (not the needle point), the skin is held taut. Within the square, ten scratches across and ten scratches down are made. (These 20 scratches will total about a meter in length)
5. Only slight capillary oozing, and not free bleeding, from each scratch is desired.
6. The contents of a vial of BCG is dropped into the square
7. The skin is held taut and the area is massaged with the flat part of the needle to mix together BCG and blood
8. A cool flow of air is directed to the area until the blood and BCG have thickened. (A blow dryer may be used without heat as heat destroys BCG)
9. The area is covered by an inverted Petri dish, which is taped in place securely but not tightly
10. The area is kept covered and dry for 48 hours

immune stimulant is levamisole hydrochloride, an oral anthelmintic that has been shown to improve immune responsiveness in a nonspecific way. The data concerning its usefulness as an immune stimulant are contradictory.

In addition to these nonspecific, broad spectrum immunostimulatory agents, many researchers are attempting to develop tumor cell vaccines that would specifically immunize a patient against his particular problem. As yet, tumor cell vaccines have not proved effective in head and neck tumors or in other human malignancies.

Finally, a note of caution should be added. Not only can immunotherapy be ineffective and toxic but, at least in animals, it may enhance tumor growth.[16] Although this has never been proved in humans, the possibility of such harm must be realized.

References

1. Chabner BA et al.: Clinical pharmacology of anticancer drugs. Semin Oncol 4:165–191, June 1977.
2. Fewer D et al.: The chemotherapy of brain tumors: Clinical experience with carmustine (BCNU) and vincristine. JAMA 222:549–552, 1972.
3. Shapiro WR: Malignant brain tumor chemotherapy: Part II. Clinical studies. Clin Bull 3:90–93, 1973.
4. Friedman MA, Carter SB: Serious toxicities associated with chemotherapy. Semin Oncol 5:193–202, June 1978.
5. Creaven PJ, Mihich E: The clinical toxicity of anticancer drugs and its prediction. Semin Oncol 4:147–163, June 1977.
6. Gralla RJ et al.: Antiemetic efficacy of high-dose metoclopramide: Randomized trials with placebo and prochloroperazine in patients with chemotherapy-induced nausea and vomiting. N Engl J Med 305:905–909, 1981.
7. Valeriote FA, Edelstein MB: The role of cell kinetics in cancer chemotherapy. Semin Oncol 4:217–226, June 1977.
8. DeVita VT: Cell kinetics and the chemotherapy of cancer. Cancer Chemother Rep 2(3):23–33, 1971.
9. Bhuyan BK et al.: Cell cycle phase specificity of antitumor agents. Cancer Res 32:398–407, 1972.
10. Barranco SC et al.: Bleomycin as a possible synchronizing agent for human tumor cells *in vivo*. Cancer Res 33:882–887, 1973.
11. Straus MJ, Moran RE: Cell cycle parameters in human solid tumors. Cancer 40:1453–1461, 1977.
12. Terz JJ et al.: Analysis of the cycling and non-cycling cell population of the human solid tumors. Cancer 40:1462–1470, 1977.
13. Klein HO, Lennartz KJ: Chemotherapy after synchronization of tumor cells. Semin Hematol 11:203–227, 1974.
14. Costanzi JJ et al.: Intravenous bleomycin infusion as a potential synchronizing agent in human disseminated malignancy: A preliminary report. Cancer 38:1503–1506, 1976.
15. Suen JY et al.: Results of BCG adjuvant immunotherapy in 100 patients with epidermoid carcinoma of the head and neck. Am J Surg 134:474–478, 1977.
16. Piessens WF et al.: Facilitation of rat mammary tumor growth by BCG. Nature 228:1210–1211, 1970.

27

Chemotherapy and Immunotherapy of Laryngeal Cancer

Frank J. Panettiere, M.D.

CHEMOTHERAPY

Epidermoid carcinomas anywhere in the head and neck region appear to have the same response to chemotherapy, regardless of site. Therefore, when discussing drug effectiveness, we can assume that drugs that have been effective against epidermoid carcinoma of other head and neck sites will be effective against laryngeal carcinoma. We would expect the typical patient receiving chemotherapy for head and neck cancer to be the least likely to respond to drug therapy. Such a patient usually has advanced disease, poor nutrition, and a large fraction of tumor cells that are metabolically inert and out of the active cell cycle. In addition, the patient usually has impaired bone marrow tolerance because of prior radiotherapy and perhaps also because of a poor nutritional state. Because of the likelihood of poor bone marrow tolerance, bleomycin sulfate (Blenoxane), a relatively nonmyelosuppressive drug, might be used. This particular drug's major toxicity is pulmonary, however, and most individuals with laryngeal cancer are heavy smokers with impaired pulmonary function. This may be further aggravated by the effects of radiotherapy to the region.

Considering all these negative factors, we find it remarkable that any drugs have proved beneficial. As their effectiveness has become better known, these agents have been used earlier in the evolution of the disease. At present, chemotherapy as a preoperative modality is being tested. Theoretically, this should prove far more effective than the usual situation in which it is used much later, in advanced disease.

Methotrexate. Historically, the first of the three major chemotherapy agents used in the management of epidermoid head and neck cancer has been methotrexate[1–4] (Table 27–1). This drug has been utilized orally, intravenously, intramuscularly, and intra-arterially. The data indicate that the intra-arterial route for methotrexate does not cause a higher response rate than the more simple routes;[5] however, it does offer a greater likelihood of complications. Obviously, those patients who in the past have been subjected to intra-arterial methotrexate have been carefully selected, favorable patients. Nevertheless, in comparison with the

Table 27–1. METHOTREXATE IN HEAD AND NECK CANCER—SYNOPSIS*

Pretherapy evaluation	Blood counts must be adequate if giving full dose Check renal function with creatinine clearance to help judge starting dose
Current regimens	40 or 50 mg IV every 4 days until toxicity, then weekly 15 mg/m^2 IM for 3 consecutive days every 3 weeks Massive doses followed by citrovorum factor (folinic acid) rescue
Toxicity	Primarily stomatitis, nausea, myelosuppression
Comments	Generally, beneficial effects do not last much more than 3 months The amount of folic acid in the normal diet does not significantly antagonize methotrexate effect, but vitamin supplements containing folic acid should be avoided Although a few enthusiasts feel that the massive dose regimens are superior, the majority feel they are not more effective despite increased monetary and toxicity costs

*This chart gives a quick overview and is not meant to replace a detailed understanding of this drug and its effects.

other routes of administration, intra-arterial methotrexate has shown no evidence of therapeutic advantage. That being the case, we could not justify utilizing methotrexate intra-arterially today.

As far as the other routes are concerned, current data indicate that intermittent methotrexate therapy is more effective and less toxic than are low daily dosages of the drug. The superiority of intermittent intravenous methotrexate was shown in 1968 by Lane and his associates.[6] More recently, intramuscular methotrexate given daily for three consecutive days and repeated every three weeks has been the most effective regimen with this drug, both in causing tumor remission and, even more importantly, in causing significant and useful prolongation of survival.[7]

A regimen utilizing very high doses of methotrexate followed by a "rescue" with its "antidote," leucovorin calcium (citrovorum factor), has been recommended.[8] The rationale for such an approach is that cells may have innate or acquired resistance to the effects of methotrexate caused by extremely high levels of methotrexate's target, the enzyme dihydrofolate reductase. Alternatively, the cells may have decreased permeability to methotrexate, which would prevent the drug from reaching the dihydrofolate reductase. The therapeutic rationale of the high-dose program is that if a massive dose of methotrexate is given, it will enter the cell by passive diffusion, without depending upon the normal transport system. Therefore, the massive amount of drug reaching the target would be adequate to overwhelm even increased amounts of the target enzyme. Citrovorum factor (folinic acid) is a substance needed in cellular metabolism that can be given to bypass the therapeutic tetrahydrofolate block caused by methotrexate. By the administration of citrovorum factor, normal cells can be "rescued" from potentially lethal toxicity much more effectively than can tumor cells.

Utilizing this technique, massive doses of methotrexate can be given. The so-called standard dose of methotrexate might be as high as 50 to 100 mg, given at intervals. When the doses are given with rescue techniques, 1000 mg, 2000 mg, or much more might be utilized. Some chemotherapists use as much as 600 mg/kg of body weight. Despite enthusiasm for high-dose methotrexate with rescue, the data do not confirm any therapeutic benefit. Capizzi and his associates have shown that the overall response rate has been in the range of 45 per cent and the median duration of the remission has been in the range of 95 days.[9]

The best regimen for utilizing methotrexate appears to be that developed at the Baylor College of Medicine and tested in a large-scale study by the Southwest Oncology Group. Methotrexate is given intramuscularly at a dose of 15 mg/m^2 daily for three days, every three weeks.[7] With this regimen, survival is markedly improved as compared with any of the other methods of using methotrexate. Moreover, it is more convenient and less expensive than the high-dose methotrexate programs.

Because methotrexate is excreted by the kidneys and standard doses produce levels that are just subtoxic to the kidney, an accurate pretreatment renal function test is necessary.[10] We should not rely upon the standard serum creatinine level alone because these patients characteristically have very little in the way of muscle mass as a result of long-term nutritional impairment. Therefore, there is little creatinine from muscle breakdown for the kidneys to excrete; thus the serum creatinine is not an adequate test of renal function in this situation. For this reason, a creatinine clearance to assess what proportion of the endogenous creatinine load is excreted is mandatory for safe utilization of methotrexate. Anyone who has treated numerous patients with epidermoid tumors of the head and neck region has seen that a serum creatinine can be normal at a time when creatinine clearance is found to be markedly decreased. These are the patients who are likely to develop severe and unexpected toxicity, which may be life-threatening or even fatal.

The major toxic effects of methotrexate are hematopoietic suppression and mucositis. Nausea and vomiting are less common but not rare. Rarely, methotrexate can cause pulmonary toxicity[11] and hepatic toxicity.[12] Since most patients treated with methotrexate for head and neck malignancies have been chronic alcohol abusers, and since those treated for other malignancies have had a high risk for liver metastases, methotrexate's propensity toward hepatic toxicity was not appreciated until it was used for patients who did not have such reasons to explain liver toxicity (mainly those treated for psoriasis).[12]

In the past, criteria for chemotherapeutic response were much looser than they are today. Minimal shrinkage of tumor size was formerly considered a response. Yet in many cases this may have represented only decreased edema or infection around the tumor. The more modern criteria require that a tumor be shrunk to half its original size or less and that such shrinkage must last for at least 30 days before a response is said to have occurred. By the older criteria (used in most of the articles in the literature pertaining to methotrexate), the response rate to this drug has been said to be 60 per cent. By the more recent and stricter criteria, the response rate to methotrexate is in the range of 40 per cent with a median response duration of approximately three months.

Table 27–2. BLEOMYCIN IN HEAD AND NECK CANCER—SYNOPSIS*

Pretherapy evaluation	Clinical, radiographic, and laboratory evaluations of pulmonary functional capacity are needed to estimate the total lifetime amount of drug that might be given with reasonable expectation of safety
Current regimens	By itself, as an antitumor agent: 10–20 units/m² IM or IV, once or twice a week In combinations, as a synchronizing agent: given by continuous infusion (see text)
Toxicity	Major toxicity is pulmonary, which may be fatal Causes allergic reactions and fever Almost completely nonmyelosuppressive
Comments	Therapeutic benefits are rather short-lived The chance for pulmonary toxicity greatly increases if a lifetime dose exceeding 400 units is given. Total lifetime doses as low as 50 units may cause pulmonary toxicity

*This chart gives a quick overview and is not meant to replace a detailed understanding of this drug and its effects.

Bleomycin Sulfate. Bleomycin was the second of the three major drugs to be widely used for head and neck cancer (Table 27–2). This drug was first developed in Japan in 1965; as early as 1969, there were reports in the Japanese literature attesting to its effectiveness in the management of head and neck tumors.[13] Soon the drug was being used all over the world. For example, Haas and his associates in the Southwest Oncology Group reported that 12 of 64 patients had objective responses, by strict criteria, when the drug was administered in twice weekly doses of 10 mg/m², either intravenously or intramuscularly.[14] The median duration of response was two months, with a range of one month through seven months. Reed, in Australia, treated 59 patients with tumors of the head and neck region with bleomycin. By strict criteria, nine of the 59 had true objective responses.[15] In the United States, Bristol Laboratories accumulated all of the American data on the drug prior to its becoming commercially available. The cumulative response data on this drug, used by itself in the management of tumors of the head and neck region, indicated that ten of 298 patients (3 per cent) had complete disappearance of the tumor. Using the strict criteria for response (at least 50 per cent shrinkage for 30 days), the total response rate was 18 per cent. Although current data do not suggest any definite superiority of intravenous bleomycin over intramuscular bleomycin, the intravenous route is generally considered preferable because any acute reaction to the drug is more likely to occur while a physician is present and a needle is in the patient's vein.

Unlike most anticancer drugs, bone marrow suppression from bleomycin is relatively minor. This drug can cause fever (which may occur three to four hours after drug administration), skin redness and thickening, and occasionally mucositis; however, the most serious effect of the drug occurs in the lung, where an interstitial pneumonitis may develop.[16, 17]

As far as the utilization of bleomycin in the management of head and neck cancers is concerned, by itself it is not very useful.[3] Although it can cause tumor regressions, such regressions are short-lived. Moreover, prolonged therapy with bleomycin markedly increases the risk of pulmonary toxicity, a special problem in this population. The population normally consists of heavy smokers who may already have had pulmonary function further compromised by radiotherapy to the area. This drug can be advantageously used (1) in the patient whose marrow cannot tolerate standard myelosuppressive drugs, (2) as a synchronizing agent (as noted previously),[18] and (3) in drug combinations. The major rationale for its use in combinations is often that its major toxicity, which is pulmonary, does not overlap with the primarily myelosuppressive toxicity of most other anticancer drugs. For this reason, bleomycin has been used often in combinations with other standard chemotherapeutic agents to add to their effectiveness.

In addition, because of its peculiar pharmacologic activities, bleomycin might be especially useful in combination with radiotherapy. Bleomycin and radiotherapy both cause single-strand scission of DNA.[19] In vitro, bleomycin prevents DNA strands that have been disrupted by radiotherapy from repairing. The problem is that bleomycin's effect in inhibiting repair of DNA might increase the toxic effects against normal cells as well.

***Cis*-Platinum (Cisplatin).** The most recently developed chemotherapeutic agent in the management of head and neck cancer appears to be the most effective agent to date. It is an inorganic platinum-containing compound known by several names: *cis*-diaminedichloride platinum II, *cis*-platinum, CACP, or cisplatin (Platinol) (Table 27–3).[20] This drug has been used in three significantly different dose regimens. The first clinically important one of these was a regimen in which the dose was divided over five days. The purpose of dividing the dose is to prevent the dose-limiting renal toxicity by offering the kidneys only a fraction of the dose at any given time. Typically, a dose of 15 to 20 mg/m^2 daily for five days has been employed.

A second regimen was developed by oncologists at Memorial–Sloan Kettering Hospital in New York. They utilized a different technique to try to prevent the drug's dose-limiting renal toxicity. Their regimen involved hospitalization for overnight intravenous hydration. The next morning, immediately before the single dose of cisplatin was administered, osmotic diuresis with mannitol, given by intravenous bolus, was accomplished. Following this, a single dose of 3 to 3.5 mg/kg of cisplatin was administered intravenously. For the next 24 hours, continued intravenous hydration was accomplished, with replacement of all fluids lost through urination and emesis, and with continuation of mannitol administration. In order to monitor renal output accurately, Foley catheterization was used and continued throughout this regimen. Hayes et al. reported that 14 of 18 patients with previously untreated epidermoid tumors of the head and neck region developed complete regression of their tumors.[21] The main disadvantage of their particular regimen is that it is quite complicated, requiring hospitalization, Foley catheterization, and continuous intravenous hydration. The regimen provides an increased dose compared to the standard program of daily doses for five days. It offers an additional advantage in that, since the typical patient treated with this drug vomits with each dose, the patient vomits on only one day rather than five per course.

Because we felt that the inpatient high-dose program with mannitol diuresis was unnecessarily complicated, inconvenient, and expensive, we developed an outpatient regimen whereby the drug dose is divided into two fractions, given one week apart.[22] In accordance with this outpatient regimen, doses of 50 mg/m^2 given twice, one week apart, and re-

Table 27–3. *CIS*-PLATINUM IN HEAD AND NECK CANCER—SYNOPSIS*

Pretherapy evaluation	A careful testing of renal function, an in-depth history as to the possibility of antecedent renal disease, and radiographic studies to document the presence of two fully functioning unobstructed kidneys are mandatory
Current regimens	Inpatient, with hydration and mannitol: 3 mg/kg monthly Outpatient, 50 mg/m^2, twice one week apart, monthly
Toxicity	Renal failure, which may be fatal Auditory toxicity, with tinnitus and high frequency loss Nausea and vomiting may be severe Rare neuropathy Minimal myelosuppression
Comments	Probably the most effective single drug against these tumors today To prevent high concentrations in the nephron, adequate hydration should be assured before each dose because drug-induced vomiting can rapidly decrease total body water with resultant impaired renal blood flow and, therefore, increased risk of nephrotoxicity

*This chart gives a quick overview and is not meant to replace a detailed understanding of this drug and its effects.

peated every four weeks proved to be both tolerable and effective. The certainty of effectiveness of this particular regimen is emphasized by the fact that it was tested not in just a few patients in a single institution but rather in some 90 patients from 22 different Southwest Oncology Group member institutions. According to strict modern criteria, the objective response rate is 27 per cent. This is especially impressive when we realize that all patients treated in accordance with this two-dose cisplatin program had previously received chemotherapy, at least with methotrexate. The median patient had received a total of three prior chemotherapy drugs. Several had received six different drugs before being offered cisplatin. All patients also had received extensive surgery and radiotherapy prior to the utilization of cisplatin. Because of this remarkable activity in heavily pretreated patients, the regimen is currently being tested in patients who have not been exposed to previous chemotherapy and even in those who have not yet had definitive surgery or radiotherapy.

Cisplatin has a number of serious toxic effects.[23] About 80 per cent of patients treated with it have vomiting, which may be severe. Metoclopramide hydrochloride (Reglan) at 2 mg/kg doses starting just before the cisplatin is given and repeated at two-hour intervals for a total of five doses can decrease the incidence of vomiting to approximately 30 per cent to 40 per cent of patients.[24] Cisplatin does offer some chance for myelosuppression, but this is much milder than with other standard chemotherapy drugs. The drug's most significant toxic effect is upon the urinary tract.[24a] It can cause severe renal dysfunction, which may be fatal. Renal toxicity is much more likely in patients who have had previous renal impairment, which clinically may have completely resolved. Those with obstructed urinary tracts or with a history of renal damage, even if clinically completely recovered, are at relatively great risk for serious renal toxicity.[25] The other distressing toxic effect of cisplatin is tinnitus and high frequency hearing loss.[26]

Most of us who utilize the platinum compound today feel that it will prove to be the most effective single agent we have in the management of epidermoid tumors of the head and neck region. It is unknown today which, if any, of the three current regimens utilizing cisplatin will become the preferable one. Each of the three programs described above has a large number of adherents. Various centers are now testing the regimen of giving the drug by continuous infusion for 24 consecutive hours, or longer.

Other Drugs. In addition to these three major drugs, several other drugs have been demonstrated to have minor degrees of effectiveness in the management of epidermoid carcinomas of the head and neck. These include (1) 5-fluorouracil (5-FU), which has only a very modest effect, (2) hydroxyurea (Hydrea), used in combination with radiotherapy to potentiate its effects,[27, 28] and (3) mitomycin C (Mutamycin) and its methyl analogue, porfiromycin, which, although effective, do offer prolonged bone marrow toxicity.[29]

Combination Therapy. Now that we have several different drugs that are effective individually in the management of head and neck cancer, it is reasonable to consider the place of combinations of drugs.[30] In fact, drugs may be used not only in combination with each other, but also in combination with other modalities such as surgery or radiotherapy. The most likely candidate for combination therapy would be bleomycin, used with one of the other drugs, because bleomycin's main toxicity, which is pulmonary, does not overlap the primarily hematopoietic or renal toxicity of the other drugs. The specific utilization of bleomycin as a synchronizing agent has already been discussed.[18]

The two primary drugs used in the management of head and neck cancer are methotrexate and cisplatin. A combination of these two drugs seems desirable, but there are problems with this. Cisplatin is a cell cycle nonspecific drug, which exerts its lethal effects on cells anywhere in the cell cycle. Theoretically, after cisplatin has exerted its effects, an enriched population of cells would be recruited into the cell cycle and, thereby, would become susceptible to the effects of an S phase drug such as methotrexate; however, cisplatin causes renal toxicity and this effect is often occult and unexpected. This causes a serious risk; the dose of methotrexate should be at the limit of tolerability, and methotrexate is excreted by the kidneys. Therefore, even a mild impairment of renal function might cause severe, and potentially lethal, toxicity. Because platinum-induced renal impairment is often unexpected, it would be quite difficult to develop a safe way to utilize these two drugs in the theoretically appropriate sequence.

Chemotherapy agents can also be used in combination with radiotherapy. We have previously mentioned that bleomycin seems to be synergistic with radiotherapy in that it inhibits the repair of radiation-induced cell damage.[19]

We also mentioned hydroxyurea as an adjuvant to radiotherapy.[27, 28] As Lustig and his associates have demonstrated, methotrexate (especially when given by the oral route prior to radiation therapy) results in a lower rate of distant metastases as well as in a statistically significant improvement in survival rate.[31] An encouraging combination approach developed by the Memorial–Sloan Kettering Cancer Institute for the initial treatment of their patients involves using high doses of cisplatin followed by an infusion of bleomycin and radiotherapy.[32] It is interesting, but not surprising, that this combination approach is far more effective as part of the initial therapy of tumors, and much less effective when used as a secondary salvage approach.

Summary of Uses of Chemotherapy. A summary of the present and anticipated functions of chemotherapy in cancer of the head and neck includes the following six clinical situations:

1. The traditional use of systemic chemotherapy in the treatment of advanced disease.

2. The use of chemotherapy as a postoperative adjuvant in treating whatever microscopic residual tumor might be present after the bulk of the tumor cell has been removed. Under these circumstances, a significant number of cells should be recruited into the cell cycle and will become susceptible to the effects of chemotherapy.

3. Chemotherapy may be used preoperatively. Classically, the major problem with chemotherapy in head and neck tumors has been the relative brevity of response duration. The response, however brief, could conceivably be utilized to achieve a more complete surgical resection. In theory, if chemotherapy is used before surgical disruption of the vascular supply, an increased drug concentration is likely to reach the cell and a greater degree of effectiveness can be expected. The effectiveness of preoperative chemotherapy is being evaluated in a multiple-institution study sponsored by the National Cancer Institute.

4. Chemotherapy may be used in combination with radiotherapy. The utilization of such drugs as bleomycin, hydroxyurea, and methotrexate in this setting has been discussed earlier in this chapter.

5. The use of chemotherapy as an adjuvant following radiotherapy is another reasonable alternative. Radiotherapy acts as a cycle nonspecific agent. Therefore, it should cause recruitment of still viable cells into the cell cycle, where they can subsequently be exposed to the lethal effects of chemotherapy drugs. This high proportion of cells in the active cell cycle should be a transient condition. It again diminishes as tumor regrowth causes greater proportions of cells to enter the G_0 phase, where they are least susceptible to the effects of chemotherapy drugs. It is for this reason that chemotherapy given soon after radiotherapy is more likely to be advantageous than the traditional situation of waiting for gross tumors to develop. Nevertheless, timing can be important because most chemotherapy drugs are myelosuppressive and may compound the immediate bone marrow toxicity of the radiotherapy.

6. Additional combined modality therapy is probably the wave of the future. As more and more chemotherapy regimens are developed and demonstrated to be effective, increased use of chemotherapy should occur. Combining modalities could conceivably lead to higher survival rates with less radical surgery or radiotherapy. At this writing, however, this is only a dream.

IMMUNOTHERAPY

Immune factors and human cancer were discussed in the previous chapter in this volume. Patients with any form of cancer are found to have impaired immune responsiveness. This is true particularly for cancer of the head and neck region. Patients bearing these tumors appear to be more profoundly immune deficient than patients with other forms of even more widespread malignancies.[33–38] As Jenkins et al. point out, radiation therapy further impairs immune responsiveness, aggravating an already inadequate situation.[36] It is well recognized that malnutrition and ethanol intake both depress immune reactivity. It is uncertain whether this impaired immune reactivity is primarily caused by such nutritional factors, or is merely aggravated by them.

Currently, there are very few meaningful reports as to the clinical effects of immunotherapy on epidermoid cancer of the head and neck region. The negative report by Suen and his associates, who found no benefit from bacille Calmette-Guérin (BCG) alone, was mentioned in the preceding chapter.[39] Other reports consider the use of BCG plus chemotherapy. Donaldson has reported twice on his uncontrolled evaluation of methotrexate plus BCG and isoniazid. His 1972 report indicated that 13 of 16 patients (81 per cent) had objective partial regressions with a mean duration of over 265 days.[40] In 1973, he reported that 20 of 32 patients (62.5 per cent) had objective partial regression with a mean duration of over 322 days.[41] These impressive, although uncontrolled, results led to a randomized controlled study by the Mayo Clinic group.[42] They found no difference in results using methotrexate alone, methotrexate plus BCG, and methotrexate plus BCG and isoniazid. The only completely positive comparative study is that of Richman and his associates at the M.D. Anderson Hospital.[43] In this study, all patients had gross tumor, and all received a five drug combination chemotherapy with the BACON regimen (bleomycin, doxorubicin hydrochloride [Adriamycin], CCNU, vincristine sulfate [Oncovin], and nitrogen mustard). The report indicates that 14 patients were randomly assigned to receive the chemotherapy alone, and 20 were entered on the same chemotherapy program plus BCG. Those receiving chemotherapy plus BCG lived significantly longer ($P = 0.014$).

The reports in the preceding paragraph are the only major published studies on the effects of immunotherapy in patients with cancer of the head and neck region. Although some of the reports are positive, the evidence is far from overwhelming that immunotherapy is effective; however, all of these reported studies pertain to patients with gross disease who, as we have already indicated, are unlikely to be benefited by immunotherapy. Moreover, chemotherapy is known to be immunosuppressive. It is believed that immunosuppression in renal transplant recipients permits such individuals to develop cancer. Perhaps the lack of definite evidence for effectiveness of chemoimmunotherapy arises partly from problems in timing—immunotherapy may be given at a time when the chemotherapy effect prevents an adequate immunologic response. It seems that the ideal sequence would be for chemotherapy to be used first in order to cause a marked reduction in the number of malignant cells, followed by immunotherapy, in the hope that the number of residual cells would be small enough for immunotherapy effectiveness.

The effectiveness of immunotherapy for cancer patients remains controversial. We can hope that over the next few years immune-stimulating drugs will be developed. The future may bring more potent immuno-stimulating agents that would be utilized following cytoreductive surgery, radiotherapy, or chemotherapy. The hope is that the total number of tumor cells remaining after that combination approach would be so small as to be within the range in which, according to animal data, nonspecific immune stimulants might be effective in eradicating cancer. Perhaps such a combination approach might serve to "kill the last cancer cell."

References

1. Bertino JR et al.: Chemotherapy of cancer of the head and neck. Cancer 31:1141–1149, 1973.
2. Bleyer WA: The clinical pharmacology of methotrexate: New applications of an old drug. Cancer 41:36–51, 1978.
3. Carter SK: The chemotherapy of head and neck cancer. Semin Oncol 4:413–424, 1977.
4. Huffman DH et al.: Pharmokinetics of methotrexate. Clin Pharmacol Ther 14:572–579, 1973.
5. Lucas RJ et al.: Prolonged intra-arterial infusion chemotherapy for advanced head and neck cancer. Grace Hosp Bull 50:3–10, 1972.
6. Lane M et al.: Methotrexate therapy for squamous cell carcinoma of the head and neck: Intermittent intravenous dose program. JAMA 204:561–564, 1968.
7. Lehane DE et al.: A comparison of methotrexate with methyl CCNU and bleomycin in patients with advanced squamous cell carcinoma of the head and neck region: A Southwest Oncology Group study. Proc Am Soc Clin Oncol 21:331, Abstract C-49, 1980.
8. Levitt M et al.: Improved therapeutic indexes of methotrexate "leucovorin rescue." Cancer Res 33:1729–1734, 1973.
9. Capizzi RL et al.: Methotrexate therapy of head and neck cancer: Improvement in therapeutic index by the use of "leucovorin rescue." Cancer Res 30: 1782–1788, 1970.
10. Ojima Y et al.: Pharmacologic studies of methotrexate in cancer patients with uropathy. Arch Surg 100:173–177, 1970.
11. Clarysse AM et al.: Pulmonary disease complicating intermittent therapy with methotrexate. JAMA 209:1861–1864, 1969.
12. Roenigk HH et al.: Hepatotoxicity of methotrexate in the treatment of psoriasis. Arch Dermatol 103: 250–261, 1971.
13. Suzuki Y et al.: Bleomycin in malignant tumors of head and neck. Keio J Med 18:153–162, 1969.
14. Haas CD et al.: Phase II evaluation of bleomycin: A Southwest Oncology Group study. Cancer 38:8–13, 1976.
15. Reed CS: Bleomycin in advanced squamous cell carcinoma of the head and neck. Med J Aust 2:742, 1972.
16. Daskal Y et al.: Ultrastructural study of pulmonary bleomycin toxicity. Cancer Res 36:1267–1272, 1976.
17. Luna MA et al.: Interstitial pneumonitis associated with bleomycin therapy. Am J Clin Pathol 58:501–510, 1972.
18. Costanzi JJ et al.: Intravenous bleomycin infusion as a potential synchronizing agent in human disseminated malignancy: A preliminary report. Cancer 38: 1503–1506, 1976.
19. Suzuki H et al.: On the mechanism of action of bleomycin: Scission of DNA strands in vitro and in vivo. J Antibiot 22:446–448, 1969.
20. Rozencweig M et al.: Investigational chemotherapeutic agents in head and neck cancer. Semin Oncol 4:425–429, 1977.

21. Hayes D et al.: Amelioration of renal toxicity with high-dose *cis*-platinum diaminodichloride (CPDD) by mannitol induced diuresis. Proc Am Assoc Cancer Res 17:169, Abstract 676, 1976.
22. Panettiere FJ et al.: Effectiveness of a new outpatient program utilizing CACP in the chemotherapy of advanced epidermoid head and neck tumors: Southwest Oncology Group study. Proc Am Assoc Clin Oncology 19:410, Abstract C-416, 1978.
23. Panettiere FJ: *Cis*-platinum (CACP) toxicity: An analysis based on three Southwest Oncology Group studies. Proc Am Assoc Cancer Res 22:157, Abstract 623, 1981.
24. Gralla RJ et al.: Antiemetic efficacy of high-dose metoclopramide: Randomized trials with placebo and prochloroperazine in patients with chemotherapy-induced nausea and vomiting. N Engl J Med 305:905–909, 1981.
24a. Dentino M et al.: Long-term effect of *cis*-diaminedichloride platinum (CDDP) on renal function and structure in man. Cancer 41:1274–1281, 1978.
25. Garnich MB, Mayer RJ: Acute renal failure associated with neoplastic disease and its treatment. Semin Oncol 5:155–165, 1978.
26. Pyle IJ et al.: Effects of *cis*-diaminedichloride platinum (NSC 119875) on hearing function in man. Cancer Chemother Rep 58:871–875, 1974.
27. Lerner HJ et al.: Concomitant hydroxyurea and radiotherapy in the management of 60 patients with head and neck cancer. Am Surg 35:525–534, 1969.
28. Richards GJ, Chambers RG: Hydroxyurea in the treatment of neoplasms of the head and neck: A resurvey. Am Surg 126:513–518, 1973.
29. Panettiere FJ et al.: Porfiromycin (NSC 56410) in the management of epidermoid and transitional cell cancer: A phase II study. Cancer Treat Rep 60:907–911, 1976.
30. Warren RD, Bender RA: Drug interactions with antineoplastic agents. Cancer Treat Rep 61:1231–1241, 1977.
31. Lustig RA et al.: Adjuvant methotrexate in the radiotherapeutic management of advanced tumors of the head and neck. Cancer 37:2703–2708, 1976.
32. Randolph VL et al.: Combination therapy of advanced head and neck cancer: Induction of remissions with diaminedichloride platinum (II), bleomycin and radiation therapy. Cancer 41:460–467, 1978.
33. Berlinger NT et al.: Immunologic assessment of regional lymph node histology in relation to survival in head and neck carcinoma. Cancer 37:697–705, 1976.
34. Browder JP, Cretien PB: Immune reactivity in head and neck squamous cell carcinoma and relevance to the design of immunotherapy trials. Semin Oncol 4:431–439, 1977.
35. Hilal EY et al.: Immunologic evaluation and prognosis in patients with head and neck cancer. Am J Surg 134:469–473, 1977.
36. Jenkins VK et al.: Lymphocyte response in patients with head and neck cancer: Effect of clinical stage and radiotherapy. Arch Otolaryngol 102:596–600, 1976.
37. Mason JM et al.: T-lymphocytes and survival of head and neck squamous cell carcinoma. Arch Otolaryngol 103:223–227, 1977.
38. Olivari A et al.: Cell-mediated immune response in head and neck cancer patients. J Surg Oncol 8:287–294, 1976.
39. Suen JY et al.: Results of BCG adjuvant immunotherapy in 100 patients with epidermoid carcinoma of the head and neck. Am J Surg 134:474–478, 1977.
40. Donaldson RC: Methotrexate plus bacillus Calmette-Guérin (BCG) and isoniazid in the treatment of cancer of the head and neck. Am J Surg 124:527–534, 1972.
41. Donaldson RC: Chemoimmunotherapy for cancer of the head and neck. Am J Surg 126:507–512, 1973.
42. Woods JE et al.: A controlled study of combined methotrexate, BCG, and INH therapy for squamous cell carcinoma of the head and neck. Surg Clin North Am 57:759–778, 1977.
43. Richman SP et al.: Chemotherapy versus chemoimmunotherapy of head and neck cancer: Report of a randomized study. Cancer Treat Rep 60:535–539, 1976.

28

Laryngeal Research

J. M. Fredrickson, M.D., D. A. Charles, M.D.,
and C. Painter, Ph.D.

Most interest in laryngeal research is centered on cancer. The major thrust has been in two areas: the reassessment of treatment protocols and modalities with a view to maximizing cure and minimizing functional disability (see the descriptions of partial laryngeal surgery in Part III of this volume), and the restoration of voice in laryngectomized patients.

AREAS WHERE STANDARDIZATION IS NEEDED

Classification. Application of proper epidemiologic techniques to studies of laryngeal cancer and treatment modalities requires common ground in classification. Introduction of the TNM joint classification of the Union Internationale Contre le Cancer (UICC) and the American Joint Committee on Cancer (AJCC) of 1962 has gone a long way towards this. The tendency of some institutions to fly in the face of world opinion and devise their own classification systems for cancer of the larynx and hypopharynx makes meaningful comparison of results impossible, as laryngeal cancer is relatively uncommon. To be significant and useful, any prospective trial of therapy will have to be multicentered. All of this presupposes a common accepted classification system that ensures that like is being compared with like. Some recent work suggests that, even within institutions, individual clinicians do not necessarily mean the same thing when using various terms to describe tumors, define their extent, and interpret the rules as laid down in classification systems.[1]

Anatomic Definition. A major difficulty in classification of laryngeal tumors has been the lack of unanimity in defining the anatomic boundaries of the various laryngeal sites and regions. A major effort was made at the Centennial Conference on laryngeal cancer to arrive at acceptable and clinically applicable definitions of laryngeal anatomic boundaries.[2] Applications of embryologic principles and knowledge of laryngeal development go part of the way in explaining patterns of tumor spread and why partial laryngectomy procedures, for instance, can be performed successfully.

Tumor Spread. Any study of tumor spread must inevitably include the examination of the neck lymph node fields, routes of spread, rates of spread, the lag phase between the histologic and clinical involvement of nodes, and the probability of lymph node involvement. All need further study and elucidation.[3]

Clinical application of the techniques of lymphangiography, well established and tried for retroperitoneal nodal involvement in malignancy, has yet to be done in a systematic fashion for the lymph node fields of the head and neck. Yet here we have one of the largest node fields in the body, housing approximately one-third of all our lymph nodes. This would seem to be an area of clinically oriented research that is ripe for development.

RESEARCH POLICIES

Policy and Priority. Research policies are to a large extent determined by the economic, social, and political climates prevailing in an area. The degree of medical–political sophistication in a given country or area will often suggest the feasibility and even advisability of a given research topic. Unique opportunities for the clinical pathologic correlation of advanced tumor behavior sometimes exist in underdeveloped countries. Research in these areas should therefore concentrate on the available material. Sophisticated equipment must here be replaced by astute clinical observation and judgment—the basic tools of most meaningful research.

Even in economically more fortunate societies, the demands of early detection, classification, and treatment leave little time for more esoteric research pursuits. Combined therapy investigations and chemotherapy were the topics most intensively studied in 27 major North American centers surveyed by Ward.[4] Cancer immunology was the next most popular research topic.

Value of Research. Research involvement by residents, either as a sideline or as a direct integrated part of training, is most important and valuable. Mandatory involvement would seem unwise, however, and is often not feasible because of service commitments and the necessity of training a competent and reliable clinician. The short-term product of the research is often overshadowed by the value of the process. Insight into the scientific process, the development of critical faculties, and the ability to evaluate a given piece of work critically all make for better clinicians. We hope that exposure to research during residency training will stimulate and encourage the small percentage who will ultimately go on to conduct useful research. It is the quality of the personnel doing research that is most important. Money and facilities do not necessarily buy good research. Basic applied and clinical research are closely related and must be integrated with medical training. Advances in technology and areas such as cell kinetics, cellular radiobiology, and immunology have meant that good research requires cooperation between clinicians who are grounded in basic sciences and full-time basic scientists. This link and cooperation are essential.

LARYNGEAL FUNCTION MEASUREMENTS

Meaningful research implies careful, objective measurement and recording of data. Spinoff from research aimed at reducing the cost of transmission of voiced messages has resulted in new insights in laryngeal physiology. Interest in disordered laryngeal function coupled with the advent of microlaryngeal surgery has stimulated interest in objective methods for detecting laryngeal pathology and vocal deviation. These investigative procedures are not designed to supplant but rather to complement the traditional methods of clinical examination. With the exception of stroboscopy and the various types of laryngeal photography, most of these methods of laryngeal measurement are still research tools. They await further refinement prior to wide clinical application.

These techniques present multiple problems for widespread clinical application in that they involve considerable initial investment and may be expensive to operate. They are not easily used with many patients. Wider clinical application would involve an increase in the number of speech scientists and speech laboratories affiliated with departments of otolaryngology throughout North America. The patient suffering from nonmalignant laryngeal disease may require more than a mirror examination and verbal reassurance that cancer is not involved. Evaluation of the problem may need to include the use of equipment that can be accommodated in a clinical setting; however, such application would involve personnel trained in the use and interpretation of these investigative procedures. Failures of communication and cooperation between laryngologists and speech scientists have often meant that each group operates in a vacuum in separate university departments.

A variety of investigative procedures have been developed to observe laryngeal function visually as well as to measure vocal output. A significant step forward was made as long ago as 1940 with a high speed motion picture of the vibrating cords produced by Bell Telephone Laboratories. Stroboscopy and electroglottography also provide information on the vibratory pattern of the vocal cords at a fraction of the cost and effort of high speed photography.

Equipment to measure airflow through the glottis and pulmonary function provides information on laryngeal aerodynamics. The spectrograph provides an analysis of the speech wave form and includes the effects of the vocal tract as well as the glottal source. Application of existing technology in electromyographic analysis of the larynx has added further dimensions to the above methods. Sophisticated radiographic methods of laryngeal imaging have been covered in Chapter 5 of this volume.

High Speed Photography. High speed motion picture photography of vocal cord movement provides a visual record of the cycle-to-cycle opening and closing movements of the vocal cords as well as the rippling movement of the mucosal covering of the vocal cords.[5, 6, 7] Abnormalities of either the adductory and abductory movements or the wavelike movements of the mucosal surface may be the earliest signals of cord pathology. The necessary equipment is expensive and any extensive analysis of the data is prohibitive in terms of time. Efforts are now under way to computerize the data from such photography. Less accurate but useful information on cord vibratory patterns can be obtained by the use of the laryngostroboscope and electroglottography.

Stroboscopy. Synchronization of the stroboscopic light with the fundamental frequency of cord vibration creates the illusion that the cords are standing still. Variation in the strobe frequency creates a slow motion effect. Both these effects, dependent on the persistence of the afterimage, enable us to observe cord vibration at any phase of the phonatory cycle. It is important to recognize that what appears to the examiner as a single opening and closing of the vocal cords is really a composite of many different openings and closings of the vocal cords over a period of time. Indirect mirror examination of the larynx is performed using a stroboscopic light. The patient's voice is monitored by a contact microphone held beside the larynx. Filtration and amplification are followed by discharge of the stroboscopic light at the fundamental frequency of cord vibration at that time. It is possible to record these results on a video system or on film for later viewing. Published reports to date indicate the usefulness of stroboscopic examination in diagnosing early pathologic lesions, confirming the early return of cord tonus in recovering palsies, and diagnosing nonorganic disorders of the larynx.[8]

Electroglottography. The basic methodology was introduced by Fabre in 1957. Electrodes are placed one on either side of the larynx. Then variations of impedance induced by vocal cord vibration are amplified and registered electrically. Some confusion still exists as to the significance of electroglottographic findings, and further work aimed at correlating these findings exactly with the phases of phonation and with laryngeal pathologic conditions remains to be done.[9, 10]

Echoglottography. In an attempt to circumvent the potentially erroneous information obtained with stroboscopy, Holmer[11] and his coworkers have used an ultrasonic pulse echo method for studying vocal fold vibrations. Echoes from the free margins of the vocal folds can be clearly identified and recorded as glottograms. It remains to be seen whether this method will be suitable for recording the complex three-dimensional movements of the vocal cords. Further problems related to the movement of the whole larynx craniocaudally with shifts in pitch and during swallowing, together with problems of reproducibility of results, need to be solved. On the positive side, echocardiography is now an accepted clinical tool, and practical problems such as these encountered in echoglottography have been surmounted.

Air Flow Studies. Instruments measuring air flow rates and air volumes may represent the most accurate objective methods of recording laryngeal function to date.[12] A laminar flow register measures flow rates. Air volume is recorded by integrating the flow rate. The slope of the integrated curve gives mean flow rate values. Relating the mean flow rate (MFR) to the vital capacity (VC) as first described by Koike and Hirano[13] gives a ratio called the vocal velocity index (VVI):

$$VVI = MFR/VC$$

Clinical evaluation of VVI in laryngeal disease shows a statistically significant difference between normal subjects and patients with organic laryngeal diseases.[14, 15] A small but significant difference is also observed between the normal subjects and the patients with functional voice disorders. It is important to realize that we cannot view airflow studies in isolation; these must be performed with a full understanding and awareness of pulmonary function.

Spectrographic Analysis. To date, the best acoustic evaluation of the sound pressure events emanating from the vocal cords (and supraglottic vocal tract) other than the trained human ear is accomplished by the sound spectrograph.[15, 16] Spectrographic analysis is dependent on high fidelity recording of the pa-

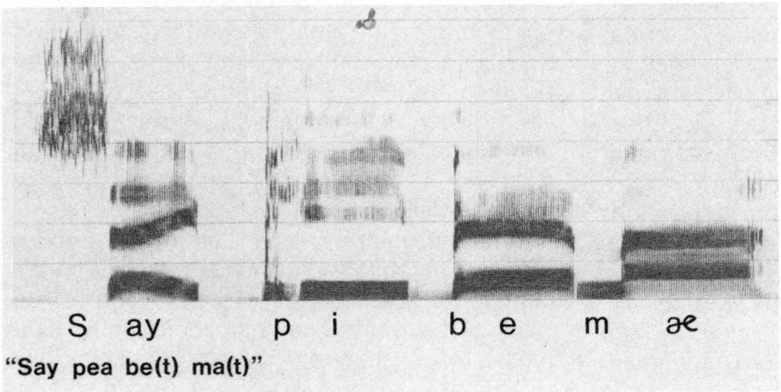

Figure 28–1. Broad-band spectrogram of an adult male saying: *"Say pea be(t) ma(t)."* This illustrates friction noise throughout *s,* after the silent period in *p,* and at the explosion in *b,* but none in *m.* This also demonstrates the different formants (bars of acoustic energy) for the four different vowels (e, *i, E,* and ae).

tient's voice in a sound isolation room. The system prints out the frequency/time and frequency/intensity spectra of the complex laryngeal tones generated by the larynx and modified by the vocal tract. Short samples of speech or sustained vowels are used for such analyses (Fig. 28–1).

Spectrographic analysis has found application in both clinical and research laboratories in the assessment and treatment of vocal disorders. A classification already exists of the acoustic properties of the hoarse voice.[15] Although the method is simple to apply and provides a permanent record that is available for independent analysis, data concerning laryngeal function are still sparse. The complex interaction of the glottal sound source and its subsequent modification by the vocal tract and articulatory mechanisms can be difficult to interpret. The exact role of spectrographic analysis remains to be defined, but it is most likely to prove beneficial in functional voice disorders and possibly in biofeedback systems for speech pathologists.

Laryngeal Electromyography. Laryngeal electromyography can be performed using the standard electromyography laboratory. A concentric needle electrode is inserted percutaneously to sample the territories supplied by the superior laryngeal nerve (cricothyroid muscle) and recurrent laryngeal nerve (thyroarytenoid muscle). Actual potentials recorded are comparable to those obtained elsewhere in the body. Electromyography is useful for the diagnosis of early denervation, reinnervation, and (to a lesser extent) primary muscle disease. Laryngeal electromyography provides useful adjunctive information for clinical diagnosis and allows the clinician to prognosticate with more confidence in cases of vocal cord paresis[17, 18, 19] (Fig. 28–2).

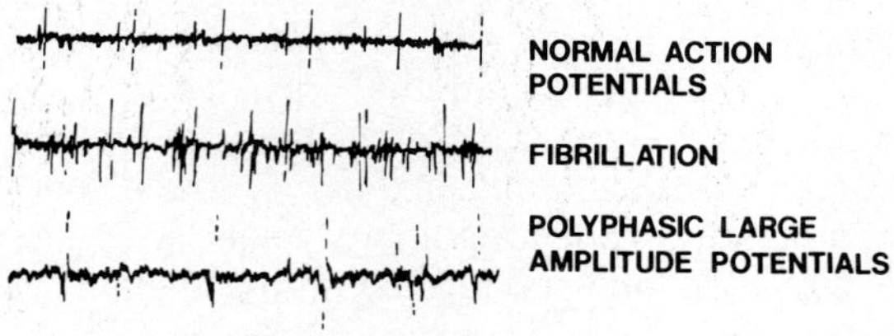

Figure 28–2. Typical electromyographic tracings.

Fiberoptics and the Larynx. Use of rigid and flexible fiberoptic endoscopes has revolutionized laryngeal examination and recording.[20, 21] Attachment of still and movie cameras has made detailed records available for teaching and research. While rigid endoscopes offer excellent lens and lighting systems, they suffer from the same disadvantages that indirect mirror examination does in those patients with an active gag reflex or an overhanging epiglottis. The transnasal flexible fiberoptic laryngoscope is superior in these areas and will often avoid hospitalization for direct examination of the larynx. The techniques and instruments are easily mastered and will complement many of the preceding methods of laryngeal measurement and quantification.

Pitch Meters. We have many ways of obtaining pitch data, but current real-time oscilloscope-displayed pitch meters are accurate, easy to use, and moderately priced. Shimmer, jitter, tremor, wide or restricted ranges, high or low registers, and unusual pitch contours are easily visualized and available for biofeedback.

Intensity Meters. Instruments to measure intensity are currently available together with pitch meters in one unit, making it equally easy to obtain data on overall intensity, range, tremor, and unusual patterns.

VOCAL RESTORATION

The numerous devices and procedures advocated for vocal restoration following total laryngectomy, since Czemak devised the first

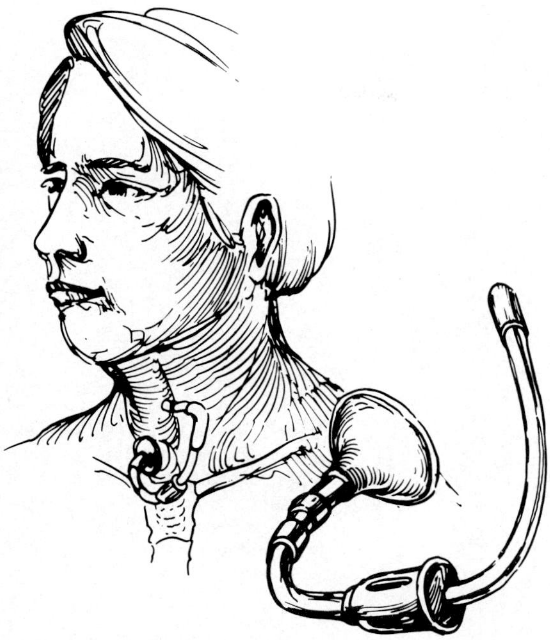

Figure 28–3. Modified Tokyo larynx. Features are mouth tube with fitted saliva cap, breathing port, and stoma cover.

known artificial larynx in 1859, are testimony to the energy and activity devoted to this problem over the years. Chapters 22 and 23 of this book discuss neoglottic reconstruction and the tracheoesophageal shunts.

Artificial larynges appropriate for patients who cannot master esophageal speech well fall into two main categories—pneumatic and electronic. Either pneumatic or electric energy is used to activate a vibrating device of some type. All pneumatic devices seek to divert exhaled air from the tracheostoma through a vibrating mechanism and back into the oral pharynx, either directly or via a pharyngocutaneous fistula.

Electronic vibrating devices (discussed later) are usually held externally to the neck skin for transcutaneous transmission of vibrations directly to the pharynx. The electronic sound can be transmitted instead via a mouth tube inserted and held in the oral cavity. There have been ingenious attempts to make the vibrator inconspicuous by incorporating it into a pipe or even a dental plate. Direct implantation of the vibrator in the retropharyngeal tissue at laryngeal level has been done successfully both in the animal laboratory and in human subjects.

Pneumatic Devices. Patients often object to the cumbersome tubes and valves of external pneumatic devices (Figs. 28–3, 28–4, and 28–5). Air leakage at the stomal end and sound leakage along the device and at the mouth of the fistula tube continue to create problems.

More recent developments have attempted to create tracheoesophageal fistulas for direct

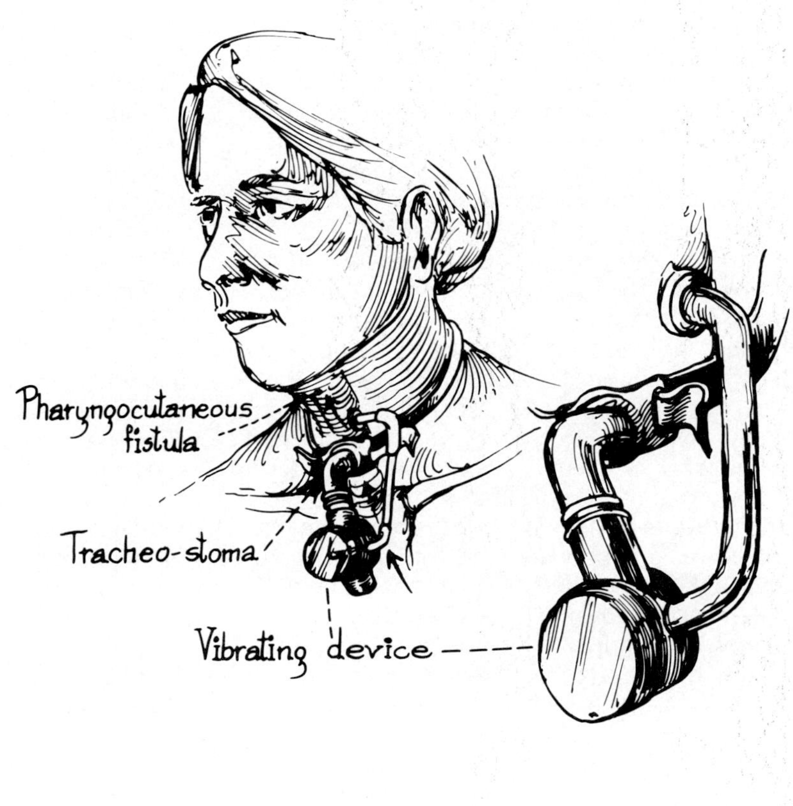

Figure 28–4. VoiceBak prosthesis. Features are tracheal connector, bypass valve, breathing port, one-way valve, and flanged Silastic fistula tube.

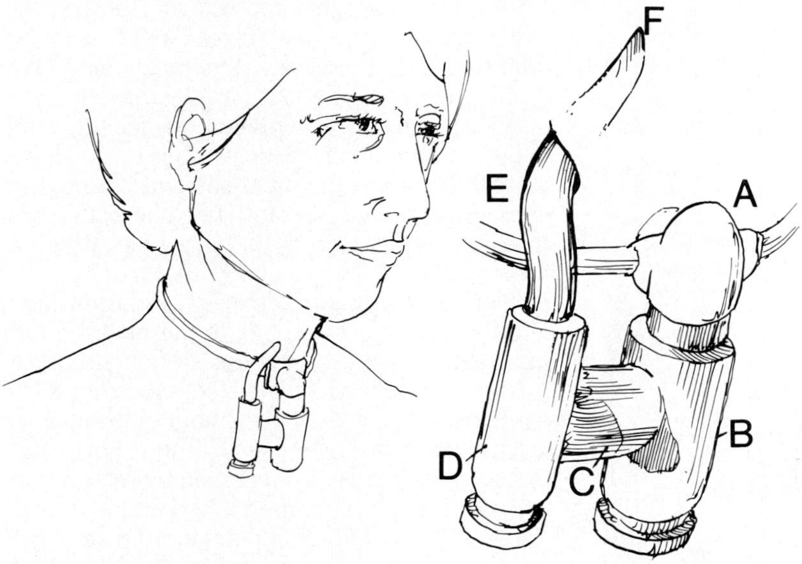

Figure 28–5. Reed fistula pneumatic device. *A,* Tracheostomy tube. *B,* Inspiratory valve. *C,* Reed housing. *D,* Saliva trap. *E,* Pharyngocutaneous fistula. *F,* Valved fistula tube.

shunting of air to the vocal tract. Another approach consists of forming a cervical esophagostomy and connecting an external bypass tract from the tracheostoma to the fistula with or without the insertion of a vibrating mechanism. Modifications have included saliva traps and valved tracheal tubes (Taub Lebarge VoiceBak, Northwestern Voice Prosthesis). If no external pseudolarynx mechanism is incorporated, then it is hoped to divert the shunted pulmonary air via the fistula to below tissue capable of excitation into audible vibration.

Taub's prosthesis (VoiceBak) is a combined surgical and prosthetic approach to vocal restoration.[22, 23] A cervical esophagostomy is created from between the heads of the sternocleidomastoid muscle to the retroesophageal area. This esophagostomy should be high enough to avoid diverting air into the stomach and low enough to allow for neoglottis formation in the esophagus. The fistula is lined with a superiorly based skin flap and allowed to become fully healed; the external prosthesis is then fitted (Fig. 28–4). Blom investigated the voice characteristics of bypass speakers and compared them favorably to superior, highly trained esophageal speakers.

Sisson's method is again a combined surgical and prosthetic method of vocal rehabilitation. It involves a hypopharyngeal fistula that is created at the time of definitive cancer surgery.[23, 24] This has the advantage of alleviating the formation of unplanned postoperative fistulas, which occur relatively frequently in heavily irradiated patients following laryngectomy. The Northwestern Voice Prosthesis consists of a stomal connector, a pressure-sensitive respiratory valve, and a conduit that ends in a saliva valve leading to the fistula fitting. The differential respiratory valve allows the patient to cough at high expiratory pressures and breathe normally at low pressures.

The Shedd method incorporates a reed vibrator in an external bypass prosthesis. This, of course, avoids the requirement of neoglottis formation in the hypopharynx or upper esophageal area and is a more predictable sound generation source[23, 25] (Fig. 28–5).

External Electronic Devices. Patient compliance for electronic speech can be difficult to obtain because of the prominent external devices. Those patients who do well with fistula bypass methods are often the same ones who are well motivated and work hard at esophageal speech. With the exceptions of the experimental implantable electrolarynx and a denture-held device, the electronic devices are basically hand-held, battery-powered transducers. Most commonly, these devices are used by holding the vibrating surface to the skin of the neck or occasionally to the cheek skin. It is often necessary to select the optimum point for application of the vibrator by trial and error. Rigid irradiated and scarred tissues, of course, are not the most suitable for this. The patient uses normal articulatory mechanisms to speak with this basic electronic sound.

Sound leakage at the interface between the vibrating surface of the device and the skin can lead to unintelligible speech. To circumvent this problem, some hand-held devices have been modified to incorporate a mouth vibrator instead of the traditional vibrating diaphragm. The presence of an intraoral vibrator may interfere with articulatory mechanisms; for that reason, the vibrator should be held to one side, away from the center of the tongue.

The most commonly used electronic hand-held device in North America is the Western Electric No. 5 electrolarynx. This is also available with modifications connecting it to a mouth vibrator. The Barts (St. Bartholomew's Hospital) electrolarynx is a commonly used British model in which a small battery-powered motor drives a spring-loaded piston against a vibrating diaphragm. The pitch can be varied by an externally adjustable locking ring. The loudness of the instrument is fixed. The Siemens-Servox is a high-quality (and expensive) German electrolarynx. A piston strikes the diaphragm at high velocity. Pitch and loudness are adjustable, and a small amount of pitch variation (5 to 20 Hz) can be achieved by varying the pressure of the vibrator on the neck.

Implantable Electromagnetic Sound Source. Retropharyngeal implantation of a vibrating sound source has been performed both in the experimental laboratory and in a limited clinical trial[26, 27] (Figs. 28–6 and 28–7). Retropharyngeal implantation facilitates full use of the remaining articulatory mechanisms. Improvement in electromechanical efficiency has eliminated the necessity for a transcutaneous connector to deliver power. The key to eventual clinical application is the goal of ongoing research—to develop an output that will result in a more human speech sound.

Choice of Method of Voice Restoration. The method of vocal rehabilitation employed should not further increase the hospital stay and

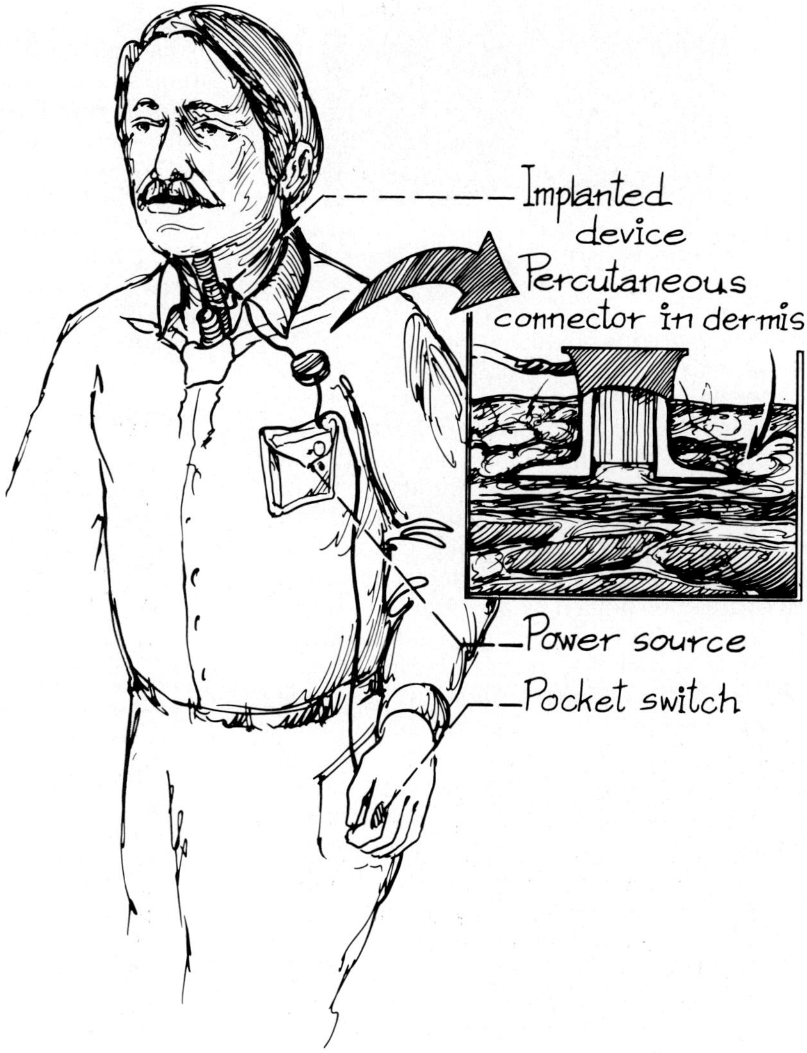

Figure 28–6. Electromagnetic implantable sound source.[26] Features are implanted device, percutaneous connector (this exteriorized connector is no longer necessary), power source, and pocket control switch.

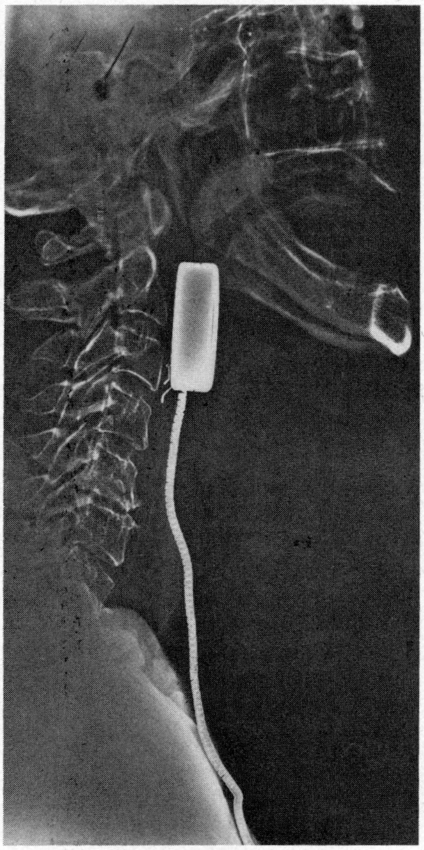

Figure 28–7. Lateral xerogram of implanted sound source in the retropharyngeal area.[26]

patient morbidity. Fistula speakers (other than those with the tracheoesophageal shunts—see Chapters 22 and 23) still face the twin problems of aspiration and stenosis. The physician should be aware of the physical and psychologic limitations of further surgical procedures on those patients who have already been traumatized by surgery, radiation, and hospitalization, often over a prolonged period. External fistula devices are often limited by poor results in achieving airtight and watertight fits over the stomata.

Fistula speech has several advantages over other methods of vocal restoration. Ideally, the fistula should be created at the time of initial definitive surgery. Speech quality, duration, and acceptability are improved and there is decreased instruction time and avoidance of the air-gulping noises of esophageal speech.

For too many surgeons and speech therapists, success for the laryngectomy patient is represented by achievement of esophageal speech. All involved should be aware of the time and effort necessary to reach this goal. Some patients are "communication losers" from the beginning because of the physical and psychologic limitations imposed by their disease. Many patients fail to achieve acceptable esophageal speech. All patients should be made aware of the alternative devices and procedures available for vocal rehabilitation, and there is no reason why a patient should not use an electrolarynx of whatever type while esophageal speech training is progressing. Centers where surgery is used only for salvage following radical radiotherapy are limited further in the use of surgical prosthetic or surgical neoglottic reconstructive methods.

There is a need for continuing support of the international group for the study of surgical and prosthetic vocal rehabilitation. Honest reporting of failures and complications as well as successes is imperative. Objective criteria for assessing alaryngeal speech are necessary. Realistic goals, individualized for each patient, must be formulated. It is unfair to a patient with a very limited life expectancy to involve him in a long series of reconstructive procedures that, in inexperienced hands, may be fraught with an unacceptably high failure rate.

Vocal Fold Physiology. Finally, it should be noted that although much of the work on vocal fold physiology carried out by speech scientists may at first appear to be remote from the day-to-day clinical work of the laryngologist, appropriate instrumental diagnostic protocols will become available only to the degree that basic research on normal and abnormal laryngeal function is pursued.

References

1. Cummings BJ, Jackson SM: Carcinoma of the larynx in Canada, 1970–74: Report of a symposium. Ann R Coll Phys Surg Can, July 1980.
2. Centennial Conference on Laryngeal Cancer, Workshop No. 1. Can J Otolaryngol 3:405–511, 1974.
3. McKelvie P: Metastatic routes in the neck. Can J Otolaryngol 3:473–479, 1974.
4. Ward P: Laryngeal cancer research in the western U.S. and Canada. Can J Otolaryngol 4:820–823, 1975.
5. VonLeden H: Ultrahigh speed photography. *In* Hinchcliffe R (ed): Scientific Foundations of Otolaryngology. Chicago, Yearbook Medical Publishers, p 577, 1976.
6. Koike Y: Highspeed photography of the larynx and film data processing. Can J Otolaryngol 4:800–805, 1975.
7. Moore GP: Ultrahigh speed photography of the larynx. Can J Otolaryngol 4:793–799, 1975.
8. Hirano M: Clinical Examination of Voice. Vienna, Springer-Verlag, 1981.
9. Lecluse FLE: Laboratory investigation in electroglottography. *In* Loebell E (ed): Proc 16th Int Congr Logopedics Phoniatrics, Interlaken, Switzerland, August 25–29, 1974. Basel, S Karger, 1976, pp 294–296.
10. Fabre M: Un procédé electrique pucutoné d'insciption

de l'accolement glottique au cours de la phonation: Glottographie de haute fréquence. Bull Acad Nat Med (Paris) 141:66–70, 1955.
11. Holmer NG et al: Ultrasonic recording of vocal fold vibrations in preparation of human larynges. Acta Otolaryngol (Stockh) 75:454–463, 1973.
12. Fourcin AJ, Abberton E: The laryngograph and the voicescope in speech therapy. *In* Loebell E (ed): Proc 16th Int Congr Logopedics Phoniatrics, Interlaken, Switzerland, August 25–29, 1974. Basel, S Karger, 1976, pp 116–122.
13. Koike Y, Hirano M: Significance of vocal velocity. Folia Phoniatr (Basel) 20:285–296, 1968.
14. Iwata S, VonLeden H: Clinical evaluation of vocal velocity index in laryngeal disease. Ann Otol Rhinol Laryngol 79:259–268, 1970.
15. Yanagihara N: Hoarseness: Investigation of the physiological mechanisms. Ann Otol Rhinol Laryngol 76:472–488, 1967.
16. Painter C: An Introduction to Instrumental Phonetics. Baltimore, University Park Press, 1979. See chapter on Acoustic Instrumentation, p 11.
17. Dedo HH: The paralyzed larynx: An electromyographic study in dogs and humans. Laryngoscope 10:1455–1517, 1970.
18. Hirose H et al.: Electrode insertion techniques for laryngeal electromyography. J Acoust Soc Am 50:1449–1450, 1971.
19. Gay T et al.: Electromyography of the intrinsic laryngeal muscles during phonation. Ann Otol Rhinol Laryngol 81:401–409, 1972.
20. Silberman HD et al.: Flexible fiberoptic nasopharyngolaryngoscope. Ann Otol Rhinol Laryngol 85: 640–645, 1976.
21. Ward P et al.: Advances in endoscopic examination of the respiratory system. Ann Otol Rhinol Laryngol 83:754–760, 1974.
22. Taub S: Air bypass voice prosthesis for vocal rehabilitation of laryngectomies. Ann Otol Rhinol Laryngol 84:45–48, 1975.
23. Proc 2nd Int Workshop Surg Prosthetic Study Group. Boston, GK Hall and Company, 1980.
24. Sisson GA et al.: Voice rehabilitation after laryngectomy. Arch Otolaryngol 101:178–181, 1975.
25. Shedd D: Reed fistula method and speech rehabilitation after laryngectomy. Am J Surg 124:510–514, 1972.
26. Fredrickson JM et al.: *In* Proc 2nd Int Workshop Surg Prosthetic Study Group. Boston, GK Hall and Company, 1980.
27. Maruzzo B et al.: A new implantable electrolarynx. Digest 34th Conf Eng Med Biol, Houston, 1981.

INDEX

Page numbers in *italic* type indicate illustrations; page numbers followed by *t* refer to tables.